Sports Nutrition

Sports Nutrition

Edited by **Pablo De Souza**

SYRAWOOD
PUBLISHING HOUSE
New York

Published by Syrawood Publishing House,
750 Third Avenue, 9th Floor,
New York, NY 10017, USA
www.syrawoodpublishinghouse.com

Sports Nutrition
Edited by Pablo De Souza

International Standard Book Number: 978-1-68286-222-3 (Hardback)

Printed in the United States of America.

Contents

Preface

This book was inspired by the evolution of our times; to answer the curiosity of inquisitive minds. Many developments have occurred across the globe in the recent past which has transformed the progress in the field.

Sports Nutrition is dedicated to the evaluation and manipulation of athletic performance through nutrition and diet. Knowledge of topics like dietary regimes, nutrition, food supplements and their impact on the overall health and performance of athletes/sportspersons, etc. is absolutely essential for the thorough understanding of sports nutrition. This book will equip the reader with a sound understanding about these topics along with the various factors influencing the nutritional requirements of athletes, like gender, age, body mass index, etc. It will successfully cater to the needs of students and healthcare professionals alike.

This book was developed from a mere concept to drafts to chapters and finally compiled together as a complete text to benefit the readers across all nations. To ensure the quality of the content we instilled two significant steps in our procedure. The first was to appoint an editorial team that would verify the data and statistics provided in the book and also select the most appropriate and valuable contributions from the plentiful contributions we received from authors worldwide. The next step was to appoint an expert of the topic as the Editor-in-Chief, who would head the project and finally make the necessary amendments and modifications to make the text reader-friendly. I was then commissioned to examine all the material to present the topics in the most comprehensible and productive format.

I would like to take this opportunity to thank all the contributing authors who were supportive enough to contribute their time and knowledge to this project. I also wish to convey my regards to my family who have been extremely supportive during the entire project.

Editor

1

Skeletal muscle metabolic gene response to carbohydrate feeding during exercise in the heat

Charles L Dumke[1*], Dustin R Slivka[2], John S Cuddy[1], Walter S Hailes[1] and Brent C Ruby[1]

Abstract

Background: Heat stress down-regulates mitochondrial function, while carbohydrate supplementation attenuates the exercise induced stimulation of mitochondrial biogenesis in humans. The effects of exogenous carbohydrate during exercise in the heat on metabolic mRNA have not been investigated in humans. The purpose of this study was to determine the impact of exercise with and without carbohydrate supplementation on skeletal muscle metabolic response in the heat.

Methods: Eight recreationally active males (4.05 ± 0.2 L·min^{-1}) completed 2 trials which included 1 hr of cycling at 70% workload max and 3 hr recovery in a hot environment. Both trials were conducted in a climate controlled environmental chamber (38°C and 40% RH). The trials differed by the consumption of either a 6% carbohydrate (CHO) containing beverage (8 ml·kg^{-1}·hr^{-1}) or placebo (P) during exercise in random order. Muscle biopsies were obtained from the *vastus lateralis* before exercise, immediately post-exercise and at the end of the 3 hr recovery period. Muscle was analyzed for muscle glycogen and mRNA related to metabolic and mitochondrial development (MFN2, PGC-1α, GLUT4, UCP3). Expired gases were measured to determine whole body substrate use during exercise.

Results: Carbohydrate oxidation and muscle glycogen utilization did not differ between trials, whereas fat oxidation was elevated during exercise in P. Exercise caused an increase in PGC-1α, and GLUT4 ($P < 0.05$) independent of exogenous carbohydrate provision. Carbohydrate consumption attenuated the mRNA response in UCP3 ($P < 0.05$).

Conclusions: This study indicates that the provision of exogenous carbohydrate attenuates the stimulation of mRNA expression of UCP3 following exercise in the heat.

Keywords: Mitochondrial biogenesis, PGC-1α, UCP3, Carbohydrate supplementation, Substrate utilization

Background

Mitochondrial adaptation is recognized as important in both health and disease. For some time it has been known that exercise induces critical adaptations in mitochondrial function within skeletal muscle [1]. More recently other factors have been considered key modifiers of mitochondrial and metabolic adaptation such as fat feeding [2], select bioflavonoids [3,4], intensity, duration and frequency of exercise [5-8], environmental temperature [9-13], and carbohydrate availability during exercise [14-16]. Acute markers for mitochondrial and metabolic alterations in fuel oxidation used in these investigations include mRNA for many different proteins involved in metabolism. These genes include the transcription regulator mitochondrial development peroxisome-proliferator- activated receptor-gamma co-activator 1 alpha (PGC-1α) [17,18], uncoupling protein 3 (UCP3) [12,19,20], the mitochondrial fusion protein mitofusin 2 [12,21], and other metabolic genes important for carbohydrate oxidation such as glucose transporter 4 (GLUT4) [22].

Carbohydrate consumption during exercise is capable of altering the stimuli for metabolic adaptation [14-16]. Cluberton et al. [14] have shown that carbohydrate consumption during exercise can attenuate the metabolic gene expression when completed in ambient temperatures. They showed that consumption of a 6% carbohydrate beverage during 1 hr of cycling at ~74% VO_{2max} lowered the exercise induced increase in mRNA of

* Correspondence: charles.dumke@umontana.edu
[1]Department of Health and Human Performance, Montana Center for Work Physiology and Exercise Metabolism, University of Montana, 32 Campus Drive, Missoula, MT 59812, USA
Full list of author information is available at the end of the article

PDK4 and UCP3 3 hr post-exercise, but not PGC-1α or GLUT4. As the authors suggest, this attenuation may be due to the increase in carbohydrate oxidation, suppression of circulating free fatty acids, and the elevation of insulin by exogenous carbohydrate consumption. Similar to carbohydrate consumption during exercise, exposure to heat in exercising humans has been shown to result in an upregulation of carbohydrate oxidation [23,24]. How carbohydrate delivery in the heat affects the metabolic adaptation to exercise remains poorly understood.

Previously we have shown in humans that PGC-1α gene expression is elevated in the cold, and attenuated following exercise in hot environments [12]. We demonstrated a ~20% reduction in PGC-1α mRNA following exercise in the heat (33°C). This attenuation in the heat is supported in other models as heat stress down-regulates mitochondrial function in yeast and broiler chickens [9-11]. In yeast, microarray genes associated with mitochondrial respiration were depressed following exposure to mild heat stress (37°C), and conversely genes associated with glycolysis were upregulated [10]. However this is not a universal finding across different experimental models [13,25]. In the absence of exercise, heat is capable of elevating expression of UCP3 in porcine muscle [25].

Since both environmental temperature and substrate availability can alter the metabolic gene response to exercise [12,14], it remains to be seen if carbohydrate ingestion in the heat attenuates the metabolic gene response following exercise and recovery in humans. Our purpose was to determine the impact of carbohydrate supplementation on select markers of exercise induced metabolic mRNA (PGC-1α, MFN2, UCP3, and GLUT4) in a hot environment (38°C).

Methods

Subjects

Eight male participants (23.5 ± 1.4 yrs, 76.6 ± 1.7 kg, 52.9 ± 2.2 ml•kg^{-1}•min^{-1}, 12.4 ± 1.6% body fat) volunteered for participation in the study. Prior to testing, participants read and signed an informed consent form approved by the University of Montana Institutional Review Board for the ethical use of human subject research and meet the standards of the Declaration of Helsinki.

Experimental design

Subjects (N = 8) completed 2 trials of 1 hr cycling at a constant load of 70% workload max (195.6 ± 11.3 watts) and 3 hr of recovery in a hot environment. Subjects arrived in the morning following an 8 hr fast. Both trials were in a controlled climate chamber at 38°C and 40% relative humidity, and separated by at least one week. Subjects were not heat acclimatized since the study was conducted in April at ~46°N latitude at the end of the northern hemisphere winter. The two counterbalanced trials for each participant differed by the provision of either a 6% carbohydrate (CHO) or placebo (P) beverage in random order. To achieve a 6% CHO solution, maltodextrin was mixed with an artificially flavored and sweetened commercially available powder (Crystal Light, Kraft Foods, Glenview, IL). Placebo contained the commercially available powder with no maltodextrin or other macronutrient energy, both P and CHO included 140 mg sodium per liter. Subjects were instructed to abstain from strenuous exercise for 48 hr, and no exercise for 24 hr before each trial. Subjects recorded diet intake for 24 hr prior to the day of the first trial and were instructed to replicate this exact diet prior to the second trial day. Muscle biopsies were collected pre ride, post ride and at the end of the 3 hr of recovery. On the morning of the trials, immediately prior to the exercise bout (< 5 min) subjects ingested 8 ml•kg^{-1} of the prescribed beverage, during exercise each beverage was consumed at a rate of 4 ml•kg^{-1}•30 min^{-1} (~37 g•hr^{-1} for CHO trial) and 4 ml•kg^{-1}•hr^{-1} (~18.4 g•hr^{-1} for CHO trial) during recovery. Body weights were recorded prior to entering the climate chamber, post ride, and at the end of the 3 hr recovery. Core temperatures were not measured since the chamber temperature was the same for both trials. Previously published reports from our lab indicate that a similar exercise protocol in the heat results in rectal temperatures exceeding 39°C [26]. Expired gases and rating of perceived exertion (RPE) were measured at 4, 24, and 54 min during the 1 hr exercise. VO_2 and VCO_2 were used determine whole-body fuel oxidation using the equation of Péronnet and Massicotte [27].

Body composition

Body density was determined using hydrodensitometry and corrected for estimated residual lung volume. Net underwater weights were recorded using load cells (Exertech, Dresbach, MN). Body density was then converted to body composition using the Siri equation [28].

Maximal exercise capacity

Maximum oxygen consumption (VO_2max) and power associated with VO_2max was measured for each fasted subject using a graded exercise protocol (starting at 95 W and increasing 35 W every three minutes) on an electronically braked cycle ergometer trainer (Velotron, RacerMate Inc., Seattle, WA). Maximum power was calculated as the highest completed stage (in W) plus the proportion of time in the last stage multiplied by the 35 W stage increment. Expired gases were measured and averaged in 15-second intervals during the test using a calibrated metabolic cart (Parvomedics, Inc., Salt Lake City, UT).

Biopsies

Biopsies were obtained pre and post exercise and following 3 h of recovery for the analysis of muscle glycogen, and metabolic gene expression (see below). Biopsies were taken from the *vastus lateralis* muscle using a 4–5 mm Bergstrom percutaneous muscle biopsy needle with the aid of suction. Biopsies were obtained from the same leg for a given trial using a separate incision 2 cm proximal to the previous biopsy. After excess blood, connective tissue, and fat were quickly removed, tissue samples (50–100 mg) were immersed in liquid nitrogen and stored at −80°C for subsequent analysis.

Glycogen

Muscle glycogen was analyzed using an enzymatic spectrophotometric method. Muscle samples were weighed (5–15 mg) upon removal from a −80°C freezer and placed in 0.5 ml, 2 N HCl solution. The sample solutions were weighed, incubated for two hours at 100°C in an oven, then re-weighed and re-constituted to their original weight using distilled water. To normalize pH, 1.5 ml of 0.67 M NaOH was added. An aliquot of this muscle extract (100 μl) was added to 1 ml of Infinity glucose (HK) liquid stable reagent (Thermo Fisher Scientific, Waltham, MA) and the absorbance read on a spectrophotometer at 340 nm. Glycogen concentration was calculated using the extinction co-efficient of NADH. Muscle glycogen concentrations are expressed in mmol · kg^{-1} wet weight of muscle tissue.

mRNA isolation

An 8–20 mg piece of skeletal muscle from the pre-exercise and 3 h recovery biopsies was homogenized in 800 μl of trizol (Invitrogen, Carlsbad CA, Cat# 15596–018) using an electric homogenizer (Tissue Tearor, Biosped Products Inc, Bartlesville OK). Samples were then incubated at room temperature for 5 minutes after which 200 μl of chloroform per 1000 μl of trizol was added and shaken vigorously. After an additional incubation at room temperature for 2–3 minutes the samples were centrifuged at 12,000 g for 15 minutes and the aqueous phase was transferred to a fresh tube. mRNA was precipitated by adding 400 μl of isopropyl alcohol and incubated overnight at −20°C. The next morning samples were centrifuged at 12,000 g for 10 minutes at 4°C and the mRNA was washed by removing the supernatant and adding 800 μl of 75% ethanol. Samples were vortexed and centrifuged at 7,500 g for 5 minutes at 4°C. mRNA was re-dissolved in 100 μl RNase-free water after the supernatant was removed and the mRNA pellet was dried. The RNA was cleaned using the RNeasy mini kit (Qiagen, Valencia CA, Cat#74104) according to the manufacturer's protocol using the additional DNase digestion step (RNase-free DNase set, Qiagen, Valencia CA, Cat# 79254). RNA purity was analyzed by the A260:A280 ratio and quantified on a nano-spectrophotometer (nanodrop ND-1000, Wilmington DE).

cDNA synthesis. First-strand cDNA synthesis was achieved using Superscript-first-strand synthesis system for RT-PCR kit (Invitrogen, Carlsbad CA, Cat #11904-0818) according to the manufacturer's protocol. Each sample within a given subject was normalized to the same amount of RNA. The resulting cDNA was then diluted two fold using RNase free water in order to have adequate volume for RT-PCR and frozen for later analysis.

Real time RT-PCR

Primer and Probe sequences are presented in Table 1. Each 25 μl reaction volume contained 500 nM primers, 250 nM probe (PrimeTime qPCR assay, Integrated DNA technologies), 1× FastStart TaqMan Probe master (Roche Applied Science, Indianapolis IN), and 2.5 μl of sample cDNA. PCR was then run using the Bio-Rad I Cycler iQ5 Real-Time PCR Detection system (Bio-Rad, Hercules CA) using a 2-step Roche protocol (1 cycle at 50°C for 10 minutes, 1 cycle at 95°C for 10 minutes, followed by 40 cycles of 95°C for 15 seconds followed by 60°C for 1 minute). Quantification of mRNA from the pre and 3 h post exercise samples was calculated using the $2^{-\Delta\Delta CT}$ as described earlier [29,30]. GAPDH was used as the reference housekeeping gene as it has been demonstrated to be the most stable among other common housekeeping genes following aerobic exercise and environmental temperature [12,31,32]. The stability of GAPDH was analyzed by the ΔCT method [29,30].

Table 1 Primers and probes used for real-time PCR

Gene	Primer 1	Primer 2	Probe
GAPDH	TGTAGTTGAGGTCAATGAAGGG	ACATCGCTCAGACACCATG	AAGGTCGGAGTCAACGGATTTGGTC
MFN2	ATGCATCCCACTTAAGCAC	CCAGAGGGCAGAACTTTCTC	AGAGGCATCAGTGAGGTGCT
PGC-1α	ATAAATCACACGGCGCTCTT	TGAGAGGGCCAAGCAAAG	AGAGGCAGAGGCAGAAGG
UCP3	CAAAATCCGGGTAGTGAGGCT	TGACTCCGTCAAGCAGGTGTAC	CCCCCAAAGGCGCGGACAAC
GLUT4	TCTTCACCTTGGTCTCGGTGTTGT	CACGAAGCCAAAGATGGCCACAAT	ATGTGTGGCTGTGCCATCCTGATGA

GAPDH Glyceraldehyde 3-phosphate dehydrogenase, *MFN2* mitofusin 2, *PGC-1α* peroxisome-proliferator- activated receptor-gamma co-activator 1 alpha, *UCP3* uncoupling protein 3, *GLUT4* glucose transporter 4.

Statistics

Dependent variables were compared using two-way repeated-measures ANOVA's (time x trial or exercise-recovery × CHO). In the event of a significant f-ratio, post hoc Fishers protected least significant difference procedure was used to determine where differences occurred. All statistics were performed using SPSS for windows Version 13 (Chicago, IL). A probability of type I error less than 5% was considered significant ($p < 0.05$). All data are reported as mean ± SE.

Results

Exercise trials

Prescribed fluid intakes were 2.16 ± 0.05 L over the course of the one hour of exercise and 3 h of recovery. Subjects lost an average of 0.63 ± 0.07 and 0.73 ± 0.13 kg body weight during the CHO and P trials respectively ($p < 0.05$), regardless of trial. This <1% of body weight loss suggests fluid intakes were sufficient to adequately meet sweat rates during the hot trials. The prescribed carbohydrate intake amounted to 129.6 ± 3.0 g of carbohydrate, or 518.4 ± 12.0 kcals over the 4 hr in the climate chamber during the CHO trial. Heart rate, RPE, oxygen consumption and carbon dioxide production increased during the exercise period ($p < 0.05$), but did not differ between trials (Table 2).

Subjects finished the exercise trial at a mean RPE of >17 (Table 2), suggesting that the combination of the heat and exercise was perceptually difficult. RER was lower by the end of the 1 hr exercise bout during P compared to CHO trial (significant trial × time interaction, $p = 0.017$), demonstrating a greater reliance on fat by the end of the P trial (Table 2). There was not a significant effect of exercise ($p = 0.5$) or trial ($p = 0.18$) on absolute carbohydrate oxidation (Figure 1A). Absolute fat oxidation was not different between trials ($p = 0.10$), but did show a significant increase ($p = 0.02$) in fat use by the end of their 1 hr bout of cycling (Figure 1B).

Muscle Glycogen Muscle glycogen did not differ between trials ($p = 0.57$), but decreased as a result of the exercise bout ($p < 0.001$) (Figure 2). This represents a 35% and 44% reduction pre and post exercise for the CHO and P trial respectively. Muscle glycogen did not significantly increase from post exercise to 3 hr of recovery in either trial.

Gene Expression There was not a significant effect of exercise in the heat on our housekeeping gene, GAPDH ($p = 0.3$). Metabolic and mitochondrial gene expression from the pre and 3 hr post exercise muscle samples using the $2^{-\Delta\Delta CT}$ method is presented in Figure 3. There was a significant effect for exercise on GLUT4 mRNA ($P = 0.04$), increasing 20% and 27% in the CHO and P trial respectively. GLUT4 expression was not altered by CHO treatment. Exercise increased PGC-1α ($P < 0.001$) 8 and 9.5 fold in the CHO and P trial respectively, but did not show a significant effect of treatment ($P = 0.15$). MFN2 did not change with exercise in the heat or carbohydrate supplementation. There was a significant effect of exercise ($P < 0.001$) and interaction (CHO × exercise) for UCP3 ($P = 0.001$), where UCP3 mRNA in the placebo trial increased over 2 fold but did not increase during the CHO trial.

Discussion

These data support previous research demonstrating the carbohydrate attenuation of metabolic adaptations to exercise. Specifically, this investigation showed the attenuation of the exercise stimulation of skeletal muscle UCP3 mRNA with carbohydrate consumption in the heat. We also confirmed exercise induced increases in GLUT4 and PGC-1α in the heat. A previous investigation demonstrated that carbohydrate consumption during exercise attenuated the mRNA expression for both UCP3 and PDK4, and only a trend towards GLUT4 in ambient conditions [14]. Similarly, we did not show a significant effect of carbohydrate consumption on GLUT4 ($p = 0.7$), but did observe an attenuation in UCP3 mRNA in the current investigation. A direct comparison between environmental temperatures would need to be performed to determine if environmental conditions alter these CHO attenuating effects.

In the current investigation carbohydrate oxidation did not differ between trials despite exercising for 1 hr at 70% workload max at 38°C and 40% RH with and without oral carbohydrate consumption. Perhaps the similar rates of carbohydrate oxidation are due to an increase in

Table 2 VO_2, VCO_2, RER, HR, and RPE during 1 h exercise trials in the heat, with and without CHO

	Placebo			CHO		
	4 min	24 min	54 min	4 min	24 min	54 min
VO_2 ($L \cdot min^{-1}$)	2.91 ± 0.10	3.21 ± 0.15	3.63 ± 0.19*	3.01 ± 0.16	3.25 ± 0.16	3.52 ± 0.22*
VCO_2 ($L \cdot min^{-1}$)	2.64 ± 0.07	2.79 ± 0.12	3.11 ± 0.17*	2.72 ± 0.13	2.87 ± 0.15	3.10 ± 0.19*
RER	0.91 ± 0.01	0.87 ± 0.01	0.86 ± 0.01†	0.90 ± 0.01	0.88 ± 0.01	0.88 ± 0.01†
HR ($beats \cdot min^{-1}$)	138.5 ± 6.7	158.9 ± 5.4	172.6 ± 4.9*	151.4 ± 5.9	162.0 ± 5.4	173.1 ± 4.4*
RPE	12.6 ± 0.3	15.0 ± 0.5	17.8 ± 0.6*	12.4 ± 0.5	15.1 ± 0.5	17.9 ± 0.4*

*$p < 0.05$ main effect of time; † $p < 0.05$ main effect of trial X time.

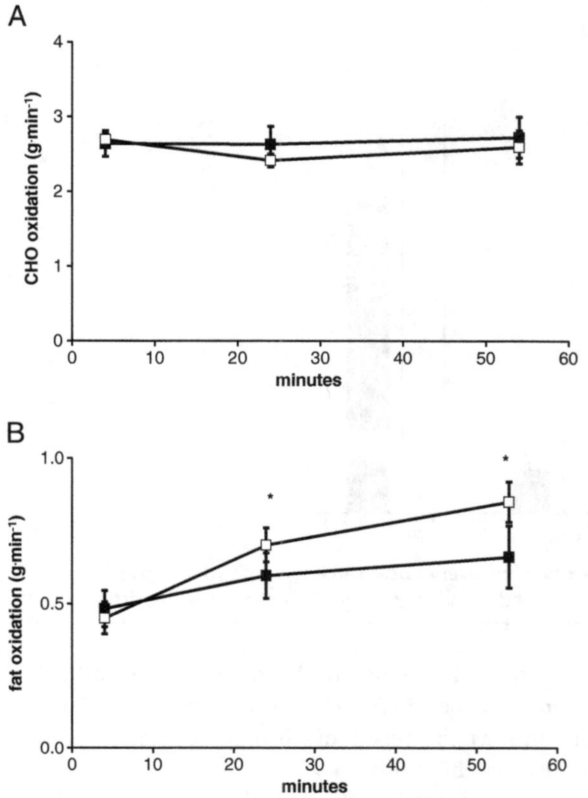

Figure 1 Substrate oxidation during exercise in the heat. A. represents carbohydrate oxidation for 1 hr in the heat with gas measurements made at 4, 24, and 54 min. **B.** represents fat oxidation for 1 hr in the heat with gas measurements made at 4, 24, and 54 min. Open and solid symbols represent the P and CHO trials respectively. * - indicates a significant main effect of time.

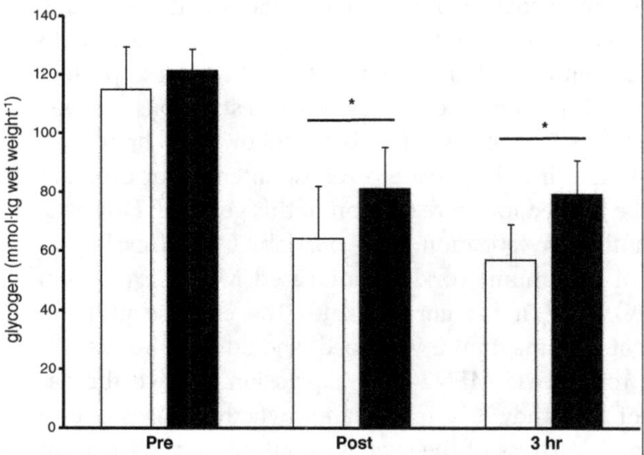

Figure 2 Muscle glycogen concentration pre, post-exercise and following 3 hr of recovery. Open and solid bars represent the P and CHO trials respectively. * - indicates a significant main effect of time.

the oxidation of endogenous carbohydrate in the heat during the P trial. Our selection of study design does not allow us to make this direct comparison, however the increase in carbohydrate oxidation in the heat is well established [23,24]. This may explain why only UCP3 was attenuated in the CHO trial in our investigation and not GLUT4. The glucose transporter GLUT4 is a gene linked to carbohydrate oxidation [33,34]. Cluberton et al. [14] showed a trend ($p = 0.09$) for carbohydrate consumption to attenuate the exercise induced increase in gene expression for GLUT4 under ambient conditions. Although they demonstrated a 2 fold increase with exercise on GLUT4 expression, it is not apparent that this reached statistical significance. In the current study, although there was a significant effect of exercise, we saw no evidence of carbohydrate ingestion on GLUT4 mRNA expression ($p = 0.7$). It is compelling to believe that this may be due to the lack of difference between CHO and P trials in absolute carbohydrate oxidation in the heat, which may mask the effects of carbohydrate ingestion on this gene. It is a limitation of the current study that there were not ambient temperature trials (with and without carbohydrate) by which to compare the effects of the heat, however this was eliminated due to the stress on the subjects (amounting to 4 trials and 12 biopsies). The purpose of this study was to provide initial insight on this topic, while relying on the previously reported effect of CHO consumption under ambient conditions on these genes [14].

Depletion of glycogen is thought to be a potential aspect of the stimulation of mitochondrial biogenesis [35]. Exercise in the current study was sufficient to lower muscle glycogen levels ~40%, which is believed to be capable of stimulating AMPK, an upstream covalent modifier of PGC-1α [5,36,37]. In the current study glycogen depletion and carbohydrate oxidation did not differ between trials during the 1 h of exercise, indirectly suggesting that AMPK activity was similar between trials. This is supported by others, as carbohydrate ingestion during cycling is not thought to alter glycogen utilization [14,38]. As well, carbohydrate ingestion during cycling does not appear to alter AMPK signaling in humans [39]. This may explain why GLUT4 was not different between trials, since AMPK is thought to be a potent simulator of GLUT4 transcription [40]. Despite this lack of effect of carbohydrate ingestion on GLUT4, UCP3 mRNA expression was attenuated by carbohydrate ingestion. This suggests that the UCP3 gene may be more sensitive to fat oxidation. We showed a significant effect of carbohydrate ingestion on RER, with the P trial demonstrating greater fat reliance by the end of the exercise bout. We unfortunately do not have substrate oxidation data for the 3 h of recovery prior to the last biopsy, when mRNA expression was sampled. However

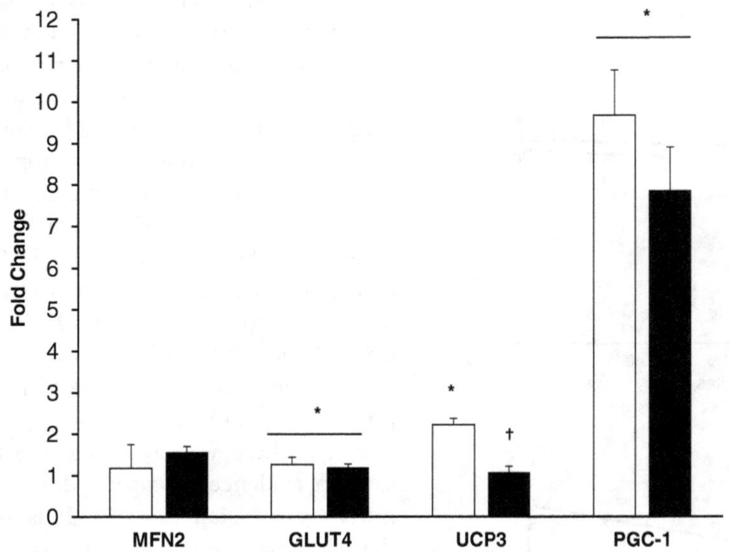

Figure 3 Muscle expression for metabolic and mitochondrial genes following 3 hr of recovery post-exercise. Open and solid bars represent the P and CHO trials respectively. * - indicates a significant main effect of time, and † - indicates a significant trial X time interaction.

since the P trial received no carbohydrate into the recovery period, it is quite possible that the greater fat oxidation during the later stages of exercise continued into recovery in the P trial and subsequently attenuated the UCP3 mRNA expression. This is supported by evidence that elevated circulating fatty acids are associated with the upregulation of skeletal muscle expression of UCP3 [14,41-43]. We do not have evidence of circulating free fatty acids (FFA) in the current study, but it is well established that fasted exercise in the absence of carbohydrate delivery elevates FFA compared to carbohydrate trials [44]. Although fat oxidation appears to coincide with UCP3 expression, the metabolic role of this protein in skeletal muscle remains unclear as it suggests a loss of exercise efficiency by uncoupling the proton gradient created in the electron transport chain from ATP synthesis. However, besides fat oxidation, UCP3 has been implicated as being important in the control of thermogenesis and the regulation of oxidative stress [45]. The long term implications of the attenuation of UCP3 expression following exercise with carbohydrate supplementation in this study and others has yet to be determined [14,43]. It is intriguing to think that lower UCP3 mRNA may play a role in previous evidence of the carbohydrate attenuating effect on fat oxidation with exercise training [44,46]. These studies demonstrated that low carbohydrate availability (fat adapted) resulted in greater rates of fat oxidation even when glycogen levels were restored with a day on a high carbohydrate diet. Our study and others have shown that UCP3 is the gene most consistently attenuated with the consumption of exogenous carbohydrate. How UCP3 expression is affected during longer periods of low carbohydrate availability remain to be seen. Acute changes in mRNA expression must be interpreted with caution, since protein amounts as the result of chronic adaptation were not the focus of this study.

For the other genes investigated, this study is consistent with previous literature which shows that the expression of GLUT4 [22] and PGC-1α mRNA is elevated following exercise [6,17,18]. More surprisingly, exercise stimulated increases in mRNA were not seen in MFN2, as these have previously been shown to be sensitive to exercise [8,12,14,21,47]. We confirmed in this study that our housekeeping gene was insensitive to both heat and exercise, and this is supported in the literature [12,31,32]. Therefore, it remains unknown why an exercise induced increase in MFN2 was not observed in the current study. MFN2 is a mitochondrial membrane protein involved in the fusion events of the mitochondrial architecture [21]. Increased expression of this gene is thought to lead to greater mitochondrial function through matrix protein mixing [48]. One of our previous investigations showed robust (~50%) increases in MFN2 following 5 hr of cycling, suggesting that greater exercise intensity or duration may be needed for up regulation of this gene [8]. However, in another investigation from our lab, 1 hr of cycling at 60% of maximum workload increased MFN2 expression (~20%) [12]. In the current study the exercise protocol (1 hr at 70% maximum workload) should have been sufficient to increase MFN2 gene expression. Due to the design of this study it is not apparent whether this is due to the modest stress of the exercise bout, modest changes in individual variability in a somewhat small sample size, or an attenuating effect of the hot environment. We previously showed that MFN2 is not significantly affected by exercise in varying environmental temperatures, with similar exercise responses in the heat (33°C), cold (7°C), and neutral (20°C) environments [12]. This suggests that small increases in variability with a sample size of eight may have affected the statistical outcome of this particular gene. Despite this, carbohydrate supplementation had no apparent attenuating effects on this mitochondrial fusion gene. To our knowledge this is the first time MFN2 has been investigated following carbohydrate supplementation in humans.

Conclusions

These data contribute to the general understanding of stimuli regulating metabolic adaptation following exercise. We found that exercise and recovery in the heat stimulates genes for PGC-1α, UCP3 and GLUT4. Carbohydrate ingestion during exercise and recovery in a hot environment attenuated mRNA expression of UCP3, but had no effect on the expression of MFN2, GLUT4 and PGC-1α. It remains to be seen through a direct comparison of environmental temperatures if this is due to similar carbohydrate oxidation rates when carbohydrate is ingested in the heat during exercise.

Regardless of environmental temperature, these data should not be interpreted as reason to avoid ingesting carbohydrate during exercise. Carbohydrate delivery during exercise bouts of >1 hr is well known to increase performance [49-51]. However, a growing body of evidence may also suggest that carbohydrate availability during training bouts can alter the metabolic response and perhaps result in increased reliance on fat stores when carbohydrate availability is low [2,7,8,52]. The concept of a 'periodized diet' to control and maximize fuel oxidation and the adaptations to specific blocks of training for both endurance and resistance exercise is an exciting new area of applied sport nutrition research.

Abbreviations

CHO: Carbohydrate; P: Placebo; VO_2: Oxygen consumption; VO_{2max}: Maximal oxygen consumption; VCO_2: Carbon dioxide production; RER: Respiratory exchange ratio; RPE: Rating of perceived exertion; mRNA: Messenger ribonucleic acid; PGC-1α: Peroxisome-proliferator- activated; receptor-gamma: Co-activator 1 alpha; UCP3: Uncoupling protein 3; MFN2: Mitofusin 2; GLUT4: Glucose transporter 4; GAPDH: Glyceraldehyde 3-phosphate dehydrogenase; PDK4: Pyruvate dehydrogenase 4.

Competing interests

The authors declare that they have no competing interests in access to these data or associations with companies involved with products used in this research. This study was supported by a grant from the Office of Naval Research Grant Award N000140910850.

The views and conclusions contained herein are those of the authors and should not be interpreted as necessarily representing the official policies or endorsements, either expressed or implied, of the Office of Naval Research or the U.S. government.

Authors' contributions

CLD participated in conception, design, and data acquisition, assisted in PCR analysis and interpretation of data, and wrote the manuscript. DRS participated in conception, design, and data acquisition, assisted in PCR analysis and interpretation of data, and aided in the drafting and revising of the manuscript. JSC participated in data acquisition, analysis and interpretation of data, and aided in the drafting and revising of the manuscript. WSH participated in data acquisition, analysis and interpretation of data, and aided in the drafting and revising of the manuscript. BCR participated in conception, design, and data acquisition, assisted in analysis and interpretation of data, and aided in the drafting and revising of the manuscript. All authors have read and given final approval of this version of the manuscript for publication.

Acknowledgments

The authors wish to thank the subjects for their investment in time and energy.

Author details

[1]Department of Health and Human Performance, Montana Center for Work Physiology and Exercise Metabolism, University of Montana, 32 Campus Drive, Missoula, MT 59812, USA. [2]School of Health, Physical Education and Recreation, University of Nebraska at Omaha, 6001 Dodge Street, Omaha, NE 68182, USA.

References

1. Holloszy JO: **Biochemical adaptations in muscle. Effects of exercise on mitochondrial oxygen uptake and respiratory enzyme activity in skeletal muscle.** *J Biol Chem* 1967, **242:**2278–2282.
2. Cameron-Smith D, Burke LM, Angus DJ, Tunstall RJ, Cox GR, Bonen A, Hawley JA, Hargreaves M: **A short-term, high-fat diet up-regulates lipid metabolism and gene expression in human skeletal muscle.** *Am J Clin Nutr* 2003, **77:**313–318.
3. Baur JA, Pearson KJ, Price NL, Jamieson HA, Lerin C, Kalra A, Prabhu W, Allard JS, Lopez-Lluch G, Lewis K, *et al*: **Resveratrol improves health and survival of mice on a high-calorie diet.** *Nature* 2006, **444:**337–342.
4. Davis JM, Murphy EA, Carmichael MD, Davis B: **Quercetin increases brain and muscle mitochondrial biogenesis and exercise tolerance.** *Am J Physiol Regul Integr Comp Physiol* 2009, **296:**R1071–1077.
5. McConell GK, Lee-Young RS, Chen ZP, Stepto NK, Huynh NN, Stephens TJ, Canny BJ, Kemp BE: **Short-term exercise training in humans reduces AMPK signalling during prolonged exercise independent of muscle glycogen.** *J Physiol* 2005, **568:**665–676.
6. Dumke CL, Mark Davis J, Angela Murphy E, Nieman DC, Carmichael MD, Quindry JC, Travis Triplett N, Utter AC, Gross Gowin SJ, Henson DA, *et al*: **Successive bouts of cycling stimulates genes associated with mitochondrial biogenesis.** *Eur J Appl Physiol* 2009, **107:**419–427.
7. Hansen AK, Fischer CP, Plomgaard P, Andersen JL, Saltin B, Pedersen BK: **Skeletal muscle adaptation: training twice every second day vs. training once daily.** *J Appl Physiol* 2005, **98:**93–99.
8. Slivka DR, Dumke CL, Hailes WS, Cuddy JS, Ruby BC: **Substrate use and biochemical response to a 3,211-km bicycle tour in trained cyclists.** *Eur J Appl Physiol*, **112:**1621–1630.
9. Azad MA, Kikusato M, Maekawa T, Shirakawa H, Toyomizu M: **Metabolic characteristics and oxidative damage to skeletal muscle in broiler chickens exposed to chronic heat stress.** *Comp Biochem Physiol A Mol Integr Physiol* 2010, **155:**401–406.
10. Sakaki K, Tashiro K, Kuhara S, Mihara K: **Response of genes associated with mitochondrial function to mild heat stress in yeast Saccharomyces cerevisiae.** *J Biochem* 2003, **134:**373–384.
11. Yang L, Tan GY, Fu YQ, Feng JH, Zhang MH: **Effects of acute heat stress and subsequent stress removal on function of hepatic mitochondrial respiration, ROS production and lipid peroxidation in broiler chickens.** *Comp Biochem Physiol C Toxicol Pharmacol* 2010, **151:**204–208.
12. Slivka DR, Dumke CL, Tucker TJ, Cuddy JS, Ruby B: **Human mRNA Response to Exercise and Temperature.** *Int J Sports Med* 2012, **33:**94–100.
13. Liu CT, Brooks GA: **Mild heat stress induces mitochondrial biogenesis in C2C12 myotubes.** *J Appl Physiol* 2012, **112:**354–361.
14. Cluberton LJ, McGee SL, Murphy RM, Hargreaves M: **Effect of carbohydrate ingestion on exercise-induced alterations in metabolic gene expression.** *J Appl Physiol* 2005, **99:**1359–1363.
15. Morton JP, Croft L, Bartlett JD, Maclaren DP, Reilly T, Evans L, McArdle A, Drust B: **Reduced carbohydrate availability does not modulate**

training-induced heat shock protein adaptations but does upregulate oxidative enzyme activity in human skeletal muscle. *J Appl Physiol* 2009, **106:**1513–1521.
16. Civitarese AE, Hesselink MK, Russell AP, Ravussin E, Schrauwen P: **Glucose ingestion during exercise blunts exercise-induced gene expression of skeletal muscle fat oxidative genes.** *Am J Physiol Endocrinol Metab* 2005, **289:**E1023–1029.
17. Pilegaard H, Saltin B, Neufer PD: **Exercise induces transient transcriptional activation of the PGC-1alpha gene in human skeletal muscle.** *J Physiol* 2003, **546:**851–858.
18. Wende AR, Schaeffer PJ, Parker GJ, Zechner C, Han DH, Chen MM, Hancock CR, Lehman JJ, Huss JM, McClain DA, *et al*: **A role for the transcriptional coactivator PGC-1α in muscle refueling.** *J Biol Chem* 2007, **282:**36642–36651.
19. Costford SR, Seifert EL, Bezaire VMFG, Bevilacqua L, Gowing A, Harper ME: **The energetic implications of uncoupling protein-3 in skeletal muscle.** *Appl Physiol Nutr Metab* 2007, **32:**884–894.
20. Bezaire V, Seifert EL, Harper ME: **Uncoupling protein-3: clues in an ongoing mitochondrial mystery.** *Faseb J* 2007, **21:**312–324.
21. Bach D, Pich S, Soriano FX, Vega N, Baumgartner B, Oriola J, Daugaard JR, Lloberas J, Camps M, Zierath JR, *et al*: **Mitofusin-2 determines mitochondrial network architecture and mitochondrial metabolism. A novel regulatory mechanism altered in obesity.** *J Biol Chem* 2003, **278:**17190–17197.
22. Neufer PD, Dohm GL: **Exercise induces a transient increase in transcription of the GLUT-4 gene in skeletal muscle.** *Am J Physiol* 1993, **265:**C1597–1603.
23. Febbraio MA, Snow RJ, Hargreaves M, Stathis CG, Martin IK, Carey MF: **Muscle metabolism during exercise and heat stress in trained men: effect of acclimation.** *J Appl Physiol* 1994, **76:**589–597.
24. Hargreaves M, Angus D, Howlett K, Conus NM, Febbraio M: **Effect of heat stress on glucose kinetics during exercise.** *J Appl Physiol* 1996, **81:**1594–1597.
25. Katsumata M, Matsumoto M, Kawakami S, Kaji Y: **Effect of heat exposure on uncoupling protein-3 mRNA abundance in porcine skeletal muscle.** *J Anim Sci* 2004, **82:**3493–3499.
26. Quindry J, Miller L, McGinnis G, Kliszczewicz B, Slivka D, Dumke C, Cuddy J, Ruby B: **Envrionmental Temperature and Exercise-Induced Blood Oxidative Stress.** *Int J Sport Nutr Exerc Metab* 2013, **23:**128–136.
27. Jeukendrup AE, Wallis GA: **Measurement of substrate oxidation during exercise by means of gas exchange measurements.** *Int J Sports Med* 2005, **26**(Suppl 1)**:**S28–37.
28. Siri WE: *Body composition from fluid space and density.* Washington, DC: National Academy of Sciences; 1961.
29. Livak KJ, Schmittgen TD: **Analysis of relative gene expression data using real-time quantitative PCR and the 2(ΔΔC(T)) Method.** *Methods* 2001, **25:**402–408.
30. Schmittgen TD, Livak KJ: **Analyzing real-time PCR data by the comparative C(T) method.** *Nat Protoc* 2008, **3:**1101–1108.
31. Jemiolo B, Trappe S: **Single muscle fiber gene expression in human skeletal muscle: validation of internal control with exercise.** *Biochem Biophys Res Commun* 2004, **320:**1043–1050.
32. Mahoney DJ, Carey K, Fu MH, Snow R, Cameron-Smith D, Parise G, Tarnopolsky MA: **Real-time RT-PCR analysis of housekeeping genes in human skeletal muscle following acute exercise.** *Physiol Genomics* 2004, **18:**226–231.
33. Wake SA, Sowden JA, Storlien LH, James DE, Clark PW, Shine J, Chisholm DJ, Kraegen EW: **Effects of exercise training and dietary manipulation on insulin-regulatable glucose-transporter mRNA in rat muscle.** *Diabetes* 1991, **40:**275–279.
34. Kuo CH, Hunt DG, Ding Z, Ivy JL: **Effect of carbohydrate supplementation on postexercise GLUT-4 protein expression in skeletal muscle.** *J Appl Physiol* 1999, **87:**2290–2295.
35. Pilegaard H, Keller C, Steensberg A, Helge JW, Pedersen BK, Saltin B, Neufer PD: **Influence of pre-exercise muscle glycogen content on exercise-induced transcriptional regulation of metabolic genes.** *J Physiol* 2002, **541:**261–271.
36. Suwa M, Nakano H, Kumagai S: **Effects of chronic AICAR treatment on fiber composition, enzyme activity, UCP3, and PGC-1 in rat muscles.** *J Appl Physiol* 2003, **95:**960–968.
37. Jorgensen SB, Richter EA, Wojtaszewski JF: **Role of AMPK in skeletal muscle metabolic regulation and adaptation in relation to exercise.** *J Physiol* 2006, **574:**17–31.
38. Coyle EF, Coggan AR, Hemmert MK, Ivy JL: **Muscle glycogen utilization during prolonged strenuous exercise when fed carbohydrate.** *J Appl Physiol* 1986, **61:**165–172.
39. Lee-Young RS, Palmer MJ, Linden KC, LePlastrier K, Canny BJ, Hargreaves M, Wadley GD, Kemp BE, McConell GK: **Carbohydrate ingestion does not alter skeletal muscle AMPK signaling during exercise in humans.** *Am J Physiol Endocrinol Metab* 2006, **291:**E566–573.
40. Ojuka EO: **Role of calcium and AMP kinase in the regulation of mitochondrial biogenesis and GLUT4 levels in muscle.** *Proc Nutr Soc* 2004, **63:**275–278.
41. Son C, Hosoda K, Matsuda J, Fujikura J, Yonemitsu S, Iwakura H, Masuzaki H, Ogawa Y, Hayashi T, Itoh H, *et al*: **Up-regulation of uncoupling protein 3 gene expression by fatty acids and agonists for PPARs in L6 myotubes.** *Endocrinology* 2001, **142:**4189–4194.
42. Weigle DS, Selfridge LE, Schwartz MW, Seeley RJ, Cummings DE, Havel PJ, Kuijper JL, BeltrandelRio H: **Elevated free fatty acids induce uncoupling protein 3 expression in muscle: a potential explanation for the effect of fasting.** *Diabetes* 1998, **47:**298–302.
43. Schrauwen P, Hesselink MK, Vaartjes I, Kornips E, Saris WH, Giacobino JP, Russell A: **Effect of acute exercise on uncoupling protein 3 is a fat metabolism-mediated effect.** *Am J Physiol Endocrinol Metab* 2002, **282:**E11–17.
44. Burke LM, Angus DJ, Cox GR, Cummings NK, Febbraio MA, Gawthorn K, Hawley JA, Minehan M, Martin DT, Hargreaves M: **Effect of fat adaptation and carbohydrate restoration on metabolism and performance during prolonged cycling.** *J Appl Physiol* 2000, **89:**2413–2421.
45. Boss O, Hagen T, Lowell BB: **Uncoupling proteins 2 and 3: potential regulators of mitochondrial energy metabolism.** *Diabetes* 2000, **49:**143–156.
46. Yeo WK, Lessard SJ, Chen ZP, Garnham AP, Burke LM, Rivas DA, Kemp BE, Hawley JA: **Fat adaptation followed by carbohydrate restoration increases AMPK activity in skeletal muscle from trained humans.** *J Appl Physiol* 2008, **105:**1519–1526.
47. Pilegaard H, Ordway GA, Saltin B, Neufer PD: **Transcriptional regulation of gene expression in human skeletal muscle during recovery from exercise.** *Am J Physiol Endocrinol Metab* 2000, **279:**E806–814.
48. Liu X, Weaver D, Shirihai O, Hajnoczky G: **Mitochondrial 'kiss-and-run': interplay between mitochondrial motility and fusion-fission dynamics.** *Embo J* 2009, **28:**3074–3089.
49. Febbraio MA, Chiu A, Angus DJ, Arkinstall MJ, Hawley JA: **Effects of carbohydrate ingestion before and during exercise on glucose kinetics and performance.** *J Appl Physiol* 2000, **89:**2220–2226.
50. Hargreaves M, Costill DL, Coggan A, Fink WJ, Nishibata I: **Effect of carbohydrate feedings on muscle glycogen utilization and exercise performance.** *Med Sci Sports Exerc* 1984, **16:**219–222.
51. Coggan AR, Coyle EF: **Effect of carbohydrate feedings during high-intensity exercise.** *J Appl Physiol* 1988, **65:**1703–1709.
52. Yeo WK, Paton CD, Garnham AP, Burke LM, Carey A, Hawley JA: **Skeletal muscle adaptation and performance responses to once a day versus twice every second day endurance training regimens.** *J Appl Physiol* 2008, **90882:**92008.

2

Additive insulinogenic action of Opuntia ficus-indica cladode and fruit skin extract and leucine after exercise in healthy males

Louise Deldicque[1†], Karen Van Proeyen[1†], Monique Ramaekers[1], Ivo Pischel[2], Hartwig Sievers[2] and Peter Hespel[1*]

Abstract

Background: Oral intake of a specific extract of *Opuntia ficus-indica* cladode and fruit skin (OpunDia™) (OFI) has been shown to increase serum insulin concentration while reducing blood glucose level for a given amount of glucose ingestion after an endurance exercise bout in healthy young volunteers. However, it is unknown whether OFI-induced insulin stimulation after exercise is of the same magnitude than the stimulation by other insulinogenic agents like leucine as well as whether OFI can interact with those agents. Therefore, the aims of the present study were: 1) to compare the degree of insulin stimulation by OFI with the effect of leucine administration; 2) to determine whether OFI and leucine have an additive action on insulin stimulation post-exercise.

Methods: Eleven subjects participated in a randomized double-blind cross-over study involving four experimental sessions. In each session the subjects successively underwent a 2-h oral glucose tolerance test (OGTT) after a 30-min cycling bout at ~70% VO_2max. At t_0 and t_{60} during the OGTT, subjects ingested 75 g glucose and capsules containing either 1) a placebo; 2) 1000 mg OFI; 3) 3 g leucine; 4) 1000 mg OFI + 3 g leucine. Blood samples were collected before and at 30-min intervals during the OGTT for determination of blood glucose and serum insulin.

Results: Whereas no effect of leucine was measured, OFI reduced blood glucose at t_{90} by ~7% and the area under the glucose curve by ~15% and increased serum insulin concentration at t_{90} by ~35% compared to placebo ($P<0.05$). From t_{60} to the end of the OGTT, serum insulin concentration was higher in OFI+leucine than in placebo which resulted in a higher area under the insulin curve (+40%, $P<0.05$).

Conclusion: Carbohydrate-induced insulin stimulation post-exercise can be further increased by the combination of OFI with leucine. OFI and leucine could be interesting ingredients to include together in recovery drinks to resynthesize muscle glycogen faster post-exercise. Still, it needs to be confirmed that such nutritional strategy effectively stimulates post-exercise muscle glycogen resynthesis.

Keywords: Nutritional supplements, Post exercise recovery, Glucose clearance, Glycogen resynthesis, Endurance athletes, Amino acids

Background

High-intensity exercise typically leads to a depletion of body carbohydrate stores, primarily muscle glycogen [1]. Hence high-dose oral carbohydrate intake during recovery after exercise is pivotal to muscle glycogen resynthesis and thus repletion of carbohydrate stores [2]. Therefore, typical sports recovery drinks include a high carbohydrate dose (~50-100 grams), composed of rapidly absorbable sugars such as maltodextrin (a D-glucose polymer) and D-glucose (~dextrose). The increased plasma insulin level due to high-dose glucose ingestion is pivotal to stimulation of muscle glucose uptake and glycogen synthesis [3,4]. Insulin, which is secreted by the pancreatic β-cells upon elevated circulating glucose concentration, stimulates glucose import in muscle cells via the GLUT4 membrane protein. It also stimulates the incorporation of the glucose molecules into the glycogen molecule via activation of the glycogen synthase enzyme [5]. In this regard it

* Correspondence: peter.hespel@faber.kuleuven.be
†Equal contributors
[1]Exercise Physiology Research Group, Department of Kinesiology, KJ Leuven, Leuven, Belgium
Full list of author information is available at the end of the article

is also important to note that muscular insulin sensitivity is markedly increased following muscle contractions [6]. Thus, any intervention that could elevate plasma insulin and/or further increase insulin sensitivity following exercise could facilitate repletion of muscle glycogen stores, and thus serve as a useful recovery agent.

In this respect, the addition of amino acids, and more particularly leucine, to a carbohydrate-rich drink is a frequent strategy used by athletes to increase insulin secretion and thereby enhance glycogen resynthesis. Leucine has a strong insulinotropic action which contributes to a faster glycogen resynthesis after exercise [7,8]. Based on recent reports [9,10], *Opuntia ficus-indica* intake could be another interesting nutritional strategy to stimulate insulin secretion and glycogen resynthesis after exercise. *Opuntia ficus-indica* is one of the approximately 200 species of the *Opuntia* genus, which belongs to the Cactaceae family [11]. *Opuntia ficus-indica* has been found to lower blood glucose and to increase basal plasma insulin levels in animals [9,12] as well as in humans [10,13,14]. This indicates a direct action on insulin secretion at the site of pancreatic β-cells rather than an indirect action via increased blood glucose levels.

Our group has recently shown that oral intake of a specific extract of *Opuntia ficus-indica* cladode and fruit skin (OFI) increases serum insulin concentration while reducing blood glucose level for a given amount of glucose ingestion after an endurance exercise bout in healthy young volunteers [10]. In a dose–response experiment we also found 1000 mg of OFI to cause a maximal increase of plasma insulin concentration. However, we did not evaluate the interaction of OFI with other insulinogenic agents like leucine. Moreover, commercial recovery drinks contain a maximal leucine dose of 3 g whereas only high doses (~7 g) have been shown to increase carbohydrate-induced insulin stimulation after exercise [7,8,15]. It is unknown whether lower doses of leucine increase carbohydrates-induced insulin stimulation as well. Against this background, the aims of the present study were: 1) to compare the degree of insulin stimulation by OFI with another prevailing strategy in sports nutrition to stimulate post exercise insulin release, i.e. 3 g oral leucine administration; 2) to determine whether OFI and leucine can have an additive action to elevate post exercise plasma insulin concentration.

Methods

Subjects

Eleven healthy, physically active males were included in the study (age: 21.1 ± 0.9 y; body weight: 74.5 ± 4.2 kg; VO_2 max: 65 ± 4 ml·min^{-1}·kg). After approval of the study protocol by the local Ethics Committee (KU Leuven), subjects were asked to give their written consent after they were informed of all experimental procedures and risks associated with the experiments. Furthermore, they were submitted to a medical screening before being enrolled in the study. Subjects who had any pathology or were taking any medication or nutritional supplements that were not compatible with the study protocol were excluded. All procedures were carried out in accordance with the Declaration of Helsinki (2000) of the World Medical Association.

Preliminary testing

Two weeks before the start of the study, the subjects performed a maximal incremental exercise test (initial load 60 Watts (W) + 35 W per 3 min) on a bicycle ergometer (Avantronic Cyclus II, Leipzig, Germany) to determine the rate of maximal oxygen uptake (VO_2max) and the corresponding workload. Heart rate (Polar, Kempele, Finland), VO_2 and VCO_2 (Cortex Metalyzer II, Leipzig, Germany) were continuously measured during the test.

Study protocol

A double–blind randomized cross-over study was performed. Subjects participated in four experimental sessions with a 1-week interval in between. Subjects abstained from any high intensity exercise for 48 hours prior to the experiments. In the evening before the experimental sessions, subjects received a standardized carbohydrate-rich dinner (860 kcal, 73% carbohydrates, 14% fat, 13% protein), after which they remained fasted. On the morning of the experiments they reported to the laboratory in the fasted state between 8:00 and 9:00a.m. to perform a 30-min endurance exercise bout at 70% of their previously determined VO_2max at a cadence fixed at 90-100 rpm. At the end of the exercise the subjects got seated in a comfortable armchair and an intravenous catheter was inserted into an arm vein for repeated blood sampling during the experiment after which a baseline blood sample was collected. The subjects received capsules containing either: 1) LUVOS Heilerde serving as placebo (PL); 2) 1000 mg *Opuntia ficus-indica* cladode and fruit skin extract (OFI) (OpunDia™, Finzelberg, Germany); 3) 3 g leucine (LEU) (Ajinomoto, Japan); 4) 1000mg *Opuntia ficus-indica* extract + 3 g leucine (OFI+ LEU). All capsules had identical appearance and the number of capsules ingested was the same for each condition. OpunDia™ is a preferred blend of *Opuntia ficus-indica* cladode and fruit skin extract containing 75% cladode extract and 25% fruit skin extract (for both extraction solvent: water; DER (drug-to-extract ratio) 2–4:1; 50% native extract, 50% collagen hydrolysate as excipient). All plant materials of *Opuntia ficus-indica* were obtained from a US American-based cultivation having breeding experience since 1923 [16]. Voucher specimens of the drug material are deposited at PhytoLab, Vestenbergsgreuth, Germany. The dose of 1000 mg OFI was selected based on preliminary dose–response data showing 1000 mg to be the lowest dose needed to maximally increase plasma insulin concentration [10]. After ingestion of the supplement together with a 75 g glucose bolus in 300 ml water, a 2-hr oral glucose tolerance test (OGTT) was started at time 0 (t_0). Thereafter, a blood sample (5 ml) was collected from the arm vein catheter into vacuum tubes containing Silica clot activator (BD Vacutainer, NJ, USA), at 30, 60, 90, and 120 min. During the OGTT, an additional dose of OFI (1000 mg) and/or LEU (3 g), together with glucose (75 g), was given at t_{60} to maintain blood glucose concentration high. Blood samples were centrifuged (1500 rpm for 15 min at 4°C) to spin down the serum which was stored at −80°C until analyzed at a later date for insulin.

Blood samples

Serum insulin was assayed by chemiluminescence using the Siemens DPC kit and according to the instructions by the manufacturer. Blood glucose concentration was determined on 10 µl blood coming from the earlobe using an automated micro-analyzer (Arkray Inc., Kyoto, Japan).

Data calculations and statistical analyses

The positive incremental area under the glucose curve and the insulin curve were calculated as previously described [17,18]. The differences between the conditions (PL, OFI, LEU and OFI+LEU) were analyzed by Student's paired T-tests using the SigmaPlot® statistical software package. A probability level of P≤0.05 was considered statistically significant. All data are expressed as means ± SE.

Results

OFI and leucine have an additive insulinogenic effect

All subjects tolerated the supplements well and none exhibited symptoms of gastrointestinal distress. Post exercise blood glucose concentration was 4.0 ± 0.1 mmol/l in all experimental conditions (Figure 1A). Thirty minutes following the initial 75 g glucose bolus together with the supplement(s), blood glucose peaked at 6.6 ± 0.1 mmol/l, to gradually decrease thereafter. Compared with PL, OFI reduced blood glucose at t_{90} by 7% (5.7 ± 0.2 in OFI vs 6.2 ± 0.3 mmol/l in PL, P<0.05, Figure 1A) and the area under the 2-h glucose curve by about 15% (190 ± 24 in OFI vs 233 ± 33mmol/l/2h in PL, P<0.05, Figure 1B). Leucine tended to decrease blood glucose concentration at t_{90} (P=0.070, Figure 1A). Post exercise serum insulin concentration was 5.7 ± 0.6 mU/l and reached 35-50 mU/l during the OGTT depending on the treatment. From t_{60} to the end of the OGTT, serum insulin concentration was higher in OFI+LEU than in PL (P<0.05, Figure 1C). OFI alone increased insulin concentration only

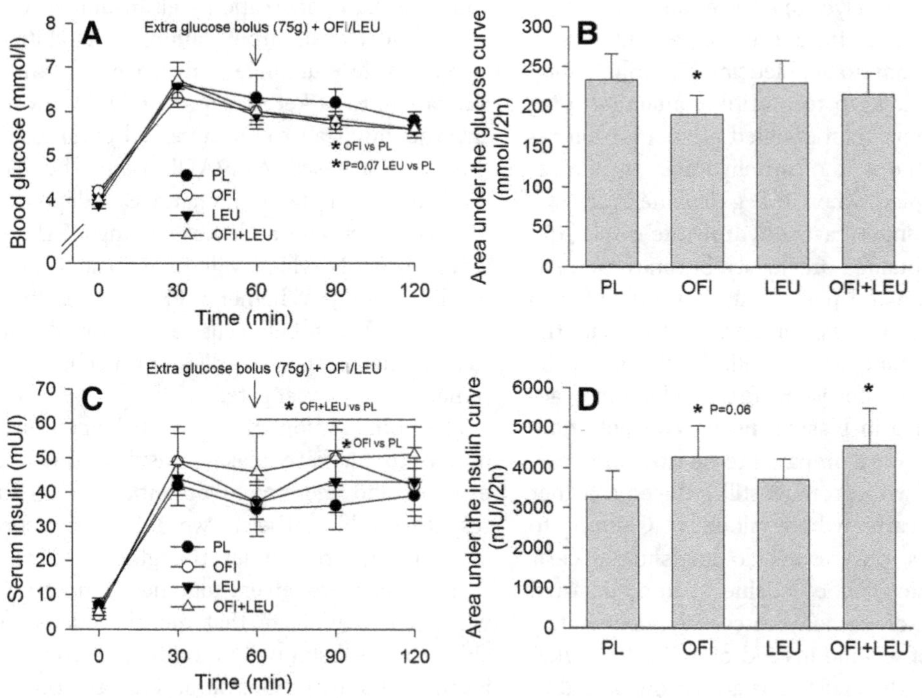

Figure 1 Effect of *Opuntia ficus-indica* cladode and fruit skin extract and/or leucine on blood glucose and serum insulin during a post exercise OGTT. Concentrations of blood glucose **(A)** and serum insulin **(C)**, as well as the calculated area under the curve for blood glucose **(B)** and serum insulin **(D)** during a 120-min OGTT after exercise and after having ingested a placebo (PL), *Opuntia ficus-indica* cladode and fruit skin extract (OFI), leucine (LEU) or *Opuntia ficus-indica* cladode and fruit skin extract + leucine (OFI+LEU). Data are means ± SE (n=11). *P<0.05 vs PL.

at t_{90} (50 ± 10 in OFI vs 36 ± 7 mU/l in PL, P<0.05). Accordingly, OFI+LEU increased by about 40% (4555 ± 923 in OFI+LEU vs 3259 ± 663 mU/l/2h in PL, P<0.05) and OFI alone tended to increase (4272 ± 761 in OFI vs 3259 ± 663 mU/l/2h in PL, P=0.059) the area under the insulin curve (Figure 1D). Leucine had no effect on insulin concentration.

Discussion

In a recent study, we showed for the first time that OFI can elevate circulating plasma insulin concentration during high rate carbohydrate ingestion in humans at rest and after exercise [10]. This finding is particularly relevant to endurance athletes seeking to restore high muscle glycogen concentration between training sessions so as to maintain training quality [19]. As muscle glycogen repletion is sensitive to insulin [3], most prominently during the initial hours following an exercise bout [20,21], it is important for athletes to establish high circulating plasma insulin concentrations during early recovery following a strenuous training. It is of note that muscle insulin sensitivity is enhanced after exercise, which facilitates glycogen resynthesis compared with rest [6]. High rate carbohydrate ingestion, up to 1.0-1.2 g/kg/h for a few hours, is the prevailing nutritional strategy to increase glucose delivery to muscles together with elevated plasma insulin concentration and thereby stimulate glycogen resynthesis [7,22]. Adding proteins to a carbohydrate load will even speed up glycogen repletion due to the insulinogenic action of proteins and more particularly due to the branched-chain amino acid leucine [7,8,15]. Adding 0.4 g casein hydrolysate/kg/h to a drink containing 0.8 g carbohydrates/kg/h more than doubled plasma insulin response compared with only the carbohydrates. Insulin response was even tripled when 0.1 g leucine/kg/h was added to the carbohydrates/casein hydrolysate drink [15]. Similar results were obtained previously, but in those earlier studies both leucine and phenylalanine were added to the supplements, which makes it impossible to isolate the actions of the two amino acids [7,8]. In the study by Kaastra [15], drinks were not isoenergetic, which may account for the difference in plasma insulin concentration. However, when drinks were prepared to be isocaloric, carbohydrates combined with proteins still induced a higher insulin response than carbohydrates alone [7]. Contrary to those previous studies, our results do not show a clear additional insulinogenic effect of leucine when co-ingested with a high amount of carbohydrates. We deliberately chose a dose of 3 g of leucine instead of ~ 7 g (0.1 g/kg) by others [7,8,15] because leucine has a very low palatability, and therefore most commercial sports supplements contain a maximum of 3 g leucine. We also based our decision on a recent report showing that 3.42 g leucine alone, in the absence of carbohydrate intake and at rest, increased plasma insulin concentration by 50% within 30 min before returning to basal levels [23]. It is thus possible that the smaller amount of leucine, compared to previous studies, added to the high amount of glucose (~1 g/kg/h) was not large enough to further enhance plasma insulin concentration in the present study.

Based on our data, 1000 mg OFI had a slightly higher insulinogenic action than 3 g leucine, certainly 30 min after ingestion of the glucose + OFI beverage. OFI seems to stimulate insulin production acutely and rapidly as serum insulin concentrations during the OGTT each time were increased 30 min after OFI ingestion but no more 60 min after OFI intake. The insulinogenic action of OFI thus clearly is short-lived. The largest effect on plasma insulin concentration was obtained by the combined ingestion of OFI plus leucine. Indeed, insulin concentration was persistently elevated during the second hour of the OGTT when OFI and leucine were administered together. In addition, a trend (P=0.09) to increase in insulin concentration was observed in OFI + LEU compared with OFI alone at 60 and 120 min. As blood glucose concentrations were not modified by OFI plus leucine, the increase in insulin did not result from higher blood glucose levels. Our results rather indicate that OFI and leucine directly stimulate pancreatic insulin release, and that the effects of both agents are additive. Whereas the physiological mechanism by which OFI facilitates glucose-induced pancreatic insulin release remains to be elucidated, it is known that leucine increases pancreatic β-cell insulin secretion through: 1) its oxidative decarboxylation; 2) its ability to allosterically activate glutamate dehydrogenase, and 3) its transamination to α-ketoisocaproate [24]. Those events will subsequently lead to an increased tricarboxylic acid-cycle flux, an increased ATP/ADP ratio, the closure of the ATP-sensitive potassium channels, a depolarization of the plasma membrane and the opening of the calcium sensitive channels which will finally cause the secretion of insulin [25-27]. Whether OFI increases the tricarboxylic acid-cycle flux in beta-cells as well, or whether it depolarizes the membrane via a different mechanism than leucine remains to be investigated.

The combination of OFI with leucine seems the best option to increase plasma insulin concentrations after exercise and thereby to potentially accelerate glycogen resynthesis. Nevertheless we did not measure any difference in the area under the glucose curve when both treatments were given together compared to placebo, which could indicate that muscle glucose uptake probably is not substantially modified by combined OFI plus leucine administration. Blood glucose concentration during an OGTT reflects the equilibrium between the rate of glucose appearance from the gut and liver, and the rate of disappearance through peripheral glucose uptake. It can be hypothesized that OFI combined with leucine actually increased both processes that resulted in unchanged blood glucose concentrations. However, this is not likely to be the case as the addition of amino acids to a carbohydrate-rich drink was previously shown to decrease the rates of appearance and disappearance of blood glucose instead [15]. As the decreases were equal in amplitude, it was suggested that amino acids-induced insulin stimulation accelerates glycogen resynthesis after exercise by increasing glycogen synthase activity rather than by increasing muscle glucose uptake [15]. Further studies should try to determine whether the higher circulating insulin levels established by combined OFI plus leucine administration together with high rate glucose uptake post exercise, effectively translate into higher glycogen synthase activity and glycogen resynthesis rate following exercise.

Conclusion

Carbohydrate-induced insulin stimulation after exercise can be further increased by the combination of *Opuntia ficus-indica* cladode and fruit skin extract with leucine. In the perspective of developing optimal nutritional strategies to recover muscle glycogen faster after high-intensity endurance exercise, OFI and leucine could be interesting ingredients to include together in recovery drinks. Still, it needs to be confirmed that such nutritional strategy effectively stimulates post exercise muscle glycogen resynthesis.

Abbreviations

GLUT4: Glucose transporter 4; LEU: Leucine; OFI: *Opuntia ficus-indica* cladode and fruit skin extract; OGTT: Oral glucose tolerance test; VO_2max: Maximal oxygen uptake.

Competing interests

Ivo Pischel and Hartwig Sievers are employees of PhytoLab GmbH & Co. KG, Germany and were involved in the study design, but not in any data generation or processing. OpunDia™ is applied for patents by Finzelberg GmbH & Co. KG, Germany, e. g. US 2010323045 (A1) - Extract Formulation of Opuntia ficus Indica (Priorities: US20080741562 20081106; EP20070120081 20071106; US20070002058P 20071106; WO2008EP65048 20081106).

Authors' contributions

PH, IP and HS were responsible for the concept of this project and for the study design. KVP, and MR were responsible for the acquisition and the analysis of the data. PH, KVP and LD were responsible for the interpretation of the data. PH and LD wrote the first version of the manuscript which was edited by the other authors. The final version was approved by all authors.

Acknowledgments

The authors thank all subjects for participating in this study. The authors also thank Dr. Ruud Van Thienen for medical assistance during the experiments. Björn Feistel and Bernd Walbroel from Finzelberg, Germany kindly supplied OpunDia™ extract. PhytoLab GmbH & Co. KG, Vestenbergsgreuth, Germany, sponsored this study.

Author details

[1]Exercise Physiology Research Group, Department of Kinesiology, KU Leuven, Leuven, Belgium. [2]PhytoLab GmbH & Co. KG, Vestenbergsgreuth, Germany.

References

1. Bergstrom J, Hultman E: **Muscle glycogen synthesis after exercise: an enhancing factor localized to the muscle cells in man.** *Nature* 1966, **210:**309–310.
2. Ivy JL, Lee MC, Brozinick JT Jr, Reed MJ: **Muscle glycogen storage after different amounts of carbohydrate ingestion.** *J Appl Physiol* 1988, **65:**2018–2023.
3. Price TB, Rothman DL, Taylor R, Avison MJ, Shulman GI, Shulman RG: **Human muscle glycogen resynthesis after exercise: insulin-dependent and -independent phases.** *J Appl Physiol* 1994, **76:**104–111.
4. Richter EA, Derave W, Wojtaszewski JF: **Glucose, exercise and insulin: emerging concepts.** *J Physiol* 2001, **535:**313–322.
5. Srivastava AK, Pandey SK: **Potential mechanism(s) involved in the regulation of glycogen synthesis by insulin.** *Mol Cell Biochem* 1998, **182:**135–141.
6. Cartee GD, Young DA, Sleeper MD, Zierath J, Wallberg-Henriksson H, Holloszy JO: **Prolonged increase in insulin-stimulated glucose transport in muscle after exercise.** *Am J Physiol* 1989, **256:**E494–E499.
7. van Loon LJ, Saris WH, Kruijshoop M, Wagenmakers AJ: **Maximizing postexercise muscle glycogen synthesis: carbohydrate supplementation and the application of amino acid or protein hydrolysate mixtures.** *Am J Clin Nutr* 2000, **72:**106–111.
8. van Loon LJ, Kruijshoop M, Verhagen H, Saris WH, Wagenmakers AJ: **Ingestion of protein hydrolysate and amino acid-carbohydrate mixtures increases postexercise plasma insulin responses in men.** *J Nutr* 2000, **130:**2508–2513.
9. Butterweck V, Semlin L, Feistel B, Pischel I, Bauer K, Verspohl EJ: **Comparative evaluation of two different Opuntia ficus-indica extracts for blood sugar lowering effects in rats.** *Phytother Res* 2011, **25:**370–375.
10. Van Proeyen K, Ramaekers M, Pischel I, Hespel P: **Opuntia ficus-indica ingestion stimulates peripheral disposal of oral glucose before and after exercise in healthy men.** *Int J Sport Nutr Exerc Metab* 2012, **22:**284–291.
11. Feugang JM, Konarski P, Zou D, Stintzing FC, Zou C: **Nutritional and medicinal use of Cactus pear (Opuntia spp.) cladodes and fruits.** *Front Biosci* 2006, **11:**2574–2589.
12. Ennouri M, Fetoui H, Bourret E, Zeghal N, Guermazi F, Attia H: **Evaluation of some biological parameters of Opuntia ficus indica. 2. Influence of seed supplemented diet on rats.** *Bioresour Technol* 2006, **97:**2136–2140.
13. Frati-Munari AC, de LC, Ariza-Andraca R, Banales-Ham MB, Lopez-Ledesma R, Lozoya X: **[Effect of a dehydrated extract of nopal (Opuntia ficus indica Mill.) on blood glucose].** *Arch Invest Med (Mex)* 1989, **20:**211–216.
14. Godard MP, Ewing BA, Pischel I, Ziegler A, Benedek B, Feistel B: **Acute blood glucose lowering effects and long-term safety of OpunDia supplementation in pre-diabetic males and females.** *J Ethnopharmacol* 2010, **130:**631–634.
15. Kaastra B, Manders RJ, Van BE, Kies A, Jeukendrup AE, Keizer HA, Kuipers H, van Loon LJ: **Effects of increasing insulin secretion on acute postexercise blood glucose disposal.** *Med Sci Sports Exerc* 2006, **38:**268–275.
16. Bunch R: **New developments in breeding and cactus pear products at D'Arrigo Bros.** *J Prof Assoc Cactus Dev* 2013, **1:**100–102.
17. Wolever TM, Jenkins DJ: **The use of the glycemic index in predicting the blood glucose response to mixed meals.** *Am J Clin Nutr* 1986, **43:**167–172.
18. Wolever TM, Jenkins DJ, Jenkins AL, Josse RG: **The glycemic index: methodology and clinical implications.** *Am J Clin Nutr* 1991, **54:**846–854.
19. Burke LM, Hawley JA, Wong SH, Jeukendrup AE: **Carbohydrates for training and competition.** *J Sports Sci* 2011, **29**(Suppl 1):S17–S27.
20. Richter EA, Mikines KJ, Galbo H, Kiens B: **Effect of exercise on insulin action in human skeletal muscle.** *J Appl Physiol* 1989, **66:**876–885.
21. Jensen TE, Richter EA: **Regulation of glucose and glycogen metabolism during and after exercise.** *J Physiol* 2012, **590:**1069–1076.
22. Beelen M, Burke LM, Gibala MJ, van Loon LJ: **Nutritional strategies to promote postexercise recovery.** *Int J Sport Nutr Exerc Metab* 2010, **20:**515–532.
23. Wilkinson DJ, Hossain T, Hill DS, Phillips BE, Crossland H, Williams J, Loughna P, Churchward-Venne TA, Breen L, Phillips SM, *et al*: **Effects of Leucine and its metabolite, beta-hydroxy-beta-methylbutyrate (HMB) on human skeletal muscle protein metabolism.** *J Physiol* 2013, **591:**2911–2923.
24. Manders RJ, Little JP, Forbes SC, Candow DG: **Insulinotropic and muscle protein synthetic effects of branched-chain amino acids: potential therapy for type 2 diabetes and sarcopenia.** *Nutrients* 2012, **4:**1664–1678.

25. Newsholme P, Brennan L, Rubi B, Maechler P: **New insights into amino acid metabolism, beta-cell function and diabetes.** *Clin Sci (Lond)* 2005, **108:**185–194.
26. Sener A, Malaisse WJ: **L-leucine and a nonmetabolized analogue activate pancreatic islet glutamate dehydrogenase.** *Nature* 1980, **288:**187–189.
27. Panten U, Kriegstein E, Poser W, Schonborn J, Hasselblatt A: **Effects of L-leucine and alpha-ketoisocaproic acid upon insulin secretion and metabolism of isolated pancreatic islets.** *FEBS Lett* 1972, **20:**225–228.

3

Effect of exercising while fasting on eating behaviors and food intake

Surabhi Bhutani, Monica C Klempel, Cynthia M Kroeger, Eleanor Aggour, Yolian Calvo, John F Trepanowski, Kristin K Hoddy and Krista A Varady*

Abstract

Background: Alternate day fasting combined with exercise is effective for weight loss.

Objective: The aim of this study was to examine the behavioral adaptations that occur when ADF is combined with exercise, and to determine how these changes affect weight loss.

Design: Obese subjects (n = 64) were randomized to 1 of 4 groups: 1) combination (ADF + endurance exercise), 2) ADF, 3) exercise, or 4) control, for 12 weeks.

Results: Body weight decreased ($P < 0.05$) in the combination group (6 ± 4 kg), ADF (3 ± 1 kg), exercise group (1 ± 0 kg), with no change in the control group (0 ± 0 kg). When given the choice, subjects chose to exercise the same amount ($P = 0.790$) on the fast days (48 ± 2%) as feed days (52 ± 2%). Percent of exercise sessions performed on fast day mornings (20 ± 6%) did not differ ($P = 0.453$) from fast day afternoons (28 ± 5%). Likeliness to cheat on the fast day was not higher if the subject exercised in the afternoon (17 ± 7%) versus the morning (10 ± 5%). Hunger decreased ($P < 0.05$) while satisfaction and fullness increased ($P < 0.05$) post-treatment in the ADF group only. Restrained eating increased ($P < 0.05$) and uncontrolled eating decreased ($P < 0.05$) in the combination and ADF groups.

Conclusion: These findings suggest that endurance exercise is an excellent adjunct therapy to ADF, as it leads to positive behavioral changes that may contribute to long-term steady weight loss.

Introduction

Alternate day fasting (ADF) is a modified form of calorie restriction comprising a fast day (25% energy intake for 24 h) alternated with a feed day (ad libitum energy intake for 24 h) [1]. Previous reports indicate that ADF is an effective strategy to reduce body weight (5% in 12 weeks) and improve body composition. More recently, it has been shown that combining ADF with exercise leads to greater weight loss (7% in 12 weeks) than what has been seen with ADF or exercise alone [2]. Although these findings are promising, it is still unclear how this combination therapy affects eating behaviors, and how these behavioral changes enhance weight loss. Recent evidence suggests that weight loss in obese individuals is attributed to an increase in cognitive restraint [3-5], reduced disinhibition, lower hunger levels [4,5] and decreased consumption of dietary fat [6]. In view of these findings, key questions that have yet to be addressed in this field include: Are obese individuals able to exercise on the fast day? If so, does exercise increase hunger in a way that causes people to cheat on the fast day? What role does the timing of the exercise session play in determining whether or not the individual will cheat? Does ADF, with or without exercise, elicit positive behavioral changes that may contribute to long-term steady weight loss?

Therefore, the aim of this study was to examine the behavioral adaptations that occur when ADF is combined with endurance training, and to investigate how these changes affect weight loss.

Materials and methods

Subjects

As described previously [2], independently living subjects were recruited from the University of Illinois at Chicago campus by means of flyers. Of the 146 interested

* Correspondence: varady@uic.edu
Department of Kinesiology and Nutrition, University of Illinois at Chicago, 1919 West Taylor Street, Room 103, Chicago, IL 60612, USA

individuals, 83 were deemed eligible to participate according to a preliminary questionnaire and body mass index (BMI) assessment. Key inclusion criteria were as follows: age 25 to 65 years; BMI between 30 and 39.9 kg/m^2; weight stable for 3 months prior to the beginning of the study (i.e. less than 5 kg weight loss or weight gain); non-diabetic; no history of cardiovascular disease; lightly active (i.e. <3 h/week of light intensity exercise at 2.5 to 4.0 metabolic equivalents (METs) for 3 months prior to the study); non-smoker; no history of bariatric surgery; and not taking weight loss, lipid or glucose lowering medications. The experimental protocol was approved by the Office for the Protection of Research Subjects at the University of Illinois, Chicago. All volunteers gave informed consent to participate in the trial.

Experimental design and randomization

A 12-week, randomized, controlled, parallel-arm feeding trial was implemented to test the effects of ADF, exercise, and ADF combined with exercise (combination group) on eating behaviors and weight loss. Eligible subjects were stratified on the basis of BMI, age, and sex, and then randomized into 1 of 4 groups: 1) combination group; 2) ADF group; 3) exercise group; 4) control group.

Diet protocol

As previously described [2], only the combination and ADF groups participated in the dietary intervention, which consisted of two periods: 1) a 4-week controlled feeding period, and 2) an 8-week self-selected feeding period. During the controlled feeding period (week 1–4) participants consumed 25% of their baseline energy needs on the fast day (24 h) and consumed food ad libitum on each feed day (24 h). Baseline energy requirements were assessed by the Mifflin equation [7]. The diet consisted of a 3-day rotating menu plan, and all fast day meals were prepared in the metabolic kitchen of the Human Nutrition Research Unit (HNRU). Fast day meals were consumed between 12.00 pm and 2.00 pm to ensure that each subject was undergoing the same duration of fasting. Meals were formulated on the basis of the American Heart Association guidelines (30% kcal from fat, 15% kcal from protein, and 55% kcal from carbohydrate). All meals were consumed outside of the research center. Participants were requested to eat only the foods provided on the fast days and to bring back any leftover foods to be weighed and recorded. Calorie-free foods, such as black coffee, tea, and diet sodas were permitted as desired. Subjects were also encouraged to drink plenty of water. During the self-selected feeding period (week 8–12) subjects continued with the ADF regimen but no fast day food was provided to them. Instead, each subject met with a dietician at the beginning of each week to learn how to maintain the ADF regimen at home. Subjects were also taught how to monitor energy intake by reading food labels, reducing portion sizes, and choosing low fat meat and dairy options. Control and exercise group subjects were asked to maintain their regular food habits, and were not provided with any food or dietary counseling.

Exercise protocol

Only the combination and exercise groups participated the exercise intervention. These subjects participated in a moderate intensity exercise program 3 times per week under supervised conditions, for 12 weeks. Exercise was performed using stationary bikes and elliptical machines at the HNRU. Training intensity was estimated for each individual using an age-predicted heart rate maximum (HRmax) equation [209 – (0.7 × age)] [8] and a Polar Heart Rate Monitor (Polar USA, Inc., NY). At the beginning of the study (weeks 1 to 4), each exercise session ran for 25 min duration and corresponded to 60% of the subject's HRmax. Training duration and intensity increased incrementally at week 4, 7 and 10 by 5 min and 5% HRmax. As such, by week 10, each subject was exercising for a 40 min duration at an intensity of 75% HRmax. ADF and control subjects were asked to maintain their regular activity habits during the study.

Weight loss assessment

Body weight was measured weekly to the nearest 0.25 kg in the fasted state using a balance beam scale (Health-OMeter, Sunbeam Products, Boca Raton, FL). Waist circumference was measured by a flexible tape to the nearest 0.1 cm, midway between the lower costal margin and super iliac crest during a period of expiration.

Adherence to the ADF diet and exercise protocol

During the controlled feeding phase (week 1–4), subjects were instructed to eat only the fast day food provided, and to report any extra food item consumed using an "Extra food log". The log was collected and reviewed by study personnel each week. If the log indicated that the subject ate an extra food item on a fast day, that day was labeled as "not adherent". Exercise compliance was assessed by recording attendance at each supervised exercise session. If an exercise session was missed, the subject was required to make up for the missed session that same week.

Physical activity maintenance assessment

Habitual, free-living physical activity was assessed by a pedometer (Digiwalker SW-200, Yamax Corporation, Tokyo, Japan SW). Subjects wore the pedometer for a 7-d period at week 1 and 12. The pedometer was worn attached to the participant's waistband during waking hours (except while bathing or swimming), and reset to zero each morning. Number of daily steps were recorded in a pedometer log provided, and the log was collected by study personnel at the weigh-in each week. No subjects were enrolled in an exercise class, and all participants were asked to refrain from joining any exercise programs during the course of the study.

Eating behavior assessment

A validated visual analog scale (VAS) [9] was used to measure hunger, fullness, and satisfaction with the ADF diet. The scale was completed on each fast day (before bedtime). In brief, the VAS consisted of 100-mm lines, and subjects were asked to make a vertical mark across the line corresponding to their feelings from 0 (not at all) to 100 (extremely) for hunger, satisfaction, or fullness. Quantification was performed by measuring the distance from the left end of the line to the vertical mark. The three-factor eating questionnaire (TFEQ-R18) [10] was used to assess restrained eating (conscious restriction of food intake in order to control body weight), uncontrolled eating (tendency to eat more than usual due to a loss of control over intake), and emotional eating (inability to resist emotional eating cues). The TFEQ consists of 18 items on a 4-point response scale (definitely true/mostly true/ mostly false/definitely false). Responses to each of the 18 items are given a score between 1 and 4. The item scores are then summated into scale scores for restrained eating, uncontrolled eating, and emotional eating. The raw scale scores are transformed to a 0–100 scale [((raw score – lowest possible raw score)/possible raw score range) – 100]. Higher scores are indicative of greater restrained, uncontrolled, or emotional eating.

Energy and macronutrient intake

Each participant completed a 3-day food record on 2 feed days during the week, and on 1 feed day during the weekend, at each week of the 12-week trial. Thus, a total of 36 feed day food records were collected for each subject. At baseline, the dietician provided 15 min of instruction to each participant on how to complete the food records. These instructions included verbal information and detailed reference guides on how to estimate portion sizes and record food items in sufficient detail to obtain an accurate estimate of dietary intake. Subjects were instructed to record food items, in as much detail as possible, in the blank food diary provided. Any mixed foods were broken down to individual food items to be recorded one per line. Food records were collected at the weigh-in each week, and were reviewed by the dietician for accuracy and completeness. All dietary information from the food records was entered into the food analysis program, Nutritionist Pro (Axxya Systems). The program was used to calculate the total daily intake of energy, protein, carbohydrate, fat, cholesterol, and fiber.

Statistical analysis

Results are presented as mean ± SEM. Differences between intervention groups at baseline were analyzed by a one-way ANOVA. Within-group differences were analyzed using repeated-measures ANOVA. An intention-to-treat analysis was performed for all variables measured. A P value of < 0.05 was used as a criterion for statistical significance in all analyses. Data were analyzed using SPSS software (version 20.0 for Mac OSX; SPSS Inc, Chicago, IL, USA).

Results

Subject baseline characteristics and weight loss

As reported previously [2], 83 subjects began the clinical trial (combination: n = 18, ADF: n = 25, exercise: n = 24, control: n = 16), and sixteen subjects finished in each intervention group (total n = 64). Additional subjects were randomized to groups with high dropout rates, such as the ADF and exercise group, to ensure that the number of subjects would be the same in each group at the end of the trial. Dropouts were primarily due to scheduling conflicts. Baseline characteristics are reported in Table 1. There were no between-group differences for age, sex, ethnicity, body weight, height, BMI, or waist circumference. Body weight decreased (P < 0.05) in the combination group (6 ± 4 kg), ADF (3 ± 1 kg) and exercise group (1 ± 0 kg), with no change in the control group (0 ± 0 kg). The decrease in waist circumference was greater (P < 0.001) in the combination group (8 ± 1 cm) compared to the ADF (5 ± 1 cm), exercise group (3 ± 1 cm), and control group (1 ± 1 cm).

ADF and exercise compliance

The combination group attended 95 ± 2% of the exercise sessions while the exercise group attended 94 ± 1% of the sessions. There was no difference (P = 0.83) in exercise compliance between groups. Adherence to the fast day diet remained high in the combination (81 ± 7%) and ADF group (80 ± 9%) throughout the course of the trial. No between-group differences were observed in fast day diet adherence when the combination group was compared to the ADF group (P = 0.23). As for regular physical activity, there were no differences in steps/d between groups or within groups from baseline to post-treatment: combination (week 1: 5566 ± 656, week 12: 6018 ± 765), ADF (week 1: 4031 ± 752, week 12: 4920 ± 664), exercise (week 1: 5381 ± 885, week 12: 5998 ± 767), and control group (week 1: 6458 ± 749, week 12: 6206 ± 736).

Timing of the fast day exercise session and impact on food intake

Subjects were given the option of scheduling their exercise sessions on feed days or fast days (morning or afternoon). Figure 1A portrays the percent of exercise sessions held on feed versus fast days. Combination group subjects showed no preference ($P = 0.790$) towards exercising on

Table 1 Subject characteristics at baseline

	Combination	ADF	Exercise	Control	P-value[1]
n	18	25	24	16	
Age (y)	45 ± 5	42 ± 2	42 ± 2	49 ± 2	0.158
Sex (F/M)	18 / 0	24 / 1	23 / 1	15 / 1	0.266
Ethnicity (n)					
African American	7	12	11	11	
Caucasian	5	7	6	3	
Hispanic	6	6	4	2	
Other	0	0	3	0	
Body weight (kg)	91 ± 6	94 ± 3	93 ± 2	93 ± 5	0.904
Height (cm)	160 ± 0	163 ± 0	162 ± 0	162 ± 1	0.896
BMI (kg/m^2)	35 ± 1	35 ± 1	35 ± 1	35 ± 1	0.934
Waist circumference	96 ± 2	100 ± 2	98 ± 2	99 ± 3	0.636

Values reported as mean ± SEM. Intention to treat analysis. BMI: Body mass index, F: Female, M: Male.
[1]P-value between groups at baseline: One-way ANOVA.

feed days (52 ± 2%) versus fast days (48 ± 2%). Furthermore, percent of exercise sessions performed on fast day mornings (20 ± 6%) did not differ (P = 0.453) from those performed on fast day afternoons (28 ± 5%). We also wanted to determine if subjects cheated more on the fast day (i.e. ate more than their prescribed amount of energy) if they exercised in the morning versus the afternoon. Results reveal that likeliness to cheat was not significantly higher if the subject chose to exercise in the afternoon (17 ± 7%) versus the morning (10 ± 5%) (Figure 1B).

Changes in eating behaviors

Changes in fast day eating behaviors are presented in Table 2. No change in hunger, satisfaction or fullness was observed in the combination group post-treatment. However in ADF subjects, hunger decreased ($P < 0.05$) while satisfaction and fullness increased ($P < 0.05$) after 12 weeks of treatment. Restrained eating increased ($P < 0.05$) by 16 ± 6 and 10 ± 2 in the combination and ADF group, respectively, after 12 weeks. Uncontrolled eating decreased ($P < 0.05$) in the combination (14 ± 4) and ADF group (6 ± 3) over the course of the trial. Emotional eating decreased ($P < 0.01$) only in the combination group (15 ± 5). No changes were observed in eating behaviors in the exercise and control group.

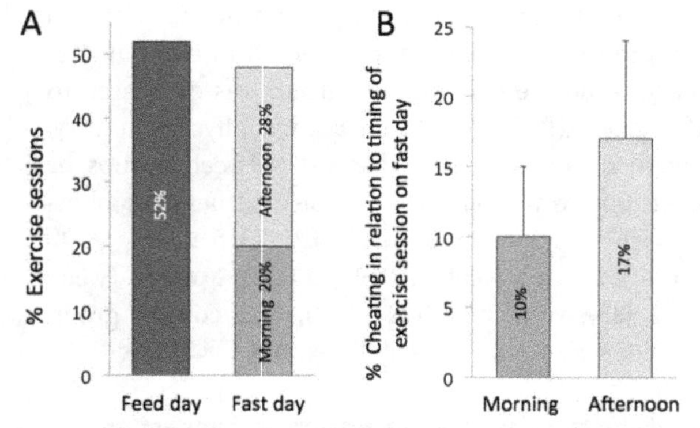

Figure 1 Timing of the fast day exercise session and impact on food intake. A. Percent of exercise sessions scheduled by subjects on feed days versus fast days (morning and afternoon). **B**. Percent of cheating on the fast day (i.e. eating more than the prescribed amount of energy) in relation to timing of the exercise session. No difference in cheating in relation to exercising in the morning versus the afternoon on the fast day (One-way ANOVA).

Impact of the fast day exercise session on eating behaviors

Hunger did not increase if the subject exercised on a fast day (week 1: 6 ± 1, week 12: 4 ± 2, P = 0.240). Fullness did not decrease if the subject exercised on a fast day (week 1: 4 ± 2, week 12: 4 ± 1, P = 0.653). Moreover, satisfaction with the ADF diet did not decrease if the subject exercised on a fast day (week 1: 4 ± 2, week 12: 4 ± 1, P = 0.549).

Changes in energy and macronutrient intake on feed days

Dietary intake for each intervention group is reported in Table 3. No changes were observed for energy, protein, carbohydrate, fat, cholesterol, and fiber after 12 weeks of treatment.

Discussion

Our findings show, for the first time, that endurance exercise can be easily incorporated into the ADF regimen. Specifically, subjects were able to exercise on the fast day, and this extra energy expenditure did not translate into increased hunger or extra food intake. We also show here that ADF combined with exercise improves several eating behaviors. For instance, after 12 weeks of treatment, restrained eating was increased while uncontrolled eating and emotional eating were decreased in obese individuals.

Table 2 Changes in eating behaviors during the 12-week study

	Intervention	Week 1	Week 12	P-value[1]	P-value[2]	Change[3]	P-value[4]
Hunger (mm)	Combination	5.7 ± 0.5	4.7 ± 0.7	0.185	0.941	−1.0 ± 0.7	0.495
	ADF	6.3 ± 0.5	4.7 ± 0.7	0.034		−1.6 ± 0.7	
Satisfaction (mm)	Combination	3.8 ± 0.8	4.1 ± 0.6	0.575	0.817	0.3 ± 0.5	0.240
	ADF	3.2 ± 0.4	4.3 ± 0.6	0.031		1.1 ± 0.5	
Fullness (mm)	Combination	3.7 ± 0.8	4.0 ± 0.7	0.564	0.967	0.3 ± 0.5	0.146
	ADF	2.4 ± 0.4	4.0 ± 0.7	0.016		1.6 ± 0.6	
Restrained eating score	Combination	40 ± 4	56 ± 7	0.029	0.207	16 ± 6 [a]	0.013
	ADF	52 ± 2	62 ± 3	0.006		10 ± 2 [a]	
	Exercise	49 ± 3	49 ± 3	0.944		0 ± 2 [b]	
	Control	47 ± 7	48 ± 6	0.828		1 ± 6 [a,b]	
Uncontrolled eating score	Combination	44 ± 3	30 ± 4	0.007	0.050	−14 ± 4 [a]	0.002
	ADF	35 ± 3	29 ± 3	0.023		−6 ± 3 [a,b]	
	Exercise	40 ± 4	39 ± 5	0.783		−1 ± 2 [b]	
	Control	23 ± 4	28 ± 6	0.152		5 ± 3 [b]	
Emotional eating score	Combination	57 ± 5	42 ± 6	0.002	0.063	−15 ± 5 [a]	0.005
	ADF	38 ± 5	35 ± 5	0.428		−3 ± 3 [b]	
	Exercise	58 ± 7	56 ± 7	0.447		−2 ± 3 [b]	
	Control	38 ± 12	38 ± 11	0.584		0 ± 5 [b]	

Values reported as mean ± SEM. Intention to treat analysis. ADF: Alternate day fasting.
[1]P-value between week 1 and week 12: Repeated-measures ANOVA.
[2]P-value between groups at week 12: One-way ANOVA.
[3]Absolute change between week 1 and 12 values.
[4]P-value between groups for absolute change: One-way ANOVA. Means not sharing a common superscript letter are significantly different (Tukey post-hoc test).

Our primary goal in this study was to see if subjects undergoing ADF can exercise on the fast day. All subjects exercised 3 times per week under supervised conditions. Throughout the study, subjects were allowed to choose the day (feed or fast day) and time (morning: 7.00-11.00 am, or afternoon: 3.00-7.00 pm) of the exercise sessions. Results reveal that the combination group showed no preference towards exercising on feed days (52%) versus fast days (48%). Moreover, the percent of exercise sessions performed on fast day mornings (20%) did not differ from those performed on fast day afternoons (28%). We also wanted to see if the negative energy balance produced by the physical activity would lead to higher energy intake on the fast day. We hypothesized that the subjects exercising on fast day afternoons would be more likely to cheat (i.e. surpass their prescribed fast day energy goal) compared to subjects exercising in the morning. We assumed that cheating would be higher in the afternoon exercisers, as hunger peaks 30–40 minutes post workout [11]. Since the morning exercisers would be able to eat their fast day meal shortly after their exercise session (12.00-2.00 pm), they would be satisfied and less likely to cheat. In contrast, the afternoon exercisers would not have another meal to eat after their exercise session, which may lead them to consume extra food to suppress the post-workout hunger. Interestingly, the likeliness to cheat was not significantly higher in the afternoon exercisers (17%) compared to the morning exercisers (10%). However, it is possible that this difference was not significant due to small sample size (n = 16). Similar to our trial, Maraki et al. studied the acute effect of one hour of morning (post breakfast) and afternoon (pre dinner) exercise on hunger and energy intake [12]. Both morning and afternoon exercisers experienced increases in hunger, but did not exhibit increased energy intake. Our findings parallel those of Maraki et al. [12] in that we also saw no increase in energy intake post-workout.

The effect of ADF with or without exercise on hunger, satisfaction and fullness was also tested. After 12 weeks of treatment, hunger decreased while satisfaction and fullness increased in the ADF group. The effect of ADF on eating behaviors was also tested by Heilbronn et al. Normal weight subjects participated in an ADF regimen (100% calorie restriction on the fast day) for 3 weeks. After this short intervention period, fullness increased, but there were no changes in the perception of hunger or satisfaction [13]. The findings of Heilbronn et al. may have differed from ours because their study employed a true ADF regimen (complete fast on the fast day) whereas we used a modified ADF regimen (75% restriction on the fast day). Since the Heilbronn et al. subjects were not allowed to eat anything on the fast day, this may explain why hunger remained

Table 3 Energy and macronutrient intake on feed days during the 12-week study

	Intervention	Week 1	Week 12	P-value[1]	P-value[2]	Change[3]	P-value[4]
Energy (kcal)	Combination	1656 ± 265	1358 ± 123	0.278	0.854	−298 ± 260	0.897
	ADF	1681 ± 155	1457 ± 204	0.228		−224 ± 173	
	Exercise	1623 ± 145	1553 ± 135	0.739		−70 ± 203	
	Control	1607 ± 307	1416 ± 207	0.360		191 ± 190	
Protein (g)	Combination	70 ± 21	63 ± 14	0.903	0.958	−7 ± 23	0.581
	ADF	65 ± 10	70 ± 10	0.115		5 ±10	
	Exercise	60 ± 5	62 ± 8	0.467		−2 ± 8	
	Control	71 ± 9	68 ± 5	0.817		3 ± 12	
Carbohydrate (g)	Combination	199 ± 35	164 ± 19	0.547	0.801	−35 ± 38	0.928
	ADF	200 ± 19	161 ± 19	0.155		−39 ± 24	
	Exercise	202 ± 25	177 ± 20	0.470		−25 ± 33	
	Control	182 ± 34	140 ± 31	0.21		−42 ± 28	
Fat (g)	Combination	64 ± 10	50 ± 7	0.454	0.793	−14 ± 11	0.983
	ADF	69 ± 8	59 ± 13	0.327		−10 ± 9	
	Exercise	64 ± 11	66 ± 6	0.717		2 ± 13	
	Control	66 ± 16	65 ± 11	0.780		−1 ± 12	
Saturated fat (g)	Combination	23 ± 3	19 ± 2	0.412	0.599	−4 ± 3	0.815
	ADF	28 ± 2	26 ± 5	0.831		−2 ± 4	
	Exercise	23 ± 3	28 ± 3	0.700		5 ± 5	
	Control	27 ± 7	26 ± 4	0.682		−1 ± 5	
Monounsaturated fat (g)	Combination	25 ± 3	20 ± 3	0.375	0.975	−5 ± 4	0.716
	ADF	24 ± 3	21 ± 6	0.969		−3 ± 5	
	Exercise	24 ± 4	22 ± 2	0.118		−2 ± 3	
	Control	23 ± 5	24 ± 4	0.915		1 ± 5	
Polyunsaturated fat (g)	Combination	16 ± 2	11 ± 2	0.309	0.725	−5 ± 3	0.930
	ADF	17 ± 2	12 ± 2	0.452		−5 ± 3	
	Exercise	17 ± 3	16 ± 2	0.294		−1 ± 3	
	Control	16 ± 3	15 ± 3	0.926		−1 ± 4	
Fiber (g)	Combination	18 ± 3	16 ± 2	0.609	0.280	−2 ± 4	0.657
	ADF	16 ± 2	11 ± 2	0.078		−5 ± 2	
	Exercise	18 ± 2	12 ± 2	0.036		−6 ± 3	
	Control	11 ± 3	10 ± 2	0.832		−1 ± 5	
Cholesterol (mg)	Combination	245 ± 34	268 ± 47	0.744	0.868	23 ± 43	0.391
	ADF	329 ± 83	225 ± 58	0.225		−104 ± 79	
	Exercise	223 ± 49	227 ± 53	0.955		4 ± 69	
	Control	380 ± 73	272 ± 25	0.120		−108 ± 57	

Values reported as mean ± SEM. Intention to treat analysis. ADF: Alternate day fasting.
[1]P-value between week 1 and week 12: Repeated-measures ANOVA.
[2]P-value between groups at week 12: One-way ANOVA.
[3]Percent change between week 1 and week 12 values.
[4]P-value between groups for percent change: One-way ANOVA. Means not sharing a common superscript letter are significantly different (Tukey post-hoc test).

elevated throughout the course of the trial. In contrast to the ADF group, the combination group did not demonstrate any changes in hunger, satisfaction or fullness in the current study. The reason for this is not clear. Blundell et al. [14] investigated the effect of medium term (7–16 d) moderate intensity endurance exercise on appetite stimulation. Findings reveal that hunger and food intake increased post-exercise in order to compensate for the negative energy balance achieved with training [14]. In contrast, Guelfi et al. demonstrated that 12 weeks of 40–60 minutes of moderate intensity exercise (70–80% HRmax) produced opposite results [15]. Specifically, Guelfi et al. showed no change in perceived hunger, while levels of perceived fullness increased [15]. It should be noted however, that subjects in the Blundell et al. [14] study were required to expend approximately 1000 kcal/d with exercise. This level of energy expenditure is far greater than that of our study (estimated to be 150–250 kcal/d). Thus, increases in hunger post-exercise may only occur if energy expenditure with exercise meets or exceeds 1000 kcal/d. Nevertheless, in light of these contradictory findings, the impact of combination diet and exercise therapies on hunger and fullness warrant further investigation.

Changes in restrained eating, uncontrolled eating, and emotional eating were also examined. In both the ADF and combination groups, restrained eating increased while uncontrolled eating decreased. These positive changes in eating behaviors are most likely due to the subjects' involvement in weekly dietary counseling [16]. As for emotional eating, only the combination group experienced decreases in this parameter. It is possible that emotional eating was not decreased in the ADF group due to the lack of the exercise intervention. Positive changes in mood have been previously reported with short bouts of exercise [12,17]. Pendleton et al. designed a trial to study the effect of cognitive behavior therapy with or without exercise on binge eating in obese women. After 16 months, only the group that was exercising experienced improvements in mood, which resulted in decreased binge eating [18]. Taken together, it is possible that the combination of ADF plus exercise may have better overall effects on these eating behaviors than each intervention alone.

We also wanted to examine the ability of our dietary counseling program to aid individuals in reducing energy intake. Subjects met with a dietician each week to learn how to ascertain the caloric content of foods, control portion sizes, read food labels, and avoid high fat foods. Dietary intake was measured using a 3-day food record that was completed each week (on feed days). After 12 weeks of treatment, energy intake decreased by approximately 300 kcal in the combination group and by 220 kcal in ADF group, though not significantly. These reported energy deficits are somewhat lower than expected given that the combination and ADF group lost 7 kg and 3 kg, respectively. These incongruences between weight loss and energy deficits are most likely due to reporting errors in the food records. In view of this, more robust measures to assess energy expenditure and intake, such as the doubly labeled water technique, should be used in future trials of ADF.

This study has several limitations. First, the effect of exercise alone on hunger, fullness and satisfaction levels was not measured in this study. This makes it impossible to tease apart the effects of ADF versus exercise on these parameters. Secondly, the sample size employed (n = 16 per group) may have been too small to detect differences between groups for certain variables such as energy intake, and likeliness to cheat post-exercise. Thirdly, we implemented food records to measure energy intake, when we should have used a more accurate method, such as the doubly labeled water technique.

In summary, our results suggest that an endurance exercise program can be easily incorporated into the ADF regimen. Adding exercise to ADF does not increase the likeness to cheat on the fast day, which ensures that weight loss will be sizeable and consistent. We also show that the combination of ADF plus exercise increases restrained eating while decreasing uncontrolled and emotional eating. Taken together, endurance exercise is an excellent adjunct therapy to ADF, as it leads to positive behavioral changes that may contribute to long-term steady weight loss.

Competing interests

The authors have no competing of interest to report.

Authors' contributions

SB designed the experiment, conducted the clinical trial, analyzed the data, and wrote the manuscript. MCK and CMK assisted with the conduction of the clinical trial. EA, YC, JFT, KKH assisted with the data analysis. KAV assisted with the design of the experiment, and wrote the manuscript. All authors read and approved the final manuscript.

Funding source

American Heart Association 12PRE8350000; University of Illinois, Chicago, Departmental funding.

References

1. Varady KA, Bhutani S, Church EC, Klempel MC: **Short-term modified alternate-day fasting: a novel dietary strategy for weight loss and cardioprotection in obese adults.** *Am J Clin Nutr* 2009, **90**(5):1138–1143. doi: 10.3945/ajcn.2009.28380.
2. Bhutani SKMC, Kroeger CM, Trepanowski JF, Varady KA: **Alternate day fasting and endurance exercise combine to reduce body weight and favorably alter plasma lipids in obese humans.** *Obesity (Silver Spring)* 2012, **21**(7):1370–1379.
3. Yanovski SZ, Sebring NG: **Recorded food intake of obese women with binge eating disorder before and after weight loss.** *Int J Eating Disord* 1994, **15**(2):135–150.
4. Foster GD, Wadden TA, Swain RM, Stunkard AJ, Platte P, Vogt RA: **The eating inventory in obese women: clinical correlates and relationship to weight loss.** *Int J Obesity Relat Metab Disord: J Int Assoc Study Obesity* 1998, **22**(8):778–785.
5. Elfhag K, Rossner S: **Who succeeds in maintaining weight loss? A conceptual review of factors associated with weight loss maintenance and weight regain.** *Obesity Rev Off J Int Assoc Study Obesity* 2005, **6**(1):85. doi: 10.1111/j.1467-789X.2005.00170.x.
6. Yao M, Roberts SB: **Dietary energy density and weight regulation.** *Nutr Rev* 2001, **59**(8 Pt 1):247–258.
7. Mifflin MD, St Jeor ST, Hill LA, Scott BJ, Daugherty SA, Koh YO: **A new predictive equation for resting energy expenditure in healthy individuals.** *Am J Clin Nutr* 1990, **51**(2):241–247.
8. Tanaka H, Monahan KD, Seals DR: **Age-predicted maximal heart rate revisited.** *J Am Coll Cardiol* 2001, **37**(1):153–156.
9. Sepple CP, Read NW: **Gastrointestinal correlates of the development of hunger in man.** *Appetite* 1989, **13**(3):183–191.
10. Karlsson J, Persson LO, Sjostrom L, Sullivan M: **Psychometric properties and factor structure of the Three-Factor Eating Questionnaire (TFEQ) in obese**

men and women. Results from the Swedish Obese Subjects (SOS) study. *Int J Obesity Relat Metab Disord: J Int Assoc Study Obesity* 2000, **24**(12):1715–1725.

11. Lofrano-Prado MC, Hill JO, Gomes Silva HJ, *et al*: **Acute effects of aerobic exercise on mood and hunger feelings in male obese adolescents: a crossover study.** *Int J Behav Nutr Phys Act* 2012, **9**(1):38. doi: 10.1186/1479-5868-9-38.
12. Maraki M, Tsofliou F, Pitsiladis YP, Malkova D, Mutrie N, Higgins S: **Acute effects of a single exercise class on appetite, energy intake and mood. Is there a time of day effect?** *Appetite* 2005, **45**(3):272–278.
13. Heilbronn LK, Smith SR, Martin CK, Anton SD, Ravussin E: **Alternate-day fasting in nonobese subjects: effects on body weight, body composition, and energy metabolism.** *Am J Clin Nutr* 2005, **81**(1):69–73.
14. Blundell JE, Stubbs RJ, Hughes DA, Whybrow S, King NA: **Cross talk between physical activity and appetite control: does physical activity stimulate appetite?** *Proc Nutr Soc* 2003, **62**(3):651–661. doi: 10.1079/PNS2003286.
15. Guelfi KJ, Donges CE, Duffield R: **Beneficial effects of 12 weeks of aerobic compared with resistance exercise training on perceived appetite in previously sedentary overweight and obese men.** *Metab Clin Exp* 2013, **62**(2):235–243. doi: 10.1016/j.metabol.2012.08.002.
16. Keranen AM, Savolainen MJ, Reponen AH, *et al*: **The effect of eating behavior on weight loss and maintenance during a lifestyle intervention.** *Prev Med* 2009, **49**(1):32–38. doi: 10.1016/j.ypmed.2009.04.011.
17. Hansen CJ, Stevens LC, Coast JR: **Exercise duration and mood state: how much is enough to feel better?** *Health Psychol: Off J Div Health Psychol, Am Psychol Assoc* 2001, **20**(4):267–275.
18. Pendleton VR, Goodrick GK, Poston WS, Reeves RS, Foreyt JP: **Exercise augments the effects of cognitive-behavioral therapy in the treatment of binge eating.** *Int J Eating Disord* 2002, **31**(2):172–184.

4

Is carbohydrate needed to further stimulate muscle protein synthesis/hypertrophy following resistance exercise?

Vandré Casagrande Figueiredo and David Cameron-Smith*

Abstract

It is now well established that protein supplementation after resistance exercise promotes increased muscle protein synthesis, which ultimately results in greater net muscle accretion, relative to exercise alone or exercise with supplementary carbohydrate ingestion. However, it is not known whether combining carbohydrate with protein produces a greater anabolic response than protein alone. Recent recommendations have been made that the composition of the ideal supplement post-exercise would be a combination of a protein source with a high glycemic index carbohydrate. This is based on the hypothesis that insulin promotes protein synthesis, thus maximising insulin secretion will maximally potentiate this action. However, it is still controversial as to whether raising insulin level, within the physiological range, has any effect to further stimulate muscle protein synthesis. The present commentary will review the evidence underpinning the recommendation to consume carbohydrates in addition to a protein supplementation after resistance exercise for the specific purpose of increasing muscle mass. The paucity of data will be discussed, thus our conclusions are that further studies are necessary prior to any conclusions that enable evidence-based recommendations to be made.

Keywords: Leucine, Insulin, Glycemic index, Skeletal muscle, Dietary supplements, Whey protein, Lean body mass

Background

In the past decade significant progress has been made in unravelling the mechanisms that regulate the complex pathways that couple gene expression to protein synthesis. Emerging from these studies has been the influence of amino acids, most predominately leucine, on protein synthesis. Leucine, over and above being a necessary amino acid in protein synthesis, also potentiates the activity of the key kinases regulating translation initiation. Far from being the only determinate of protein synthesis, leucine along with energy status, mechano-sensing, ionic and hormonal mediators all converge to dictate the rate of protein synthesis. Insulin also plays an important role in protein synthesis, as a potent stimulator of PI-3K/Akt/mTOR axis, coupling growth with nutritional availability.

In a recent review by Stark et al. [1] published in the *Journal of the International Society of Sports Nutrition*, it was stated that fast-acting carbohydrates (e.g., glucose or maltodextrin) should be consumed together with proteins after resistance exercise to promote muscle hypertrophy. The two primary reasons cited for the necessity of adding carbohydrates to the post exercise meal/supplement were; 1), acutely, there is a synergistic effect of insulin and leucine on protein synthesis; and, 2) chronically, the addition of carbohydrate to a protein supplement would increase Lean Body Mass (LBM) to a greater extent than when protein is consumed alone. These assumptions require careful analysis, given the almost total absence of clinical data and the unsupported statements that have been made.

* Correspondence: d.cameron-smith@auckland.ac.nz
The Liggins Institute, Faculty of Medical and Science Health, University of Auckland, 85 Park Road, Grafton, Private Bag 92019, Auckland 1023, New Zealand

Does leucine require insulin to stimulate protein synthesis?

It is physiologically relevant to state that "leucine cannot modulate protein synthesis as effectively without the presence of insulin" as Stark et al. [1] claimed. However, the cited supportive data [2,3] are both cell culture in vitro models where it is possible to exclude insulin entirely from the treatment conditions. Results from cell culture studies are therefore not necessarily transferable to the *in vivo* conditions, without consideration of the differences. In one of these studies the cells were deprived of serum overnight (12+ hours) prior to stimulation with insulin [2]. Both studies [2,3] compared insulin treated cells with untreated cells. This contrasts the physiological state, in which even short-term (overnight) fasting conditions have low, but measurable levels of circulating insulin (~5 mU/L). At these low levels, protein synthesis can be elicited by amino acids [4]. More importantly, increasing insulin levels more than 30 times over fasting levels has no further effect on protein synthesis even while aminoacidemia is kept at high levels [4]. Thus, technically it is true that insulin is needed to increase protein synthesis when amino acids delivery are increased, however even very low levels of insulin are able to act in concert with leucine to enable protein synthesis. Moreover, it should be noted that leucine ingestion has the ability to stimulate insulin secretion [5,6] and that the majority of protein supplementation studies report a marked increase in circulating insulin concentrations, at a minimum 2–3 fold above fasting values [7,8].

Does insulin act to inhibit protein degradation?

Given that at physiological concentrations, increased insulin is unlikely to augment protein synthesis *in vivo*, it is also necessary to consider whether this also applied for protein degradation. Indeed, Børsheim et al. [9] demonstrated that carbohydrate supplementation (100 g) alone following resistance exercise is capable of improving net muscle protein balance through reduction at protein degradation rates rather than through increasing protein synthesis. However, the resultant small increase in insulinemia due to protein ingestion alone is also sufficient to inhibit the increased protein breakdown measured after resistance exercise [10].

Absence of clinical data on muscle gain

It has been further stated by Stark et al. [1] that "(...) studies using protein sources with a carbohydrate source tended to increase LBM more than did a protein source alone" (herein cited as references 11, 12, 13, 14, 15, 16). This fails to adequately reflect the data within these cited studies. The majority of those studies compared the co-ingestion of protein and carbohydrate versus carbohydrate alone [11,12] or versus a different source of protein whilst maintaining similar amounts of carbohydrates [13-15]. Moreover, the last cited study [16] analysed the impact of supplementation timing, not supplement composition. To date there are no clinical studies comparing the impact of the co-ingestion of carbohydrate-protein with just protein supplement on LBM. Interestingly, Wilkinson et al. [14] and Hartman et al. [13] both compared different sources of protein (milk versus soy) which also contained appreciable levels of carbohydrate. Both beverages had similar amounts of carbohydrate but the glycemic index (GI) differed: soy group contained maltrodextrin while milk group had lactose (as expected). Yet it was the lower GI supplement (milk) which generated the greatest net gain in lean mass [13] and higher fractional synthesis rate [14]. In these studies, at least, GI was not positively associated with muscle gains.

To date only three studies [10,17,18] have addressed the impact of combined carbohydrate with protein/amino acids versus protein/amino acids alone on acute protein synthesis in young adults. These studies demonstrate that adding carbohydrate to a protein dose that alone is known to maximally stimulate protein synthesis (20-25 g of high-quality protein rich in leucine) has no additive or synergic effect on muscle protein synthesis and breakdown. The same result has recently also been demonstrated in older subjects [19]. Converging with those data, the addition of 30 g or 90 g of carbohydrates to 20 g of essential amino acids produces the same effect on protein synthesis and protein breakdown, regardless the great difference in insulinemia in both groups [20]. Insulin seems to only further increase protein synthesis at pharmacological doses [21], which means that it is not achievable by carbohydrate supplementation.

There remain valid reasons for the inclusion of carbohydrates into protein supplements that are to be consumed following resistance exercise. These included the maximization of glycogen restoration, especially when the time period between exercise sessions is short [22]. However, based on the available clinical data, there is no evidence that the addition of carbohydrates to a protein supplement will increase, acutely, muscle protein synthesis and, chronically, LBM to a greater extent than protein alone, which is in contrast to the statements of Stark and colleagues [1].

Conclusion and perspectives

There is a growing body of literature analysing the impact that co-ingestion of protein-carbohydrate versus carbohydrate alone has on protein synthesis. However, there are far fewer studies examining the actions of co-ingested carbohydrate-protein compared to protein alone. More importantly, no chronic study has addressed the effects of adding carbohydrate to protein compared to protein alone on muscle hypertrophy.

In conclusion, whilst it cannot be excluded that carbohydrate addition may provide benefits for recovering athletes, on the basis of available data, no further beneficial actions of carbohydrates, irrespective of GI, are evident concerning muscle hypertrophy when a protein supplement that maximally stimulate muscle protein synthesis is ingested. Further studies are required before conclusions and recommendations can be made.

Abbreviations
LBM: Lean body mass; GI: Glycemic index; mU/L: milliunits per liter; PI-3K: Phosphoinositide 3-kinase; Akt: Protein kinase B; mTOR: Mammalian target of rapamycin.

Competing interests
The authors declare that they have no competing interests.

Authors' contributions
VCF and DCS wrote the manuscript. Both authors read and approved the final version.

Acknowledgements
We thank Dr. James Markworth for his valuable comments and suggestions during manuscript preparation. We also would like to thank the anonymous reviewers for the constructive criticism on the manuscripts.

References
1. Stark M, Lukaszuk J, Prawitz A, Salacinski A: **Protein timing and its effects on muscular hypertrophy and strength in individuals engaged in weight-training.** *J Int Soc Sports Nutr* 2012, **9**(1):54.
2. Nobukuni T, Joaquin M, Roccio M, Dann SG, Kim SY, Gulati P, Byfield MP, Backer JM, Natt F, Bos JL, Zwartkruis FJ, Thomas G: **Amino acids mediate mTOR/raptor signaling through activation of class 3 phosphatidylinositol 3OH-kinase.** *Proc Natl Acad Sci USA* 2005, **102:**14238–14243.
3. Byfield MP, Murray JT, Backer JM: **hVps34 is a nutrient-regulated lipid kinase required for activation of p70 S6 kinase.** *J Biol Chem* 2005, **280:**33076–33082.
4. Greenhaff PL, Karagounis LG, Peirce N, Simpson EJ, Hazell M, Layfield R, Wackerhage H, Smith K, Atherton P, Selby A, Rennie MJ: **Disassociation between the effects of amino acids and insulin on signaling, ubiquitin ligases, and protein turnover in human muscle.** *Am J Physiol Endocrinol Metab* 2008, **295**(3):E595–604.
5. Floyd JC Jr, Fajans SS, Knopf RF, Conn JW: **Evidence that insulin release is the mechanism for experimentally induced leucine hypoglycemia in man.** *J Clin Invest* 1963, **42:**1714–1719.
6. Anthony JC, Lang CH, Crozier SJ, Anthony TG, MacLean DA, Kimball SR, Jefferson LS: **Contribution of insulin to the translational control of protein synthesis in skeletal muscle by leucine.** *Am J Physiol Endocrinol Metab* 2002, **282**(5):E1092–1101.
7. Akhavan T, Luhovyy BL, Brown PH, Cho CE, Anderson GH: **Effect of premeal consumption of whey protein and its hydrolysate on food intake and postmeal glycemia and insulin responses in young adults.** *Am J Clin Nutr* 2010, **91**(4):966–975.
8. Morifuji M, Ishizaka M, Baba S, Fukuda K, Matsumoto H, Koga J, Kanegae M, Higuchi M: **Comparison of different sources and degrees of hydrolysis of dietary protein: effect on plasma amino acids, dipeptides, and insulin responses in human subjects.** *J Agric Food Chem* 2010, **58**(15):8788–8797.
9. Børsheim E, Cree MG, Tipton KD, Elliott TA, Aarsland A, Wolfe RR: **Effect of carbohydrate intake on net muscle protein synthesis during recovery from resistance exercise.** *J Appl Physiol* 2004, **96**(2):674–678.
10. Staples AW, Burd NA, West DW, Currie KD, Atherton PJ, Moore DR, Rennie MJ, Macdonald MJ, Baker SK, Phillips SM: **Carbohydrate does not augment exercise-induced protein accretion versus protein alone.** *Med Sci Sports Exerc* 2011, **43**(7):1154–1161.
11. Josse AR, Tang JE, Tarnopolsky MA, Phillips SM: **Body composition and strength changes in women with milk and resistance exercise.** *Med Sci Sports Exerc* 2010, **42**(6):1122–1130.
12. Rankin JW, Goldman LP, Puglisi MJ, Nickols-Richardson SM, Earthman CP, Gwazdauskas FC: **Effect of post-exercise supplement consumption on adaptations to resistance training.** *J Am Coll Nutr* 2004, **23**(4):322–330.
13. Hartman JW, Tang JE, Wilkinson SB, Tarnopolsky MA, Lawrence RL, Fullerton AV, Phillips SM: **Consumption of fat-free fluid milk after resistance exercise promotes greater lean mass accretion than does consumption of soy or carbohydrate in young, novice, male weightlifters.** *Am J Clin Nutr* 2007, **86**(2):373–381.
14. Wilkinson SB, Tarnopolsky MA, Macdonald MJ, Macdonald JR, Armstrong D, Phillips SM: **Consumption of fluid skim milk promotes greater muscle protein accretion after resistance exercise than does consumption of an isonitrogenous and isoenergetic soy-protein beverage.** *Am J Clin Nutr* 2007, **85**(4):1031–1040.
15. Elliot TA, Cree MG, Sanford AP, Wolfe RR, Tipton KD: **Milk ingestion stimulates net muscle protein synthesis following resistance exercise.** *Med Sci Sports Exerc* 2006, **38**(4):667–674.
16. Cribb PJ, Hayes A: **Effects of supplement timing and resistance exercise on skeletal muscle hypertrophy.** *Med Sci Sports Exerc* 2006, **38**(11):1918–1925.
17. Koopman R, Beelen M, Stellingwerff T, Pennings B, Saris WH, Kies AK, Kuipers H, Van Loon LJ: **Coingestion of carbohydrate with protein does not further augment postexercise muscle protein synthesis.** *Am J Physiol Endocrinol Metab* 2007, **293**(3):E833–842.
18. Glynn EL, Fry CS, Timmerman KL, Drummond MJ, Volpi E, Rasmussen BB: **Addition of carbohydrate or alanine to an essential amino acid mixture does not enhance human skeletal muscle protein anabolism.** *J Nutr* 2013, **143**(3):307–314.
19. Hamer HM, Wall BT, Kiskini A, De Lange A, Groen BBL, Bakker JA, Gijsen AP, Verdijk LB, Van Loon LJC: **Carbohydrate co-ingestion with protein does not further augment post-prandial muscle protein accretion in older men.** *Nutr Metab (Lond)* 2013, **10**(1):15.
20. Glynn EL, Fry CS, Drummond MJ, Dreyer HC, Dhanani S, Volpi E, Rasmussen BB: **Muscle protein breakdown has a minor role in the protein anabolic response to essential amino acid and carbohydrate intake following resistance exercise.** *Am J Physiol Regul Integr Comp Physiol* 2010, **299**(2):R533–540.
21. Hillier TA, Fryburg DA, Jahn LA, Barrett EJ: **Extreme hyperinsulinemia unmasks insulin's effect to stimulate protein synthesis in the human forearm.** *Am J Physiol* 1998, **274**(6 Pt 1):E1067–1074.
22. Slater G, Phillips SM: **Nutrition guidelines for strength sports: sprinting, weightlifting, throwing events, and bodybuilding.** *J Sports Sci* 2011, **29**(1):S67–77.

5

Assessing a commercially available sports drink on exogenous carbohydrate oxidation, fluid delivery and sustained exercise performance

Justin D Roberts*, Michael D Tarpey†, Lindsy S Kass†, Richard J Tarpey† and Michael G Roberts†

Abstract

Background: Whilst exogenous carbohydrate oxidation (CHO_{EXO}) is influenced by mono- and disaccharide combinations, debate exists whether such beverages enhance fluid delivery and exercise performance. Therefore, this study aimed to ascertain CHO_{EXO}, fluid delivery and performance times of a commercially available maltodextrin/fructose beverage in comparison to an isocaloric maltodextrin beverage and placebo.

Methods: Fourteen club level cyclists (age: 31.79 ± 10.02 years; height: 1.79 ± 0.06 m; weight: 73.69 ± 9.24 kg; VO_{2max}: 60.38 ± 9.36 mL · kg^{-1} min^{-1}) performed three trials involving 2.5 hours continuous exercise at 50% maximum power output (W_{max}: 176.71 ± 25.92 W) followed by a 60 km cycling performance test. Throughout each trial, athletes were randomly assigned, in a double-blind manner, either: (1) 1.1 g · min^{-1} maltodextrin + 0.6 g · min^{-1} fructose (MD + F), (2) 1.7 g · min^{-1} of maltodextrin (MD) or (3) flavoured water (P). In addition, the test beverage at 60 minutes contained 5.0 g of deuterium oxide (^2H_2O) to assess quantification of fluid delivery. Expired air samples were analysed for CHO_{EXO} according to the $^{13}C/^{12}C$ ratio method using gas chromatography continuous flow isotope ratio mass spectrometry.

Results: Peak CHO_{EXO} was significantly greater in the final 30 minutes of submaximal exercise with MD + F and MD compared to P (1.45 ± 0.09 g · min^{-1}, 1.07 ± 0.03 g · min^{-1}and 0.00 ± 0.01 g · min^{-1} respectively, $P < 0.0001$), and significantly greater for MD + F compared to MD (P = 0.005). The overall appearance of ^2H_2O in plasma was significantly greater in both P and MD + F compared to MD (100.27 ± 3.57 ppm, 92.57 ± 2.94 ppm and 78.18 ± 4.07 ppm respectively, $P < 0.003$). There was no significant difference in fluid delivery between P and MD + F ($P = 0.078$). Performance times significantly improved with MD + F compared with both MD (by 7 min 22 s ± 1 min 56 s, or 7.2%) and P (by 6 min 35 s ± 2 min 33 s, or 6.5%, $P < 0.05$) over 60 km.

Conclusions: A commercially available maltodextrin-fructose beverage improves CHO_{EXO} and fluid delivery, which may benefit individuals during sustained moderate intensity exercise. The greater CHO_{EXO} observed when consuming a maltodextrin-fructose beverage may support improved performance times.

Keywords: Fructose, Maltodextrin, Exogenous carbohydrate oxidation, Fluid delivery, Performance

* Correspondence: j.d.roberts@herts.ac.uk
†Equal contributors
School of Life & Medical Sciences, University of Hertfordshire, College Lane, Hatfield, Hertfordshire, UK

Introduction

It has long been established that carbohydrate (CHO) ingestion at frequent intervals, or late into submaximal aerobic exercise can maintain plasma glucose concentrations [1], and support performance through a number of mechanisms including glycogen preservation, increased total carbohydrate oxidation rates (CHO_{TOT}), lowered subjective perception of fatigue and prevention of acute onset hypoglycaemia [1-3].

When exercise is of a prolonged nature (ie: >3 hours), CHO_{TOT} plays a significant role in sustaining power output (particularly if the exercise is considered strenuous). It is well established that exogenous carbohydrate oxidation rates (CHO_{EXO}) may be limited at 1.0 $g.min^{-1}$ when single sugars eg: glucose, are consumed, due to saturation of the intestinal sodium glucose cotransporter (SGLT1). The resulting contribution from endogenous carbohydrate sources to maintain CHO_{TOT} may therefore limit performance.

However, combinations of glucose, fructose and sucrose have yielded 20-55% greater CHO_{EXO} than glucose alone, through additional utilisation of a separate GLUT5 transport mechanism [4-8]. Whilst optimal CHO ingestion rates of 30–80 $g.hr^{-1}$ have been recommended for events lasting up to 2.5 hours, no differences in CHO_{EXO} have been observed between combined and single sugar beverages at moderate CHO intakes (0.80 $g.min^{-1}$ [9]). Therefore, optimal CHO_{EXO} are likely to coincide with higher total ingestion rates of mixed sugar beverages.

Indeed, CHO_{EXO} with combined glucose and fructose beverages have been reported at 1.26 $g.min^{-1}$ up to 1.75 $g.min^{-1}$ with ingestion rates of 1.80 to 2.40 $g.min^{-1}$ respectively [4]. Case study assessment of world class triathletes in our laboratory have indicated high CHO_{EXO} values of >1.75 $g.min^{-1}$ after 3 hours of competitive paced cycling with sustained ingestion rates of 2.00 $g.min^{-1}$ indicating potential training tolerance to carbohydrate ingestion (unpublished observations). However, such high intakes may not be practical, or indeed tolerable, by club level and recreational athletes, and may exacerbate gastrointestinal distress [10] which could be detrimental to both sustained performance and beverage delivery.

The use of maltodextrin-fructose formulas have been shown to elicit equally high CHO_{EXO} [11], and may maintain gastrointestinal comfort [12]. Whilst the benefit of sports drinks on fluid delivery has been contested [13], with higher carbohydrate delivery, there is recent evidence to suggest that combined transportable sugar beverages may enhance fluid delivery [8,14-16], which may benefit the athlete when net fluid loss may impede late stage exercise performance. Less is known about commercially available sports drinks [17], particularly maltodextrin-fructose formulas, on fluid delivery.

Of key interest is the effect of sports drinks on exercise performance. The inclusion of CHO beverages has been shown to improve exercise performance and time to fatigue during relatively short laboratory [18-20] and field based assessments [21]. More recently, studies have demonstrated an effect of multiple transportable carbohydrates on sustained time trial performance [22,23] and power output [22,24]. However, this is not supported elsewhere [25], especially when commercially available carbohydrate beverages have been used [26].

With recent public interest in the accuracy of marketing claims, and whether commercially available sports drinks are indeed beneficial for performance [27,28], we were invited to undertake an independent assessment of a commercial maltodextrin/ fructose beverage (MD + F: Energy Source™, High 5 Ltd.) on total and exogenous carbohydrate oxidation, and fluid delivery in comparison to a maltodextrin only beverage (MD) and placebo (P). A further aim was to assess the influence of the three beverages on cycling performance following a period of sustained steady state exercise. It was hypothesised that the MD + F commercial formula would lead to greater exogenous oxidation and fluid delivery rates, resulting in a specific performance gains.

Materials and methods

Participants

Fourteen club level male cyclists were recruited for participation following power calculation assessment (G*Power3, Dusseldorf [29]). All participants had an endurance training background of at least two years, and did not suffer from diabetes or have known dysglycemia. Before undertaking the study, participants were required to provide written informed consent and satisfactorily complete a health screen questionnaire. Additionally, participants were excluded if consuming other nutritional supplements. Ethical approval for the study was provided by the University of Hertfordshire Life and Medical Sciences Ethics Committee.

Procedures

Preliminary testing

At least one week prior to experimental trials, participants completed an incremental exercise test to volitional exhaustion for assessment of maximal power output (W_{max}) and maximal oxygen consumption (VO_{2max}). All testing was undertaken in the Human Physiology Laboratory, Division of Sport, Health and Exercise, University of Hertfordshire. Upon reporting to the laboratory, the participants' nude body mass (Seca, model 780, Hamburg, Germany) and height were recorded. Following this, maximal tests were performed on a Computrainer (RaceMate Inc, Seattle, USA) and related Coaching Software program (Comp CS, RaceMate Inc, Seattle,

USA). The Computrainer was pre-calibrated and standardised to the body mass and cycle of the participant.

Following a 10 minute standardised warm-up at 100 W, an incremental step protocol was then undertaken, with power output progressing by 30 W each 3 minutes until volitional exhaustion. Participants were fitted with an oro-nasal face mask (7920 series, Hans Rudolph Inc., Kansas City, USA) attached to a triple-V digital volume transducer. Respiratory data was recorded throughout exercise using a Metalyzer 3B system online automated gas-analyser in conjunction with Metasoft version 3 software (Cortex Biophysik, Leipzig, Germany). Heart rate (HR) was recorded continuously via radio-telemetry (Polar Electro Oy, Kempele, Finland). Ratings of perceived exertion (RPE) were collected in the final minute of each stage, using the Borg 6–20 subjective exertion scale [30]. The test concluded when participants reached volitional exhaustion or were unable to maintain the required power output.

Maximal power was calculated by adding the final completed workload to the fraction of time spent in the non-completed workload, multiplied by 30 W. Oxygen consumption (VO_2) was defined as maximal when two of the following criteria were met: 1) a levelling off of VO_2 with increasing workload (increase of no more than 2 $ml \cdot kg^{-1} \cdot min^{-1}$); 2) attainment of maximal predicted heart rate (±10 $beats.min^{-1}$); and 3) a respiratory exchange ratio (RER) of >1.05. The highest attained VO_2, maintained for 20 seconds, was determined to be the VO_{2max}. Participants also undertook a separate habituation trial for both steady state and performance conditions. The characteristics of the participants are shown in Table 1.

Experimental trials

All experimental trials were undertaken in the Human Physiology Laboratory, Division of Sport, Health and Exercise, University of Hertfordshire under controlled conditions (temperature: 22.4 ± 0.9°C; barometric pressure – range: 979–1023 mBar; and relative humidity – range: 21–56%). No differences were reported between trials ($P > 0.05$) for any of the environmental variables.

The study employed a randomised, placebo-controlled, double-blind cross over design for beverage condition. Participants were required to perform three exercise trials separated by one week, each comprising a 2.5 hour cycle at 50% W_{max} (oxidation trial), followed by a 60 km cycling test (performance trial). Trials were undertaken at the same time of day to minimise the potential for diurnal variance. Participants reported to the laboratory following a 12 hour overnight fast. Upon arrival, nude body mass was measured and participants rested for 5 minutes before baseline measurements (for expired air and blood analytes) were undertaken. All trials were performed on a pre-calibrated Computrainer (RaceMate Inc, Seattle, USA), as employed in preliminary testing.

Sub-maximal oxidation trial

Following a 10 minute warm up at 100 W, participants began a 2.5 hour oxidation trial at 50% W_{max}. Steady state power output was based on individual quantification of W_{max} from pre-experimental assessment. Expired air samples were collected via the Douglas bag method at 30 and 60 minutes, and then 15 minute intervals thereafter, and analysed for percentage O_2 and CO_2, using a Servomex 1440 gas analyser (Servomex Group Ltd, Crowborough, UK). Total Douglas bag volume was measured using a dry gas meter (Harvard Apparatus, Holliston, USA). Standardised measurements for minute ventilation (V_E, $L.min^{-1}$), oxygen uptake (VO_2, $L.min^{-1}$), carbon dioxide (VCO_2, $L.min^{-1}$) and respiratory exchange ratio (RER) were recorded at 0, 30 and 60 minutes, and every 15 minutes thereafter during the oxidation trial.

In addition, immediately following each Douglas bag collection, duplicate 10 ml expired air samples were extracted into vacuumed Exetainer tubes (Labco Ltd, High Wycombe, UK) for the determination of expired gas $^{13}C{:}^{12}C$ ratio. Exetainer samples were analysed independently (Iso-Analytical Ltd., Crewe, UK) for $^{13}C{:}^{12}C$ ratio by gas chromatography continuous flow isotope ratio mass spectrometry (GC-IRMS, Europa Scientific 20–20 IRMS). Stable isotope measurements and indirect calorimetry were used to calculate rates of CHO_{EXO}, CHO_{TOT} (total carbohydrate oxidation) and FAT_{TOT} (total fat oxidation).

At rest, and at 15 minute intervals throughout the oxidation trial, 30 µl of capillarised wholeblood was collected in heparinised tubes and frozen at −8°C for subsequent analysis of blood glucose using an Analox micro-stat PGM7 (Analox Instruments Ltd, London, UK). Telemetric HR was recorded at 15 minute intervals throughout the oxidation trial. Ratings of perceived exertion (RPE_{TOTAL} and RPE_{LEGS}) using the 6–20 and 0–10 Borg scales respectively were recorded every 30 minutes during submaximal exercise. Participants also verbally completed an adapted 14 point gastrointestinal (GI) symptom assessment questionnaire [31] every 30 minutes, grading the degree of subjective discomfort on a 0–10 visual analogue scale. Particular attention was given to symptoms categorised as both 'moderate' (4–6) and 'severe' (7–10).

Beverage administration

In a double-blind random order manner, participants were assigned the following beverages across trials: maltodextrin only (MD), isoenergetic maltodextrin with fructose (MD + F) or aspartame sweetened, citrus flavoured water (P). All CHO beverages were supplied by

Table 1 Summary of participant characteristics and pre-experimental data collection

Age (years)	Height (m)	Weight (kg)	VO_{2max} (L.min^{-1})	VO_{2max} (ml.kg^{-1}.min^{-1})	W_{max} (watts)	50% W_{max} (watts)
31.79 ± 10.02	1.79 ± 0.06	73.69 ± 9.24	4.40 ± 0.56	60.38 ± 9.36	352.64 ± 52.39	176.71 ± 25.92

Table 1 shows the key characteristics of all participants, including data for maximal power output from pre-experimental assessment. Values are presented as mean ± SD; n = 14; VO_{2max}, maximal oxygen uptake; W_{max}, maximal power output.

High 5 Ltd., and prepared as 10% concentrated formulas in opaque drinks bottles. The test beverages provided an average CHO delivery rate of 1.7 $g \cdot min^{-1}$ for MD (corn-derived glucose monohydrate), and 1.1 $g \cdot min^{-1}$ maltodextrin with 0.6 $g \cdot min^{-1}$ fructose for MD + F (using corn-derived glucose monohydrate and crystalline fructose, Energy Source™, High 5 Ltd.). This was based on discussion with the manufacturer to provide a realistic, but high ingestion rate (102 g total carbohydrate per hour in line with high dosages recommended for longer duration exercise).

Beverages were administered as controlled 270 ml doses at the start of the oxidation trial and every 15 minutes (until completion of the performance trial), providing a fluid intake of 1.08 $L \cdot h^{-1}$. In terms of content, the test beverages per 100 g comprised: i) for MD + F – 96.7 g of total carbohydrate (of which 59.7 g from maltodextrin, 31.5 g from fructose); 0.0 g of protein and fat; and delivered 388 kcal; ii) for MD - 96.0 g of total carbohydrate (of which 90.9 g from maltodextrin, 4.0 g from fructose); 0.0 g of protein and fat; and delivered 384 kcal; and P – 0.3 g of total carbohydrate (of which 0.3 g total sugars); 0.2 g of protein and 0.0 g of fat; and delivered 10 kcal.

All CHO beverages contained 816 mg per 100 g (~35.5 mmol.L^{-1}) of sodium (as tri-sodium citrate and sodium chloride). Corn-derived glucose monohydrate and crystalline fructose were used due to their naturally high ^{13}C content, allowing for the quantification of CHO_{EXO}. The ingested glucose and fructose were subject to elemental analyser-isotope ratio mass spectrometry (EA-IRMS; Europa Scientific 20–20) for the determination of ^{13}C-enrichment (MD: −11.41 δ‰, MD + F: −11.84 δ‰ vs. Pee Dee Bellemnitella (PDB)).

Assessment of fluid delivery

The quantification of plasma deuterium enrichment has previously been validated for qualitative assessment of fluid delivery [8,14]. Based on both sample size power determination (G*Power 3, Dusseldorf) and cost, it was deemed that only 7 participants were required for assessment of fluid delivery. Prior to the oxidation trial, an intravenous 20 gauge cannula was inserted by a qualified phlebotomist into an antecubital vein for 7 of the participants, to allow repeated blood sampling. Sample lines were kept patent after each blood collection with a 2 ml isotonic saline flush (0.9% sodium chloride saline, Baxter, Norfolk, UK).

Participants received 5 g of deuterium oxide (^2H_2O, Sigma Aldrich, Dorset, UK), included in the beverage administered at 60 minutes, for assessment of fluid delivery. Blood samples were collected in 10 ml Vacutainer tubes, containing sodium fluoride/K_3EDTA as an anticoagulant (Beckton Dickinson, Plymouth, UK), at 15 minute intervals from the 60 minute time point into the oxidation trial. Blood samples were analyzed for plasma ^2H_2O enrichment via equilibration (Europa 20–20 continuous-flow isotope ratio mass spectrometry) by an independent laboratory (Iso-Analytical Ltd., Crewe, UK). Indwelling cannulas were removed at the end of the oxidation trial.

Performance trial

Upon completion of the oxidation trial, participants performed a 60 km performance trial using the same Computrainer (RaceMate Inc, Seattle, USA). This was based on manufacturer recommendation to simulate durations encountered during sportive level events. Treatment beverages continued to be ingested every 15 minutes in the same quantity as for the oxidation trial. Participants were instructed to complete the 60 km cycle course in the fastest possible time, and were given verbal encouragement throughout the test coinciding with beverage administration.

Telemetric HR and capillarised wholebood (for glucose analysis as previously described) were assessed at 15 minute intervals. In line with laboratory safety regulations, participants were required to stop exercising if blood glucose dropped below 2.5 mmol·L^{-1}. Gastrointestinal symptom assessment was undertaken every 30 minutes as previously described. Speed (km.hr^{-1}), power output (W) and distance covered (km) were recorded during the performance trial at 15 minute intervals, but with an adapted monitor only permitting sight of distance covered. At the cessation of the test, participants cooled down for 5 minutes at 100 W.

Trial control measures

All participants were required to maintain a food and exercise diary for 7 days prior to the first exercise trial, and maintain these patterns before each subsequent trial. Participants were provided with a list of foods naturally abundant in ^{13}C (CHO derived from C4 plants, e.g.: corn and sugar cane) and instructed to avoid them for the 7 days prior to the first exercise trial and for the duration of the experimental period to reduce background ^{13}C from endogenous stores. Food lists also provided a number of alternative high CHO foods to prevent a reduction in CHO intake. Additionally, to reduce background interference from ^{13}C-enriched glycogen stores, participants performed a 150–180 minute glycogen-depleting ride 5 days before each trial. Previous studies have employed similar interventions to limit the effects of background ^{13}C-levels [5,7,8]. Participants were asked to refrain from caffeine, alcohol ingestion and intense exercise for 24 hours before each trial.

Calculations

Total oxidation rates:

Rates of CHO_{TOT} and FAT_{TOT} ($g \cdot min^{-1}$) were calculated from absolute VO_2 and VCO_2 ($L \cdot min^{-1}$) utilising the following stoichiometric equations [32], with protein oxidation during exercise assumed negligible:

$$CHO_{TOT} = 4.585(VCO_2)\text{-}3.226(VO_2)$$

$$FAT_{TOT} = 1.695(VO_2)\text{-}1.701(VCO_2)$$

Exogenous carbohydrate oxidation rates:

The rate of CHO_{EXO} ($g \cdot min^{-1}$) was calculated using the following formula [33]:

$$CHOEXO = VCO2 \cdot \left(\frac{Exp\text{-}Exp_{BKG}}{Ing\text{-}Exp_{BKG}}\right) \cdot \left(\frac{1}{k}\right)$$

Where δExp is the ^{13}C-enrichment of expired air throughout the oxidation trial, δIng is the ^{13}C-enrichment of the CHO solution, Exp_{BKG} is the ^{13}C-enrichment of expired air throughout the placebo trial (P) and k is the CO_2 produced via the oxidation of 1 g of glucose ($k = 0.7467$ litres of CO_2 per gram of glucose [8]).

The ^{13}C-enrichment was expressed as δ‰ difference between the ^{13}C:^{12}C ratio of the sample and a known laboratory reference standard (PDB) according to the following formula [34]:

$$\delta^{13}C = \left[\left(\frac{\frac{^{13}C}{^{12}C}\text{ of sample}}{\frac{^{13}C}{^{12}C}\text{ of standard}}\right)\text{-}1\right] \cdot 10^3$$

The rate of CHO_{ENDO} was calculated by subtracting CHO_{EXO} from CHO_{TOT}. Substrate oxidation was calculated over the final 90 minutes of exercise (60–150 minutes) due to the earlier capture of $^{13}CO_2$ in the bicarbonate (HCO_3^-) pool. It has been reported that dilution in the bicarbonate pool becomes negligible after 60 minutes of exercise, when 100% of the $^{13}CO_2$ from oxidation is retrieved [8,35,36].

Carbohydrate oxidation efficiency:

Estimation of carbohydrate oxidation efficiency was determined using the following formula [7]:

$$CHOEXO\ efficiency = 100 \cdot \left(\frac{CHOEXO}{CHO\ ingestion\ rate}\right)$$

Statistical analyses:

Statistical analyses were performed using SPSS Statistics for Windows version 19 (SPSS, Chicago, USA). A two-way analysis of variance (ANOVA) with repeated measures design was used to assess for interaction effects between conditions, trials and over time. Where appropriate, a one-way ANOVA was used to assess for differences for relevant experimental measures (e.g.: mean CHO_{EXO}) between trials only. Significant differences were assessed with a student t-test with Bonferoni post hoc adjustments. Where pertinent, pearson chi squared assessment was undertaken (e.g.: gastrointestinal responses). An alpha level of 0.05 was employed for assessment of statistical significance. All data are reported as means ± SE.

Results

Submaximal oxidation trial

Total carbohydrate oxidation

Data for total carbohydrate oxidation rates are represented in Figures 1 and 2. During steady state aerobic exercise performed at 50% W_{max}, mean CHO_{TOT} between 60–150 minutes were significantly different between treatment conditions ($F = 20.601$; $P = 0.0001$). Mean CHO_{TOT} were significantly greater for both MD + F and MD compared with P throughout the last 90 minutes of steady state exercise ($2.74 \pm 0.07\ g.min^{-1}$ for MD + F and $2.50 \pm 0.11\ g.min^{-1}$ for MD v $1.98 \pm 0.12\ g.min^{-1}$ for P respectively; $P = 0.0001$). Mean

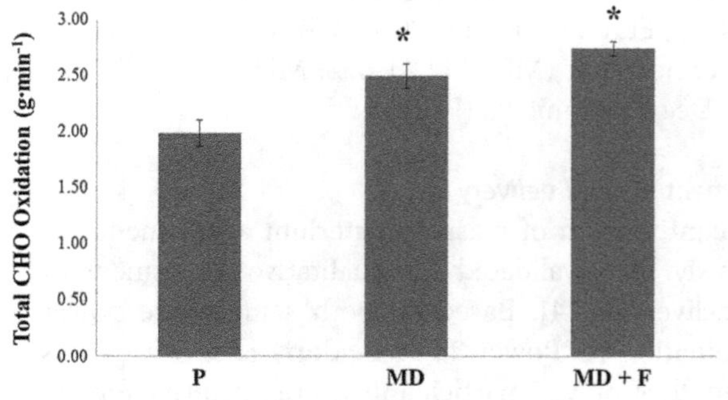

Figure 1 Assessment of test beverages on mean CHO_{TOT} oxidation rates between 60–150 minutes of the submaximal exercise trial. Figure 1 demonstrates the influence of all test beverages on mean total carbohydrate oxidation rates in the final 90 minutes of the oxidation trial. Data are presented as mean ± SE; n = 14. P, Placebo; MD, maltodextrin beverage; MD + F, maltodextrin-fructose beverage; CHO_{TOT}, total carbohydrate oxidation rates. *denotes significant difference ($P < 0.001$) to P.

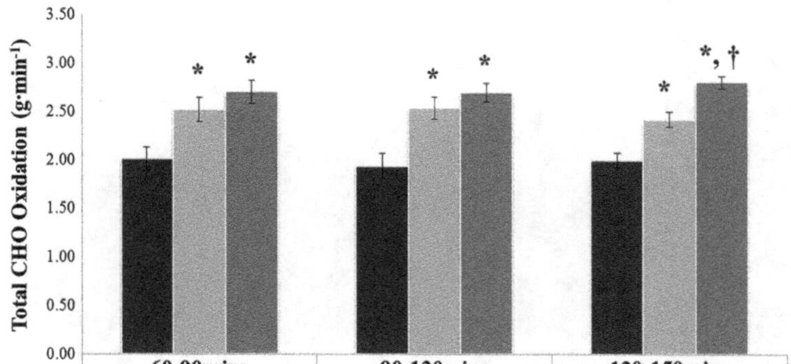

	60-90mins	90-120mins	120-150mins
P	2.01	1.94	2.00
MD	2.52	2.54	2.42
MD + F	2.71	2.70	2.81

Figure 2 Assessment of test beverages on mean CHO_{TOT} oxidation rates at various timepoints during the submaximal exercise trial. Figure 2 shows the difference between test beverages for total carbohydrate oxidation rates at specific 30 minute time periods in the final 90 minutes of the oxidation trial. Data are presented as mean ± SE; n = 14. P, Placebo; MD, maltodextrin beverage; MD + F, maltodextrin-fructose beverage; CHO_{TOT}, total carbohydrate oxidation rates. *denotes significant difference ($P < 0.005$) to P within timepoint assessment. † denotes significant difference between MD and MD + F within timepoint assessment ($P = 0.004$).

CHO_{TOT} were not shown to be statistically different between MD + F and MD ($P > 0.05$).

When assessing specific intervals during the oxidation trial, between 60–90 minutes and 90–120 minutes of submaximal exercise performed at 50%W_{max}, both carbohydrate test beverages demonstrated higher mean CHO_{TOT} compared to P ($P < 0.005$). Whilst this observation continued in the last 30 minutes of the oxidation trial, a significant difference was also found between MD + F and MD between 120–150 minutes of the test (2.81 ± 0.06 $g.min^{-1}$ v 2.42 ± 0.10 $g.min^{-1}$ respectively; $P = 0.004$).

Exogenous carbohydrate oxidation

Data for CHO_{EXO} are represented in Figure 3 and Table 2. A significant interaction effect was found for both time and beverage (F = 31.659; $P = 0.0001$). Whilst no differences were observed between conditions at rest ($P > 0.05$), both carbohydrate beverages displayed significantly higher CHO_{EXO} at all timepoints from 30 minutes in comparison to P ($P < 0.0001$). Mean CHO_{EXO} between 60–150 minutes was significantly different between test conditions (F = 180.077; $P = 0.0001$). Both carbohydrate beverages displayed significantly greater mean CHO_{EXO} compared with P ($P = 0.0001$). However, throughout the final 90 minutes of steady state exercise, CHO_{EXO} was significantly higher with MD + F compared with MD (1.27 ± 0.07 $g.min^{-1}$ v 0.98 ± 0.04 $g.min^{-1}$ respectively; $P = 0.019$). When analysed for respective 30 minute time periods, CHO_{EXO} was significantly higher for MD + F compared with MD between 90–120 minutes and 120–150 minutes only ($P < 0.025$). Peak CHO_{EXO} was significantly greater in the final 30 minutes of submaximal exercise with MD + F and MD compared to P (1.45 ± 0.09 $g \cdot min^{-1}$, 1.07 ± 0.03 $g \cdot min^{-1}$ and 0.00 ± 0.01 $g \cdot min^{-1}$ respectively, $P < 0.0001$), and significantly greater for MD + F compared to MD (P = 0.005).

Assessment of exogenous carbohydrate efficiency ($CHO_{EXO\ Eff}$%) was additionally undertaken across the oxidation trial. Mean $CHO_{EXO\ Eff}$% was significantly greater with MD + F and MD compared to P for all assessed time periods ($P < 0.0001$). Additionally $CHO_{EXO\ Eff}$% was significantly greater with MD + F compared to MD overall (74.7 ± 4.4% v 57.9 ± 2.1% respectively; $P = 0.019$), and at respective assessed timepoints from 90 minutes ($P < 0.025$).

Endogenous carbohydrate oxidation

Data for mean CHO_{ENDO} are represented in Table 2. In a similar pattern to mean CHO_{TOT}, a significant interaction effect was found between treatment conditions for mean CHO_{ENDO} between 60–150 minutes of the oxidation trial (F = 13.822; $P = 0.0001$). Both MD + F and MD conditions demonstrated lower mean CHO_{ENDO} during the last 90 minutes of continuous exercise compared to P (1.47 ± 0.07 $g.min^{-1}$, 1.51 ± 0.10 $g.min^{-1}$ and 1.97 ± 0.12 $g.min^{-1}$ respectively; $P < 0.004$). Whilst mean CHO_{ENDO} progressively declined for each averaged 30 minute period within treatment condition, the same pattern was observed with both carbohydrate beverages demonstrating significantly lower CHO_{ENDO} in comparison to P ($P < 0.038$). No differences were observed between MD + F and MD ($P > 0.05$).

Total fat oxidation

Data for mean FAT_{TOT} are shown in Table 2. Over the final 90 minutes of the oxidation trial, mean FAT_{TOT} was statistically different between conditions (F = 10.494; $P = 0.0001$). Specifically, both carbohydrate beverages

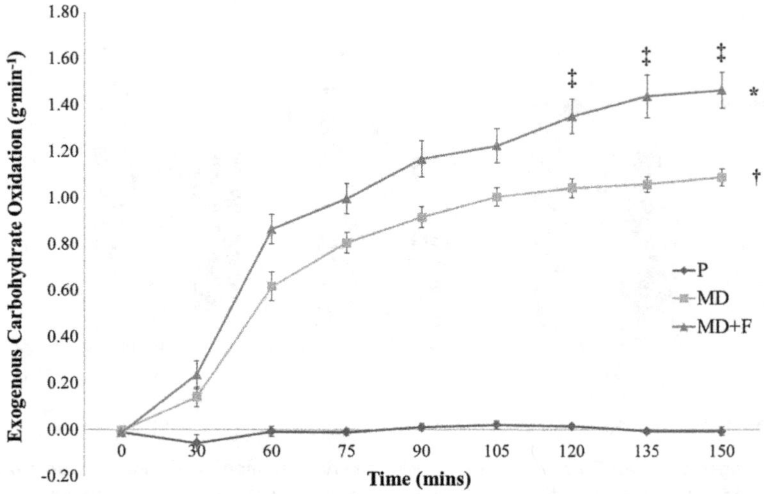

Figure 3 Assessment of test beverages on exogenous CHO oxidation rates during the submaximal exercise trial. Figure 3 demonstrates the time course effect of the test beverages on exogenous carbohydrate oxidation rates. Data are presented as mean ± SE; n = 14. P, Placebo; MD, maltodextrin beverage; MD + F, maltodextrin-fructose beverage. *denotes an overall significant difference between MD + F and P ($P = 0.0001$). † denotes an overall significant difference between MD and P ($P = 0.0001$). ‡denotes a significant difference between MD and MD + F at specific timepoint ($P < 0.008$).

demonstrated lower mean FAT_{TOT} in comparison to P ($P = 0.008$). Whilst absolute values were lower for MD + F in relation to MD, mean FAT_{TOT} was not statistically different between carbohydrate beverages (0.33 ± 0.04 $g.min^{-1}$ for MD + F v 0.41 ± 0.05 $g.min^{-1}$ for MD, $P > 0.05$) over the final 90 minutes of the oxidation trial. The same observation was noted for all 30 minute intervals, with both carbohydrate beverages demonstrating significantly lower mean FAT_{TOT} in comparison to P only ($P < 0.021$).

Assessment of exercise intensity was deemed comparable during the oxidation trial, with no significant differences observed for mean absolute VO_2 ($L.min^{-1}$) and power output (W) between test conditions – see Table 3.

Table 2 Influence of test beverages on carbohydrate and fat oxidation rates during a submaximal exercise test

		Overall	Respective time period assessed		
		60-150 mins	60-90 mins	90-120 mins	120-150 mins
CHO_{ENDO}	P	1.97 ± 0.12	2.00 ± 0.12	1.92 ± 0.12	1.99 ± 0.12
($g.min^{-1}$)	MD	1.51 ± 0.10*	1.66 ± 0.12*	1.52 ± 0.10*	1.35 ± 0.10*
	MD + F	1.47 ± 0.07*	1.62 ± 0.08*	1.41 ± 0.07*	1.36 ± 0.07*
CHO_{EXO}	P	0.00 ± 0.00	−0.00 ± 0.01	0.02 ± 0.01	−0.00 ± 0.01
($g.min^{-1}$)	MD	0.98 ± 0.04*	0.86 ± 0.04*	1.02 ± 0.04*	1.07 ± 0.03*
	MD + F	1.27 ± 0.07*†	1.08 ± 0.07*	1.28 ± 0.07*†	1.45 ± 0.09*†
$CHO_{EXO\ Eff}$	P	0.1 ± 0.3	−0.1 ± 0.05	0.9 ± 0.8	−0.6 ± 0.8
(%)	MD	57.9 ± 2.1*	50.5 ± 2.5*	60.1 ± 2.3*	63.0 ± 1.9*
	MD + F	74.7 ± 4.4*†	63.5 ± 4.2*	75.5 ± 4.3*†	85.2 ± 5.0*†
FAT_{TOT}	P	0.59 ± 0.06	0.58 ± 0.06	0.60 ± 0.06	0.58 ± 0.06
($g.min^{-1}$)	MD	0.41 ± 0.05*	0.42 ± 0.05*	0.41 ± 0.05*	0.41 ± 0.05*
	MD + F	0.33 ± 0.04*	0.34 ± 0.03*	0.34 ± 0.04*	0.32 ± 0.04*

Table 2 demonstrates the influence of the test beverages on endogenous and exogenous carbohydrate and fat oxidation rates during the submaximal exercise trial. Data for carbohydrate oxidation efficiency are also shown to demonstrate the progressive benefit of a combined sugar beverage overall and at 30 minute averaged timepoints. Data are presented as mean ± SE; n = 14. P, Placebo; MD, maltodextrin beverage; MD + F, maltodextrin-fructose beverage. CHO_{ENDO}, endogenous carbohydrate oxidation; FAT_{TOT}, total fat oxidation; CHO_{EXO}, exogenous carbohydrate oxidation; $CHO_{EXO\ Eff}$, carbohydrate oxidation efficiency *denotes a significant difference ($P < 0.038$) to P within respective time period. † denotes a significant difference between MD and MD + F ($P < 0.025$) within respective time period.

Table 3 Assessment of oxygen uptake, power output, mean heart rate, blood glucose and perceived exertion during both the oxidation and performance trials

		Oxidation trial	Performance trial
VO_2 ($L.min^{-1}$)	P	2.65 ± 0.07	N/A
	MD	2.69 ± 0.06	N/A
	MD + F	2.70 ± 0.09	N/A
Power (W)	P	176.3 ± 6.95	201.0 ± 22.4
	MD	175.0 ± 6.67	197.6 ± 21.6
	MD + F	174.4 ± 6.59	227.0 ± 23.2*
Heart rate ($b.min^{-1}$)	P	128.7 ± 4.7	149.0 ± 6.3
	MD	132.4 ± 3.7	151.9 ± 6.3
	MD + F	133.1 ± 4.4†	160.7 ± 5.0*
Blood glucose ($mmol.L^{-1}$)	P	3.90 ± 0.11	3.24 ± 0.25
	MD	4.77 ± 0.12†	4.17 ± 0.22†
	MD + F	4.97 ± 0.12†	4.18 ± 0.23†
RPE_{TOTAL} (6–20 scale)	P	11.9 ± 0.6	15.6 ± 0.6
	MD	12.2 ± 0.5	16.3 ± 0.5
	MD + F	11.6 ± 0.6	16.4 ± 0.7
RPE_{LEGS} (0–10 scale)	P	3.8 ± 0.4	7.1 ± 0.4
	MD	4.2 ± 0.5	7.1 ± 0.3
	MD + F	3.3 ± 0.4‡	6.9 ± 0.6

Table 3 shows the average data for key physiological, power output and subjective perception of exertion vaiables over both the oxidation and performance trials. Data are presented as mean ± SE; (n = 14 for oxidation trial; n = 6 for performance trial finishers). P, Placebo; MD, maltodextrin beverage; MD + F, maltodextrin-fructose beverage; RPE, Rating of Perceived Exertion. *denotes a significant difference to MD and P ($P < 0.03$). † denotes significant difference to P ($P < 0.05$).‡ denotes a significant difference to MD ($P = 0.021$) within trial only.

Fluid delivery assessment

Estimation of total fluid delivery, as assessed via plasma ^2H_2O enrichment is demonstrated in Figure 4. As the deuterium oxide was provided within the 60 minute beverage, this timepoint was employed for baseline comparisons. The increase in plasma ^2H_2O enrichment from 60 minutes served to quantify total fluid delivery both within treatment condition and in comparison to P. Plasma ^2H_2O enrichment increased in all conditions over time (F = 55.491; $P = 0.0001$), demonstrating the greatest increase in the P condition, with a peak of 101.67 ± 3.87 ppm by 120 minutes of the oxidation trial, and thereafter plateauing with an end value of 100.27 ± 3.56 ppm.

Plasma ^2H_2O enrichment was significantly lower in the MD condition from 75 minutes in comparison to P ($P < 0.025$), and from 90 minutes in comparison to MD + F ($P < 0.05$). In contrast, values for plasma ^2H_2O enrichment were statistically lower for MD + F compared to P at the 90 and 105 minute timepoints only ($P < 0.039$). The ingestion of MD + F resulted in a peak plasma ^2H_2O enrichment of 92.57 ± 2.94 ppm by the end of the oxidation trial, and was comparable to values obtained for P (100.27 ± 3.56 ppm; $P > 0.05$).

60 km performance trial

Performance trial measures

Whilst all participants attempted the 60 km performance trial, during the P condition, 8 athletes were unable to finish demonstrating the exhaustive nature of the protocol. In contrast, all participants completed the performance trial whilst consuming both carbohydrate test beverages. Statistical analysis was therefore carried out on all finishers (n = 6) for comparison across trials. Relative differences in performance times between beverages are shown in Figure 5. Additionally, inclusion of all finishers (n = 14) for the two test beverages are shown for interest.

Performance times were significantly faster with MD + F compared with MD and P (5722.8 ± 284.1 seconds v 6165.0 ± 257.9 seconds v 6117.5 ± 358.0 seconds respectively; $P < 0.05$). In absolute terms, performance times significantly improved with MD + F compared with both MD (by 7 min 22 s ± 1 min 56 s, or 7.2%) and P (by 6 min 35 s ± 2 min 33 s, or 6.5%, $P < 0.05$) over 60 km. No difference was observed for performance times between MD and P ($P > 0.05$). The difference observed between MD + F and MD was further noted when assessment of all 14 finishers was separately undertaken (5868.36 ± 151.31 seconds for MD + F v 6217.14 ± 150.93 seconds for MD; $P = 0.001$).

In a similar manner, relative differences in mean power output was significantly different for MD + F compared to both MD and P for the performance trial ($P < 0.03$; Figure 6). Mean power output was 14.9% greater with MD + F compared to MD (227.0 ± 23.2 W v 197.6 ± 21.6 W, $P = 0.029$), and 13.0% greater with MD + F compared to P (227.0 ± 23.2 W v 201.0 ± 22.4 W, $P = 0.025$). No difference was observed for performance times between MD and P ($P > 0.05$). The difference observed between MD + F and MD was further noted when assessment of all 14 finishers was separately undertaken (234.0 ± 12.0 W for MD + F v 204.3 ± 11.1 W for MD; $P = 0.001$).

Other physiological and subjective measures during both trials

Heart rate, perceived exertion, blood glucose and gastrointestinal distress assessment

Data for mean heart rate ($b.min^{-1}$), blood glucose and subjective perceived exertion are shown in Table 3. During the oxidation trial, mean heart rate was marginally lower with P (F = 4.059; $P = 0.029$), but only statistically different to MD + F ($P = 0.045$). However, as no differences were observed for RPE_{TOT}, absolute VO_2 or power output ($P > 0.05$) compliance to the exercise intensity

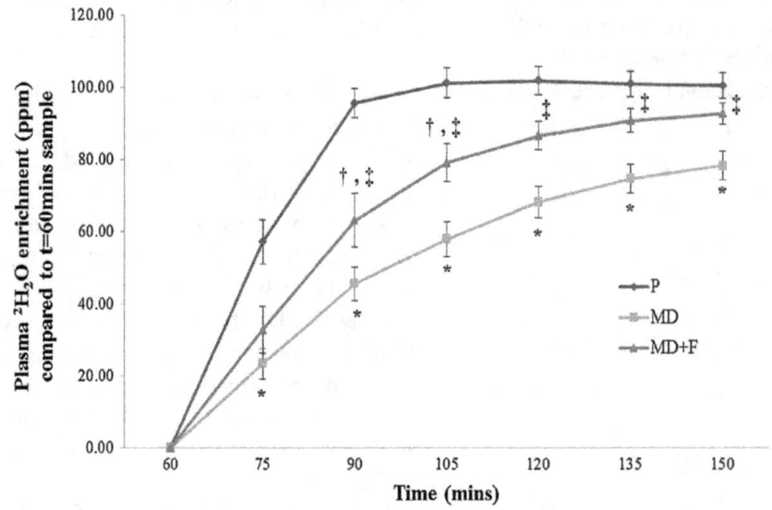

Figure 4 Influence of beverage administration on plasma deuterium enrichment (ppm). Figure 4 shows the impact of the test beverages on plasma deuterium enrichment, which was employed as a semi-quantitative method for assessing fluid delivery. Data are presented as mean ± SE; n = 7. P, Placebo; MD, maltodextrin beverage; MD + F, maltodextrin-fructose beverage. *denotes significant difference ($P < 0.025$) to P. † denotes significant difference ($P < 0.039$) to P. ‡ denotes significant difference between MD and MD + F ($P < 0.05$).

was deemed appropriate. Blood glucose was significantly greater with both test beverages in comparison to P during the oxidation trial (F = 26.505; $P = 0.0001$), although no differences existed between MD and MD + F (4.77 ± 0.12 mmol.L^{-1} and 4.97 ± 0.12 mmol.L^{-1} respectively, $P > 0.05$). Mean subjective RPE_{LEGS} (using a 0–10 Borg Scale) was significantly lower for MD + F compared with MD ($P = 0.021$) over the course of the oxidation trial.

During the performance trial, greater participant effort was demonstrated via increases in mean heart rate, RPE_{TOTAL} and RPE_{LEGS} in comparison to the oxidation trial. However, as 8 athletes could not complete the performance trial for P, comparisons were made for finishers of all trials only. Mean heart rate was significantly higher with MD + F (160.7 ± 5.0 b.min^{-1}) compared to both MD and P (151.9 ± 6.3 b.min^{-1} and 149.0 ± 6.3 b.min^{-1} respectively, $P < 0.03$). Mean blood glucose was similar between test beverages during the performance trial (4.18 ± 0.23 mmol.L^{-1} for MD + F and 4.17 ± 0.22 mmol.L^{-1} for MD), with both being significantly greater than P (3.24 ± 0.25 mmol.L^{-1}) only ($P < 0.05$). No differences were observed between test conditions for

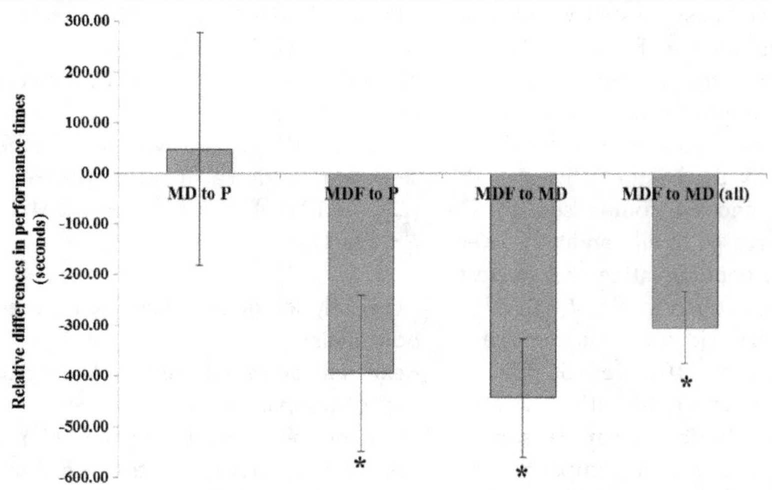

Figure 5 Relative differences in 60 km performance times between beverages. Figure 5 indicates the difference in performance times during the preloaded 60 km time trial when test beverages were compared for all finishers. The final column is included to demonstrate that all participants completed the test when consuming carbohydrate beverages. P, Placebo; MD, maltodextrin beverage; MD + F, maltodextrin-fructose beverage. Data are presented as mean ± SE; comparisons made for finishers of all trials (first three columns: n = 6) and between test beverages for all finishers (end column: n = 14) *denotes significant difference between relative beverages ($P < 0.05$).

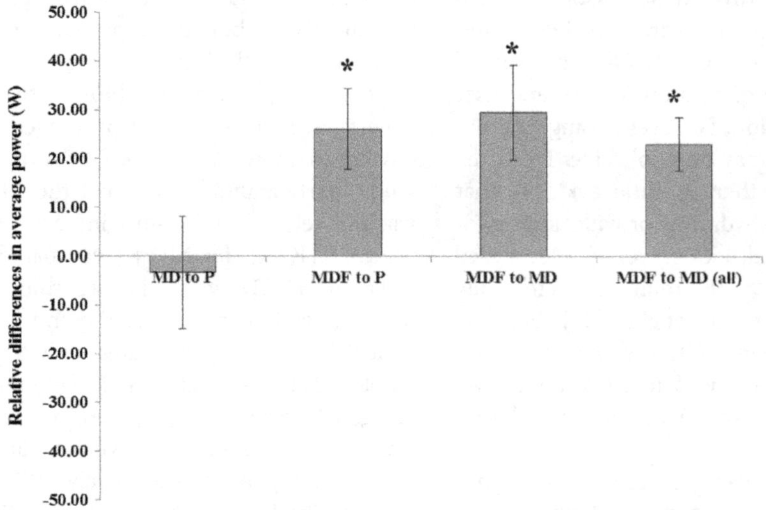

Figure 6 Relative differences in average power output between beverages during the performance trial. Figure 6 indicates the difference in average power measured in watts, during the preloaded 60 km time trial when test beverages were compared for all finishers. The final column is included to demonstrate that all participants completed the test when consuming carbohydrate beverages. P, Placebo; MD, maltodextrin beverage; MD + F, maltodextrin-fructose beverage. Data are presented as mean ± SE; comparisons mace for finishers of all trials (first three columns: n = 6) and between test beverages for all finishers (end column: n = 14) * denotes significant difference between relative beverages ($P < 0.05$).

RPE_{TOTAL} or RPE_{LEGS} during the performance trial ($P > 0.05$).

Overall responses to the gastrointestinal distress questionnaire are shown in Table 4. A higher number of significantly positive responses were noted for MD. Bloating and belching severity were considerably greater with MD (22.2% and 19.0%) compared to MD + F (<4.8%) and P (<1.6%) respectively ($P < 0.05$). Whilst responses for other symptoms were considered minor ie: <7% of all responses, it was noted that symptoms of nausea, stomach problems, and urge to vomit or defecate were observed in the MD trial.

Discussion

The aim of this study was to carry out an independent assessment of a commercially available sports drink on carbohydrate oxidation, fluid delivery and sustained performance. Whilst previous research has indicated benefits of consuming multiple transportable carbohydrates [11,12,16,22], there is minimal research on commercial formulas demonstrating such mechanisms in line with performance gains. Additionally, there is continued interest as to whether sports drinks are indeed beneficial to recreational and club level athletes, with implications that moderately higher dosing strategies may yield effective results for longer duration events. With current dosage recommendations for events lasting longer than 2 hours being >90 $g.hr^{-1}$ [4], we were asked to investigate the potential influence of a commercial MD + F beverage provided at a relatively high carbohydrate delivery rate (102 $g.hr^{-1}$) on club level athletes.

The main finding from the study was that a commercial MD + F beverage significantly enhanced both CHO_{EXO} and fluid delivery during steady state exercise compared to both MD and P. This resulted in an average higher power output and time to complete the subsequent 60 km time trial. The findings support previous research that

Table 4 Influence of test beverages on overall gastrointestinal distress responses

Symptom	P	MD	MD + F
Urge to urinate	33 (26.2)*	17 (13.5)	19 (15.1)
Bloating severity	2 (1.6)	28 (22.2)*	6 (4.8)
Belching severity	2 (1.6)	24 (19.0)*	5 (4.0)
Nausea	1 (0.8)	8 (6.3)*	0 (0.0)
Stomach problems	1 (0.8)	7 (5.6)*	0 (0.0)
Stomach cramps	0 (0.0)	1 (0.8)	0 (0.0)
Headaches	1 (0.8)	2 (1.6)	0 (0.0)
Intestinal cramps	0 (0.0)	0 (0.0)	0 (0.0)
Stomach burning	1 (0.8)	2 (1.6)	0 (0.0)
Flatulence severity	0 (0.0)	2 (1.6)	0 (0.0)
Left & right side aches	3 (2.4)	0 (0.0)	1 (0.8)
Dizziness	8 (6.3)*	1 (0.8)	2 (1.6)
Urge to defecate	0 (0.0)	4 (3.2)*	0 (0.0)
Urge to vomit	0 (0.0)	4 (3.2)*	0 (0.0)

Table 4 shows the overall data for responses to the gastrointestinal distress questionnaire, with particular attention given to responses rated moderate to severe. Data are presented as total number of responses (rated moderate to severe) for both oxidation and performance trials. Numbers in brackets represent data expressed as a percentage of maximum number of responses. P, Placebo; MD, maltodextrin beverage; MD + F, maltodextrin-fructose beverage. *denotes a significant difference to other test conditions ($P < 0.05$).

combined sugar beverages provided at reasonably high concentrations (~10%) and carbohydrate delivery rates may enhance exercise performance [22,24]. This should be interpreted with a degree of caution for the end-user based on total exercise duration. For events ranging from 2 to 6 hours, such findings may be applicable. However, for shorter duration events, there is little evidence that 'multiple transportable carbohydrates' provide any ergogenic benefit over that of maltodextrin or glucose based beverages. Indeed, for events < 90 minutes, water only strategies may offer equally valid benefits [37]. Furthermore, as the duration exceeds 6 hours, beverage and gastrointestinal tolerance may have a negative impact on performance, indicating a potential need for lower dosing and fluid delivery strategies [10,38].

In this study, both test beverages resulted in higher CHO_{TOT} compared with P during exercise undertaken at 50% W_{max}. As steady state exercise intensity was comparable across trials (for oxygen uptake, power output and perceived exertion), the use of P resulted in a higher rate of CHO_{ENDO} and FAT_{TOT}, which was expected. The inclusion of the two test beverages resulted in lower CHO_{ENDO}, potentially decreasing reliance on hepatic glucose utilisation, and permitting glycogen sparing, particularly in type I muscle fibres, during continuous aerobic exercise. Indeed, as the use of carbohydrate beverages has been shown to spare glycogen early into exercise [39], this may provide a subtle benefit late into exercise if CHO_{TOT} is enhanced.

Whilst CHO sparing from endogenous sources was apparent with both test beverages across all time points, it was specifically noted that CHO_{TOT} was 16.1% greater with MD + F compared to MD in the final 30 minutes of the oxidation trial. This differs from previous research utilising similar dosing strategies of fructose: maltodextrin [11], which is surprising considering CHO_{EXO} rates during the same time frame were significantly increased and comparable to values observed in the current study. As there was a progressive increase in CHO_{EXO} with MD + F throughout the oxidation trial (with mean CHO_{EXO} of 1.27 $g.min^{-1}$ being significantly greater than MD), this implies that intestinal saturation was not a limiting factor at this dosage, as supported elsewhere [5,11]. During the MD trial, CHO_{EXO} was maintained from 90 minutes indicating potential saturation of the SGLT1 transporter mechanism. As there was no significant difference in either average CHO_{EXO} or carbohydrate oxidation efficiency between the test beverages prior to this, the use of combined sugar beverages may be more applicable for events lasting longer than 90 minutes, supporting current recommendations [4].

It should also be noted that participants in this study undertook the oxidation trial following an overnight fast. Whilst this is not normal practice for trained athletes competing, it has been shown that the influence of low dietary carbohydrate availability prior to sustained exercise has little impact on accumulated CHO_{EXO} and steady state performance [40] in the presence of CHO beverages. However, more prolonged states of starvation have been shown to reduce CHO_{EXO} [41]. In the current study, participants maintained their habitual diet which was unlikely to significantly impact on CHO_{EXO}.

Peak CHO_{EXO} for MD + F compared well with previous research [5,8,11], with values reaching 1.45 ± 0.09 $g.min^{-1}$, 35.5% greater than MD, by the end of the oxidation trial. When lower ingestion rates of 0.8 $g.min^{-1}$ have been employed to replicate practices employed by athletes (48 $g.hr^{-1}$), peak CHO_{EXO} were not significantly different between glucose + fructose versus glucose only beverages (0.56 v 0.58 $g.min^{-1}$ respectively, [9]). Therefore, benefits of combined sugar beverages, particularly for longer duration events, are more likely with higher ingestion rates >1.0 $g.min^{-1}$. Interestingly, when higher ratios of fructose to maltodextrin have been employed [12], it has been suggested that peak CHO_{EXO} may occur with a 0.8 F: MD ratio compared to 0.5 or 1.25 ratios at ingestion rates of 1.8 $g.min^{-1}$. However, as the relative concentrations of the beverages employed were >10%, CHO_{TOT} was considerably lower than the current study, and short duration performance gains observed [12] may not be replicated with longer duration events.

In the current study, the ratio of F: MD was 0.54 delivered at an ingestion rate of 1.7 $g.min^{-1}$ (based on product analysis). This resulted in a higher CHO_{TOT} than previously observed with a 0.8 ratio [12], most likely based on higher CHO_{EXO} and lower beverage concentration, which may not have limited gastric emptying rates or intestinal beverage delivery. It is unknown whether peak CHO_{EXO} during this study would have been greater if the oxidation trial had been extended. However previous research has indicated a relative maintenance so long as ingestion rates are maintained and tolerated [42]. The ingestion of a commercially available MD + F sports drink used in this study supports the general contention that the inclusion of fructose to a glucose/maltodextrin beverage will involve both SGLT1 and GLUT5 transport mechanisms leading to an increased rate of total carbohydrate delivery across the intestinal lumen.

Although higher ingestion rates of 2.4 $g.min^{-1}$ have been previously employed, leading to higher peak CHO_{EXO} rates of 1.75 $g.min^{-1}$ [7], it is likely that a higher beverage concentration, or total fluid consumption, would have led to progressive gastrointestinal disturbances within this cohort based on subjective reporting of drink tolerance at the end of the study. At the ingestion rates employed, it was apparent that gastrointestinal issues were less evident with MD + F compared to MD, but also that relative tolerance was being reached by the end of the performance trial. Higher ingestion rates may be better tolerated by well-trained athletes, as supported elsewhere [7] and from observations of world class triathletes in our laboratory in which peak CHO_{EXO} have exceeded 1.75 $g.min^{-1}$ with CHO ingestion rates of 2.0 $g.min^{-1}$. Whether this indicates a training adaptation or tolerance to beverage consumption, or full saturation of SGLT1 and GLUT5 is unknown. More likely, as trained endurance athletes are encouraged to consume high carbohydrate diets to facilitate recovery and repetitive training bouts, higher CHO_{EXO} may be the result of high carbohydrate availability, irrespective of total muscle glycogen and GLUT4 expression [40].

An important finding from the study was that plasma ^2H_2O enrichment was significantly enhanced with the inclusion of the MD + F formula, and statistically no different to P in the last 30 minutes of the oxidation trial. As plasma ^2H_2O enrichment has been used elsewhere as a semi-quantitative method [14,16], the finding indicates that MD + F did not restrict fluid delivery. However, findings for the MD beverage were significantly lower than P at all timepoints. The most likely explanation is that the ingestion of MD + F resulted in higher overall CHO_{TOT} and CHO_{EXO}, particularly in the final 30 minutes of the oxidation trial. As saturation of the SGLT1 transporter may have occurred with MD, fluid uptake across of the intestinal lumen may have been restricted. The inclusion of fructose, however, may have prevented complete intestinal SGLT1 saturation, hence allowing continued fluid uptake.

Our results are comparable to previous research [8,14,16], although plasma ^2H_2O enrichment values were deemed higher in the current study where an MD + F beverage was used. In previous studies, increasing beverage concentration above 6% resulted in reduced fluid delivery based on a glucose only beverage [14]. Whilst this may, in part, explain findings for the MD beverage, it would appear that the combined use of MD + F at a 10% concentration did not restrict fluid delivery. During events lasting longer than 2 hours where acute dehydration and carbohydrate depletion may limit sustained performance, the use of a commercial MD + F beverage may therefore support both high fluid delivery and CHO_{EXO} rates.

The use of combined carbohydrate beverages has been shown to enhance exercise performance [22-24]. However, several of these studies did not assess CHO_{EXO} to support conclusions, or use commercial formulas more applicable to the end user. Recent studies have indicated that running performance may not be enhanced when commercial beverages are employed [26]. In the current study, 8 participants were unable to complete the 60 km performance test, demonstrating the demanding nature of the protocol. However, data for finishers of all trials indicated that performance times and corresponding mean power outputs were significantly improved with MD + F. Mean power output was 14.9% higher during the MD + F trial compared to MD, and 13% higher compared to P.

This observation compares with previous findings [22], and may be a consequence of the higher CHO_{TOT} and CHO_{EXO} at the end of the oxidation trial with MD + F. Surprisingly mean power output was comparable between MD and P, which may indicate subjective perception of the test beverages and hence relative effort, despite being randomly assigned to trial order. As all participants were able to complete the performance trial when consuming the test beverages, this demonstrates the benefit of regularly consuming CHO during sustained exercise. However, in a similar manner, performance times and mean power output was significantly improved with MD + F compared with MD for all participants (n = 14).

Whilst RPE_{TOTAL} and RPE_{LEGS} were comparable during the performance test between conditions, it was noted that mean blood glucose was higher with both MD and MD + F compared to P. As power output was higher in the MD + F condition, this correlated with greater cardiovascular exertion despite similar perceived effort. As both test drinks were matched for electrolyte content, the buffering of endogenous acids is unlikely to be a key mechanism explaining greater power output with MD + F. Instead, higher CHO_{TOT} and potential for liver glycogen sparing with MD + F most likely explains the significant increase in performance.

It is difficult to compare data from previous research when different types of performance tests have been employed. When shorter distance preloaded time trials have been assessed, the use of glucose only beverages resulted in a dose response effect, with 60 $g.hr^{-1}$ leading to a 10.7% increase in mean power over 20 km compared to lower dosages [43]. However, as a limiting factor for longer duration events may be CHO_{EXO}, such results may not extend to longer time trials when single carbohydrate beverages are used. Furthermore, performance times during sustained endurance events, such as Ironman Triathlon, have been shown to correlate with higher total CHO intakes ranging from 90–120 $g.hr^{-1}$ [10], despite also relating to a higher incidence of gastrointestinal responses. In the current study, gastrointestinal responses did not impede performance, although it was observed that underlying responses were lower with MD + F compared to MD, similar to previous studies [5].

Where longer time trials (>100 km) have been performed (without prior steady state exercise), findings are mixed [44-46] both for low (0.62 $g.min^{-1}$ [44]) and moderate (1.10 $g.min^{-1}$) ingestion rates [45]. As a higher ingestion rate was employed in the current study, along with greater beverage concentration, the high CHO_{TOT}

and CHO_{EXO} rates observed with MD + F may explain the improved performance during a 60 km time trial in comparison to these studies. Additionally, if ergogenic effects occur following peak CHO_{EXO}, then overall trials lasting <120 minutes may not be sufficient to observe performance benefits from combined sugar beverages.

Conclusions

The use of a commercially available MD + F formula resulted in greater increases in total and exogenous carbohydrate oxidation rates during sustained steady state exercise compared to an isoenergetic MD beverage, and P. Additionally, the inclusion of fructose resulted in matched fluid delivery compared with P, and resulted in performance gains in direct comparison to MD. Athletes undertaking sustained exercise greater than 2 hours should consider strategies utilising combined carbohydrate formulas to maximise carbohydrate and fluid delivery, which may support enhanced exercise performance.

Abbreviations

CHO: Carbohydrate; CHO_{TOT}: Total carbohydrate oxidation rate (measured in $g.min^{-1}$); CHO_{EXO}: Exogenous carbohydrate oxidation rate (measured in $g.min^{-1}$); CHO_{ENDO}: Endogenous carbohydrate oxidation rate (measured in $g.min^{-1}$); FAT_{TOT}: Total fat oxidation rate (measured in $g.min^{-1}$); GLUT5: Glucose transporter 5; MD: Isoenergetic maltodextrin formula used in the study; MD + F: Maltodextrin plus fructose formula used in the study; P: Placebo formula used in the study; RER: Respiratory exchange ratio, the ratio from dividing expired carbon dioxide with oxygen uptake; RPE: Rating of perceived exertion (subscript relates to total or leg related exertion); SGLT1: Sodium dependent glucose transporter 1; V_E: Minute ventilation, the amount of air breathed in one minute ($L.min^{-1}$); VO_2: Volume of oxygen uptake (measured in $L.min^{-1}$); VO_{2max}: Maximal oxygen uptake (measured in $L.min^{-1}$); VCO_2: Volume of expired carbon dioxide (measured in $L.min^{-1}$); W_{max}: Maximal power output determined from an incremental protocol to volitional exhaustion (measured in W).

Competing interests

Research funding and product supply to support this study was received from High 5 Ltd. All data was collected, analysed and reported by the investigatory team fully independently of the company.

Authors' contributions

All authors were involved in the study. JDR was the principal researcher, involved with liaison with the company, participant assessment, data collection, statistical analysis and manuscript generation; MDT was co-researcher involved with cohort organization, data collection and blood analyses, confirmation of statistical analyses, and manuscript editing; LSK was involved with monitoring of data collection including collation of performance data, and test beverage administration, as well as manuscript editing; RJT was involved with data collection and analysis; MGR was involved in quality control, data collection, and technical accuracy in preparation of the manuscript. All authors read and approved the final manuscript.

Acknowledgements

The authors wish to acknowledge High5 Ltd. for providing the support and funding to undertake this study. All products used for test beverages were supplied by High 5 Ltd. independently of the investigatory team. The authors also wish to acknowledge the support and external collaboration with Iso-Analytical Ltd., for independent assessment of expired air and blood samples.

References

1. Jeukendrup AE: **Carbohydrate intake during exercise and performance.** *Nutrition* 2004, **20**:669–677.
2. Bosch AN, Dennis SC, Noakes TD: **Influence of carbohydrate ingestion on fuel substrate turnover and oxidation during prolonged exercise.** *J Appl Physiol* 1994, **76**(6):2364–2372.
3. Coggan AR, Coyle EF: **Reversal of fatigue during prolonged exercise by carbohydrate infusion or ingestion.** *J Appl Physiol* 1987, **63**(6):2388–2395.
4. Jeukendrup AE: **Multiple transportable carbohydrates and their benefits.** *Sports Sci Exchange* 2013, **26**(108):1–5.
5. Jentjens RLPG, Moseley L, Waring RH, Harding LK, Jeukendrup AE: **Oxidation of combined ingestion of glucose and fructose during exercise.** *J Appl Physiol* 2004, **96**(4):1277–1284.
6. Jentjens RLPG, Shaw C, Birtles T, Waring RH, Harding LK, Jeukendrup AE: **Oxidation of combined ingestion of glucose and sucrose during exercise.** *Metab Clin Exp* 2005, **54**:610–618.
7. Jentjens RLPG, Jeukendrup AE: **High rates of exogenous carbohydrate oxidation from a mixture of glucose and fructose ingested during prolonged cycling exercise.** *Br J Nutr* 2005, **93**(4):485–492.
8. Jentjens RLPG, Underwood K, Achten J, Currell K, Mann CH, Jeukendrup AE: **Exogenous carbohydrate oxidation rates are elevated following combined ingestion of glucose and fructose during exercise in the heat.** *J Appl Physiol* 2006, **100**(3):807–816.
9. Hulston CJ, Wallis GA, Jeukendrup AE: **Exogenous CHO oxidation with glucose plus fructose intake during exercise.** *Med Sci Sports Exerc* 2009, **41**(2):357–363.
10. Pfeiffer B, Stellingwerff T, Hodgson AB, Randell R, Pottgen K, Res P, Jeukendrup AE: **Nutritional intake and gastrointestinal problems during competitive endurance events.** *Med Sci Sports Exerc* 2012, **44**(2):344–351.
11. Wallis GA, Rowlands DS, Shaw C, Jentjens RLPG, Jeukendrup AE: **Oxidation of combined ingestion of maltodextrins and fructose during exercise.** *Med Sci Sports Exerc* 2005, **37**(3):426–432.
12. O'Brien WJ, Rowlands DS: **Fructose-maltodextrin ratio in a carbohydrate-electrolyte solution differentially affects exogenous carbohydrate oxidation rate, gut comfort, and performance.** *Am J Physiol Gastrointest Liver Physiol* 2011, **300**:G181–G189.
13. Davis JM, Burgess WA, Slentz CA, Bartoli WP: **Fluid availability and sports drinks differing in carbohydrate type and concentration.** *Am J Clin Nutr* 1990, **51**:1054–1057.
14. Jeukendrup AE, Currell K, Clarke J, Cole J, Blannin AK: **Effect of beverage glucose and sodium content on fluid delivery.** *Nutr & Metabol* 2009, **6**(9):1–7.
15. Jeukendrup AE: **Carbohydrate and exercise performance: the role of multiple transportable carbohydrates.** *Cur Opin Clin Nutr Metab Care* 2010, **13**(4):452–457.
16. Jeukendrup AE, Moseley L: **Multiple transportable carbohydrates enhance gastric emptying and fluid delivery.** *Scan J Med Sci Sports* 2010, **20**(1):112–121.
17. Rowlands DS, Bonetti DL, Hopkins WG: **Unilateral fluid absorption and effects on peak power after ingestion of commercially available hypotonic, isotonic, and hypertonic sports drinks.** *Int J Sport Nutr Exerc Metab* 2011, **21**(6):480–491.
18. Rollo I, Williams C: **Influence of ingesting a carbohydrate-electrolyte solution before and during a 1-hr running performance test.** *Int J Sport Nutr Exerc Metab* 2009, **19**:645–658.
19. El-sayed MS, Balmer J, Rattu AJM: **Carbohydrate ingestion improves endurance performance during a 1 h simulated cycling time trial.** *J Sports Sci* 1997, **15**:223–230.
20. Coggan AR, Coyle EF: **Carbohydrate ingestion during prolonged exercise: effects on metabolism and performance.** *Exerc Sport Sci Rev* 1991, **19**:1–40.
21. Ali A, Williams C, Nicholas CW, Foskett A: **The influence of carbohydrate-electrolyte ingestion on soccer skill performance.** *Med Sci Sports Exerc* 2007, **39**(11):1969–1976.
22. Currell K, Jeukendrup AE: **Superior endurance performance with ingestion of multiple transportable carbohydrates.** *Med Sci Sports Exerc* 2008, **40**(2):275–281.
23. Triplett D, Doyle JA, Rupp JC, Benardot D: **An isocaloric glucose-fructose beverages effect on simulated 100-km cycling performance compared with a glucose-only beverage.** *Int J Sport Nutr Exerc Metab* 2010, **20**(2):122–131.
24. Rowlands DS, Swift M, Ros M, Green JG: **Composite versus single transportable carbohydrate solution enhances race and laboratory cycling performance.** *Appl Physiol Nutr Metab* 2012, **37**:425–436.

25. Colombani PC, Mannhart C, Mettler S: **Carbohydrates and exercise performance in nonfasted athletes: a systematic review of studies mimicking real-life.** *Nutrition J* 2013, **12:**1–6.
26. Coletta A, Thompson DL, Raynor HA: **The influence of commercially-available carbohydrate and carbohydrate-protein supplements on endurance running performance in recreational athletes during a field trial.** *J Int Soc Sports Nutr* 2013, **10**(17):1–7.
27. Cohen D: **The truth about sports drinks.** *BMJ* 2012, **345:**e4737. 1–8.
28. Thompson M, Heneghan C, Cohen D: **How valid is the European food safety authority's assessment of sports drinks?** *BMJ* 2012, **345:**e4753. 1–6.
29. Faul F, Erdfelder E, Lang A-G, Buchner A: **G*power 3: a flexible statistical power analysis program for the social, behavioral, and biomedical sciences.** *Behav Res Meth* 2007, **39**(2):175–191.
30. Borg G: **Ratings of perceived exertion and heart rates during short term cycle exercise and their use in a new strength test.** *Int J Sports Med* 1982, **3**(3):153–158.
31. Jeukendrup AE, Vet-Joop K, Sturk A, Stegen JHJC, Senden J, Saris WHM, Wagenmakers AJM: **Relationship between gastro-intestinal complaints and endotoxemia, cytokine release and the acute-phase reaction during and after a long-distance triathlon in highly trained men.** *Clin Sci* 2000, **98:**47–55.
32. Péronnet F, Massicotte D: **Table of nonprotein respiratory quotient: an update.** *Can J Sport Sci* 1991, **16**(1):23–29.
33. Pirnay F, Lacroix M, Mosora F: **Glucose oxidation during prolonged exercise evaluated with naturally labeled [^{13}C] glucose.** *J Appl Physiol Resp Environ & Exerc Physiol* 1977, **43**(2):258–261.
34. Craig H: **Isotopic standards for carbon and oxygen and correction factors for mass-spectrometric analysis of carbon dioxide.** *Geochim Cosmochim Acta* 1957, **12:**133–149.
35. Roberts JJ, Koziet J, Chauvet D, Darmaun D, Desjeux JF, Young VR: **Use of ^{13}C-labeled glucose for estimating glucose oxidation: some design considerations.** *J Appl Physiol* 1987, **63**(5):1725–1732.
36. Pallikarakis N, Sphiris N, Lefebvre P: **Influence of the bicarbonate pool on the occurrence of $^{13}CO_2$ in exhaled air.** *Eur J Appl Physiol* 1991, **63**(3–4):179–183.
37. Below PR, Mora-Rodriguez R, Gonzalez-Alonso J, Coyle EF: **Fluid and carbohydrate ingestion independently improve performance during 1 h of intense exercise.** *Med Sci Sports Exerc* 1995, **27**(2):200–210.
38. Rehrer NJ: **Fluid and electrolyte balance in ultra-endurance sport.** *Sports Med* 2001, **31**(10):701–715.
39. Stellingwerff R, Boon H, Gijsen AP, Stegen JHCH, Kuipers H, van Loon LJC: **Carbohydrate supplementation during prolonged cycling spares muscle glycogen but does not affect intramyocellular lipid use.** *Eur J Physiol* 2007, **454:**635–647.
40. Cox GR, Clark SA, Cox AJ, Halson SL, Hargreaves M, Hawley JA, Jeacocke N, Snow RJ, Yeo WK, Burke LM: **Daily training with high carbohydrate availability increases exogenous carbohydrate oxidation during endurance cycling.** *J Appl Physiol* 2010, **109:**126–134.
41. Rowlands DS, Johnson NA, Thomson JA, Chapman P, Stannard SR: **Exogenous glucose oxidation is reduced with carbohydrate feeding during exercise after starvation.** *Metab Clin Exp* 2009, **58:**1161–1169.
42. Jeukendrup AE, Moseley L, Mainwaring GI, Samuels S, Perry S, Mann CH: **Exogenous carbohydrate oxidation during ultraendurance exercise.** *J Appl Physiol* 2006, **100:**1134–1141.
43. Smith JW, Zachwieja JJ, Peronnet F, Passe DH, Massicotte D, Lavoie C, Pascoe DD: **Fuel selection and cycling endurance performance with ingestion of [$_{13}$C] glucose: evidence for a carbohydrate dose response.** *J Appl Physiol* 2010, **108:**1520–1529.
44. Langenfeld ME, Seifert JG, Rudge SR, Bucher RJ: **Effect of carbohydrate ingestion on performance of non-fasted cyclists during a simulated 80-mile time trial.** *J Sports Med Phys Fitness* 1994, **34**(3):263–270.
45. Madsen K, Maclean DA, Kiens B, Christensen D: **Effects of glucose, glucose plus branched-chain amino acids, or placebo on bike performance over 100 km.** *J Appl Physiol* 1996, **81**(6):2644–2650.
46. Angus DJ, Hargreaves M, Dancey J, Febbraio MA: **Effect of carbohydrate or carbohydrate plus medium-chain triglyceride ingestion on cycling time trial performance.** *J Appl Physiol* 2000, **88**(1):113–119.

Hydrolyzed protein supplementation improves protein content and peroxidation of skeletal muscle by adjusting the plasma amino acid spectrums in rats after exhaustive swimming exercise: a pilot study

Xinying Wang[1†], Chenglin Niu[2†], Jun Lu[3], Ning Li[1] and Jieshou Li[1*]

Abstract

Background: This study was designed to evaluate the effects of hydrolyzed protein supplementation upon skeletal muscle total protein and peroxidation in rats following exhaustive swimming exercise.

Methods: Twenty-four rats were randomized to 4 experimental groups (n = 6 per group): control group fed standard diet without exercise (SD), exercise (EX), exercise plus standard diet for 72 hours (EX + SD), and exercise plus standard diet supplemented with hydrolyzed protein (2 g/kg/d) for 72 hours (EX + HP). Immediately following exercise, the EX group was euthanized for collecting plasma and skeletal muscle samples. The EX + SD and EX + HP groups were fed their respective diets for 72 hour still plasma and skeletal muscle collection. Skeletal muscle samples were used to measure levels of total protein (TP), malondialdehyde (MDA), and protein carbonyl (PC). Plasma samples were used to analyze the amino acids spectrum.

Results: Compared with the EX + SD, EX + HP presented the significantly increased TP ($P = 0.02$) and decreased MDA and PC levels ($P = 0.035$). MDA was negatively correlated with the methionine levels. Moreover, EX + HP maintained higher levels of plasmaleucine, isoleucine, and methionine than EX + SD, which may be associated with the increased skeletal muscle TP levels observed ($P < 0.05$).

Conclusions: These results collectively suggest that hydrolyzed protein supplementation can improve skeletal muscle TP and ameliorate peroxidation damage in rats subjected to exhaustive exercise stress, which may be, at least in part, related with the maintenance of plasma leucine, isoleucine, and methionine levels.

Keywords: Protein hydrolysates, Oxidative stress, Amino acid spectrum, Physical training

Background

Exercise promotes muscle protein turnover, resulting in the specific morphological and metabolic skeletal muscle adaptation [1,2]. Exhaustive exercise leads to myofibrillar degradation and is associated with the decreased force generating capabilities of muscle at fatigue [3]. Muscle protein loss following exhaustive exercise is accompanied by a direct detection of free-radical generation in whole body and skeletal muscle [4,5]. The elevated lipid and protein peroxidation, malondialdehyde (MDA) and protein carbonyl (PC) have been observed in different tissues including skeletal muscle in rats following exhaustive exercise [6,7]. As a result, excessive reactive oxygen species (ROS) can attack the vital biomolecules, such as plasma membrane lipids and proteins, and further deteriorates normal cellular functions and delays recovery from fatigue. Hence, adequate amino acid is required for skeletal muscle to meet the increasing demand of protein retention and reduce the peroxidation following exhaustive

* Correspondence: feonix@163.com
†Equal contributors
[1]Research Institute of General Surgery, Jinling Hospital, Medical School, Nanjing University, 305 East Zhongshan Road, Nanjing 210002, Jiangsu Province, People's Republic of China
Full list of author information is available at the end of the article

exercise. It is beneficial for the fast recovery from athletes during competition season. However, promoting positive muscle protein balance is dependent upon the availability of nutrient metabolites and the lack of appropriate nutrient intake can lead to a net negative protein balance and ROS accumulation [8,9]. This loss leads to a decrease in muscular strength, delayed recovery from fatigue, and decreased resistance to stress (disease or trauma) [3].

Previous studies suggest that standard diets cannot supply enough nutrients after exercise due to metabolic derangement in tissues [10,11]. Exogenous nutrients or nutritional supplements may help to improve muscle protein content and counteract the oxidative stress of exercise in subjects unaccustomed to physical activity [12-14]. Supplementations provide a nonpharmacological therapy, and has been gradually received attention in literatures. Protein hydrolysates can stimulate protein synthesis and inhibit protein breakdown, and therefore, improve the net muscle protein balance after exercise [10,15]. It is also reported that whey protein hydrolysate can ameliorate drug-induced oxidative stress [16]. However, it remains to be elucidated whether the protein hydrolysates supplementation in a short term improves the protein retention and oxidative stress of skeletal muscle following exhaustive exercise. Therefore, we hypothesized that an additional hydrolyzed protein supplementation could enhance the muscle protein content and eliminate the oxidative stress products by regulating the plasma amino acid spectrums in rats following exhaustive exercise.

Methods

Experimental design

Rats were randomly divided into four groups (n = 6 per group): a control group fed standard diet without exercise (SD), exercise (EX), exercise plus standard diet for 72 h (EX + SD), or exercise plus standard diet supplemented with hydrolyzed protein (2 g/kg/d) for 72 h (EX + HP). Animals were maintained in individual cages and fed a standard chow diet and water *ad libitum.* All rats of the EX, EX + SD and EX + HP groups received a single bout of exhaustive swimming on the first day in the experimental period (time 0 hour). EX was sacrificed immediately following exercise. The animals of the other groups had open access to a standard rodent chow diet and water *ad libitum* throughout the study. A standard lab rat diet was rich in dietary fiber, trace elements, and intact protein (18 g/100 g fodder) including 1.76 g leucine and 5 g crude fiber per 100 g fodder.

Additionally, the EX + HP group received a supplementation of protein hydrolysate (6.67 ml/kg body weight) by oral gavage once per day, while EX + SD received the same value of purified water via oral gavage. The protein hydrolysates (HYDROPROTEIN, Shen Yi Food Nutrition, Zhuji, ZJ.) contain 60% hydrolyzed whey protein as its source of nitrogen, providing a rich source of leucine (4.67 g/100 g powder) (powder, 50 g/per bag). The protein consists of 100% content of di- and tripeptides. It was dissolved in purified water (Nestle Company, USA) and the final protein concentration was 0.3 g/ml. After 72 hours of feeding following exercise, both EX + SD and EX + HP groups were sacrificed for sample collection.

Subjects

Twenty-four 7-week-old (250 g) specific pathogen-free male Sprague Dawley male rats were used and individually housed in a metabolic cage at the Jinling hospital Animal Research facility at Nanjing, Jiangsu province. They were placed in a room maintained at 22°C with a 12: 12-hour light: dark cycle and provided with rodent chow and water *ad libitum.* This experimental study was approved and performed in strict accordance with the guidelines for the Institutional Animal Care and Use committee, Jinling hospital trial registration (2010NKY062). The experimental model was conducted in a manner consistent with the relevant ethical guidelines for animal research, Jinling hospital. All surgery was performed under pentobarbital anesthesia, and all efforts were made to minimize suffering.

Exhaustive exercise model

We chose the swimming model as an exhaustive physical training model. The rats were hanging a heavy object which accounted for 3% of their weight, then were placed into a 40 cm × 40 cm × 100 cm container filled with water (30°C) [17]. In our preliminary test, we examined the swimming time period and the appropriate load weight of swimming rats. It was found that rats would float if the hanging weight was lower than 3% of body weight and would easily sink if it was more than 6% of body weight. So we chose the 3% of body weight as load weight tied to their tails. Animals were removed from the swimming chamber when they were exhausted, as determined by their inability to surface after repeated attempts, or their remaining below the water surface for 10 s. The average swimming time was is about 140 min in the rat model. And so the exercise intensity was similar among the three groups. The rats were wiped up by dry and warm towels in the warm room to prevent the thermoregulatory response.

Procedures

The rats were anesthetized with pentobarbital (50 mg/kg body weight). Blood was rapidly collected from the abdominal aorta and plasma was immediately separated after centrifugation at 5000 g for 5 minutes (Ningbo Hinotek Technology Co., Ltd., China) at 4°C, then placed in -80°C until assay. The gastrocnemius was removed and washed in 0.9% cold saline and placed immediately in liquid nitrogen.

Body weight, food intake and excrement measurement

All rats were weighed before and after experiment with electronic scale (Furi FEJ-2000B, Shenzhen, China) and the body weight was recorded. Daily food intake and excrement were also recorded.

Tissue preparation for total protein, MDA and PC determination

To carry out the assays, the gastrocnemius was weighed and homogenized by adding a 9 times of the volume of 0.9% saline. The 10% homogenate was centrifuged for 10 minutes (1800 g/min) and the supernatant was diluted with 10 times of the volume of 0.9% saline to 1% concentration. All procedures were done in accordance with the manufacturer's instructions. The 1% supernatant was assayed spectrophotometrically for total protein (TP), malondialdehyde (MDA) and protein carbonyl (PC) activity level with commercial kits (A045-2, A003-1, A087, respectively, Nanjing Jiancheng Bio-engineering Institute, Nanjing, China).

Analyses of plasma amino acid spectrum

The plasma amino acids spectrum was quantified by high performance liquid chromatography (HPLC) (Waters 2695, MA, USA). Sample extracts were chromatographed on a column that was kept at 85°C and monitored by fluorescence-detection. H_2O was used in the mobile phase at a flow-rate of 1.0 ml/min. In brief, 20 μL plasma was mixed uniformly with 100 μL derivative regent (containing phenylisothiocyanate, triethylamine, dehydrated alcohol, deionized water) after thawing, and 20 μL mixed liquid was injected into HPLC pump to measure the plasma concentrations of amino acids. The measurement for all plasma samples were repeated in triplicate [18].

Statistical analyses

The data are presented as means ± SEM. SPSS16.0 software was applied for statistical analysis of all data (SPPS Inc., Chicago, IL, USA). Differences between groups were examined for statistical significance using one-way analysis of variance (ANOVA) and then determined with the Student-Newman-Keuls test. The correlation was determined by stepwise multiple linear regression. The criterion for significance was $P < 0.05$.

Results

Food intake, excrement and body weight

Groups EX + SD and EX + HP consumed 30 grams of standard diet daily. No significant differences in food intake were observed between groups (SD: 31.0 ± 2.5 g, EX: 33.0 ± 3.1 g, EX + SD: 30.0 ± 1.9 g, EX + HP: 32.0 ± 2.8 g), suggesting protein supplementation did not influence food intake within the 72 hours period. Supplementation of protein hydrolysate or water did not increase the frequency of diarrhea in the EX + SD group and EX + HP group, compared with SD group during the duration of the study (SD: 2.2 ± 0.5 g, EX + SD: 2.5 ± 0.8 g, EX + HP: 2.8 ± 0.6 g).

Before the experiment, there was no difference in body weight among the four groups (SD: 255.7 ± 14.4 g, EX: 265.5 ± 8.5 g, EX + SD: 257.3 ± 8.1 g, EX + HP: 259.7 ± 23.7 g). Following exhaustive swimming exercise, body weights of EX group, EX + SD group and EX + HP group were significantly decreased compared with their initial body weights (EX: 257.5 ± 9.2 g, EX + SD: 253.5 ± 6.4 g, EX + HP: 252.7 ± 19.6 g). At 72 hours after feeding, the body weights of EX + SD group and EX + HP group were higher than immediately following exercise ($P < 0.05$). The body weight increase observed in EX + HP group was higher compared with EX + SD group (269.7 ± 29.0 g vs 263.0 ± 7.8 g), but the difference did not reach significance ($P > 0.05$).

Total protein, PC and MDA levels in rat skeletal muscle

As illustrated in Figure 1, the total protein amount of skeletal muscle was significantly increased in EX + HP group, compared with EX + SD group ($P = 0.02$). The level of MDA was significantly lower in EX + HP group compared with EX + SD group ($P = 0.035$), meanwhile it was elevated in EX + SD group compared with EX group ($P = 0.014$) (Figure 2). The mean level of PC was increased in EX + SD group compared with SD group ($p < 0.001$), but it was ameliorated significantly in EX + HP group compared with EX + SD group ($p < 0.001$) (Figure 3).

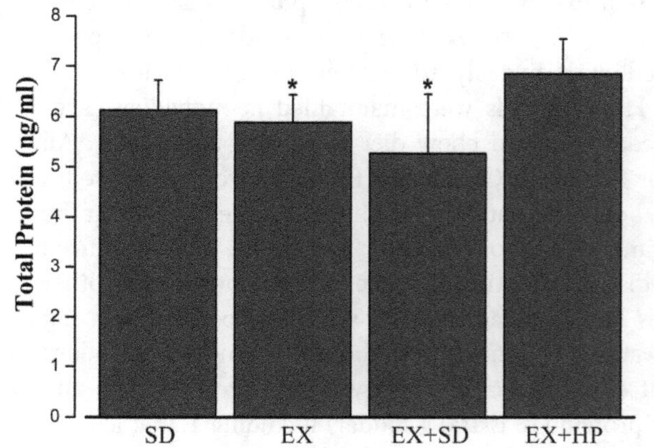

Figure 1 Concentrations of skeletal muscle total protein levels in standard diet (SD), exercise (EX), exercise plus standard diet for 72 hours (EX + SD), and exercise plus standard diet supplemented with hydrolyzed protein (2 g/kg/d) for 72 hours (EX + HP). EX + HP group presented significantly higher values than did the EX + SD and EX groups. *P < 0.05: Different from the EX + HP group.

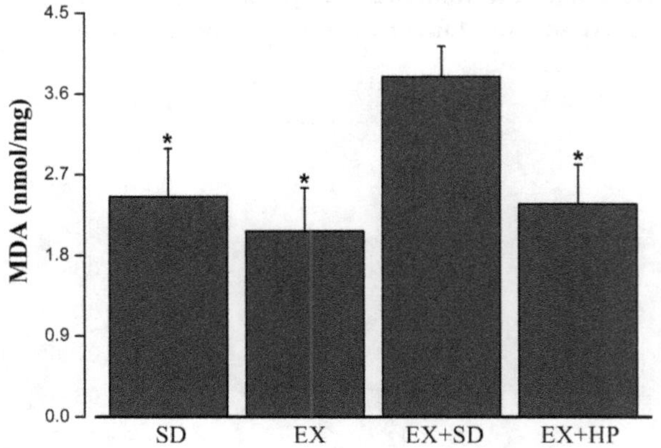

Figure 2 Concentrations of skeletal muscle malondialdehyde (MDA) levels in standard diet (SD), exercise (EX), exercise plus standard diet for 72 hours (EX + SD), and exercise plus standard diet supplemented with hydrolyzed protein (2 g/kg/d) for 72 hours (EX + HP). SD, EX and EX + HP groups presented significantly lower values than did the EX + SD group. *P < 0.05: Different from the EX + SD group.

Plasma concentrations of amino acids

The plasma levels of leucine, methionine, phenylalanine, histidine, threonine, arginine, lysine, glycine, valine, serine and cysteine were significantly higher following exercise, compared with SD group ($p < 0.05$, Table 1). Conversely, the plasma concentration of isoleucine significantly declined in EX + SD during the 72 hours recovery period, compared with groups SD and EX ($P < 0.001$). Meanwhile, the concentrations of leucine ($P = 0.049$), isoleucine ($P < 0.01$) and methionine ($P = 0.046$) were significantly increased in group EX + HP, compared with group EX + SD.

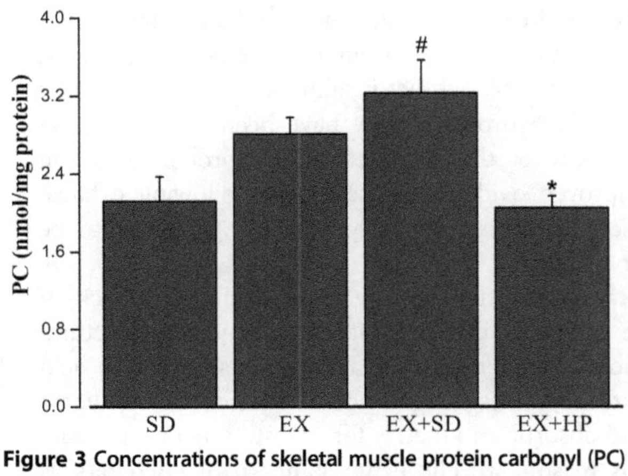

Figure 3 Concentrations of skeletal muscle protein carbonyl (PC) levels in standard diet (SD), exercise (EX), exercise plus standard diet for 72 hours (EX + SD), and exercise plus standard diet supplemented with hydrolyzed protein (2 g/kg/d) for 72 hours (EX + HP). EX + HP group presented significantly lower values than did the EX and EX + SD groups. EX + SD group presented significantly higher values than did the SD group.* P < 0.001: Different from the EX and EX + SD groups. # P < 0.001: Different from the SD group.

Moreover, there were significant positive correlations between total protein content and leucine ($r = 0.993$, $P < 0.001$), isoleucine ($r = 0.945$, $P = 0.004$) and methionine ($r = 0.902$, $P = 0.014$) levels. Furthermore, significant negative correlation was found between plasma methionine concentration and MDA levels ($r = 0.59$, $P = 0.02$) (Table 1).

Discussion

The purpose of this study was to investigate whether hydrolyzed protein supplementation, in a short term, could improve the protein retention and eliminate peroxidation products of skeletal muscle in rats following exhaustive exercise. Our results showed that the protein hydrolysate supplementation improved skeletal muscle protein content and reduced oxidative stress following exhaustive swimming.

Following exhaustive swimming exercise, body weights were dramatically decreased for reasons that were likely multivariable. Acute high intensity swimming can result in energy substrate exhaustion with hepatic glycogen mobilization and skeletal muscle protein catabolism. In addition, catabolism produces water, which is lost during exercise through the skin, respiratory tract and urinary system, to maintain metabolic balance and regulate body temperature. In the present study, there were significant increases in body weight for groups EX + SD and EX + HP after 72 h of feeding, implicating these changes following exercise were temporary and could been restored after post-exercise feeding.

Exercise modifies protein and amino acid metabolism, which is reflected from altered plasma amino acid concentrations [19,20]. Our data demonstrate the levels of leucine, valine, methionine, phenylalanine, histidine, threonine, arginine and lysine were significantly elevated in rats immediately following exhaustive swimming compared with non-exercised controls. It was reported that the increase of plasma amino acid concentrations, particularly leucine and essential amino acids, could activate the key signaling proteins to accelerate the protein anabolism [21-23]. However, significantly reduced levels of leucine, isoleucine, methionine, histidine, threonine, arginine, lysine, glutamate and alanine were observed after 72 hours of recovery and standard diet feeding, which suggest standard diet was insufficient to restore these amino acid levels following exhaustive exercise. In contrast, hydrolyzed protein supplementation not only elevated the levels of leucine, isoleucine and methionine, but also augmented the skeletal muscle protein retention compared with standard diet. Moreover, there were significant positive correlations between the total protein content and leucine, isoleucine and methionine levels. It indicates that the improvement of protein content in skeletal muscle may be a consequence of enhanced plasma leucine, isoleucine and methionine levels

Table 1 The concentrations of plasma free amino acids (AA) of the rats among the standard diet group (SD), exercise group (EX), exercise plus standard diet for 72 h group (EX + SD), and exercise plus standard diet supplemented with hydrolyzed protein (2 g/kg/d) for 72 h group (EX + HP)

AA (uM)	SD	EX	EX + SD	EX + HP
Aspartic acid	0.146 ± 0.150	0.204 ± 0.061	0.141 ± 0.026	0.127 ± 0.140
Glutamate	0.398 ± 0.126	0.399 ± 0.114	0.283 ± 0.050	0.303 ± 0.036
Serine	0.764 ± 0.131	1.499 ± 0.221*	0.861 ± 0.285	0.938 ± 0.177
Glycine	0.960 ± 0.292	1.815 ± 0.176*	1.037 ± 0.298	1.112 ± 0.359
Histidine	0.259 ± 0.041	0.519 ± 0.033*	0.241 ± 0.057	0.263 ± 0.032
Threonine	0.894 ± 0.298	2.398 ± 0.405*	0.668 ± 0.148	1.239 ± 0.708
Alanine	2.092 ± 0.372	2.167 ± 0.343	1.651 ± 0.403	1.990 ± 0.356
Arginine	0.578 ± 0.101	0.924 ± 0.071*	0.509 ± 0.122	0.539 ± 0.183
Proline	0.835 ± 0.271	1.035 ± 0.077	0.601 ± 0.030	0.754 ± 0.199
Tyrosine	0.144 ± 0.038	0.177 ± 0.252	0.139 ± 0.063	0.134 ± 0.101
Valine	0.175 ± 0.079	0.923 ± 0.770*	0.350 ± 0.062	0.397 ± 0.077#
Methionine	0.132 ± 0.019	0.335 ± 0.017*	0.081 ± 0.028	0.127 ± 0.041&
Cysteine	1.158 ± 0.083	1.582 ± 0.306*	1.204 ± 0.130	1.242 ± 0.047
Isoleucine	0.359 ± 0.018&	0.450 ± 0.136	0.172 ± 0.042#	0.368 ± 0.031&
Leucine	0.340 ± 0.190	1.533 ± 0.195*	0.284 ± 0.056	0.365 ± 0.070&
Phenylalanine	0.229 ± 0.032	0.507 ± 0.059*	0.206 ± 0.015	0.223 ± 0.042
Lysine	1.459 ± 0.443	4.466 ± 0.361*	1.251 ± 0.135	1.311 ± 0.405

Note: *P < 0.05 significantly increased compared with SD group; #P < 0.05 significantly decreased compared with SD group; & P < 0.05 significantly increased compared with EX + SD group.

following protein hydrolysate supplementation. The present study provides the first evidence that following exhaustive swimming exercise, protein retention was more efficiently improved by supplementation of additional hydrolyzed protein administered in a short term, compared with feeding a standard diet alone in rats.

MDA is suggested to be a biomarker of oxidative stress associated with tissue injury. In addition to MDA, PC may serve as a biomarker of oxidative stress because the oxidation process may be accelerated by the formation and accumulation of carbonylated protein [24,25]. In the present study, a higher level of MDA and PC appeared in rats at 72 hours after exercise, suggesting oxidative stress persists for up to 72 hours following exhaustive exercise. Exercise induced oxidative damage may lead to protein denaturation and loss of essential biological, which causes muscle damage and decreased muscle performance [26,27]. Nutrients can regulate oxidative stress and prevent muscular damage [12,28]. Supplementation of hydrolyzed protein was found to accompany with the reduction of MDA and PC levels, indicating that protein hydrolysate ingestion might ameliorate the peroxidation products of skeletal muscle following exhaustive exercise.

It has demonstrated that methionine, which is distinct from other amino acids, plays a significant role in controlling oxidative stress [29]. In our study, significant negative correlation between plasma methionine concentration and MDA levels was observed. The higher content of methionine (14.2 μg/mg) in our protein hydrolysate might represent a possible mechanism through which hydrolyzed protein supplementation reduces peroxidation damage. In addition, amino acid, especially leucine, was demonstrated to stimulate insulin secretion [30]. An emerging body of evidence suggests that insulin can suppress the inflammatory process through modulating key inflammatory molecules in addition to acting as an anabolic hormone [31]. It thus can be speculated that insulin secretion after feeding with protein hydrolysate may have been responsible, at least in part, for the increased muscle protein retention and improved oxidative stress in rats following exhaust exercise in the present study; however, it needs to be further explored.

Limitations of the current study included a lack of muscle biopsy and morphological assay for structural alterations. Furthermore, measuring plasma amino acid concentration does not provide a measure of the digestion and absorption kinetics for ingested dietary protein. For this reason, we chose the standard diet fed rats as the control to compare the discrimination of amino acid concentrations following 72 hours of post-exercise feeding. Our future research plans include the use of labeled amino acids to accurately assess the appearance rate of amino acids derived from dietary protein in plasma and skeletal muscle.

Conclusions

In conclusion, the short-term oral supplementation of hydrolyzed protein to standard diet may be an efficacious option in improving protein retention and eliminating reactive oxygen species in rats following exhaustive exercise. Our findings strengthen the importance of protein hydrolysate supplementation in exhaustive exercise-stress situations.

Abbreviations

SD: Standard diet without exercise; EX: Exercise; EX + SD: Exercise plus standard diet; EX + HP: Exercise plus standard diet supplemented with hydrolyzed protein; TP: Total protein; MDA: Malondialdehyde; PC: Protein carbonyl; ROS: Reactive oxygen species; HPLC: High performance liquid chromatography.

Competing interests

The authors declare that they have no competing interests.

Authors' contributions

XW and CN carried out the animal studies and participated in the samples measurement. XW drafted the manuscript. JL performed the statistical analysis and helped to draft the manuscript. NL and JL sconceived of the study, and participated in its design and coordination. All authors read and approved the final manuscript.

Funding

This work was supported by National Natural Science Foundation of China (81070282), Natural Science Foundation of Jiangsu Province (BK2010460) and The Six Personnel Peak of Jiangsu Province (079).

Author details

[1]Research Institute of General Surgery, Jinling Hospital, Medical School, Nanjing University, 305 East Zhongshan Road, Nanjing 210002, Jiangsu Province, People's Republic of China. [2]Department of ICU, Brain Hospital, Nanjing Medical University, 264 Guangzhou Road, Nanjing 210029, Jiangsu Province, China. [3]Department of Orthopedics, Zhongda Hospital, Southeast University, 87 Dingjiaqiao, Nanjing 210009, Jiangsu Province, China.

References

1. Koopman R, van Loon LJ: **Aging, exercise, and muscle protein metabolism.** *J Appl Physiol* 2009, **106**(6):2040–2048.
2. Ebbeling CB, Clarkson PM: **Exercise-induced muscle damage and adaptation.** *Sports Med* 1989, **7**(4):207–234.
3. Parkhouse WS: **Regulation of skeletal muscle myofibrillar protein degradation: relationships to fatigue and exercise.** *Int J Biochem* 1988, **20**(8):769–775.
4. Venditti P, Di Meo S: **Effect of training on antioxidant capacity, tissue damage, and endurance of adult male rats.** *Int J Sports Med* 1997, **18**(7):497–502.
5. Venditti P, Di Meo S: **Antioxidants, tissue damage, and endurance in trained and untrained young male rats.** *Arch Biochem Biophys* 1996, **331**(1):63–68.
6. Huang C-C, Lin TJ, Lu YF, Chen CC, Huang CY, Lin WT: **Protective effects of L-arginine supplementation against exhaustive exercise-induced oxidative stress in young rat tissues.** *Chin J Physiol* 2009, **52**(5):306–315.
7. Powers SK, Jackson MJ: **Exercise-induced oxidative stress: cellular mechanisms and impact on muscle force production.** *Physiol Rev* 2008, **88**(4):1243–1276.
8. Dangin M, Boirie Y, Garcia-Rodenas C, Gachon P, Fauquant J, Callier P, Ballèvre O, Beaufrère B: **The digestion rate of protein is an independent regulating factor of postprandial protein retention.** *Am J Physiol Endocrinol Metab* 2001, **280**(2):E340–E348.
9. Anand T, Phani Kumar G, Pandareesh MD, Swamy MS, Khanum F, Bawa AS: **Effect of bacoside extract from Bacopa monniera on physical fatigue induced by forced swimming.** *Phytother Res* 2012, **26**(4):587–593.
10. Mero A: **Leucine supplementation and intensive training.** *Sports Med* 1999, **27**(6):347–358.
11. Arnal MA, Mosoni L, Boirie Y, Houlier ML, Morin L, Verdier E, Ritz P, Antoine JM, Prugnaud J, Beaufrère B, Mirand PP: **Protein pulse feeding improves protein retention in elderly women.** *Am J Clin Nutr* 1999, **69**(6):1202–1208.
12. Thomas C, Perrey S, Ben Saad H, Delage M, Dupuy AM, Cristol JP, Mercier J: **Effects of a supplementation during exercise and recovery.** *Int J Sports Med* 2007, **28**(8):703–712.
13. Malaguti M, Angeloni C, Garatachea N, Baldini M, Leoncini E, Collado PS, Teti G, Falconi M, Gonzalez-Gallego J, Hrelia S: **Sulforaphane treatment protects skeletal muscle against damage induced by exhaustive exercise in rats.** *J Appl Physiol* 2009, **107**(4):1028–1036.
14. Kim S, Park SH, Lee HN, Park T: **Prunus mume extract ameliorates exercise-induced fatigue in trained rats.** *J Med Food* 2008, **11**(3):460–468.
15. van Loon LJ: **Application of protein or protein hydrolysates to improve postexercise recovery.** *Int J Sport Nutr Exerc Metab* 2007, **17**(Suppl):S104–S117.
16. Athira S, Mann B, Sharma R, Kumar R: **Ameliorative potential of whey protein hydrolysate against paracetamol-induced oxidative stress.** *J Dairy Sci* 2013, **96**(3):1431–1437.
17. Thomas D, Marshall KI: **Effects of repeated exhaustive exercise on myocardial subcellular membrane structures.** *Int J Sports Med* 1988, **9**(4):257–260.
18. Harder U, Koletzko B, Peissner W: **Quantification of 22 plasma amino acids combining derivatization and ion-pair LC–MS/MS.** *J Chromatogr B Analyt Technol Biomed Life Sci* 2011, **879**(7–8):495–504.
19. Cuisinier C, Ward RJ, Francaux M, Sturbois X, de Witte P: **Changes in plasma and urinary taurine and amino acids in runners immediately and 24 h after a marathon.** *Amino Acids* 2001, **20**(1):13–23.
20. Blomstrand E, Murakami T, Nakai N, Nagasaki M, Harris RA: **Effect of branched-chain amino acid and carbohydrate supplementation on the exercise-induced change in plasma and muscle concentration of amino acids in human subjects.** *Acta Physiol Scand* 1995, **153**(2):87–96.
21. Norton LE, Layman DK: **Leucine regulates translation initiation of protein synthesis in skeletal muscle after exercise.** *J Nutr* 2006, **136**(2):533S–537S.
22. Shimomura Y, Murakami T, Nakai N, Nagasaki M, Harris RA: **Exercise promotes BCAA catabolism: effects of BCAA supplementation on skeletal muscle during exercise.** *J Nutr* 2004, **134**(6S):1583S–1587S.
23. Børsheim E, Tipton KD, Wolf SE, Wolfe RR: **Essential amino acids and muscle protein recovery from resistance exercise.** *Am J Physiol Endocrinol Metab* 2002, **283**(4):E648–E657.
24. Dalle-Donne I, Rossi R, Giustarini D, Milzani A, Colombo R: **Protein carbonyl groups as biomarkers of oxidative stress.** *Clin Chim Acta* 2003, **329**(1–2):23–38.
25. Pirinccioglu AG, Gökalp D, Pirinccioglu M, Kizil G, Kizil M: **Malondialdehyde (MDA) and protein carbonyl (PCO) levels as biomarkers of oxidative stress in subjects with familial hypercholesterolemia.** *Clin Biochem* 2010, **43**(15):1220–1224.
26. Sen CK: **Antioxidants in exercise nutrition.** *Sports Med* 2001, **31**(13):891–908.
27. Xu J, Li Y: **Effects of salidroside on exhaustive exercise-induced oxidative stress in rats.** *Mol Med Report* 2012, **6**(5):1195–1198.
28. Jackson MJ: **Control of reactive oxygen species production in contracting skeletal muscle.** *Antioxid Redox Signal* 2011, **15**(9):2477–2486.
29. Moundras C, Rémésy C, Levrat MA, Demigné C: **Methionine deficiency in rats fed soy protein induces hypercholesterolemia and potentiates lipoprotein susceptibility to peroxidation.** *Metabolism* 1995, **44**(9):1146–1152.
30. Yang J, Dolinger M, Ritaccio G, Mazurkiewicz J, Conti D, Zhu X, Huang Y: **Leucine stimulates insulin secretion via down-regulation of surface expression of adrenergic α2A receptor through the mTOR (mammalian target of rapamycin) pathway: implication in new-onset diabetes in renal transplantation.** *J Biol Chem* 2012, **287**(29):24795–24806.
31. Hyun E, Ramachandran R, Hollenberg MD, Vergnolle N: **Mechanisms behind the anti-inflammatory actions of insulin.** *Crit Rev Immunol* 2011, **31**(4):307–340.

7

The prevalence of exercise-associated hyponatremia in 24-hour ultra-mountain bikers, 24-hour ultra-runners and multi-stage ultra-mountain bikers in the Czech Republic

Daniela Chlíbková[1†], Beat Knechtle[2,5*], Thomas Rosemann[2†], Alena Žákovská[3†] and Ivana Tomášková[4†]

Abstract

Background: To assess the prevalence of exercise-associated hyponatremia (EAH) in two 24-hour mountain bike (MTB) (R1,R2), one 24-hour running (R3) and one multi-stage MTB (R4) races held in the Czech Republic in a cluster of four cross-sectional studies.

Methods: In 27 ultra-mountain bikers (ultra-MTBers), 12 ultra-runners, and 14 multi-stage MTBers, fluid intake, changes (Δ) in body mass, hematocrit, plasma volume, plasma [Na^+], plasma [K^+], plasma osmolality, urine [Na^+], urine [K^+], urine specific gravity, urine osmolality, K^+/Na^+ ratio in urine, transtubular potassium gradient and glomerular filtration rate were measured and calculated. The use of non-steroidal anti-inflammatory drugs and symptoms of EAH were recorded using post-race questionnaires.

Results: Of the 53 finishers, three (5.7%) developed post-race EAH, thereof one (3.7%) ultra-MTBer, one (8.3%) ultra-runner and one (7.1%) multi-stage MTBer. Plasma [Na^+] decreased significantly ($p < 0.001$) only in R4. Urine osmolality (R1, R3, R4 $p < 0.001$; R2 $p < 0.05$) and glomerular filtration rate ($p < 0.001$) increased, and body mass decreased in all races ($p < 0.05$). Δ body mass was inversely related to the number of kilometers achieved ($p < 0.001$) in R2 where better ultra-MTBers tended to lose more weight. Δ body mass ($p < 0.001$) and %Δ body mass ($p = 0.05$) were positively related to lower post-race plasma [Na^+] in R3 that was associated with increased loss in body mass. Fluid intake was positively related to race performance in R1 and R2 (R1: $p = 0.04$; R2: $p = 0.01$) where ultra-MTBers in R1 and R2 who drank more finished ahead of those who drank less. Post-race plasma [Na^+] was negatively associated with race performance in ultra-MTBers in R2 ($p < 0.05$), similarly ultra-runners in R3 ($p < 0.05$) where finishers with more kilometres had lower post-race plasma [Na^+].

Conclusions: The prevalence of EAH in the Czech Republic was no higher compared to existing reports on ultra-endurance athletes in other countries. Lower plasma [Na^+] and development of EAH may be attributed to overdrinking, a pituitary secretion of vasopressin, an impaired mobilization of osmotically inactive sodium stores, and/or an inappropriate inactivation of osmotically active sodium.

Keywords: 24-hour race, Multi-stage race, Fluid intake, Body mass, Sodium

* Correspondence: beat.knechtle@hispeed.ch
[†]Equal contributors
[2]Institute of General Practise and for Health Services Research, University of Zurich, Zurich, Switzerland
[5]Facharzt FMH für Allgemeinmedizin, Gesundheitszentrum St. Gallen, Vadianstrasse 26, 9001 St. Gallen, Switzerland
Full list of author information is available at the end of the article

Background

Hydration status and its role in endurance performance is an important topic in exercise physiology. Recent studies investigated the changes in hydration status and the development of exercise-associated hyponatremia (EAH) in ultra-distance running races [1-15], in triathlon races [16-20], in mountain bike (MTB) multi-stage races [21-24], in single ultra-distance road cycling races [8,25,26], and in single ultra-distance MTB races [8,27,28]. However, 24-hour races have been investigated to a lesser extent [29-36]. Prior to 2010 there had been only one published study [9] investigating the prevalence of EAH in a single-stage ultra-marathon held in Europe.

Excessive fluid consumption leading to weight gain is thought to be the principal cause of reduced plasma [Na^+] and previous studies in ultra-endurance events have shown an association between fluid intake, changes in body mass and plasma [Na^+] [16,29,37-40]. However, in some studies a significant relationship between post-race plasma [Na^+] and losses in body mass was reported [11,41]. EAH is most commonly found in athletes competing in ultra-endurance events and it is defined as plasma [Na^+] < 135 mmol/l [39]. Signs and symptoms of EAH include nausea, vomiting, confusion, headache, seizures, pulmonary and cerebral oedema (hyponatremic encephalopathy), and possibly death [39]. Risk factors for EAH include low race pace, prolonged exercise with duration of more than four hours, female gender, a low body mass, pre-exercise hyperhydration, the use of non-steroidal anti-inflammatory drugs (NSAIDs), non-elite status, and extremely hot or cold environment [12,20,39,40].

Aside from the excessive fluid consumption associated with a high fluid availability and a sustained intake, EAH occurs due to an increased retention of fluid brought on by non-osmotic secretion of arginine vasopressin [12,42,43], elevated sweat sodium loss, the inability to mobilise exchangeable internal sodium stores, an inappropriate inactivation of osmotically-active sodium, metabolic water production, and an impaired renal blood flow or glomerular filtration [11,40].

Previous data on regular distance marathons have shown the prevalence of this fluid and electrolyte disorder to be at 22% [39]. However, in general, in ultra-endurance athletes, the prevalence of EAH should not exceed 10% [30], although there have been variable results in studies investigating the prevalence of EAH in ultra-marathons and other ultra-endurance events. Knechtle et al. reported that the prevalence of EAH was no higher in ultra-endurance athletes compared with existing reports on marathoners and Ironman triathletes [8], while studies of a single-stage mountain ultra-marathoner race [10], a 1,600-km multi-stage race [13] in Australia and a European 24-hour race showed no cases of EAH [10,30]. Conversely, in a recent study of 45 male ultra-marathoners in a 161-km ultra-marathon held in the USA, 51.2% of the finishers presented with EAH [7]. The longer nature of the 161-km ultra-marathon coupled with the prolonged period spent on the trail were assumed to be the main reasons for the increased prevalence of EAH, though when the data for five consecutive years were combined, the prevalence of EAH was shown to be 15.1% and positively related to ambient temperature [11]. In another study, 8% of mountain ultra-marathoners competing in a 7-stage race (350 km) in Switzerland developed EAH [8], while mild asymptomatic EAH was found to occur in 4% of the volunteer ultra-endurance mountain runners in New Zealand [9].

Studies investigating fluid intake and electrolyte metabolism balance have also been conducted in mountain ultra-endurance bike races. Studies of a single stage MTB race held in Switzerland [27,28] and multi-stage races in South Africa, the Alps (*i.e.* Germany, Austria, Switzerland and Italy) [21,22]. Similarly, no case of EAH was found in 65 ultra-endurance road cyclists competing in a 720-km ultra-cycling marathon in Switzerland [25]. On the contrary, 50% of the participants in an Alaskan cold weather race presented symptoms of EAH upon finishing the race [24].

Knechtle et al. described for 200 athletes competing in different disciplines in Switzerland that 12 finishers (6%) developed EAH [8]. The prevalence of EAH was 13% in swimmers, 10.7% for road cyclists, 8% for both ultra-marathoners and mountain ultra-marathoners and no case in mountain bikers. Regarding different disciplines, EAH was higher in running [1,3,4,6-12,38,39,44,45] compared to cycling [8,22,25,27,28]. However, according to recent findings the comparison of cyclists and runners is problematic because there are fewer studies of bike races [8].

There is a dearth of data on the prevalence of EAH in races held in Europe. Therefore, the aim of the current study was to investigate a series of ultra-endurance races held in the Czech Republic. Twenty-four-hour races held in different disciplines such as cycling and running are an ideal occasion to compare a prevalence of EAH between ultra-cyclists and ultra-runners. We intended to assess the prevalence of EAH in ultra-MTBers and ultra-runners in 24-hour races as single ultra-marathons and nearly non-stop performances without defined breaks with a specific load, and in a multi-stage race with an intermittent load with possibility of regeneration. We hypothesized an increased fluid intake during a 24-hour race for both cyclists and runners due to the large amount of fluids available at the refreshment stations in every lap. Since a slow running [31] or a slow cycling pace were considered as a main risk factor for fluid overload and development of EAH [21,25,29,38] we hypothesized that the prevalence of EAH would be higher in 24-hour races compared to a MTB stage race because there is a possibility of excessive drinking behavior and the duration of exercise is nearly

24 hours. Regarding recent studies, we hypothesized that the prevalence of EAH would be higher in runners compared to cyclists. Finally, it was hypothesized, that body mass loss in all races would have no influence on race performance [18,38,46,47]. In cases of fluid overload, we would expect post-race an increase in body mass [39] and a decrease in plasma [Na$^+$] [12,39,48].

Methods

Ethics

Research within the project proceeded in accordance with the law (No. 96/2001 Coll. M. S. on Human Rights and Biomedicine and Act No. 101/2000 Coll. Privacy) and the study was approved by the local institutional ethics committee.

Subjects (a cluster of four races)

Data were collected during four ultra-endurance races in the Czech Republic, were derived from four observational, cross-sectional studies and comprised athletes (*i.e.* ultra-MTBers, ultra-runners, and mountain bikers) participating in the, Czech Championship 24-hour MTB race' in Jihlava city (R1), in the, Bike Race Marathon Rohozec 24 hours' in Liberec city (R2), in the, Sri Chinmoy Self-Transcendence Marathon 24-hour race' in Kladno city (R3) and in the Trilogy Mountain Bike Stage Race' in Teplice nad Metují (R4) (see Tables 1 and 2).

Race participants were notified of the study approximately three months before the race start via an e-mail and were informed about the planned investigation with indication that participation was voluntary. Those who volunteered were instructed to keep a training diary until the start of the race. The training three months before the race, (*i.e.* number and duration of training units, training distance in kilometers and hours pre-race experience) were recorded.

A total of 58 athletes, thirteen recreational ultra-MTBers from 91 participants in solo category (R1), seventeen ultra-MTBers from 116 participants in solo category (R2), thirteen ultra-runners from 48 participants in solo category (R3) and fifteen MTBers from 206 participants (R4), all originating from the Czech Republic, agreed to participate (Table 2).

Races (R1,R2,R3,R4)

The first measurement was performed at the, Czech Championship 24-hour MTB race' in Jihlava (R1), the race with the highest number of participants from the series of 24-hour MTB races held in the Czech Republic. The ultra-MTBers started at 12:00 on May 19th 2012 and finished at 12:00 on May 20th 2012. The course was comprised of a 9.5 km single-track with an elevation of 220 m. A single aid station, located at the start/finish area was provided by the organizer where a variety of food and beverages such as hypotonic sports drinks, tea, soup, caffenaited drinks, water, fruit, vegetables, energy bars, bread, soup, sausages, cheese, bread, chocolate and biscuits were available. The ultra-MTBers could also use their own supplies in their pitstops. The maximum temperature was +30°C, the minimum temperature was +6°C during the night on some places of the route and the average temperature was +18 (6)°C. No precipitation was recorded and relative humidity was at 43 (12)% over the duration of the race.

The largest and the oldest (18th edition) 24-hour cycling race in the Czech Republic with the longest tradition, the, Bike Race Marathon Rohozec' in Liberec (R2), took place from June 9th 2012 to June 10th 2012. The course was comprised of a 12.6 km track with an elevation of 250 m. The track surface consisted of paved and unpaved roads and paths. There was one aid station located at the start and finish with food and beverages similar to those mentioned above. The maximum temperature was +23°C, the minimum temperature was +6°C during the night and the average temperature was +15 (4)°C. Over the duration of the race, 3 (1.5) mm of precipitation was recorded and relative humidity varied from 44% till 98%.

The, Sri Chinmoy Self-transcendence Running Marathon 24- hour race' (R3) took place from July 21st 2012 to July 22nd 2012 in Kladno. We chose this race because it was the largest 24-hour running race in the Czech Republic with the highest number of participants and we also wanted to compare ultra-runners with ultra-MTBers. The lap was 1 km, situated around an athletic stadium on asphalt with 1 m rise. The athletes could consume food and beverages *ad libitum* from a buffet provided by the organizer with warm and cool food like apples, ananas, oranges, dried fruit, potatoes, rice, cookies, bread, pasta, porridge, soup, water, tea, isotonic drinks, fruit juices, cola, broth, and coffee. Runners could place their own camping tables and chairs with personal belongings, food and drinks in a

Table 1 Description of races, Nr – number of race, TR – temperature range, AT – average temperature, AH – average relative humidity, weather, P – precipitation, F - finishers, prevalence of EAH (R1,R2,R3,R4)

Nr	Type of race	TR (°C)	AT (°C)	AH (%)	Weather	P (mm)	F	Prevalence of EAH
R1	24-h MTB race	6 – 30	18 (6)	43 (1)	Sun	—	12	0 (0%)
R2	24-h MTB race	6 – 23	15 (4)	72 (2)	Clouds	3 (2)	15	1 (6.7%)
R3	24-h running race	10 – 18	12 (3)	62 (3)	Rain	15(5)	12	1 (8.3%)
R4	Multi-stage race	22 – 33	26 (7)	55 (9)	Sun	—	14	1 (7.1%)

Table 2 Age, anthropometry, training, pre-race experience, and race performance of subjects (R1,R2,R3,R4), n = 53

	Race 1 n = 12	Race 2 n = 15	Race 3 n = 12	Race 4 n = 14
Type of race	**24-h MTB race**	**24-h MTB race**	**24-hour RUN race**	**Stage MTB race**
Age, y	40.3 (9.1)	36.8 (6.4)	38.3 (7.7)	38.0 (6.1)
Body mass, kg	75.2 (12.9)	72.1 (11.0)	66.3 (8.8)	75.3 (8.2)
Body height, m	178.1 (11.6)	176.7 (9.5)	174.8 (10.9)	176.6 (5.5)
BMI, kg/m^2	23.5 (2.0)	23.0 (1.9)	21.7 (1.2)	24.1 (2.0)
Years as active cyclist or runner	10.3 (5.7)	8.6 (6.2)	9.8 (7.2)	11.4 (8.0)
Number of finished ultra-marathons	9.3 (7.2)	8.3 (7.3)	15.7 (19.3)	5.6 (6.6)
Total training hours weekly, h	12.3 (7.0)	12.1 (3.2)	10.6 (4.2)	10.7 (5.0)
Training cycle or run hours weekly, h	11.6 (6.2)	11.4 (3.2)	8.2 (3.4)	9.6 (3.9)
Training intensity, b/min	139.2 (6.7)	140.0 (9.3)	141.3 (18.8)	131.4 (12.3)
Cases of EAH, absolute	0	1	1	1
Prevalence of EAH, %	0	6.7	8.3	7.1

Results are presented as mean (SD). EAH = exercise-associated hyponatremia. R1: ‚Czech Championship 24-hour MTB race' in Jihlava city, 24-hour MTB race, R2: Bike Race Marathon Rohozec 24 hours' in Liberec city, 24-hour MTB race, R3: Sri Chinmoy Self-transcendence Marathon 24-h race' in Kladno city, 24-hour RUN race, R4: Trilogy Mountain Bike Stage Race' in Teplice nad Metují, multi-stage MTB race (prolog: 3 km with 300 m difference in elevation, Stage 1: 66 km with 2,200 m, Stage 2: 63 km with 2,300 m and Stage 3: 78.8 km with 3,593 m).

designated area. The maximum temperature was +18°C, the minimum temperature was +10°C, and the average temperature was +12 (3)°C. On average 15 (5) mm of precipitation was recorded and relative humidity changed from 58 till 94% over the duration of the race.

The ‚Trilogy Mountain Bike Stage Race' (R4), the first MTB stage race held in the Czech Republic, took place from July 4th 2012 till July 8th 2012 in Teplice nad Metují. This four day race consisted of a prologue and three stages, each of which had a completely different character. We chose this race to compare 24-hour races with a stage race. The difficulty of this race was similar to other stage MTB races in Europe. The prologue covered 3 km with 300 m difference in elevation, Stage 1 covered 66 km with 2,200 m of altitude to climb, Stage 2 was 63 km in length with 2,300 m difference in elevation and Stage 3 was 78.8 km with 3,593 m. Stage routes were characterized by a large number of individual trails which only interrupted by a necessary minimum of road sections. Aid stations located along the routes offered beverages such as hypotonic sports drinks, tea, soup, caffenaited drinks, water, fruit, vegetables, energy bars, bread, soup, sausages, cheese, bread, chocolate and biscuits. During the prologue the average temperature was +32 (1)°C and relative humidity was 55 (2)% over the duration of the race. At Stage 1 the maximum temperature was +33°C, the minimum +22°C, the average temperature was +27 (7)°C and relative humidity changed from 80% at the start till 48% at the end of the race. At Stage 2 the maximum temperature was +30°C, the minimum +22°C, the average temperature +25 (3)°C and relative humidity changed from 83% till 60% over the duration of the race. At Stage 3 the maximum temperature was +31°C, the minimum +19°C, the average temperature was +25 (2)°C and relative humidity changed from 85% till 37% over the duration of the race.

Procedures and calculations

The procedures of pre- and post-race measurements were identical. At first, pre-race anthropometry of the subjects was assessed. Athletes were measured after voiding their urinary bladder. Body mass was measured using a calibrated commercial scale (Tanita BC-351, Tanita corporation of America, Inc.) to the nearest 0.1 kg. Subjects were barefoot and generally clothed in cycling attire for both the pre- and post-race measurements. Body height was determined using a stadiometer (Harpenden Stadiometer, Baty International Ltd) to the nearest 0.01 m. Body mass index was calculated using body mass and body height. Blood samples were drawn from an antecubital vein. Standardization of the sitting position prior to blood collection was respected since postural changes can influence blood volume and concentration of hematocrit. One Sarstedt S-Monovette (plasma gel, 7.5 ml) for chemical and one Sarstedt S-Monovette (EDTA, 2.7 ml) for hematological analysis were cooled and sent to the laboratory and were analysed within 6 hours. Blood samples were obtained to determine pre- and post-race hematocrit, plasma [Na^+], plasma [K^+], and plasma osmolality. Hematocrit was determined using Sysmex XE 2100 (Sysmex Corporation, Japan), plasma [Na^+] and plasma [K^+] were determined using biochemical analyzer Modula SWA, Modul P + ISE (Hitachi High Technologies Corporation, Japan, Roche Diagnostic), and plasma osmolality was determined using Arkray Osmotation (Arkray Factory, Inc., Japan). Samples of urine were collected in one Sarstedt monovett for urine (10 ml) and sent to the laboratory. In urine samples, pre- and post-race [Na^+], [K^+], specific gravity and osmolality were determined. Urine [Na^+], urine [K^+] and urine urea were determined using biochemical analyzer Modula SWA, Modul P + ISE (Hitachi High Technologies Corporation, Japan, Roche Diagnostic), urine specific gravity was determined using Au Max-4030 (Arkray Factory, Inc., Japan), and osmolality was determined using Arkray Osmotation (Arkray Factory, Inc., Japan). Transtubular potassium gradient was calculated using the formula ($potassium_{urine} \times osmolality_{serum}$)/($potassium_{serum} \times osmolality_{urine}$) [49]. Glomerular filtration rate was calculated using the formula of Levey et al. [50]. K^+/Na^+ ratio in urine was calculated. Percentage change in plasma volume was calculated from pre- and post-race values of hematocrit using the equation of van Beaumont [51]. In an effort to maintain impartial interpretation, the results were not reviewed at the time and no opportunity existed to recommend for or against participation in the races.

Pre-race testing took place during the event's registration in the morning before the race between 07:00 a.m. and 11:00 a.m. in the morning in 24-hour races and three hours before the start of the prolog in the multi-stage race. The athletes were informed of the procedures and gave their informed written consent. No measurements were taken during the race. During the race fluid consumption was recorded by the athlete or by one of the support team on a recording sheet. At each aid station, they marked the number of cups of fluid consumed. In addition, all fluid intake provided by the support crew was recorded. The athletes primarily ate and drank as they ran or cycled. Fluid intake was estimated according to the reports of the athletes. The organizer provided no special advice on the web site about what and how much the athletes should drink during the race. Post-race measurements were taken immediately after the races and were finished within two hours in the 24-hour races, when all finishers ended the race and some of them were finally able to hand in urine samples due to problems with antidiuresis. Post-race measurements were taken directly after arrival at the finish line after every stage in the multi-stage MTB race. Questionnaires were also issued at these times and athletes gave information of the use of non-steroidal anti-inflammatory drugs [9] during the races and symptoms of EAH [12,40].

Statistical analysis

Results are presented as mean and standard deviation (SD) as appropriate. The Shapiro-Wilk test was applied to check for normal distribution of data. Paired sample *t*-tests or the Wilcoxon signed-rank tests were used to compare laboratory parameters before and after the race as appropriate and to compare continuous measures. The results were compared using the Mann-Whitney *U* -test. The correlations of the changes in parameters during the race were evaluated using Pearson product-moment to assess the univariate associations. For all statistical tests, significance was set at a level of 0.05.

Results

Out of the 58 athletes recruited, 53 (91.4%), such as 12 ultra-MTBers (R1), 15 ultra-MTBers (R2), 12 ultra-runners (R3), and 14 MTBers (R4) successfully completed one of the four races (R1-R4) and passed both pre- and post-race measurements (Table 1). One cyclist had to give up due to an equipment failure, while four others had to quit the race because of medical complications or physical exhaustion. Hyponatremia was not evident in those who failed to complete their respective race. Table 2 summarizes anthropometric and training characteristics of the 50 finishers without EAH from all races (R1-R4).

Prevalence of exercise-associated hyponatremia

In three subjects (EAH-A-R2, EAH-B-R3, EAH-C-R4), post-race plasma [Na^+] varied between 129 and 134 mmol/l corresponding biochemically to a mild to medium hyponatremia (Table 3). Based on the classification by Noakes et al. [39], hypernatremia is defined as a serum [Na^+] ≥ 145 mmol/l, normonatremia as a serum [Na^+] = 135 - 144.9 mmol/l, biochemical hyponatremia as a serum [Na^+] = 129 - 134.9 mmol/l, and clinical hyponatremia as a serum [Na^+] ≤ 129 mmol/l. The prevalence of post-race EAH in 24-hour MTB races (R1, R2) in the Czech Republic was 3.7% from 27 ultra-MTBers. No ultra-MTBer in R1 developed post-race EAH. One ultra-MTBer in R2 (EAH-A-R2) showed post-race EAH, where plasma [Na^+] dropped from 138 mmol/l pre-race to 129 mmol/l post-race. Two other ultra-MTBers - one each from R1 and R2 - started their races with plasma [Na^+] indicating hyponatremia (132 mmol/l), however they developed no post-race hyponatremia. No ultra-MTBer (R1,R2) showed pre-race or post-race hypernatremia. The estimated prevalence of EAH in the 24-hour running race (R3) was 8.3% from 12 ultra-runners. One ultra-runner (EAH-B-R3) developed EAH, as his plasma [Na^+] dropped from 137 mmol/l pre-race to 133 mmol/l post-race. No ultra-runner showed pre-race or post-race hypernatremia. The estimated prevalence of EAH in the multi-stage MTB race was 7.1% from 14 MTBers. One MTBer (EAH-C-R4) developed EAH, as his plasma [Na^+] dropped from 142 mmol/l pre-race to 134 mmol/l post-race. No MTBer developed pre-race or post-race hypernatremia.

The intake of NSAIDs was reported by 3 (25%) of 12 ultra-runners and by no cyclist (from 41) in any race. Regarding symptoms associated with race performance

Table 3 Characteristics of the three cases (EAH-A-R2, EAH-B-R3, EAH-C-R4) with exercise-associated hyponatremia (n = 3)

	EAH-A-R2	EAH-B-R3	EAH-C-R4
Type of race	24-h MTB race	24-h RUN race	Multi-stage MTB race
Age (years)	39	38	42
Body height (m)	196	168	177
BMI (kg/m^2)	23.4	18.8	23.6
Pre-race body mass (kg)	90.0	54.6	73.9
Post-race body mass (kg)	88.2	53.2	71.7
Δ body mass (kg)	−1.8	−1.4	−2.2
Δ body mass (%)	−2.0	−2.6	−3.0
Pre-race plasma sodium (mmol/l)	138.0	137.0	142.0
Post-race plasma sodium (mmol/l)	129.0	133.0	134.0
Δ haematocrit (%)	−7.6	−9.4	3.8
Δ plasma potassium (mmol/l)	32.6	−29.2	3.6
Δ plasma osmolality (mosmol/kg H_2O)	−0.7	−1.1	1.7
Pre-race urine specific gravity (g/ml)	1.015	1.010	1.007
Post-race urine specific gravity (g/ml)	1.025	1.025	1.028
Δ urine osmolality (mosmol/kg H_2O)	338.9	163.5	228.0
Δ urine potassium (mmol/l)	323.2	90.5	1282.0
Δ urine sodium (mmol/l)	108.3	25.9	−71.4
Δ K/Na in urine (%)	103.1	51.2	4737.0
Δ Transtubular potassium gradient (%)	1262.5	611.4	4340.0
Years as active cyclist or runner	5	15	5
Number of finished ultra-marathons	4	30	2
Total training hours weekly, h	12	13	10
Training cycle or run hours weekly, h	10	30	10
Training intensity, b/min	140	130	140

in R1, most of ultra-MTBers without EAH noted in the post-race questionnaires muscle weakness (41.7%), problems with antidiuresis (33.3%), and breathing problems (33.3%). Muscle weakness (46.7%), problems with antidiuresis (40%), headache (26.7%), and breathing problems (26.7%) were the most reported post-race symptoms associated with race performance in R2 by finishers without EAH. Chills (50.8%), stomach pain (33.3%) and irritability (33.3%) were the most noted post-race symptoms associated with race performance in R3 by ultra-runners without EAH. MTBers without EAH reported muscle weakness (50%), swelling (42.9%) and myalgia (35.7%) in R4.

Subjects who exhibited hyponatremia reported no intake of NSAIDs during the study period. The ultra-MTBer (EAH-A-R2) reported muscle weakness. The ultra-runner (EAH-B-R3) in a 24-hour running race R3 with EAH reported symptoms like antidiuresis, headache, flushing, irritability, dizziness, myalgia, disorientation, lethargy, swelling and mental status change. The MTBer (EAH-C-R4) in the multi-stage MTB race (R4) with EAH reported symptoms like antidiuresis, muscle weakness, myalgia and swelling. EAH-A-R2, EAH-B-R3 and EAH-C-R4 developed a post-race biochemical EAH.

Hyponatremic finishers (n = 3) and their anthropometric parameters, parameters of hydration status, and fluid intake

Anthropometric parameters, blood and urine parameters, pre-race training logs of hyponatremic cases EAH-A-R2, EAH-B-R3 and EAH-C-R4 are summarized in Table 3. Pre and post-race results for physical, blood and urine parameters are shown in Table 4. For comparison purposes, we used cut-off points for hydration state based upon Δ body mass by Noakes et al. [39], where ≥ 0 Δ body mass is overhydration, < 0 to -3% Δ body mass is euhydration, and < -3% Δ body mass is dehydration. A decrease was seen in both body mass and Δ body mass, respectively, in EAH-A-R2 (1.8 kg, 2.0%) and EAH-B-R3 (1.4 kg, 2.6%). In EAH-C-R4, decreases in body mass (2.2, 2.8, 2.2 kg) and Δ body mass (3.0%, 3.8%, 3.0%)

Table 4 Physical, blood and urine parameters before and after the race (n = 3)

	Pre-race	Post-race	Change (absolute)	Change (%)
Body mass (kg)	72.8 (12.5)	71.0 (12.4)	−1.8 (0.4)*	−2.5 (0.5)*
Haematocrit (%)	42.7 (1.1)	40.9 (3.2)	−1.8 (3.1)	−4.4 (7.2)
Plasma sodium (mmol/l)	139 (1.9)	132 (1.9)	−7 (2.6)*	−5 (1.9)*
Plasma potassium (mmol/l)	5.5 (0.7)	5.5 (0.5)	−0.1 (1.7)	−2.3 (30.9)
Plasma osmolality (mosmol/kg H_2O)	287.7 (3.6)	287.7 (5.5)	0.0 (4.4)	0.0 (1.5)
Urine specific gravity (g/ml)	1.011 (0.003)	1.026 (0.001)	0.020 (0.010)*	1.520 (0.550)*
Urine osmolality (mosmol/kg H_2O)	204.0 (36.9)	681.0 (97.2)	477.0 (132.9)*	243.5 (88.7)*
Urine potassium (mmol/l)	17.2 (8.1)	81.2 (35.1)	64.0 (55.8)	565.2 (631.6)
Urine sodium (mmol/l)	40.0 (10.7)	43.3 (20.2)	3.3 (29.5)	20.9 (90.0)
K/Na ratio in urine	0.4 (0.1)	4.4 (0.1)	4.0 (6.3)	1630.5 (2690.5)
Transtubular potassium gradient	2.3 (1.3)	32.5 (8.0)	30.2 (11.9)*	2071.3 (1991.6)*
Glomerular filtration rate (ml/min)	91.9 (6.6)	64.2 (13.3)	−27.8 (28.1)	−28.5 (26.1)

Results are presented as mean (SD), *= p ≤ 0.05.

were seen after Stage 1, 2 and 3 respectively. EAH-A-R2 consumed 0.90 l/h, EAH-B-R3 and EAH-C-R4 each consumed 0.75 l/h, which equated to 0.010 l/kg in EAH-A-R2, 0.014 l/kg in EAH-B-R3, 0.010 l/kg in EAH-C-R4; which was not related to race speed, ambient temperature or relative humidity during the race ($p > 0.05$).

Normonatremic finishers (n = 50) and their anthropometric parameters, parameters of hydration status, and fluid intake

Race 1 - R1 (24-hour MTB race)

For all finishers body mass significantly decreased ($p < 0.001$) in R1, Δ body mass was -2.0 kg (2.7%). In the one (8.3%) ultra-MTBer, body mass increased by 0.1 kg. In the remaining 11 cyclists, body mass decreased between 1.0 kg and 5.1 kg. Three of them (25.0%) were dehydrated according to Noakes et al. [39]. The Δ body mass or % Δ body mass were neither related to plasma [NA^+], Δ plasma [Na^+] or race performance. Finishers showed a significantly increase in urine specific gravity ($p < 0.001$). Increased post-race urine osmolality ($p < 0.001$) was significantly related to increased post-race urine [K^+] ($p < 0.001$) (r = 0.61, $p < 0.05$). K^+/Na^+ ratio in urine significantly increased ($p < 0.001$) and it was > 1. Plasma volume decreased by 3.9% (12.6%); Δ plasma volume was not related to post-race plasma osmolality, or to post-race urine osmolality. Hematocrit, plasma [Na^+], plasma [K^+], plasma osmolality, and urine [Na^+] remained stable (see Table 5). Post-race plasma [Na^+] was significantly and positively related to Δ plasma [Na^+] ($r = 0.78$, $p < 0.001$). Transtubular potassium gradient significantly increased ($p < 0.001$), and glomerular filtration race significantly decreased ($p < 0.001$). Ultra-MTBers consumed a total of 0.49 (0.15) l/h during the 24-hour MTB race. Fluid intake varied between 0.30 l/h and 0.70 l/h and was positively related to the number of achieved kilometers (race performance) during the 24-hour MTB race ($r = 0.58$, $p = 0.04$) (Figure 1). Fluid intake showed no correlation to body mass, Δ body mass, post-race plasma [Na^+], Δ plasma [Na^+], Δ plasma volume or USG.

Race 2 - R2 (24-hour MTB race)

BM decreased ($p < 0.05$), Δ BM was -1.3 kg (1.9%), finishers were euhydrated following the definition of Noakes et al. [39]. In four (26.7%) ultra-MTBers, body mass increased between 0.2 kg and 2.0 kg. In the remaining 11 ultra-MTBers, body mass decreased between 0.7 kg and 5.0 kg, indicating that five (33.3%) were dehydrated. Δ body mass was negatively and significantly related to race performance ($r = -0.69$, $p < 0.001$). Neither Δ body mass nor% Δ body mass were related to post-race plasma [Na^+] or Δ plasma [Na^+]. Hematocrit, plasma [Na^+], plasma [K^+], plasma osmolality, and transtubular potassium gradient remained stable (see Table 5). Post-race plasma [Na^+] was significantly and positively related to Δ plasma [Na^+] ($r = 0.72$, $p < 0.001$). Plasma volume increased by 4.9% (11.3%) and Δ plasma volume was not related to an increased K^+/Na^+ ratio in urine > 1 ($p < 0.05$), plasma osmolality, or to urine osmolality. Urine [Na^+] and glomerular filtration race significantly decreased ($p < 0.001$), and urine specific gravity increased ($p < 0.001$). Ultra-MTBers consumed a total of 0.55 (0.19) l/h during the 24-hour MTB race. Fluid intake varied between 0.20 l/h and 0.95 l/h and correlated significantly and positively to race performance ($r = 0.62$, $p = 0.01$) (Figure 1) as in ultra-MTBers in R1. Fluid intake showed no correlation to post-race body mass, Δ body mass, Δ plasma volume or urine specific gravity. However, post-race plasma [Na^+] was negatively associated with race performance in ultra-MTBers ($r = -0.53$, $p < 0.05$) (Figure 1), as in ultra-runners in R3. Also, fluid

Table 5 (A,B,C,D) - Changes in blood and urine parameters (R1,R2,R3,R4) in subjects without EAH, n = 50

A	Pre-race			
Parameter	**R1**	**R2**	**R3**	**R4**
Haematocrit (%)	41.7 (3.7)	41.8 (3.0)	42.1 (3.2)	41.7 (2.3)
Plasma sodium (mmol/l)	138.0 (2.7)	137.7 (2.1)	140.0 (1.7)	141.8 (1.9)
Plasma potassium (mmol/l)	6.5 (1.5)	4.6 (0.3)	6.6 (0.9)	5.1 (0.4)
Plasma osmolality (mosmol/kg H_2O)	289.9 (5.0)	289.4 (4.7)	288.6 (3.4)	288.7 (3.4)
Urine specific gravity (g/ml)	1.015 (0.004)	1.016 (0.004)	1.013 (0.005)	1.015 (0.007)
Urine osmolality (mosmol/kg H_2O)	485.01 (219.1)	530.01 (272.3)	364.8 (163.3)	444.4 (273.0)
Urine potassium (mmol/l)	28.3 (28.9)	50.4 (37.7)	28.3 (15.8)	37.0 (28.9)
Urine sodium (mmol/l)	58.7 (46.1)	82.8 (40.8)	81.3 (39.5)	94.2 (52.3)
K/Na ratio in urine	0.5 (0.4)	0.6 (0.4)	0.4 (0.2)	0.5 (0.4)
Transtubular potassium gradient	6.9 (6.7)	25.7 (28.9)	7.0 (7.0)	15.5 (22.1)
Glomerular filtration rate (ml/min)	86.9 (15.0)	82.9 (8.6)	93.0 (7.6)	86.9 (8.2)
B	Post-race			
Parameter	**R1**	**R2**	**R3**	**R4**
Haematocrit (%)	42.8 (3.0)	40.8 (2.8)	40.8 (2.9)	39.7 (2.9)
Plasma sodium (mmol/l)	137.4 (2.6)	136.8 (2.8)	138.7 (2.5)	139.2 (2.5)
Plasma potassium (mmol/l)	6.1 (1.0)	4.6 (0.9)	5.0 (0.6)	5.1 (0.5)
Plasma osmolality (mosmol/kg H_2O)	292.7 (4.2)	291.8 (5.0)	290.4 (6.0)	290.1 (4.4)
Urine specific gravity (g/ml)	1.021 (0.004)	1.022 (0.004)	1.019 (0.010)	1.025 (0.007)
Urine osmolality (mosmol/kg H_2O)	764.3 (196.9)	730.9 (241.4)	505.0 (312.0)	763.4 (291.4)
Urine potassium (mmol/l)	77.8 (25.4)	61.9 (47.9)	44.2 (27.8)	76.3 (31.2)
Urine sodium (mmol/l)	43.2 (30.6)	44.4 (44.9)	51.2 (34.7)	80.4 (58.9)
K/Na ratio in urine	2.3 (1.0)	2.3 (2.7)	0.9 (0.6)	2.2 (3.0)
Transtubular potassium gradient	35.6 (19.7)	40.3 (41.4)	20.5 (17.7)	42.8 (22.6)
Glomerular filtration rate (ml/min)	69.6 (12.4)	71.2 (9.9)	86.2 (9.5)	72.3 (12.2)
C	Change (absolute)			
Parameter	**R1**	**R2**	**R3**	**R4**
Haematocrit (%)	1.1 (3.2)	−1.0 (2.6)	−1.3 (2.0)*	−2.0 (2.2)
Plasma sodium (mmol/l)	−0.6 (3.9)	−0.9 (2.8)	−1.3 (2.6)	−2.6 (2.4)**
Plasma potassium (mmol/l)	−0.4 (1.7)	−0.1 (1.0)	−1.6 (1.1)**	−0.0 (0.5)
Plasma osmolality (mosmol/kg H_2O)	2.8 (4.2)	2.4 (6.2)	1.8 (5.8)	1.4 (5.5)
Urine specific gravity (g/ml)	0.006 (0.004)**	0.006 (0.006)**	0.006 (0.011)	0.010 (0.009)**
Urine osmolality (mosmol/kg H_2O)	279.3 (195.1)**	200.8 (342.4)*	114.2 (355.8)**	319.0 (326.9)**
Urine potassium (mmol/l)	49.5 (39.0)**	11.5 (22.9)	15.9 (35.9)	39.3 (40.6)**
Urine sodium (mmol/l)	−15.6 (37.5)	−37.8 (46.0)**	−30.1 (38.4)*	−13.8 (70.3)
K/Na ratio in urine	1.7 (0.7)**	1.7 (2.4)*	0.56 (0.7)*	1.7 (3.1)
Transtubular potassium gradient	28.7 (14.1)**	14.6 (46.4)	13.5 (20.0)*	27.3 (23.7)**
Glomerular filtration rate (ml/min)	−17.2 (14.7)**	−11.7 (9.8)**	−6.8 (6.1)**	−14.6 (14.2)**
D	Change (%)			
Parameter	**R1**	**R2**	**R3**	**R4**
Haematocrit (%)	2.8 (8.0)	−2.4 (6.1)	−3.1 (4.8)*	−4.8 (5.1)
Plasma sodium (mmol/l)	−0.4 (2.8)	−0.6 (2.0)	−0.9 (1.9)	−1.8 (1.7)**
Plasma potassium (mmol/l)	−6.3 (27.8)	−0.6 (22.9)	−24.6 (14.1)**	−1.0 (9.2)
Plasma osmolality (mosmol/kg H_2O)	0.9 (1.5)	0.8 (2.1)	0.6 (2.0)	0.5 (1.9)

Table 5 (A,B,C,D) - Changes in blood and urine parameters (R1,R2,R3,R4) in subjects without EAH, n = 50 *(Continued)*

Urine specific gravity (g/ml)	0.7 (0.4)**	0.5 (0.6)**	0.6 (1.1)	1.0 (0.9)**
Urine osmolality (mosmol/kg H_2O)	57.6 (85.3)**	37.9 (161.2)*	38.4 (195.6)**	71.8 (185.1)**
Urine potassium (mmol/l)	174.8 (458.2)**	22.9 (22.0)	56.3 (191.8)	106.2 (422.9)**
Urine sodium (mmol/l)	−26.5 (81.6)	−46.0 (118.1)**	−37.0 (36.1)*	−14.6 (105.2)
K/Na ratio in urine	359.9 (187.2)**	281.7 (327.6)*	148.7 (222.3)*	366.6 (347.9)
Transtubular potassium gradient	417.7 (575.1)**	56.9 (1185.7)	192.7 (2133.5)*	176.6 (1196.2)**
Glomerular filtration rate (ml/min)	−19.8 (14.7)**	−14.1 (11.7)**	−7.3 (6.7)**	−16.8 (13.9)**

Results are presented as mean (SD), *= p ≤ 0.05, **= p < 0.01.

intake was negatively related to post-race plasma [Na^+] ($r = 0.56, p < 0.05$).

Race 3 - R3 (24-hour running race)

Body mass decreased ($p < 0.05$), Δ body mass was -0.9 kg (1.4%). In two (16.7%) ultra-runners body mass increased by 0.1 kg and 1.0 kg, indicating overhydration according to Noakes et al. [39]. In the remaining 10 ultra-runners, body mass decreased between 0.3 kg and 2.7 kg, two (16.7%) ultra-runners were dehydrated. Δ body mass was neither related to Δ plasma [Na^+] nor race performance. Δ body mass ($r = 0.78, p < 0.001$), and % body mass ($r = 0.58, p = 0.05$) were positively related to post-race plasma [Na^+]. Race performance was negatively associated with post-race plasma [Na^+] ($r = -0.64, p < 0.05$), similarly as in R2. Post-race plasma [Na^+] was significantly and positively related to Δ plasma [Na^+] ($r = 0.78, p < 0.001$). Plasma volume increased by 5.9% (8.7%) ($p < 0.05$), while Δ plasma volume was not related to post-race plasma osmolality, or to post-race urine osmolality. Hematocrit and urine [Na^+] ($p < 0.05$), glomerular filtration race and plasma [K^+] ($p < 0.001$) significantly decreased. K^+/Na^+ ratio in urine increased ($p <$ 0.05), but was < 1. In contrast, urine osmolality increased significantly ($p < 0.001$) (Table 5). Ultra-runners consumed a total of 0.58 (0.38) l/h during a 24-hour running race. Fluid intake varied between 0.15-0.90 l/h and showed no association with race performance, body mass, Δ body mass, post-race plasma [Na^+], Δ plasma [Na^+], Δ plasma volume or post-race urine specific gravity.

Race 4 - R4 (multi-stage MTB race)

Body mass decreased ($p < 0.05$), Δ body mass was -1.6 kg (2.1%) after Stage 1 ($p < 0.001$); -1.7 kg (-2.3%) after Stage 2 ($p < 0.001$), and -1.3 kg (-1.7%) after Stage 3 ($p < 0.05$). Body mass decreased in all MTBers after Stage 1, three (21.4%) were dehydrated according to Noakes et al. [39]. In one (7.9%) MTBer, body mass remained stable, in another (7.9%) MTBer body mass increased by 0.1 kg, indicating overhydration, while in the remaining 12 MTBers body mass decreased between 0.3 kg and 3.9 kg, five (35.7%) MTBers were dehydrated after Stage 2. In three (21.4%) MTBers, body mass increased between 0.5 kg and 2.4 kg, they were overhydrated, and in the remaining 11 MTBers body mass

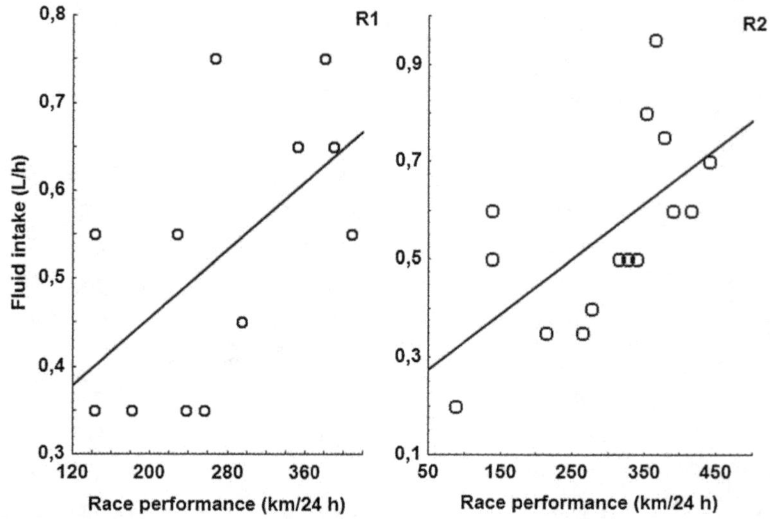

Figure 1 Fluid intake was positively related to race performance (R1: $r = 0.58, p = 0.05$; R2: $r = 0.63, p = 0.01$). R1: Czech Championship 24-hour MTB race' in Jihlava city, 24-hour MTB race, R2: ‚Bike Race Marathon Rohozec 24 hours' in Liberec city, 24-hour MTB race.

decreased between 0.6 kg and 3.4 kg, six (42.9%) MTBers were dehydrated after Stage 3. Δ body mass or % Δ body mass were neither related to Δ plasma [Na^+], post-race plasma [Na^+], nor race performance. Plasma [Na^+], and glomerular filtration race decreased significantly ($p < 0.001$), and plasma volume increased by 5.3% (5.7%), Δ plasma volume was not related to post-race plasma osmolality, or to post-race urine osmolality. Post-race plasma [Na^+] was significantly and positively related to Δ plasma [Na^+] ($r = 0.71$, $p < 0.001$). In contrast, urine specific gravity, urine osmolality and urine [K^+] increased significantly ($p < 0.001$), K^+/Na^+ ratio in urine did not increase significantly and was > 1 post-race. Urine specific gravity was associated with urine [K^+] ($r = 0.70$, $p < 0.001$). Transtubular potassium gradient increased significantly ($p < 0.001$) (Table 5). Multi-stage ultra-MTBers consumed approximately a total of 0.43 (0.3) l/h during every stage. Fluid intake varied between 0.2-0.85 l/h and showed no association with achieved race time from all stages. Fluid intake showed no correlation to post-race body mass, Δ body mass, post-race plasma [Na^+], Δ plasma [Na^+], Δ plasma volume or Δ urine specific gravity.

Discussion

The aim of the study was to investigate the prevalence of EAH in ultra-endurance athletes such as ultra-MTBers, ultra-runners and MTBers in four races held in the Czech Republic, Europe. The most important finding was that three (5.7%) of the 53 finishers developed post-race EAH with post-race plasma [Na^+] < 135 mmol/l. The prevalence of EAH in the Czech Republic was not higher than in other reports from Europe. Moreover, symptoms typical of EAH were also reported in normonatremic competitors.

Prevalence of EAH in all races (R1,R2,R3,R4)

The prevalence of post-race EAH varied from 0% to 8.3% in the individual races. No ultra-MTBer developed EAH in the 24-hour MTB race R1. One ultra-MTBer in the 24-hour MTB race (R2), one ultra-runner in the 24-hour running race (R3) and one MTBer in the multi-stage MTB race (R4) showed EAH with mild clinical symptoms. Furthermore, two (3.7%) athletes (R2) presented with pre-race EAH, and no finisher was pre- or post race hypernatremic. The work herein failed to support the hypothesis that the prevalence of EAH would be higher in 24-hour races compared with the multi-stage MTB race. The prevalence of EAH in all 24-hour races (R1,R2,R3) was 5.4% for 39 athletes and 7.1% for 14 athletes in the multi-stage MTB race (R4). The prevalence of EAH was lower in ultra-MTBers compared to ultra-runners and MTBers. The current work also demonstrated that the prevalence of EAH was higher in ultra-runners compared to ultra-MTBers. In contrast with the results of the current study, EAH occurred in more than 50% of the finishers of a 161-km ultramarathon in California which took place on single track mountain trails similar those in R1 and R2 in the present study [7]. Studies on EAH in ultra-running events in Switzerland [30] and New Zealand [9] reported prevalences of 0% and 4% respectively compared to the 8.3% reported here. The prevalence of EAH in ultra-MTBers (3.7%) and MTBers (7.1%) in the current study was also similar to studies of multi-stage MTB races in South Africa and the Alps [21,22], as well as single ultra-distance road cycling and MTB races in Switzerland [8,25-28]. On average, post-race EAH in the Czech Republic amounted to 5.7% and did not exceed 10%. Regarding existing reports on EAH in single ultra-distance running races [1,3,4,6-12,38,39], in MTB multi-stage races [21,22], in single ultra-distance MTB races [8,22,25,28] the prevalence rates in the Czech Republic were no higher in the present athletes.

An interesting finding was that the normonatremic group reported also symptoms typical for EAH. Muscle weakness, antidiuresis and breathing problems were the most reported post-race symptoms in finishers in the 24-hour cycling races (R1, R2). Moreover, swelling and myalgia occurred in the multi-stage race alongside reported muscle weakness. The presented problems with antidiuresis could be associated with dehydration and SIADH (syndrome of inappropriate secretion of antidiuretic hormone). On the contrary, symptoms like chills, stomach pain and irritability in runners (R3) were probably more associated with race performance and were influenced by weather conditions. Post-race, all finishers, both hyponatremic and normonatremic, presented without symptoms of altered mental status. No subject required medical attention for hyponatremia.

Regarding post-race symptoms associated with race performance reported by finishers with EAH, the ultra-MTBer EAH-A-R2 reported muscle weakness. This symptom was frequent in all cycling races (R1,R2,R4). We assume that it could be related to higher race intensity during the races since EAH-A-R2 was also in the top finishers of the race and a more difficult racing terrain compared to the flat course in a 24-hour ultra-running event. Muscle weakness could be also associated with hypovolemia [52]. The myalgia reported in EAH-B-R3 and EAH-C-R4 may have been attributed to the extreme physical demands of the respective races, in all hyponatremic cases TTKG gradient increased and was > 10, presumably indicating an increased activity of aldosterone [2,53]. We assume that athletes suffered a great stress. The swelling and antidiuresis in EAH-B-R3 and EAH-C-R4 may have been a result of fluid overload, thus further investigation is warranted. The consensus on EAH states that it left untreated, symptoms of EAH can digress rapidly [48], in the current study however, reported symptoms were left untreated in the aftermath of the races. Nonetheless, no severe symptomatic case of EAH encephalopathy associated with dehydration has been reported in literature [52]. Subjects EAH-A-R2, EAH-B-R3 and EAH-C-R4 were contacted 24 h and 72 h after their races. Each reported that they all were fully oriented and without evidence of altered mental status and they did not require medical attention for hyponatremia. Since no hyponatremic athlete used NSAIDs we propose that NSAIDs did not influence an prevalence of EAH in the present subjects. Because both groups with and without EAH reported similar symptoms, no subject required medical attention for post-race hyponatremia, and no finisher had seizures or respiratory mistress during or within 24 h of the race finishing, we conclude that no hyponatremic finisher had EAH encephalopathy or pulmonary edema.

Blood and urine parameters in hyponatremic finishers (n = 3)

Plasma volume increased in EAH-A-R2 and EAH-B-R3 and decreased in EAH-C-R4. Plasma osmolality remained stable and urine osmolality increased in all cases. In all hyponatremic cases (*i.e.* EAH-A-R2, EAH-B-R3 and EAH-C-R4) the transtubular potassium gradient increased and was > 10, presumably indicating an increased activity in aldosterone [54-56]. Previous work has suggested that EAH could promote rhabdomyolysis through changes in intracellular potassium or calcium concentrations [23]. Therefore, rhabdomyolysis could be a stimulus for EAH via the syndrome of SIADH mechanism [12,57] given the physiological demands of these races. EAH-A-R2 and EAH-B-R3 were hyperhydrated and EAH-C-R4 was dehydrated according to blood parameters. Hyponatremic cases EAH-A-R2 and EAH-B-R3 were dehydrated according to urinary parameters, however increased urinary sodium losses could be compatible with SIADH and they were overhydrated. Urine [Na^+] decreased only in EAH-C-R4 possibly due to stimulation of the RAAS. The lower plasma [Na^+] and the subsequent development of EAH in EAH-A-R2, EAH-B-R3 and EAH-C-R4 may be attributed to overdrinking, the retention of fluid because of inadequate suppression of vasopressin secretion, impaired mobilization of osmotically inactive sodium stores, and/or inappropriate inactivation of osmotically active sodium.

Changes in plasma [Na^+], plasma [K^+], hematocrit, plasma volume, and plasma osmolality in normonatremic finishers (n = 50)

Plasma [Na^+] remained stable with a non-significant decrease in all normonatremic finishers in the 24-hour races (R1-R3), but significantly decreased in the multi-stage race (R4). In the multi-stage race (R4) we must consider the possibility of interstitial swelling that does not dissipate between stages. Hematocrit was stable in R1, R2, R4, and decreased in R3, and was not related to fluid intake in either race. Furthermore, plasma [K^+] decreased in R3, although plasma [Na^+] did non-significantly decrease in this race. Plasma volume decreased in R1 and increased in R2, R3 and R4, and Δ plasma volume was not related to post-race plasma [Na^+] or Δ plasma [Na^+] in either race. The hemodilution seen in R2, R3 and R4 may have been a result of prolonged stress [23]. In longer ultra-endurance races plasma volume might increase, because ultra-athletes may retain a fluid reserve in the interstitial fluid of the extracellular fluid compartment [20,24], an increased plasma volume can be due to shift in body fluid. On the contrary, the reduction of plasma volume in R1 reflected in body mass reduction might be caused by dehydration, although the decreased plasma volume could be shown as a hemoconcentration due to the acute effect of strenuous endurance on hematological parameters [23]. The activation of the RAAS (renin-angiotensin-aldosterone-system) could lead to an enhanced retention of Na^+ and free water, resulting in an increase in plasma volume and a decrease in plasma [Na^+] [2,58]. Presumably, the increase in plasma volume in R2-R4 and the retention of water was due to an increased activity of both vasopressin and aldosterone [1,2,12,16,19,57,59].

Urinary indices are suggested as parameters of hydration status [53,60,61], however several studies have documented that they are not accurate measures of hydration status immediately following exercise activity [62] and plasma osmolality would be a better marker of hydration status in the situation of acute dehydration [58,63]. Plasma osmolality remained stable in all races with a non-significant increase despite a decrease in plasma [K^+] in R3 and a decrease in plasma [Na^+] in R4. An increase in transtubular potassium gradient could be responsible for a preservation of both plasma [Na^+] and body water during ultra-endurance exercise due to an increased activity of aldosterone [8]. We assume that this may explain why plasma osmolality was stable in all races despite a loss in body mass. These findings support recent findings in Tam et al. [63] that the body primarily defends plasma [Na^+] and aids at maintaining [Na^+] and osmolality in plasma, but not body mass during endurance performance. In ultra-marathoners, plasma [Na^+] and plasma osmolality are well regulated and do not change while drinking *ad libitum* [58].

Changes in urine [Na^+], urine [K^+], urine specific gravity and urine osmolality in normonatremic finishers (n = 50)

Since hematological parameters such as plasma [Na^+] or hematocrit were not valid indicators for the detection of mild hypohydration [61], urine parameters such as colour, urine specific gravity, and urine osmolality were considered to be valid indices of hydration status [61]. The decrease in body mass might be due to dehydration since urine specific gravity as a sign of dehydration [60,61] significantly increased in all cycling races (R1,R2, R4), and non-significantly increased in R3. Cyclists (R1, R2,R4) lost approximately 2.3% of body mass, with urine specific gravity of > 1.020 mg/l indicating dehydration [64], ultra-runners (R3) were minimally dehydrated according to changes in urine specific gravity.

On the contrary, the use of urine specific gravity as a marker of hydration status is time-dependent and shows only chronic dehydration, but not acute dehydration [53]. In ultra-endurance races, chronic dehydration seemed to result in a reduced renal function [8,55,56], because during long endurance performances renal blood flow and glomerular filtration rates decrease and limit the delivery of filtrate to the diluting segments of the kidney [55]. The increase in urine osmolality in all races (R1-R4) might be due to an increase in water permeability in the kidney, matching the fact that athletes urinated less frequently [2]. This could lead to impairments of free water excretion in R1, R2 and R4 with indicators of a more chronic than an acute dehydration. Post-race symptoms reported by finishers in all races indicated this hypothesis. Glomerular filtration race significantly decreased and urine osmolality increased and it seemed to be a result in a change in renal function.

Arginine vasopressin secretion, aldosterone activity and the prevalence of EAH

SIADH is also considered as a potentional mechanism to develop EAH [39], because arginine vasopressin (AVP) regulates body's retention of water. Changes in sodium and potassium concentrations and osmolality in plasma and urine are also indirect markers for the activity of aldosterone [2,4,16,19,45] and AVP-secretion [12,42,43,45,57,59]. Urine [K^+] significantly increased in R1 and R4, and urine specific gravity was associated with post-race urine [K^+] in R4. On the contrary, urine [K^+] in R2 and R3 remained stable, and urine [Na^+] significantly decreased in R2 and R3, although the K^+/Na^+ ratio in urine was < 1 only in R3.

The increased urinary [Na^+] losses could be compatible with SIADH in R2 and R3. In all races, the transtubular potassium gradient increased and was > 10 in R1, R3 and R4, probably due to an increased aldosterone activity. This change in aldosterone is associated with a change in the K^+/Na^+-ratio in urine, a positive ratio suggests an increased aldosterone activity [16,18]. In all races (R1-R4), the K^+/Na^+-ratio in urine increased. The K^+/Na^+-ratio in urine was < 1.0 only in R3, suggesting that more potassium than sodium was excreted through the kidney, however the K^+/Na^+-ratio in urine was > 1 in R1, R2 and R4. Body water increase with simultaneous dehydration (R2-R4) might be possibly due to endocrine-induced renal water retention, in order to maintain the metabolic processes that are required for energy supply and blood flow during prolonged exercise [54].

Finishers were more hyperhydrated than dehydrated in R3. Apart from fluid overload, however, other mechanisms may have lead to water retention in R3, such as protein catabolism [54]. In a 24-hour running race, Fellmann et al. [59] found an increase in plasma volume, aldosterone and AVP. Stuempfle et al. [24] showed an increased activity of both aldosterone and AVP after an ultra-endurance race. Alternatively, there might be also an impairment in mobilization of osmotically-inactive sodium stores or inappropriate inactivation of osmotically-active sodium [11,18]. These cannot be determined from the present study.

Fluid overload and the prevalence of EAH

Fluid overload is considered as the main risk factor for EAH [39,48]. We observed a higher than recommended fluid intake in EAH-A-R2. Fluid intake rates in EAH-B-R3 and EAH-C-R4 were at the upper limits of recommended fluid intakes. However, we did not observe the combination of overhydration and hyponatremia in the present work.

We expected that the prevalence of EAH would be higher in the 24-hour races (R1-R3) compared with the multi-stage MTB race (R4) due to the higher possibility of excessive drinking and their duration. This hypothesis was not supported in the present subjects since relative fluid consumption was similar in all groups (R1-R4) despite the different length of the races and the different weather conditions. Considering the aid stations and the nutrition provided, the races were comparable and only one ultra-MTBer in R1 and two MTBers in R4 used backpack type hydration packs. The average fluid intake in all races was 0.51 (0.1%) l/h which was in accordance with the International Marathon Medical Directors Association (IMMDA) [65] which recommends drinking *ad libitum* between 0.4 l/h and 0.8 l/h.

Fluid intake was the highest in R3 which had the coldest weather conditions and the highest prevalence of EAH (8.3%). In single stage ultra-distance races, Stuempfle et al. [24] reported a fluid overload caused by excessive fluid consumption during cold weather in a 161-km race in Alaska leading to both an increase in plasma volume and a decrease in plasma [Na^+], although no athletes were classified as hyponatremic. Similar findings were also reported in 100-km ultra-marathoners [3] where the prevalence of EAH (4.8%) was in line with the findings of a study on 24-hour ultra-marathon runners [30]. Paradoxically, in R4 taking place in the warmest conditions, the finishers had the lowest fluid intake. In studies of multi-stage MTB races [21,22] fluid intake also did not exceed 0.75 l/h and was between 0.34 l/h and 0.55 l/h in the respective races. Although in both multi-stage races [21,22] no case of EAH was documented, we found one hyponatremic case in R4 (EAH-C-R4). In another study investigating 196 road cyclists in a 109-km cycling race one athlete developed hyponatremic encephalopathy despite a modest fluid intake [64].

Fluid intake was inversely related to post-race plasma [Na^+] in R2, and also the highest number of overhydrated but normonatremic finishers from all races according to Noakes et al. [39] occurred in this race, although an average overall fluid intake was in line with IMMDA recommendations. Regarding these findings, fluid intake was probably responsible for hyperhydration in four normonatremic finishers in R2. This finding underlines the classic hypothesis of the pathogenesis of EAH as reported by Noakes at al. [39]. On the contrary, only one overhydrated normonatremic finisher occurred in R1 with no prevalence of EAH. In agreement with the findings of Knechtle et al. [3], there was a decrease in body mass, plasma [Na^+] showed no changes, and Δ body mass was not related to fluid intake in R1. The hourly fluid intake of 0.49 l (0.30 l - 0.70 l) in R1 was not sufficient to prevent dehydration, but with regards to *ad libitum* fluid intake, body fluid homeostasis was maintained. Since fluid intake was not related to Δ plasma volume nor to Δ plasma [Na^+] in R1, the effective homeostasis must result from the buffering effect of the exchangeable osmotically inactive body sodium stores [39]. Regardless of the modest fluid consumption in all groups (R1-R4), finishers in R2, R3 and R4 were more hyperhydrated than euhydrated, and factors other than fluid intake seemed responsible for fluid regulation in ultra-athletes, such as a hormonal regulation by aldosterone [2,19,21,24,57] and inappropriate levels of the hormone vasopressin [42,43] and the exchangeable osmotically inactive body sodium stores [39].

Changes in body mass and prevalence in EAH

An important finding of this study was that of the three participants who were hyponatremic post-race, no finisher showed an increase in body mass. Both EAH-A-R2 and EAH-B-R3 were euhydrated, while EAH-C-R4 was dehydrated as defined by Noakes et al. [39]. Another observation from our study was that body mass decreased in all normonatremic ultra-endurance athletes (ultra-MTBers, ultra-runners and MTBers) in the 24-hour races (R1-R3), and in the multi-stage MTB race (R4). Δ body mass varied from a 6.6% loss in body mass to a 3.4% gain in body mass. EAH is more commonly associated with overhydration. In a recent study by Hoffman et al. [11], 18.5% of the finishers were dehydrated. Of those with EAH, 35.6% were euhydrated, and 35.6% were dehydrated. In 887 finishers of a 161-km ultramarathon, Δ body mass varied from an 8% loss to a 10% gain [11]. Top finishers in the ultra-MTBers (R1,R2) and the ultra-runners (R3) varied in Δ body mass from a 0.7% gain to a 6.6% loss and in the MTBers (R4) from a 3.4% gain in body mass to a 4.3% loss in body mass. On average, finishers in R1-R4 were euhydrated as defined by Noakes [39].

An extremely hot or cold environment is considered as a risk factor for EAH [12,40], however we found no relationship between the prevalence of EAH and the ambient temperature in the present study. The 24-hour MTB race (R1) was held in a warm weather with low humidity during the whole race and the multi-stage race (R4) was held in typical hot summer weather, however with higher humidity (Table 1). The 24-hour MTB race (R2) was in more variable weather conditions with some precipitations, higher temperature fluctuations and high humidity (Table 1). The 24-h running race (R3) was held in colder weather with heavy precipitations compared with races R1, R2 or R4. In a recent study with 887 observations of weight change in a 161-km running race, Hoffman et al. [11] found significant correlations for percentage Δ body mass and percentage of dehydrated runners with ambient temperature. In the 24-hour races R1 and R2 large differences in ambient temperature appeared during the day and night, which are similar to the changes seen by Lebus et al. in the ultra-runners in a 161-km ultra-marathon [7]. The lowest Δ body mass in R3 might be also due to a colder temperature than in other races, because of a wind chill and heavy raining during the race, there was probably less sweat loss. R1 and R4 were held in favorable weather conditions in contrast with the colder ambient temperatures in R2 and R3, moreover accompanied with rain during the whole race. The highest number of dehydrated athletes was in R4 (the multi-stage race), on the contrary, the least number of overhydrated finishers was in R1 (the 24-hour MTB race) with no case of EAH. Higher Δ body mass were seen in R1 and R4 compared to races held under colder conditions (R2,R3). Although there were large differences in ambient temperatures during the day and night, EAH did not occur in R1 in very high ambient temperature. Therefore we concluded that like in Hoffman et al. [11] and Knechtle et al. [15] the environmental conditions probably had an influence on race performance, but not on the prevalence of EAH in our subjects in these concrete races. The present work is also in agreement with previous studies [11,38] showing that while a greater ambient temperature was associated with the number of dehydrated finishers, it was not associated with a larger number of overhydrated finishers.

The hypothesis that body mass losses would have no influence on race performance [11] was supported in R2 (the 24-hour MTB race). Δ body mass was negatively related to race performance, finishers with the greatest body mass losses tended to have a better race performance such as a higher number of achieved kilometers. The significant relationship between percentage Δ body mass and race time showed that the fastest runners tended to lose more body mass as observed by Hoffman et al. [11] in a 161-km ultra-marathon and Kao et al. [32] in a 24-hour running race. Also, in Zouhal et al. [47] a loss in body mass did not affect performance, and in Knechtle et al. [15] faster runners in a 100-km ultra-marathon lost more body mass than slower runners. These data support the finding that Δ body mass during exercise may not reflect exact changes in hydration status [20,60], and a loss in body mass did not impair race performance. Presumably, the decrease in body mass in the present athletes in R2 could also be due to dehydration [60], or changes in body mass representing a balance of fluid and energy intake and fluid and energy losses from external and internal sources with significant fat mass losses during the race [26,37]. We assume that the loss in body mass could be also due to a substrate losses as well as fluid losses.

The additional finding that in any race post-race body mass or Δ body mass was negatively related to post-race plasma [Na^+] warrants further investigation. These findings contrast with those from previous studies of other endurance events where post-race plasma [Na^+] has been found to be negatively related to percentage Δ body mass [1,3,44,53]. Moreover, Δ body mass and % Δ body mass were positively related to post-race plasma [Na^+] in ultra-runners (R3). Finishers with lower levels of plasma [Na^+] had higher losses in body mass. A direct positive relationship between post-race plasma [Na^+] and Δ body mass was reported by Hoffman et al. [11,38], Lebus et al. [7] and by Reid et al. [66], in contrast to what has been observed for many other races. Hoffman et al. [11] provided in the latest study the other side of the inverted-U curve to support the depletional model of EAH. Sodium losses, impairment in mobilization of osmotically inactive sodium stores and/or inappropriate inactivation of osmotically active sodium are alternative explanations. The relative importance of each of these factors cannot be determined from the present study.

Race pace and prevalence of EAH

Despite other influences, a lower race pace could also increase the risk of EAH [39]. We hypothesized that the prevalence of EAH would be higher in ultra-runners in a 24-hour race, since they compete at a slower pace compared to ultra-cyclists in a 24-hour race. The important finding was that two (4.9%) of all 41 cyclists and one (8.3%) of 12 runners in our study developed EAH which was consistent with our premises. It should be taken into account that race speed and the number of achieved kilometers (*i.e.* race performance) during a 24-hour race might depend on physical condition, motivation, tactics or other factors [35,36,66].

The performance of the best athletes in a 24-hour MTB race was as fast at the end as at the beginning of a race, and the decrease or the increase in race speed has to do with tactics in the race, not overall pace [66]. It is difficult to compare race speed between cyclists and runners. However, the comparison of race performance of cases with EAH showed different results. In the 24-hour MTB races, EAH-A-R2 was a cyclist with a higher speed (18.4 km/h) and a better race performance (*i.e.* 9th place from 116 participants in solo category) in comparison with the other finishers in R2 (Table 2). EAH-B-R3 was even the best in absolute ranking (*i.e.* 1st place from 48 participants) with an average running speed of 9.2 km/h. Moreover, in R2 and R3, race performance was negatively associated with post-race plasma [Na^+]. Finishers with lower post-race [Na^+] in R2 and R3 achieved more kilometers during the 24 hours. These findings supported our results, where two of three hyponatremic athletes in our study were among the top finishers in our races. Presumably, the specific character of 24-hour races might explain this contradictory finding. The better performance seen in the faster runners is influenced by numerous reasons, such as the motivation to achieve a higher number of kilometers or better race time [35,36,66]. On the contrary, EAH-C-R4 was one of the slower cyclists with the absolute ranking 158th place from 160 finishers, and with an average cycling speed of 6.5 km/h. Therefore, only in EAH-C-R4 we can assume that race speed was one of the factors which influenced EAH in our tested group.

Fluid intake and race performance

An important finding was the fact that in the ultra-MTBers (R1,R2), fluid intake was positively related to the number of kilometers achieved during 24-hour MTB race, which is in agreement with previous studies [3,15,25,30,47]. The ultra-MTBers in the 24-hour MTB races R1 and R2 who drank more finished ahead of those who drank less. Furthermore, the ultra-MTBers in 24-hour MTB R2 with greater body mass losses achieved more kilometers in the race than those with lower body mass losses.

In a recent study, Knechtle et al. showed similar findings in 24-hour ultra-runners [30]. In contrast to the ultra-MTBers in R1 and R2, in the ultra-runners in R3 fluid intake was not related to race performance. We assume that the ultra-MTBers in R1 and R2 with a better race performance who did not develop EAH drank more than the others, however, still in accordance with IMMDA. In 219 runners in a 100-km ultra-marathon, the faster runners had a support crew to provide drinks in contrast to the slower runners with no support crew [15]. Presumably, also our faster ultra-MTBers used this possibility of an additional fluid intake. In Knechtle et al. [15], the faster athletes who probably had a higher sweating rate lost more fluids and consequently drank more fluids. The finding that fluid intake was positively correlated with race performance suggests that athletes in R1 and R2 were drinking appropriately. Faster athletes were working harder and required more water than slower athletes. We hypothesised that in cases of fluid overload, fluid intake would be related to post-race body mass, Δ body mass, post-race plasma [Na^+], and Δ plasma [Na^+], respectively. In none of the races was fluid intake associated with post-race body mass, Δ body mass, Δ plasma [Na^+], Δ plasma volume, or Δ urine specific gravity.

Another finding was that the finishers with a better race performance had lower post-race plasma [Na^+] in R2 and R3, and a higher body mass loss in R2. Also in Hoffman et al. [11], Knechtle et al. [15] and Noakes [63] faster runners tended to lose more body mass. Likewise, fluid intake was negatively associated with Δ body mass in a recent study [25]. In a 24-hour running race Δ body mass showed no association with post-race plasma [Na^+], however, no subject developed EAH [31]. Moreover, fluid intake correlated negatively to average running speed [31].

However, it is difficult to explain the decrease in body mass despite the increased fluid intake and the lower post-race plasma [Na^+]. In a recent study, faster runners lost more body mass, and faster runners drank more fluid than slower runners [65]. Also, faster ultra-MTBers in R2 lost more body mass although they drank more. We assume that the present ultra-athletes who ingested more fluid probably had a higher sweat loss during the race than the slower ones. The athletes who run the fastest will have the highest sweat rates. If they do not drink more than others they will finish with the greatest levels of body mass loss and hence the highest levels of dehydration [42]. In some instances fluid may have taken the place of food in terms of energy consumed. In a study of 2,135 endurance athletes including marathon runners and triathletes, plasma [Na^+] decreased despite of an increased fluid intake, however body mass also decreased [39].

Limitations

It was not possible in these races to determine urinary excretion of the finishers precisely since the athletes were not able to correctly record it during the race. Since ultra-endurance performance is associated with skeletal muscle damage [67], we have to investigate also the role of muscle damage in causing a decrease in skeletal muscle mass or fat mass.

Conclusions

Overall prevalence of EAH was 5.7% and was not higher compared to existing reports for other ultra-endurance athletes competing in other countries. No ultra-MTBer developed EAH in the 24-hour MTB race (R1). One ultra-MTBer in the 24-hour MTB race (R2), one ultra-runner in the 24-hour running race (R3) and one MTBer in the multi-stage MTB race (R4) developed EAH with mild symptoms. To support the trend of the prevalence of EAH in the Czech Republic and to clarify the cause it is necessary to observe ultra-endurance athletes in a number of different races or a long time and repeatedly. The lower plasma sodium and the subsequent development of EAH may be attributed to overdrinking, a pituitary secretion of the hormone vasopressin, impaired mobilization of osmotically inactive sodium stores, and/or inappropriate inactivation of osmotically active sodium. Future studies need to investigate the change in body composition. A loss in body mass of >3% does not appear to adversely affect performance despite *ad libitum* fluid consumption being advised.

Competing interests

The authors declare that they have no competing interests.

Authors' contributions

DCH and BK developed the objectives of the study and intervention, DCH managed recruitment and data collection, DCH and AZ participated in the practical measurement in all field studies, DCH and IT performed statistical analysis, DCH, BK and TR lead the drafting of the manuscript, interpreted the findings and critically reviewed the manuscript. All authors read and approved the final manuscript.

Acknowledgements

The authors gratefully acknowledge the athletes for their splendid cooperation without which this study could not have been done. We thank the organizers and the medical crew of the ‚Czech Championship 24-hour MTB race' in Jihlava (R1), the ‚Bike Race Marathon Rohozec' in Liberec (R2), the ‚Sri Chinmoy Self-transcendence Running Marathon 24-hour race' in Kladno (R3) and the 'Trilogy Mountain Bike Stage Race' in Teplice nad Metují (R4) for their generous support. A special thank goes to the laboratory staff of the University Hospital ‚U Svaté Anny' in Brno, Czech Republic, for their efforts in analyzing hematological and biochemical samples even during the night-times. A special thank goes to Marcus Shortall from the Institute of Technology Tallaght for his help with translation and the extensively correction of the whole text.

Author details

[1]Centre of Sports Activities, Brno University of Technology, Brno, Czech Republic. [2]Institute of General Practise and for Health Services Research, University of Zurich, Zurich, Switzerland. [3]Institute of Experimental Biology, Faculty of Science, Masaryk University, Brno, Czech Republic. [4]Faculty of Forestry and Wood Sciences, Czech University of Life Sciences, Prague, Czech Republic. [5]Facharzt FMH für Allgemeinmedizin, Gesundheitszentrum St. Gallen, Vadianstrasse 26, 9001 St. Gallen, Switzerland.

References

1. Bűrge J, Knechtle B, Knechtle P, Gnädinger M, Rűst CA, Rosemann T: **Maintained serum sodium in male ultra-marathoners – the role of fluid intake, vasopressin, and aldosterone in fluid and electrolyte regulation.** *Horm Metab Res* 2011, **43**(9):646–652.

2. Bracher A, Knechtle B, Gnädinger M, Bürge J, Rüst CA, Knechtle P, Rosemann T: **Fluid intake and changes in limb volumes in male ultra-marathoners: does fluid overload lead to peripheral oedema?** *Eur J Appl Physiol* 2011, **112**(3):991–1003.
3. Knechtle B, Knechtle P, Rosemann T: **Do male 100-km ultra-marathoners over drink?** *Int J Sports Physiol Perform* 2011, **6**(2):195–207.
4. Knechtle B, Senn O, Imoberdorf R, Joleska I, Wirth A, Knechtle P, Rosemann T: **Maintained total body water content and serum sodium concentrations despite body mass loss in female ultra-runners drinking ad libitum during a 100 km race.** *Asia Pac J Clin Nutr* 2010, **19**(1):83–90.
5. Knechtle B, Wirth A, Knechtle P, Rosemann T: **Increase of total body water with decrease of body mass while running 100 km nonstop – formation of edema?** *Res Q Exerc Sport* 2009, **80**(3):593–603.
6. Knechtle B, Knechtle P, Rosemann T: **Low prevalence of exercise associated hyponatremia in male 100 km ultra-marathon runners in Switzerland.** *Eur J Appl Physiol* 2011, **111**(6):1007–1016.
7. Lebus DK, Casazza GA, Hoffman MD, Van Loan MD: **Can changes in body mass and total body water accurately predict hyponatremia after a 161-km running race?** *Clin J Sport Med* 2010, **20**(3):193–199.
8. Knechtle B, Gnädinger M, Knechtle P, Imoberdorf R, Kohler G, Ballmer P, Rosemann T, Senn O: **Prevalence of exercise-associated hyponatremia in male ultra endurance athletes.** *Clin J Sport Med* 2011, **21**(3):226–232.
9. Page AJ, Reid SA, Speedy DB, Mulligan GP, Thompson J: **Exercise-associated hyponatremia, renal function, and nonsteroidal anti-inflammatory drug use in an ultra endurance mountain run.** *Clin J Sport Med* 2007, **17**(1):43–48.
10. Reid SA, King MJ: **Serum biochemistry and morbidity among runners presenting for medical care after an Australian mountain ultramarathon.** *Clin J Sport Med* 2007, **17**(4):307–310.
11. Hoffman MD, Hew-Butler T, Stuempfle KJ: **Exercise-associated hyponatremia and hydration status in 161-km ultramarathoners.** *Med Sci Sports Exerc* 2013, **45**(4):784–791.
12. Hew-Butler T, Jordaan E, Stuempfle KJ, Speedy DB, Siegel AJ, Noakes TD, Soldin SJ, Verbalis JG: **Osmotic and nonosmotic regulative of arginine vasopressin during prolonged endurance exercise.** *J Clin Endocrinol Metab* 2008, **93**(6):2072–2078.
13. Fallon KE, Sivyer G, Sivyer K, Dare A: **The biochemistry of runners in a 1600 km ultramarathon.** *Br J Sports Med* 1999, **33**(4):264–269.
14. Cejka C, Knechtle B, Knechtle P, Rüst CA, Rosemann T: **An increased fluid intake leads to feet swelling in 100-km ultra-marathoners – an observational field study.** *J Int Soc Sports Nutr* 2012, **9**(11):1–10.
15. Knechtle B, Knechtle P, Wirth A, Rüst CA, Rosemann T: **A faster running speed is associated with a greater body weight loss in 100-km ultra-marathoners.** *J Sports Sci* 2012, **30**(11):1131–1140.
16. Knechtle B, Morales NP, Gonzáles ER, Gutierrez AA, Sevilla JN, Gómez RA, Robledo AR, Rodríguez AL, Fraire OS, Antonie JL, Lopez LC, Kohler G, Rosemann T: **Effects of a multistage ultraendurance triathlon on aldosterone, vasopressin, extracellular water and urine electrolytes.** *Scot Med J* 2012, **57**(1):26–32.
17. Meyer M, Knechtle B, Bürge J, Knechtle P, Mrazek C, Wirth A, Ellenrieder B, Rüst CA, Rosemann T: **Ad libitum intake leads to no leg swelling in male Ironman triathletes – an observational field study.** *J Int Soc Sports Nutr* 2012, **9**(1):1–13.
18. Rüst CA, Knechtle B, Knechtle P, Rosemann T: **Higher prevalence of exercise-associated hyponatremia in Triple iron ultra-triathletes than reported for Ironman triathletes.** *Chin J Physiol* 2012, **55**(3):147–155.
19. Fellmann N, Sagnol M, Bedu M, Falgairette G, Van Praagh E, Gaillard G, Jouanel P, Coudert J: **Enzymatic and hormonal responses following a 24 h endurance run and a 10 h triathlon race.** *Eur J Appl Physiol* 1988, **57**:545–553.
20. Hew-Butler T, Collins M, Bosh A, Sharwood K, Wilson G, Armstrong M, Jennings C, Swart J, Noakes T: **Maintenance of plasma volume and serum sodium concentration despite body weight loss in ironman triathletes.** *Clin J Sport Med* 2007, **17**(2):116–122.
21. Rose SC, Peters-Futre EM: **Ad libitum adjustments to fluid intake during cool environmental conditions maintain hydration status during a 3-day mountain bike race.** *Brit J Sports Med* 2010, **44**:430–436.
22. Schenk K, Gatterer H, Ferrari M, Ferrari P, Cascio VL, Burtscher M: **Bike Transalp 2008: liquid intake and its effect on the body's fluid homeostasis in the course of a multistage, cross country, MTB marathon race in the central Alps.** *Clin J Sport Med* 2010, **20**(1):47–52.
23. Wirnitzer C, Faulhaber M: **Hemoglobin and hematocrit during an 8 day mountain bike race.** *J Sports Sci Med* 2007, **6**:265–266.
24. Stuempfle KJ, Lehmann DR, Case HS, Hughes SL, Evans D: **Change in serum sodium concentration during a cold weather ultradistance race.** *Clin J Sport Med* 2003, **13**(3):171–175.
25. Rüst CA, Knechtle B, Knechtle P, Rosemann T: **No case of exercise-associated hyponatraemia in top male ultra-endurance cyclists: the 'Swiss Cycling Marathon'.** *Eur J Appl Physiol* 2012, **112**(2):689–697.
26. Knechtle B, Wirth A, Knechtle P, Rosemann T: **An ultra-cycling race leads to no decrease in skeletal muscle mass.** *Int J Sports Med* 2009, **30**(3):163–167.
27. Knechtle B, Knechtle P, Rosemann T, Senn O: **No dehydration in mountain bike ultra-marathoners.** *Clin J Sport Med* 2009, **19**(5):415–420.
28. Knechtle B, Knechtle P, Roseman T: **No case of exercise-associated hyponatraemia in male ultra-endurance mountain bikers in the 'Swiss Bike Masters'.** *Chin J Physiol* 2011, **54**(6):379–384.
29. Knechtle B, Knechtle P, Müller G, Zwyssig D: **Energieumsatz an einem 24 stunden Radrennen: Verhalten von Körpergewicht und Subkutanfett.** *Österreichisches J für Sportmedizin* 2003, **33**:11–18.
30. Knechtle B, Knechtle P, Rosemann T: **No exercise-associated hyponatremia found in an observational field study of male ultra-marathoners participating in a 24-hour ultra-run.** *Phys Sportsmed* 2010, **38**(4):94–100.
31. Knechtle B, Wirth A, Knechtle P, Rosemann T, Senn O: **Do ultra-runners in a 24-h run really dehydrate?** *Irish J Med Sci* 2011, **180**(1):129–134.
32. Kao WF, Shyu CL, Yang XW, Hsu TF, Chen JJ, Kao WC, Polun C, Huang YJ, Kuo FC, Huang CI, Lee CH: **Athletic performance and serial weight changes during 12- and 24-hour ultra-marathons.** *Clin J Sports Med* 2008, **18**(2):155–158.
33. Knechtle B, Knechtle P, Kohler G, Rosemann T: **Does a 24-hour ultra-swim lead to dehydration?** *J Hum Sport Exerc* 2011, **6**(1):68–79.
34. Rüst CA, Knechtle B, Knechtle P, Rosemann T: **A comparison of anthropometric and training characteristics between recreational male marathoners and 24-hour ultra-marathoners.** *Open Access J Sports Med* 2012, **3**:121–129.
35. Knechtle B, Knechtle P, Rosemann T: **No association of skin-fold thicknesses and training with race performance in male ultraendurance runners in a 24-hour run.** *J Hum Sport Exerc* 2011, **6**(1):94–100.
36. Knechtle B, Knechtle P, Rüst CA, Rosemann T: **Leg skinfold thicknesses and race performance in male 24-hour ultra-marathoners.** *Proc (Bayl Univ Med Cent)* 2011, **24**(2):110–114.
37. Raschka C, Plath M: **Body fat compartment and its relationship to food intake and clinical chemical parameters during extreme endurance performance.** *Schweiz Z Sportmed* 1992, **40**(1):13–25.
38. Hoffman MD, Stuempfle KJ, Rogers IR, Weschler LB, Hew-Butler T: **Hyponatremia in the 2009 161-km Western States Endurance Run.** *Int J Sports Physiol Perform* 2012, **7**(1):6–10.
39. Noakes TD, Sharwood K, Speedy D, Hew T, Reid S, Dugas J, Almond C, Wharam P, Weschler L: **Three independent biological mechanisms cause exercise-associated hyponatremia:evidence from 2, 135 weighed competitive athletic performances.** *Proc Natl Acad Sci USA* 2005, **102**(51):18550–18555.
40. Rosner MH: **Exercise-associated hyponatremia.** *Semin Nephrol* 2009, **29**(3):271–281.
41. Reid SA, Speedy DB, Thompson JM, Noakes TD, Mulligan G, Page T, Campbell RG, Milne C: **Study of hematological and biochemical parameters in runners competing a standard marathon.** *Clin J Sport Med* 2004, **14**(6):344–353.
42. Noakes T: *Waterlogged. The Serious Problem of Over Hydration in Endurance Sports.* New Zealand: Human Kinetics; 2012.
43. Verbalis JG: **Disorders of body water homeostasis.** *Best Pract Res Clin Endocrinol Metab* 2003, **17**(4):471–503.
44. Knechtle B, Duff B, Schulze I, Kohler G: **A multi-stage ultra-endurance run over 1,200 km leads to a continuous accumulation of total body water.** *J Sports Sci Med* 2008, **7**:357–364.
45. Knechtle B, Kiouplidis K, Knechtle P, Imoberdorf R, Ballmer P: **Does a multi-stage ultra-endurance run cause de-or hyperhydration?** *J Hum Sport Exerc* 2010, **5**(1):59–70.
46. Rüst CA, Knechtle B, Knechtle P, Wirth A, Rosemann T: **Body mass change and ultraendurance performance: a decrease in body mass is associated with an increased running speed in male 100-km ultramarathoners.** *J Strength Cond Res* 2012, **26**(6):1505–1516.
47. Zouhal H, Groussard C, Minter G, Vincent S, Cretual A, Gratas-Delamarche A, Delamarche P, Noakes TD: **Inverse relationship between percentage body**

weight change and finishing time in 643 forty-two kilometer marathon runners. *Br J Sports Med* 2011, **45**(14):1101–1105.

48. Hew-Butler T, Almond C, Ayus JC, Dugas J, Meeuwisse W, Noakes T, Reid S, Siegel A, Speedy D, Stuempfle K, Verbalis J, Weschler L: **Exercise-associated hyponatremia (EAH) consensus panel. Consensus statement of the 1st International exercise-associated hyponatremia consensus development conference, Cape Town, South Africa 2005.** *Clin J Sport Med* 2005, **15**(4):208–213.
49. West ML, Marsden PA, Richardson RM, Zettle RM, Halperin ML: **New clinical approach to evaluate disorders of potassium excretion.** *Miner Electrolyte Metab* 1986, **12**(4):234–238.
50. Levey AS, Bosh JP, Lewis JB, Greene T, Rogers N, Roth D: **A more accurate method to estimate glomerular filtration rate from serum creatinine: a new prediction equation. Modification of diet in renal disease study group.** *Ann Intern Med* 1999, **130**(6):461–470.
51. Van Beaumont W: **Evaluation of hemoconcentration from hematocrit measurements.** *J Appl Physiol* 1972, **32:**712–713.
52. Gordillo R, Kumar J, Woroniecki RP: **Disorders of sodium homeostasis.** In *Fluids and Electrolytes in Pediatrics.* 1st edition. Edited by Feld LG, Kaskel FJ, Frederick J. New York: Humana Press; 2010:47–53.
53. American College of Sports Medicine, Sawka MN, Burke LM, Eichner ER, Maughan RJ, Montain SJ, Stachenfeld NS: **American college of sports medicine position stand. Exercise and fluid replacement.** *Med Sci Sports Exerc* 2007, **39**(2):377–390.
54. Knechtle B, Knechtle P, Kohler G: **The effects of 1,000 km nonstop cycling on fat mass and skeletal muscle mass.** *Res Sports Med* 2011, **19**(3):170–185.
55. Irving RA, Noakes TD, Irving GA, Van Zyl-Smit R: **The immediate and delayed effects of marathon running on renal function.** *J Urol* 1986, **136**(6):1176–1180.
56. Nagashima K, Wu J, Kavouras SA, Mack GW: **Increased renal tubular sodium reabsorption during exercise-induced hypervolemia in humans.** *J Appl Physiol* 2001, **91**(3):1129–1236.
57. Siegel AJ, Verbalis JG, Clement S, Mendelson JH, Mello NK, Adner M, Shirey T, Glowacki J, Lewandrowski EL: **Hyponatremia in marathon runners due to inappropriate arginine vasopressin secretion.** *Am J Med* 2007, **120:**11–17.
58. Tam N, Hew-Butler T, Papadopoulou E, Nolte H, Noakes TD: **Fluid intake and changes in blood chemistry, running speed and body mass during an 80 km mountain trail race.** *Med Sport* 2009, **13**(2):108–115.
59. Fellmann N, Ritz P, Ribeyre J, Beaufrère B, Delaître M, Coudert J: **Intracellular hyperhydration induced by a 7-day endurance race.** *Eur J Appl Physiol Occup Physiol* 1999, **80**(4):353–359.
60. Kavouras SA: **Assessing hydration status.** *Curr Opin Clin Nutr Metab Care* 2002, **5**(5):519–524.
61. Shirreffs SM: **Markers of hydration status.** *Eur J Clin Nutr* 2003, **57**(2):56–59.
62. Popowski LA, Oppliger RA, Lambert PG, Johnson RF, Gisolf CV: **Blood and urinary measures of hydration status during progressive acute dehydration.** *Med Sci Sports Exerc* 2001, **33**(5):747–753.
63. Tam N, Nolte HW, Noakes TD: **Changes in total body water content during running races of 21.1 km and 56 km in athletes drinking ad libitum.** *Clin J Sport Med* 2011, **21**(3):218–225.
64. Dugas JP, Noakes TD: **Hyponatremic encelophathy despite a modest rate of fluid intake during a 109 km cycle race.** *Br J Sports Med* 2005, **39**(10):1–3.
65. Hew-Butler T, Verbalis JG, Noakes TD: **Updated fluid recommendation: position statement from the International marathon medical directors association (IMMDA).** *Clin J Sport Med* 2006, **16**(4):283–292.
66. Chlíbková D, Žákovská A, Tomášková I: **Predictor variables for 7-day race in ultra-marathoners.** *Procedia - Soc Behav Sci* 2012, **46:**2362–2366.
67. Skenderi KP, Kavouras SA, Anastasiou CA, Yiannakouris N, Matalas AL: **Exertional rhabdomyolysis during a 246-km continuous race.** *Med Sci Sports Exerc* 2005, **38**(6):1054–1057.

Cardiovascular and ride time-to-exhaustion effects of an energy drink

Michael T Nelson[1*], George R Biltz[1] and Donald R Dengel[1,2]

Abstract

Background: Currently, there are few studies on the cardiovascular and fatigue effects of commercially available energy drinks. This study investigated the effects of Monster energy drink (Monster Beverage Corporation, Corona, California), on resting heart rate (HR), heart rate variability (HRV), ride time-to-exhaustion, peak exercise HR, respiratory exchange ratio (RER), and peak rating of perceived exertion (RPE).

Methods: The study used a double-blind, randomized, placebo controlled, crossover design. After an 8-hr fast, 15 subjects consumed Monster Energy Drink (ED standardized to 2.0 mg * kg^{-1} caffeine) or a flavor-matched placebo preexercise. Resting HR and HRV were determined. After an initial submaximal workload for 30 minutes, subjects completed 10 min at 80% ventilatory threshold (VT) and rode until volitional fatigue at 100% VT.

Results: Resting HR was significantly different (ED: 65+/−10 bpm vs. placebo: 58+/−8 bpm, p = 0.02), but resting HRV was not different between the energy drink and placebo trials. Ride time-to-exhaustion was not significantly different between trials (ED: 45.5+/− 9.8 vs. placebo: 43.8+/−9.3 min, p = 0.62). No difference in peak RPE (ED: 9.1 +/− 0.5 vs. placebo: 9.0 +/− 0.8, p = 1.00) nor peak HR (ED: 177 +/− 11 vs. placebo: 175 +/− 12, p = 0.73) was seen. The RER at 30% of VT was significantly different (ED: 0.94 +/− 0.06 vs. placebo: 0.91 +/− 0.05, p = 0.046), but no difference between the two conditions were seen at the other intensities.

Conclusion: Although preexercise ingestion of the energy drink does increase resting HR there was no alteration in HRV parameters. Ride time-to-exhaustion was not enhanced.

Background

After a multivitamin, energy drinks (ED) are the most popular dietary supplement in the young adult population [1,2]. Despite their popularity, sparse data exists to support the efficacy and cardiovascular effects, especially in younger adults, which is the target audience [3]. In a small meta-analysis, Shah et al. [4] found that subjects had a 10 mm Hg increase in systolic blood pressure. The main ingredients in most commercially available energy drinks are carbohydrates, B vitamins, caffeine, taurine, herbs, and flavorings.

Caffeine and carbohydrates taken separately have been previously shown to increase exercise duration and capacity [5-9]. A limited number of published studies on preexercise ingestion of energy drinks, however have produced mixed results [10-15]. Some studies showed positive effects such as increased cycling time-trial performance [10], increased bench-press muscle endurance [11], decreased sprint times [13], and increased exercise time at 65-75% of maximum heart rate (HR) on a cycle ergometer [12]. Other studies though [11,14,15], have failed to show any beneficial effect.

Currently there are little data on the cardiovascular effects of energy drinks [16,17]. In addition to caffeine the amino acid taurine, a common energy drink ingredient, is theorized to have potential cardiac effects [18,19]. Bichler and colleagues [20] investigated the combination of caffeine and taurine vs. a placebo and found it actually caused a significant *decline* in heart rate.

The purpose of this study was to investigate a preexercise ingestion of Monster energy drink (Monster Beverage Corporation, Corona, California) on resting HR and HR variability in addition to ride time-to-exhaustion (TTE) in recreationally active young adults. We hypothesize that resting HR and HR variability preexercise will be altered and the ride TTE will be increased after the subjects consume the energy drink (ED standardized to 2.0 mg per

* Correspondence: michaeltnelson@yahoo.com
[1]School of Kinesiology, University of Minnesota, Minneapolis, MN, USA
Full list of author information is available at the end of the article

kilogram of body mass of caffeine) compared to a taste-matched placebo.

Methods

Participants

There were 15 recreationally active subjects (8 male and 7 female). They averaged (mean ± SD) 25.5 ± 4.1 years of age (men 24.1 ± 2.7, women 27.1 ± 5.0), weighed an average of 77.9 ± 18.4 kg (men 86.7 ± 17.6, women 67.9 ± 4.4), had an average body mass index of 25.1 ± 4.0 kg/m^2 (men 26.6 ± 3.6, women 23.4 ± 3.8), with an average percent body fat of 22.3 ± 8.4% (men 18.0 ± 7.4, women 27.3 ± 6.7), and had an average peak oxygen uptake of 39.5 ± 7.0 ml • kg^{-1} • min^{-1} (men 41.3 ± 3.0, women 37.6 ± 9.7).

Prior to testing, all participants were informed of the study details and procedures including all the potential risks. Participants completed the Physical Activity Readiness Questionnaire which assess their health history [21] and were excluded if they had any significant injury or illness in the previous two weeks. The protocol, informed consent, and related documentation were reviewed by the University of Minnesota Institutional Review Board for approval before the study started and conducted in accordance with their requirements.

Preliminary testing

Subjects were asked to make three visits to the Laboratory of Integrative Human Physiology (LIHP) on non-consecutive days. The three trips consisted of an initial peak aerobic capacity test and two ride time-to-exhaustion tests, all performed on a stationary electronically braked cycle ergometer (Lode Corival, Groningen, The Netherlands). Subjects were instructed to fast for a minimum of 8 hours previous to all exercise tests, to avoid any caffeine for 48 hours prior, and to not participate in exercise during the previous 24 hours. The 48 hour withdrawal of caffeine was considered adequate given the half-life of caffeine is about 4–6 hours [22]. An overnight fast was done to minimize any effect of the previous meal on respiratory exchange ratio (RER) [23-25]. Subjects were instructed to not change their diet or exercise during the study.

Prior to the first exercise assessment, height and weight were measured using a wall-mounted stadiometer (Ayrton Stadiometer, Model S100, Prior Lake, MN) and digital weight scale (Model 5002, Scale-Tronix Inc., Wheaton, IL). Each measurement was done three times and the mean recorded. Body mass index was calculated as the body weight (kg) divided by height squared (m^2). Air displacement plethysmography (Bod Pod® Life Measurement Inc., Concord, CA) was used to obtain initial visit body fat percentages. Subjects were instructed to sit still and breathe normally while the body volume measurement was conducted. Thoracic gas volume was estimated according to the methods described by Dempster and Aitkens [26]. Body fat percentage was calculated by computer software using the Siri equation and the collected data [27].

Heart rate was collected prior to exercise to further characterize resting cardiovascular parameters via heart rate variability (HRV) analysis. Participants were prepped for electrode placement for measurement of HR via a 3-lead electrocardiograph (ECG). The ECG (Lead II) was continuously recorded via an automated tonometer (Colin Pilot 7000; Colin Medical Instruments Corp., San Antonio, TX). Participants were asked to pace their breathing at 0.25 Hz (approximately 15 breaths per min) using a computer metronome (Crystal Metronome 1.4.4, MIL software & Matthew Lloyd) cadence. Participants were instructed to lay flat on their backs on a cushioned bed for 10 minutes to ensure that a resting state was attained. After the initial rest period, participants continued to lie relaxed for an additional 10 minutes to record resting ECG measures.

Following resting measures of HR, subjects were fitted with headgear and mouthpiece for collection of expired air by a calibrated open-circuit spirometry metabolic cart (CPX-D, MedGraphics Corporation, St. Paul, MN). Then subjects were fitted with a HR monitor (Polar, Polar Electro Oy, Finland) placed around their chest at the level of the xiphoid process to ensure a quality heart rate signal. Seat and handlebar height were recorded and were replicated for subsequent experimental trials. After warm-up on the bicycle ergometer for 5 minutes at 25 Watts, subjects were asked to complete a progressive resistance exercise test. Subjects rode at a cadence of 60–90 rpm against an increasing resistance of 50 Watts every 2 minutes until volitional exhaustion. Rating of perceived exertion (RPE) was obtained at the end of each stage using the 10-point Borg category scale [28]. All subjects met at least two of the following criteria to be considered a maximal test: 1) increase in VO_2 between the last 2 stages of less than half the expected increase, 2) RER ≥ 1.10, or 3) RPE ≥ 9 on the Borg 1–10 scale. Analyzed gas samples were used to determine peak aerobic capacity ($VO_{2\ peak}$) and the ventilatory threshold (VT) by the D_{max} method [29].

Experimental design

This study used a randomized, double-blind, placebo controlled, crossover design. Subjects were randomized for preexercise intake with the ED or placebo and received the opposite treatment a minimum of 7 days later (see Table 1 for ingredients). Regular version Monster ED was standardized at 2.0 mg per kilogram of body mass ($mg \cdot kgBM^{-1}$) of caffeine and the placebo was prepared from noncaffeinated diet Mountain Dew and lemon juice by a lab staff member. Both drinks were

Table 1 Monster energy drink ingredients

Ingredient	Amount (per kg body mass)
Carbohydrate	0.65 mg $kgBM^{-1}$
Cafeine	2 mg $kgBM^{-1}$
Taurine	25 mg $kgBM^{-1}$
Pana-ginseng	5 mg $kgBM^{-1}$
Vitamin C	1.5 mg $kgBM^{-1}$
Ribiflavin	0.04 mg $kgBM^{-1}$
Niacin	0.50 mg $kgBM^{-1}$
Vitamin B6	0.05 mg $kgBM^{-1}$
Vitamin B12	0.15 mg $kgBM^{-1}$

served in a dark, opaque container and consumed 60 minutes before testing started. The beverage was consumed within a 10-minute period from the time it was received. The mean total beverage volume was 467 ± 109 mL (about one 16 oz can). Resting HR data were obtained as explained above followed by exercise. After a minimum of 7 days from preliminary testing, subjects returned to LIHP for their initial energy drink trial. They observed the same pre-testing criteria with respect to fasting, caffeine, and exercise. All testing was performed in a climate controlled environment between 6:00 to 8:00 am at a minimum of 1 week apart. Participants were informed that they would receive either an energy drink or a taste-matched placebo before experimental testing and a small amount of water (75 mL total) at the 15 minute and 30 minute mark during exercise. Participants were instructed to not discuss the characteristics of the beverages with other participants and were asked at the end of the experimental trial which beverage they received.

Experimental protocol

After a minimum of 7 days from preliminary testing, subjects returned to LIHP for their initial energy drink trial. They were fitted with headgear and mouthpiece for collection of ventilation, oxygen consumption (VO_2), carbon dioxide production (VCO_2), and RER on a breath-by-breath basis. They were also fitted with a HR monitor as described above. After a 5 minute warm up on a bicycle ergometer at 25 Watts, subjects pedaled at a workload corresponding to 30% of their pre-determined VT for 15 minutes, then pedaled at a workload corresponding to 60% of their VT for an additional 15 minutes.

For the ride TTE portion, subjects continued to pedal at 80% of their VT for 10 minutes and then an additional 10 minutes at a workload equal to 100% of VT until volitional fatigue. The total time ride TTE was recorded. Heart rate and RPE were recorded every 2 minutes during exercise. Constant verbal encouragement by the same tester was given to the subjects during each trial to elicit a maximal effort.

The second drink trial was conducted a minimum of 7 days afterwards. Subjects received the opposite assigned preexercise drink from their first exercise trial. The cycle ergometer test protocol and data collection methods remained the same.

Heart rate variability data analyses

Lead II ECG data for HRV preexercise was collected as described above and were digitally recorded continuously using a desktop computer with WinDaq Pro data collection software (DATAQ Instruments Inc., Akron, OH). The signal was sampled at 500 Hz throughout all testing. The WinDaq Pro software allowed for instantaneous analog to digital conversion of the ECG signal with recordings stored for latter off-line analysis (Kubios Heart Rate Variability software version 2.0 beta 3; Biosignal Analysis and Medical Imaging Group, Kuopio, Finland). Standard time domain parameters [the root mean square of successive differences (RMSSD), the standard deviation of all NN (normal RR) intervals (SDNN) and the percentage of successive NN intervals differing >50 ms (pNN50)] and frequency domain parameters [low frequency power (LF, (0.04 – 0.15 Hz)), high frequency power (HF, (0.15 – 0.4 Hz)) and the ratio of LF/HF] in addition to mean resting HR were calculated. All analysis was performed according to the standards set by the Task Force of the European Society of Cardiology and the North American Society of Pacing and Electrophysiology [30]. The time points from 2 to 8 minutes of the last 10 minute resting period were utilized for calculation of all resting HRV variables. Each 5-minute segment was manually reviewed for ectopic beats or arrhythmias. Segments containing such alterations of normal electrophysiological function were excluded from analysis.

The power spectral density of the RR interval data was calculated using a fast-Fourier transform for the frequency domain parameters. This was based on Welch's periodogram method to reduce noise in the estimated power spectra with a sampling rate of 4 Hz, and a window width of 256 seconds with an overlap of 50%, corresponding to 128 seconds. Paced breathing was performed to reduce the potential confounding effects of respiratory variation on HRV measures [31].

Statistical analyses

Beat-by-beat resting HR data was analyzed using Kubios Heart Rate Variability software to obtain the mean HR, time domain, frequency domain, and sample entropy scores for both the supplement and placebo trial. They were compared via a two sample Student's t test. Exercise ride TTE, HR during exercise, and RPE were also analyzed using a two sample Student's *t* test. Differences were considered significant at $p < 0.05$. Data are expressed as mean ± SD and were analyzed using SPSS software (version 13.0; SPSS, Inc., Chicago, IL) and Prism® Graphpad Software version 6.0 (Graphpad Software, Inc., San Diego, CA).

Results

Preliminary testing

A total of 16 participants completed the study, but one was excluded from the analysis due to heavy exercise prior to testing. Resting HR was significantly higher following the ED than the placebo (ED: 65 ± 10 bpm vs. placebo: 58 ± 8 bpm, p = 0.02). Heart rate variability as calculated via RMSSD, SDNN, pNN50, HF power, LF power, LF/HF ratio, and sample entropy however were not significantly different (see Table 2).

Experimental testing

Exercise TTE between the ED and the placebo condition was not statistically different between trials (ED: 45.5 ± 9.8 vs. placebo: 43.8 ± 9.3 min p = 0.62). There was no significant difference in peak RPE (ED: 9.1 ± 0.5 vs. placebo: 9.0 ± 0.8, p = 1.00) or peak HR (ED: 177 ± 11 bpm vs. placebo: 175 ± 12 bpm, p = 0.73) during exercise in either the supplement or placebo condition. The RER at 60% VT (ED: 0.99 ± 0.05 vs. placebo: 0.98 ± 0.05, p =0.60), 80% of VT (ED: 1.02 ± 0.07 vs. placebo: 1.03 ± 0.07, p = 0.51), and 100% of VT (ED: 1.04 ± 0.09 vs. placebo: 1.04 ± 0.08, p = 0.62) were not significantly different between the two conditions (Figure 1). The RER at 30% of VT however was significantly higher following the ingestion of ED vs. the placebo (0.94 ± 0.06 vs. 0.91 ± 0.05, p = 0.046). There were no side effects reported from the exercise testing, ED, or placebo. Only one subject dropped out after the initial baseline. At the completion of the experimental trial, six subjects correctly identified the order of ED vs. placebo, four did not, and five were not sure.

Table 2 Comparison of resting heart rate variability parameters under energy drink and placebo conditions

Parameter	Energy drink	Placebo	p-value
RMSSD (ms)	76.1 (46.0)	83.7 (54.5)	0.33
SDNN (ms)	94.1 (34.3)	102.0 (51.9)	0.28
pNN50 (%)	38.8 (24.7)	38.8 (21.2)	1.00
LF (ms^2)	1319 (756)	2295 (2593)	0.12
HF (ms^2)	4047 (4569)	4235 (5317)	0.79
LF/HF ratio	0.93 (1.15)	0.91 (0.93)	0.90
SampEn	1.33 (0.37)	1.44 (0.37)	0.22

Data are presented as mean (standard deviation). RMSSD - root-mean square differences of successive R-R intervals, SDNN- standard deviation of normal-to-normal intervals, pNN50 percentage of successive NN intervals differing >50 ms, LF - low frequency, HF - high frequency, LF/HF ratio low frequency to high frequency ratio (no units), SampEn - Sample Entropy (no units).

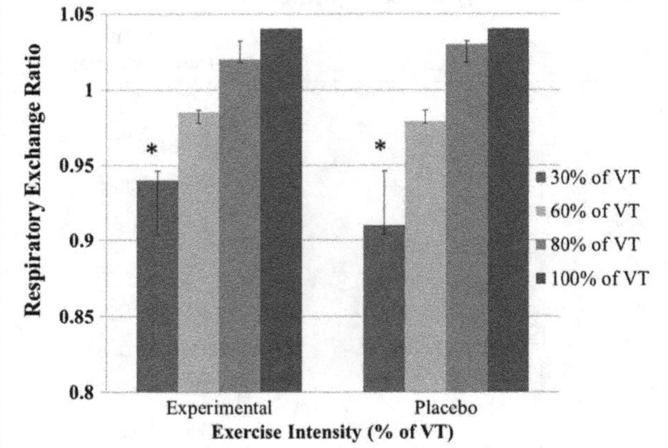

Figure 1 Respiratory exchange ratio vs. exercise intensity as a percentage of ventilatory threshold (% of VT) for energy drink and placebo conditions. Values are mean ± standard deviation. Only 30% of VT intensity was different from experimental vs. placebo (*p < 0.046).

Discussion

This was the first study to investigate preexercise ingestion of the ED Monster in relation to ride TTE and cardiovascular parameters. Cardiovascular parameters at rest did show an increase in HR after consuming the ED, but there were no changes in any HRV parameters. Ride TTE during cycle ergometery testing, peak RPE, and peak HR during exercise were not different between the two conditions. The RER measurements during each intensity were not different between the two conditions, except for the RER at 30% of VT where the placebo condition was lower.

Exercise effects

The main finding in this study is consistent with data by Candow et al. [14] who conducted a high-intensity run TTE study in young adults (VO_{2max} of 45.5 ± 6.3 ml • kg^{-1} • min^{-1}) using a double-blind, crossover, repeated-measures method. They showed no increase in run time or change in RPE with the energy drink Red Bull given preexercise. However, Ivy et al. [10] did see an improvement with preexercise Red Bull. Their study also used a double-blind, randomized, crossover design, but was conducted in athletes with a higher VO_{2max} (54.9 ± 2.3 ml • kg^{-1} • min^{-1}) and employed a time trial format. Kazemi et al. [32] demonstrated that Phantom and Dragon energy drinks also significantly increased TTE vs. placebo by 9.3% and 6.5% respectively during a Bruce treadmill test.

Caffeine

One reason for the lack of increased ride time was possibly the lower dose of caffeine standardized at 2 mg · $kgBM^{-1}$. The recent International Society of Sports Nutrition (ISSN) position stand on energy drinks [33] concluded that although they contain a number of nutrients, the primary ergogenic nutrients appear to be carbohydrate and/or caffeine. The exact mechanism of how caffeine works is still debated, but it is believed to primarily function by acting as an adenosine receptor antagonist, increasing release of free fatty acids, and increasing calcium release and uptake [34]. The track record of positive effects of caffeine is quite good and most studies showed an improvement in exercise capacity in the range of 3–13 mg · $kgBM^{-1}$ [9,33,35-40], although Cox et al. [41] did show a decreased time during a time trial performance undertaken at the end of a prolonged cycling bout with a low dose at approximately 1.5 mg · $kgBM^{-1}$. Denadai, et al. [39] used a dose of around 3 mg · $kgBM^{-1}$ and showed that in untrained subjects who exercised below their anaerobic threshold, caffeine increased ride TTE and reduced perceived exertion. Further enhancement in performance does not result when caffeine is consumed in higher dosages (≥ 9 mg · $kgBM^{-1}$).

This study used a standardized dose of 2.0 mg · $kgBM^{-1}$, which is on the lower end for a dose to increase ride TTE. Subjects had to consume the entire ED amount prior to testing, therefore a higher amount may have resulted in gastrointestinal issues due to the increased level of fluid. Subjects were fasted and asked to abstain from caffeine for 48 hours prior to testing, but no other diet controls were applied to make it as applicable to free living subjects as possible.

Rating of perceived exertion

In the current study, there was no significant difference between peak RPEs when supplementing with an ED or placebo. A meta-analysis in 2005 [42] on caffeine found that it reduced RPE during exercise by 5.6%. Our results are in agreement with Candow et al. [14] and Ivy et al. [10] who did not show any difference in RPE during a high-intensity run time-to-exhaustion and a simulated cycling time trial, respectively.

Heart rate

Surprisingly, there are little data on the effects of energy drinks on heart rate. No difference was found for peak HR during exercise in this study, but resting HR was higher under the ED condition. Willoughby et al. [16] found HR was unaffected one hour after 50 young adults consumed one 250 ml (8 oz) can of sugar-free Red Bull (approximately 80 mg of caffeine). Steinke et al. [17] however demonstrated that HR was reduced 30 minutes after subjects consumed 75 mg of caffeine. Bichler and colleagues [20] studied a combination of caffeine and taurine, two common ingredients in energy drinks, which resulted in a significant decline in HR.

Heart rate variability

Heart rate variability may serve as a method to further investigate the cardiac effects of these drinks as it allows quantification of sympathovagal balance [43,44]. Some subjects may be more sensitive to energy drinks resulting in a more sympathetic response, thus altered HRV. In this study, we did not find any difference in time domain, frequency domain, or sample entropy HRV analysis. Since their inception, energy drinks have been suspected of leading to an increased risk of cardiac issues [45]. A recent review on energy drinks [46] regarding safety concluded that there is not enough data currently to allow a definitive dietary recommendation to be made regarding safe levels of ED consumption, and recommended caution. The ISSN Position Stand [33] stated that indiscriminant use of energy drinks, especially if more than one serving per day, may lead to adverse events and harmful side effects.

The only other study on HRV and energy drinks done by Wiklund et al. [47] showed a decreased LF/HF ratio and a tendency to increased HF power (increased vagal modulation). The dose used was high as subjects consumed 3 cans of Red Bull, which represents a dose of 3000 mg of taurine and 240 mg of caffeine after an overnight fast. They also measured RR intervals for the HRV analysis at 30 minutes after the intake of the ED compared to the 60 minute timeframe here. These differences may account for the variance in the results obtained.

As mentioned, the two ingredients in energy drinks that could affect HRV are taurine and caffeine. Taurine has been shown to moderate the flow of cations, especially calcium, across the cell membranes, thus protecting the heart muscle from both high and low concentrations [18,19]. Caffeine is known to increase vagal autonomic nerve activity in resting subjects [48,49]. Ingestion of caffeine preexercise has also been associated with exaggerated vagal withdrawal during post-exercise recovery because of higher baseline level of vagal activity before exercise [49]. However, Rauh et al. [50] did not find any significant differences in respective HRV parameters (HR, RMSSD, SDNN, pNN50, LF, HF and LF/HF) conducted at rest 30, 60, and 90 minutes after 100 and 200 mg caffeine doses were taken and compared to a placebo. They concluded that caffeine at a dose up to 200 mg does not influence HRV [50].

Conclusion

In conclusion, the results of this present study indicate that consuming Monster ED increases resting HR, but does not increase ride time-to-exhaustion. The ED did not have an impact on parasympathetic and sympathetic balance at rest via HRV analysis. RER was higher after the ED demonstrating a greater reliance on glucose during exercise, but this was only seen at the lowest intensity. The ED did not change the perception of exercise intensity as measured by peak RPE. Future research should compare the effects of regular energy drinks at various caffeine dosages during a ride time-to-exhaustion and a time trial format.

Abbreviations

ED: Energy drink; BM: Body mass; TTE: Time-to-exhaustion; RPE: Rating of perceived exertion; RER: Respiratory exchange ratio; VO_{2max}: Maximal oxygen consumption; HR: Heart rate; LIHP: Laboratory of Integrative Human Physiology; VO_2: Oxygen consumption; CO_2: Carbon dioxide; HRV: Heart rate variably; ECG: Electrocardiograph; $VO_{2\ peak}$: Peak aerobic capacity; VT: Ventilatory threshold; SD: Standard deviation; RMSSD: Root mean square of successive differences; SDNN: Standard deviation of all NN (normal RR) intervals; pNN50: Percentage of successive NN intervals differing >50 ms; LF: Low frequency power; HF: High frequency power; LF/HF: Ratio of low frequency to high frequency; ISSN: International Society of Sports Nutrition.

Competing interest

The authors declare that they have no competing interests.

Authors' contributions

MN developed the study design, collected data, conducted statistical analysis, and drafted and submitted the manuscript. DD and GB assisted in the study design, interpretation of data, and critically reviewed the manuscript. All authors read and approved the final manuscript.

Acknowledgements

We would like to thank everyone that volunteered to participant in this study. Without your help this study would not have been possible.

Author details

[1]School of Kinesiology, University of Minnesota, Minneapolis, MN, USA.
[2]Department of Pediatrics, University of Minnesota Medical School, Minneapolis, MN, USA.

References

1. Hoffman JR, Faigenbaum AD, Ratamess NA, Ross R, Kang J, Tenenbaum G: **Nutritional supplementation and anabolic steroid use in adolescents.** *Med Sci Sports Exerc* 2008, **40**(1):15–24.
2. Froiland K, Koszewski W, Hingst J, Kopecky L: **Nutritional supplement use among college athletes and their sources of information.** *Int J Sport Nutr Exerc Metab* 2004, **14**(1):104–120.
3. Clauson KA, Shields KM, McQueen CE, Persad N: **Safety issues associated with commercially available energy drinks.** *J Am Pharm Assoc (2003)* 2008, **48**(3):e55–e63. quiz e64-7.
4. Shah S, Lacey C, Riddock I: **Impact of energy drinks on electrocardiographic and blood pressure parameters: A meta-analysis of clinical studies [abstract].** *Circulation* 2013, **127**(AP324).
5. Noakes TD, Lambert EV, Lambert MI, McArthur PS, Myburgh KH, Benade AJ: **Carbohydrate ingestion and muscle glycogen depletion during marathon and ultramarathon racing.** *Eur J Appl Physiol Occup Physiol* 1988, **57**(4):482–489.
6. Jeukendrup AE: **Carbohydrate intake during exercise and performance.** *Nutrition* 2004, **20**(7–8):669–677.
7. Kang J, Robertson RJ, Goss FL, DaSilva SG, Visich P, Suminski RR, Utter AC, Denys BC: **Effect of carbohydrate substrate availability on ratings of perceived exertion during prolonged exercise of moderate intensity.** *Percept Mot Skills* 1996, **82**(2):495–506.
8. Costill DL, Dalsky GP, Fink WJ: **Effects of caffeine ingestion on metabolism and exercise performance.** *Med Sci Sports* 1978, **10**(3):155–158.
9. Graham TE, Spriet LL: **Performance and metabolic responses to a high caffeine dose during prolonged exercise.** *J Appl Physiol* 1991, **71**(6):2292–2298.
10. Ivy JL, Kammer L, Ding Z, Wang B, Bernard JR, Liao YH, Hwang J: **Improved cycling time-trial performance after ingestion of a caffeine energy drink.** *Int J Sport Nutr Exerc Metab* 2009, **19**(1):61–78.
11. Forbes SC, Candow DG, Little JP, Magnus C, Chilibeck PD: **Effect of Red Bull energy drink on repeated Wingate cycle performance and bench-press muscle endurance.** *Int J Sport Nutr Exerc Metab* 2007, **17**(5):433–444.
12. Alford C, Cox H, Wescott R: **The effects of red bull energy drink on human performance and mood.** *Amino Acids* 2001, **21**(2):139–150.
13. Del Coso J, Portillo J, Munoz G, Abian-Vicen J, Gonzalez-Millan C, Munoz-Guerra J: **Caffeine-containing energy drink improves sprint performance during an international rugby sevens competition.** *Amino Acids* 2013, **44**(6):1511–1519.
14. Candow DG, Kleisinger AK, Grenier S, Dorsch KD: **Effect of sugar-free Red Bull energy drink on high-intensity run time-to-exhaustion in young adults.** *J Strength Cond Res* 2009, **23**(4):1271–1275.
15. Astorino TA, Matera AJ, Basinger J, Evans M, Schurman T, Marquez R: **Effects of red bull energy drink on repeated sprint performance in women athletes.** *Amino Acids* 2011, **42**(5):1803–1808.
16. Willoughby SR: **Energy drink effects platelet aggregation and endothelial function: A possible link to increased cardiovascular risk.** *Heart Lung Circ* 2009, **18:**S265.
17. Steinke L, Lanfear DE, Dhanapal V, Kalus JS: **Effect of "energy drink" consumption on hemodynamic and electrocardiographic parameters in healthy young adults.** *Ann Pharmacother* 2009, **43**(4):596–602.
18. Huxtable RJ: **Physiological actions of taurine.** *Physiol Rev* 1992, **72**(1):101–163.
19. Schaffer SW, Azuma J: **Review: myocardial physiological effects of taurine and their significance.** *Adv Exp Med Biol* 1992, **315:**105–120.
20. Bichler A, Swenson A, Harris MA: **A combination of caffeine and taurine has no effect on short term memory but induces changes in heart rate and mean arterial blood pressure.** *Amino Acids* 2006, **31**(4):471–476.
21. Adams R: **Revised physical activity readiness questionnaire.** *Can Fam Physician* 1999, **45:**992–995. 1004–5.
22. Graham TE: **Caffeine and exercise: metabolism, endurance and performance.** *Sports Med* 2001, **31**(11):785–807.
23. Brooks GH, Fahey TD, Baldwin KDS: *Exercise Physiology: Human Bioenergetics and its Applications.* Boston: McGraw-Hill; 2005.
24. Wilmore JH, Costill DL: *Physiology of Sport and Exercise.* 4th edition. Champaign, Illinois: Human Kinetics Publishers; 2007.
25. Miller SL, Maresh CM, Armstrong LE, Ebbeling CB, Lennon S, Rodriguez NR: **Metabolic response to provision of mixed protein-carbohydrate supplementation during endurance exercise.** *Int J Sport Nutr Exerc Metab* 2002, **12**(4):384–397.
26. Dempster P, Aitkens S: **A new air displacement method for the determination of human body composition.** *Med Sci Sports Exerc* 1995, **27**(12):1692–1697.
27. Siri WE: **Body composition from fluid spaces and density: analysis of methods. 1961.** *Nutrition* 1993, **9**(5):480–491.
28. Borg GA: **Psychophysical bases of perceived exertion.** *Med Sci Sports Exerc* 1982, **14**(5):377–381.
29. Cheng B, Kuipers H, Snyder AC, Keizer HA, Jeukendrup A, Hesselink M: **A new approach for the determination of ventilatory and lactate thresholds.** *Int J Sports Med* 1992, **13**(7):518–522.
30. Task Force of the European Society of Cardiology and the North American Society of Pacing and Electrophysiology: **Heart rate variability: standards of measurement, physiological interpretation and clinical use.** *Circulation* 1996, **93**(5):1043–1065.
31. Katona PG, Jih F: **Respiratory sinus arrhythmia: noninvasive measure of parasympathetic cardiac control.** *J Appl Physiol* 1975, **39**(5):801–805.
32. Kazemi F, Gaeini A, Kordi M, Rahnama N: **The acute effects of two energy drinks on endurance performance in female athlete students.** *Sport Sci Health* 2009, **5**(2):55–60.
33. Campbell B, Wilborn C, La Bounty P, Taylor L, Nelson MT, Greenwood M, Ziegenfuss TN, Lopez HL, Hoffman JR, Stout JR, Schmitz S, Collins R, Kalman DS, Antonio J, Kreider RB: **International Society of Sports Nutrition position stand: energy drinks.** *J Int Soc Sports Nutr* 2013, **10**(1):1–2783. 10-1.
34. Davis JK, Green JM: **Caffeine and anaerobic performance: ergogenic value and mechanisms of action.** *Sports Med* 2009, **39**(10):813–832.
35. Kovacs EM, Stegen JHCH, Brouns F: **Effect of caffeinated drinks on substrate metabolism, caffeine excretion, and performance.** *J Appl Physiol* 1998, **85**(2):709–715.
36. Spriet LL, MacLean DA, Dyck DJ, Hultman E, Cederblad G, Graham TE: **Caffeine ingestion and muscle metabolism during prolonged exercise in humans.** *Am J Physiol* 1992, **262**(6 Pt 1):E891–E898.
37. Graham TE, Spriet LL: **Metabolic, catecholamine, and exercise performance responses to various doses of caffeine.** *J Appl Physiol* 1995, **78**(3):867–874.
38. Pasman WJ, van Baak MA, Jeukendrup AE, de Haan A: **The effect of different dosages of caffeine on endurance performance time.** *Int J Sports Med* 1995, **16**(4):225–230.

39. Denadai BS, Denadai ML: **Effects of caffeine on time to exhaustion in exercise performed below and above the anaerobic threshold.** *Braz J Med Biol Res* 1998, **31**(4):581–585.
40. Burke LM: **Caffeine and sports performance.** *Appl Physiol Nutr Metab* 2008, **33**(6):1319–1334.
41. Cox GR, Desbrow B, Montgomery PG, Anderson ME, Bruce CR, Macrides TA, Martin DT, Moquin A, Roberts A, Hawley JA, Burke LM: **Effect of different protocols of caffeine intake on metabolism and endurance performance.** *J Appl Physiol* 2002, **93**(3):990–999.
42. Doherty M, Smith PM: **Effects of caffeine ingestion on rating of perceived exertion during and after exercise: a meta-analysis.** *Scand J Med Sci Sports* 2005, **15**(2):69–78.
43. Montano N, Ruscone TG, Porta A, Lombardi F, Pagani M, Malliani A: **Power spectrum analysis of heart rate variability to assess the changes in sympathovagal balance during graded orthostatic tilt.** *Circulation* 1994, **90**(4):1826–1831.
44. Eckberg DL: **Sympathovagal balance: a critical appraisal.** *Circulation* 1997, **96**(9):3224–3232.
45. Finnegan D: **The health effects of stimulant drinks.** *Br Nutr Found Nutr Bull* 2003, **28:**147–155.
46. Burrows T, Pursey K, Neve M, Stanwell P: **What are the health implications associated with the consumption of energy drinks? A systematic review.** *Nutr Rev* 2013, **71**(3):135–148.
47. Wiklund U, Karlsson M, Ostrom M, Messner T: **Influence of energy drinks and alcohol on post-exercise heart rate recovery and heart rate variability.** *Clin Physiol Funct Imaging* 2009, **29**(1):74–80.
48. Hibino G, Moritani T, Kawada T, Fushiki T: **Caffeine enhances modulation of parasympathetic nerve activity in humans: quantification using power spectral analysis.** *J Nutr* 1997, **127**(7):1422–1427.
49. Yeragani VK, Krishnan S, Engels HJ, Gretebeck R: **Effects of caffeine on linear and nonlinear measures of heart rate variability before and after exercise.** *Depress Anxiety* 2005, **21**(3):130–134.
50. Rauh R, Burkert M, Siepmann M, Mueck-Weymann M: **Acute effects of caffeine on heart rate variability in habitual caffeine consumers.** *Clin Physiol Funct Imaging* 2006, **26**(3):163–166.

9

A seven day running training period increases basal urinary hepcidin levels as compared to cycling

Marc Sim[1*], Brian Dawson[1], Grant J Landers[1], Dorine W Swinkels[2], Harold Tjalsma[2], Erwin T Wiegerinck[2], Debbie Trinder[3,4] and Peter Peeling[1]

Abstract

Background: This investigation compared the effects of an extended period of weight-bearing (running) vs. non-weight-bearing (cycling) exercise on hepcidin production and its implications for iron status.

Methods: Ten active males performed two separate exercise training blocks with either running (RTB) or cycling (CTB) as the exercise mode. Each block consisted of five training sessions (Day 1, 2, 4, 5, 6) performed over a seven day period that were matched for exercise intensity. Basal venous blood samples were obtained on Day 1 (D1), and on Recovery Days 3 (R3) and 7 (R7) to assess iron status, while basal and 3 h post-exercise urinary hepcidin levels were measured on D1, D2, D6, as well as R3 and R7 (basal levels only) for each condition.

Results: Basal urinary hepcidin levels were significantly elevated ($p \leq 0.05$) at D2, R3 and R7 as compared to D1 in RTB. Furthermore, 3 h post-exercise urinary hepcidin levels on D1 were also significantly higher in RTB compared to CTB ($p \leq 0.05$). In CTB, urinary hepcidin levels were not statistically different on D1 as compared to R7. Iron parameters were not significantly different at D1 compared to R3 and R7 during both conditions.

Conclusions: These results suggest that basal hepcidin levels may increase over the course of an extended training program, especially if a weight-bearing exercise modality is undertaken. However, despite any variations in hepcidin production, serum iron parameters in both RTB and CTB were unaffected, possibly due to the short duration of each training block. In comparing running to cycling, non-weight-bearing activity may require more training sessions, or sessions of extended duration, before any significant changes in basal hepcidin levels appear. Chronic elevations in hepcidin levels may help to explain the high incidence of iron deficiency in athletes.

Keywords: Iron deficiency, Weight-bearing exercise, Non-weight-bearing exercise, Cytokines

Introduction

Iron plays a number of critical roles within the body, including oxygen (O_2) transport and energy production [1]. Specific to athletes, iron status may be compromised as a result of exercise-induced sweating, hemolysis, hematuria and gastrointestinal bleeding (see [2] for review). Recent work has suggested that post-exercise increases in the iron regulatory hormone hepcidin may also alter iron metabolism [3-9]. Hepcidin is a peptide hormone that plays a key role in regulating iron metabolism. Elevated hepcidin levels degrade the ferroportin export channels on the surface of macrophages and the intestinal duodenum, resulting in a reduction in iron recycling (by macrophages from senescent erythrocytes) and absorption from the intestine, respectively [10,11]. Presently, numerous studies have reported that hepcidin levels peak 3 h post-exercise [3-9]. These studies have attributed such a response to exercise-induced increases in the inflammatory cytokine interleukin-6 (IL-6).

To date, most studies have used running-based protocols to investigate the post-exercise hepcidin response [3-6,8,9]. Until recently, the use of alternate modalities such as cycling remained unclear. However, Troadec et al. [12] recently reported that a 45 min low intensity

* Correspondence: marc.sim@uwa.edu.au
[1]School of Sport Science, Exercise and Health, The University of Western Australia, Crawley, Western Australia, Australia
Full list of author information is available at the end of the article

cycling trial (60% of heart rate reserve) did not influence post-exercise IL-6 and hepcidin levels. Subsequently, Sim et al. [7] reported that IL-6 and hepcidin levels were significantly elevated in the post-exercise period after high (interval) and low (continuous) intensity running and cycling. Of interest, serum iron was not significantly elevated immediately after low intensity cycling, suggesting that non-weight bearing exercise may have the potential to reduce the degree of exercise-induced hemolysis, similar to the findings of Telford et al. [13]. Although these studies have provided some insight into the benefits of using cycling as an alternate exercise modality, it remains unclear whether such differences may improve iron status over an extended training period.

Currently, limited studies have attempted to examine how exercise might affect post-exercise hepcidin production over an extended period, and what the implications may be for iron status. Recently, Auersperger et al. [14] reported that serum hepcidin and ferritin decreased in athletes adopting an eight week interval running program. In addition, McClung et al. [15] showed that nine weeks of basic combat training (BCT) compromised numerous iron parameters in female soldiers. On the contrary, McClung et al. [16] reported that seven days of training (military specific exercise and ski marching) elevated hepcidin levels without affecting iron status in male soldiers. Of importance, the iron status of an athlete may also dictate both the pre-exercise levels of hepcidin, and the magnitude of hepcidin response to an acute exercise stimulus (e.g. serum ferritin <30 $\mu g.L^{-1}$, hepcidin suppressed) [17].

Considering that the aforementioned investigations used mainly weight-bearing activity (that may have increased the degree of exercise-induced hemolysis), it remains to be investigated how accumulated bouts of weight-bearing (running) vs. non-weight-bearing (cycling) exercise may impact iron status over time. Additionally, previous investigations [14-16] have only measured basal hepcidin levels; however, the acute post-exercise hepcidin response over consecutive exercise bouts currently remains unknown. As such, this study set out to compare the effects of a seven day period of running vs. cycling exercise on hepcidin production and iron status in active individuals.

Methods

Ten active males participated in this study [age = 24 ± 1 y, body mass = 70.5 ± 3.2 kg, stature = 175.9 ± 2.6 cm, running peak oxygen uptake (VO_{2peak}) = 58.0 ± 2.0 $ml.kg^{-1}.min^{-1}$, cycling VO_{2peak} = 49.7 ± 1.8 $ml.kg^{-1}.min^{-1}$]. At the time of recruitment, participants were performing a minimum of three exercise training sessions per week. The sample size was determined via customised computer software (GPOWER Version 2, Department of Psychology, Bonn University, Bonn, Germany) using effect sizes (ES) attained from similar research [3-7,18]. A sample size of 10 was recommended to yield a power of 0.90 at a significance level of $p \leq 0.05$. When recruited, all participants had a healthy iron status (serum ferritin = 79.3 ± 15.0 $\mu g.L^{-1}$, transferrin saturation = 33 ± 3%), and were not taking any iron supplements. Prior to participation, written consent was obtained with approval granted by the Human Ethics Committee of The University of Western Australia (RA/4/1/5636).

Experimental overview

Participants attended the laboratory for two separate running (RTB) and cycling (CTB) exercise training blocks over a three week period. Each training block lasted for seven days, consisting of five exercise training sessions and two rest days. The training sessions were designed to engage both the aerobic and anaerobic energy systems, and consisted of a variety of training types (e.g. low intensity aerobic, fartlek, and intervals). Participants were assigned to RTB or CTB in a randomised, counter-balanced order. Subsequently, in the week prior to each training block, a familiarisation session consisting of a graded exercise test (GXT) was performed on a motorised treadmill or cycle ergometer to determine each individual's running and cycling VO_{2peak}, maximum HR (HR_{max}), and the corresponding velocity (vVO_{2peak}) or power output (pVO_{2peak}). During each seven day period, exercise training was performed on Day One (D1), Two (D2), Four (D4), Five (D5) and Six (D6), while Days Three (R3) and Seven (R7) were recovery days (Figure 1). After completing their first training block, participants had a seven day recovery period before they started the subsequent condition. In addition, no manual labour or exercise training was performed outside of the experimental protocol, and participants were asked to keep their physical activity levels to a minimum during the seven days of recovery between conditions.

For the duration of both conditions, all exercise sessions started between 0700–0800 each day, and participants were provided with 300 ml of water to be consumed *ad libitum.* For RTB and CTB, baseline venous blood samples were taken on three separate occasions, which included D1, R3 and R7. Finally, urine samples were obtained on arrival (baseline) and 3 h post-exercise on D1, D2 and D6, as well as R3 and R7 (baseline only). All baseline venous and urine samples were obtained between 0700 and 0800 to minimise diurnal variation.

Experimental procedures

Graded exercise test

The running GXT was conducted on a motorised treadmill (VR 3000, NuryTech Inc, Germany) utilising 3 min exercise and 1 min rest periods. The initial speed was 10 $km.h^{-1}$, with subsequent 1 $km.h^{-1}$ increments over

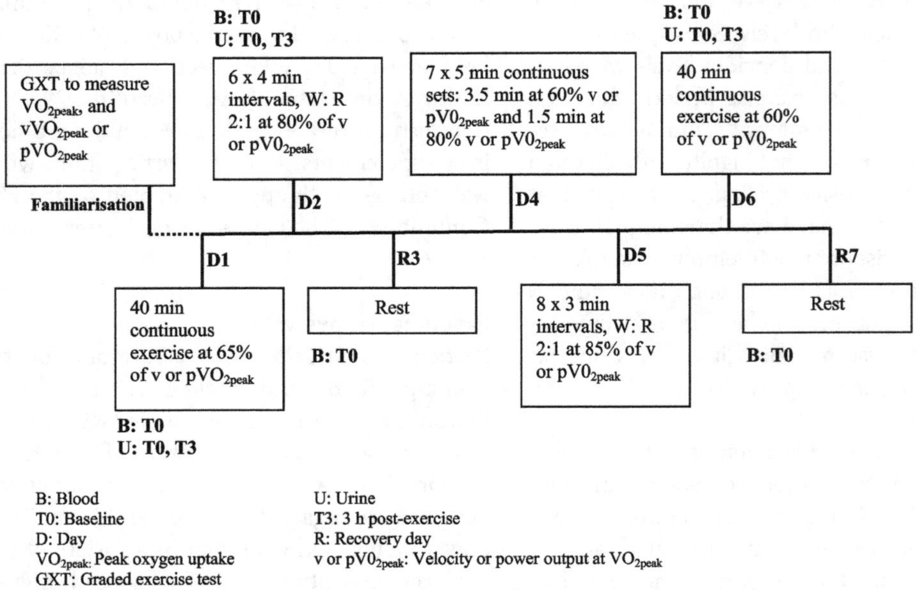

Figure 1 Diagrammatic representation of the running and cycling training blocks.

each exercise period until volitional exhaustion. The cycle GXT was conducted in a similar fashion (3 min exercise: 1 min rest), and performed on a calibrated wind-braked ergometer (Evolution Pty. Ltd., Melbourne, Australia), using customised data collection software (Cyclemax, School of Sport Science, Exercise & Health, The University of Western Australia). The initial workload was 100 W, with increments by 40 W every 3 min. Both HR and ratings of perceived exertion (RPE) were recorded during the final 10 s of each workload. Expired air was analysed for O_2 and CO_2 concentrations (Ametek Gas Analysers, Applied Electrochemistry, SOV S-3A/1 and COV CD-3A, Pittsburgh, PA), with the analysers calibrated pre-test and verified post-test using certified gravimetric gas mixtures (BOC Gases, Chatswood, Australia). Ventilation was recorded every 15 s via a turbine ventilometer (Vacumed Universal Ventilation Meter, 17125, Ventura, CA), calibrated before, and verified after exercise using a 1 L syringe in accordance with the manufacturer's specifications. Peak oxygen consumption was determined by summing the four highest consecutive 15 s VO_2 values.

Exercise trials

Running training

All running sessions were conducted outdoors on a marked ~600 m track, consisting of grass (300 m) and bitumen road (300 m) surface. Participants were provided with a Global Positioning System (GPS) enabled watch (Garmin Forerunner 110, Garmin International Inc, Kansas, USA) to assist in pace-maintenance, and strictly adhered to the stipulated velocity for each session based on their predetermined vVO_{2peak} (see Table 1) attained during the GXT (mean vVO_{2peak}: 15.0 ± 0.3 $km.h^{-1}$,

Table 1 Mean (±SEM) heart rate (HR) expressed as a percentage of the maximum HR (%HR_{max}) attained during each respective graded exercise test, ratings of perceived exertion (RPE) and the prescribed intensity for each exercise trial during the running (RTB) and cycling (CTB) training blocks

	Day 1		Day 2		Day 4		Day 5		Day 6	
	RTB	CTB	RTB	CTB	RTB	CTB	RTB	CTB	RTB	CTB
%HR_{max}	84	84	89	89	86	85	89	89	78	78
	(1)	(1)	(1)	(2)	(1)	(1)	(1)	(1)	(1)	(2)
RPE	12[a]	14	13[a]	15	12[a]	14	14[a]	16	11[a]	12
	(1)	(0)	(0)	(0)	(0)	(0)	(0)	(0)	(0)	(0)
Prescribed exercise intensity (kph or watts)	9.8	198	12.0	243	9.0/12.0[+]	182/243[+]	12.8	258	9.0	182
	(0.2)	(7)	(0.3)	(8)	(0.2/0.3)	(6/8)	(0.3)	(9)	(0.2)	(6)

[a]Significantly different to CTB on the corresponding day.
[+](recovery/effort speed or power).

see Figure 1 for a comprehensive breakdown of each running session). These sessions were performed under comfortable environmental conditions (Dry Globe temperature: 27.0 ± 0.8°C, Relative Humidity: 58 ± 3%, Wind Speed 4.9 ± 0.8 $km.h^{-1}$).

Cycling training

All cycling sessions were performed in a laboratory (Dry Bulb Temperature: 25.1 ± 0.1°C, Relative Humidity: 52 ± 0%) on a calibrated wind-braked ergometer (Evolution Pty. Ltd., Melbourne, Australia), using customised data collection software (Cyclemax, School of Sport Science, Exercise & Health, The University of Western Australia). This software program provided instantaneous and mean power feedback, which enabled participants to perform the training sessions based on their pVO_{2peak} (Table 1) attained during the GXT (mean pVO_{2peak}: 304 ± 10 W, see Figure 1 for a comprehensive breakdown of each cycle session).

Heart rate, ratings of perceived exertion

Heart rate and RPE were collected at 5 min intervals (when the exercise task was of a continuous nature; D1, D4 and D6) or at the end of each interval effort (for days where interval training was performed; D2 and D5) during the training sessions for RTB and CTB. Heart rate was measured using a Garmin HR monitor (Garmin Forerunner 110, Garmin International Inc, Kansas, USA), while RPE adopted Borg's 6–20 scale (6 = no exertion to 20 = maximal exertion) [19].

Food intake

Participants completed a food diary for the entire seven days of RTB and CTB. They were required to record detailed information on food type and serving size. To standardise the food intake between the different training weeks, participants were instructed to replicate their daily eating habits for the duration of the study. This data was then entered into a commercial software program (Foodworks 2007, Version 5, Service-pack 1) to obtain the percentage of macronutrient (carbohydrates, fats, protein), food iron content and total kilojoule (kj) intake.

Blood collection and analysis

After participants lay down for a minimum of 5 min, venous blood was collected via venepuncture of an antecubital forearm vein into two 8.5 ml SST II gel vacutainers (BD, PL6 7BP, United Kingdom). Subsequently, the blood clotted for 60 min at room temperature, before being centrifuged at 10°C and 3000 rpm for 10 min. The serum supernatant was divided into 1 ml aliquots and stored at −80°C until analysis. Serum iron studies and high sensitivity C-reactive protein (CRP) were measured at Royal Perth Hospital Pathology Laboratory (Pathwest, Perth, Western Australia, Australia). Serum iron was measured using the Architect analyser (c1600210), and determined using an Iron Reagent (Sentinel Diagnostics, Milano, Italy). Coefficient of variation (CV) for iron determination at 12.01 and 43.35 $\mu mol.L^{-1}$ was 1.73 and 0.61%, respectively. Serum ferritin levels were determined using an Architect analyser (1SR06055) and a Ferritin Reagent (Abbott Diagnostics, Illinois, USA). The CV for ferritin determination at 28.62, 223.05 and 497.85 $\mu g.L^{-1}$ was 4.58, 4.46 and 4.36%, respectively. Transferrin was measured using Architect analyser (c1600210), and determined using a Transferrin Reagent (Abbott Diagnostics, Abbott Laboratories Abbott Park, IL 60064 USA). The CV for transferrin determination at 19.29, 32.23, 42.60 $\mu mol.L^{-1}$ was 1.78 and 1.19, 1.39%, respectively. The CRP was measured using an Architect analyser (c16000), and determined using a CRP Vario Reagent (Abbott Diagnostics, Abbott Laboratories, Abbott Park, IL 60064, USA). The CV for CRP determination at 5.89 and 24.76 $mg.L^{-1}$ was 2.08 and 2.03%, respectively.

Urine collection and analysis

Urine samples were collected in 75 ml sterilised containers and were centrifuged at 10°C and 3000 rpm for 10 min. The supernatant was divided into 1 ml aliquots and stored at −80°C until analysis. Urinary hepcidin-25 was measured at the Department of Clinical Chemistry, Radboud University Nijmegen Medical Centre, the Netherlands, by a combination of weak cation exchange chromatography and time-of-flight mass spectrometry (WCX-TOF MS) [20,21]. An internal standard (synthetic hepcidin-24; custom made Peptide International Inc.) was used for quantification. Peptide spectra were generated on a Microflex LT matrix-assisted laser desorption/ionisation TOF MS platform (Bruker Daltonics). Values were normalised to urine creatinine values and reported in nmol/mmol creatinine. The lower limit of detection was 0.1 $nmol.L^{-1}$ with an intra-run and inter-run CV of 3 to 7% and 10 to 13%, respectively [22].

Statistical analysis

Results are expressed as mean and standard error of the mean ± SEM. Repeated measures ANOVA analysed time, trial and time*trial effects of the different RTB and CTB sessions on various serum iron and inflammatory parameters, as well as urinary hepcidin levels. Post-hoc paired samples t-tests were used to determine where specific trial differences existed, using an alpha level set at $p \leq 0.05$. Cohens-d ES were also calculated (<0.4 = *small*, 0.4-0.8 = *moderate*, >0.8 = *large*).

Results

Heart rate and ratings of perceived exertion

Mean HR for each trial was expressed as a percentage of the maximum HR (HR_{max}) attained during the running and cycling GXT; which were 193 ± 3 and 186 ± 3 bpm, respectively. Mean percentage of HR_{max} was not significantly different between any of the running and cycling training sessions on their corresponding days (Table 1). Mean RPE was significantly higher ($p \leq 0.05$) in all cycle training sessions as compared to running on their corresponding days (Table 1).

Food intake

Daily kJ for RTB and CTB was 10,171 ± 305 and 10,027 ± 268 kJ, respectively. For RTB, the percentage composition of daily kJ intake for carbohydrates, fats and proteins was 47 ± 2, 27 ± 2 and 22 ± 1%, respectively. For CTB, the percentage composition of daily kJ intake for carbohydrates, fats and proteins was 49 ± 2, 25 ± 2 and 22 ± 1%, respectively. The daily food iron content for RTB and CTB was 6.7 ± 0.5 and 6.7 ± 0.6 mg, respectively. Daily energy intake, the percentage composition of carbohydrates, fats and proteins, as well as food iron content were not different between conditions ($p > 0.05$).

Blood parameters

Blood parameters are displayed in Table 2. No time or trial effects were recorded for serum ferritin and iron, as well as transferrin saturation on D1, R3 and R7 for both RTB and CTB. Although no trial effects existed for CRP, time effects revealed that CRP levels were significantly lower ($p \leq 0.05$) at R7 as compared to D1 during CTB.

Urinary hepcidin

Urinary hepcidin levels on the exercise days (D1, D2, D6) are displayed in Table 3. On D1, significant time and interaction effects ($p \leq 0.05$) were demonstrated, with post-hoc analysis revealing that hepcidin levels were significantly higher 3 h post-exercise as compared to baseline during RTB ($p \leq 0.05$), which was supported by a large ES ($d = 1.68$). Furthermore, 3 h post-exercise hepcidin levels were significantly higher ($p \leq 0.05$) during RTB as compared to CTB ($d = 0.68$, *moderate*). For D2, there were no significant main effects, although a large ES ($d = 0.99$) suggested that hepcidin levels may be increased 3 h post-exercise when compared to baseline for RTB. Additionally, baseline hepcidin levels were significantly higher at D2 as compared to D1 for RTB ($p \leq 0.05$). For D6, no significant main effects were again recorded. However, large ES suggested hepcidin levels may increase 3 h post-exercise as compared to baseline in both RTB ($d = 1.69$) and CTB ($d = 0.99$). Basal urinary hepcidin levels for D1, R3 and R7 are displayed in Table 4. No trial effects were recorded between days, but time effects revealed that hepcidin levels were significantly higher at R3 ($p = 0.010$; $d = 0.79$, *moderate*) and R7 ($p = 0.016$; $d = 0.49$, *moderate*) as compared to baseline in RTB. Additionally, a large ES ($d = 1.26$) suggested that basal hepcidin levels were higher at R7 than D1 during CTB.

Discussion

The results of this investigation suggest that acute bouts of running (as compared to cycling) performed over a seven day period have the ability to significantly increase basal urinary hepcidin levels. Hepcidin levels were also significantly elevated 3 h post-exercise compared to baseline on D1 of RTB, with strong ES evident to suggest acute increases in hepcidin levels in the post-exercise recovery period after the majority of all training sessions. Such findings concur with the results of previous research [3-9]. Despite this, it should also be considered that any changes in basal hepcidin levels at R7 as compared to D1 did not appear to directly impact any iron parameters in either condition.

Hepcidin and inflammation

Previously, it has been suggested that elevated hepcidin levels in the post-exercise recovery period may alter iron metabolism in athletes [3-9]. These studies have highlighted the role of the inflammatory cytokine IL-6

Table 2 Mean (±SEM) baseline serum ferritin, iron, transferrin saturation and C-reactive protein (CRP) at Day 1, Recovery Days 3 and 7 in the running (RTB) and cycling (CTB) training blocks

Blood Parameters	RTB			CTB		
	Day 1	Recovery 3	Recovery 7	Day 1	Recovery 3	Recovery 7
Serum Ferritin ($\mu g.L^{-1}$)	79.3 (15.0)	82.6 (16.0)	84.2 (13.7)	84.7 (17.4)	82.4 (15.5)	77.9 (15.5)
Serum Iron ($\mu mol.L^{-1}$)	19.6 (2.0)	20.3 (1.5)	17.5 (2.0)	15.8 (1.0)	22.6 (2.8)	17.5 (1.6)
Transferrin Saturation (%)	33 (5)	34 (2)	30 (4)	26 (2)	37 (4)	29 (2)
CRP ($mg.L^{-1}$)	1.08 (0.35)	1.10 (0.34)	0.91 (0.33)	1.17 (0.38)	1.12 (0.38)	0.75[a] (0.28)

[a]Significantly different to CTB Day1.

Table 3 Mean (±SEM) for urinary hepcidin levels at baseline (T0) and 3 h post-exercise (T3) during the exercise days for the running (RTB) and cycling (CTB) training blocks

		Urinary hepcidin (nM.mmol Cr^{-1})		p-values			Effect sizes		
		T0	T3	Trial	Time	Interaction	T0-T3	T0: RTB-CTB	T3: RTB-CTB
Day 1	RTB	0.46 (0.14)	1.19[a] (0.26)	0.179	0.002	0.014	1.68	0.15	0.68
	CTB	0.52 (0.06)	0.64[b] (0.10)				0.63		
Day 2	RTB	0.76[c] (0.20)	1.38 (0.37)	0.524	0.245	0.190	0.99	0.14	0.54
	CTB	0.85 (0.24)	0.84 (0.28)				0.02		
Day 6	RTB	0.71 (0.04)	0.93 (0.16)	0.173	0.171	0.505	1.69	0.29	0.25
	CTB	0.43 (0.12)	0.80 (0.28)				0.99		

[a]Significantly different to T0.
[b]Significantly different to RTB Day 1, T3.
[c]Significantly different to RTB Day 1, T0.

and hemolysis in this process, suggesting that chronically elevated hepcidin levels may explain the high incidence of iron deficiency commonly reported in athletes. Such a proposition appears plausible based on the results of the current investigation, since basal hepcidin levels were significantly higher during RTB at D2, R3 and R7, compared to D1. Furthermore, although not statistically significant, moderate to large ES suggest basal hepcidin levels appeared higher at R3 (d = 0.64) and R7 (d = 1.26) compared to baseline in CTB.

Despite the large ES for hepcidin to increase, the inflammatory marker CRP was not significantly higher at R3 and R7 as compared to D1 in both conditions, suggesting no accumulated increases in inflammation. Typically, exercise-induced hepcidin production has been linked specifically to elevations in IL-6, which peaks immediately post-exercise [3-9,18]. Although IL-6 was not measured here, CRP synthesis can be stimulated by increases in pro-inflammatory cytokines such as IL-6, IL-1 and tumor necrosis factor (TNF)-alpha [23,24], and as such, CRP was selected as a surrogate measure of inflammation. Despite CRP levels being previously reported to be elevated up to 24 h post-exercise [6], this was not observed in the current investigation. However,

Table 4 Mean (±SEM) urinary hepcidin levels at baseline (T0) on Day 1 and Recovery days 3 and 7 for the running (RTB) and cycling (CTB) training blocks

		Urinary hepcidin (nM.mmol Cr^{-1})	p-values			Effect sizes		
		T0	Trial	Time	Interaction	RTB -CTB	Day 1-Recovery 3, 7	Recovery 3-7
Day 1	RTB	0.62 (0.20)				0.15	-	-
	CTB	0.56 (0.10)						
Recovery 3	RTB	0.80[a] (0.17)	1.000	0.047	0.365	0.28	0.79	-
	CTB	0.64 (0.18)					0.64	
Recovery 7	RTB	0.67[a] (0.14)				0.20	0.49	0.24
	CTB	0.76 (0.18)					1.26	0.21

[a]Significantly different to RTB Day1.

in agreement with these results, previous investigations have shown IL-6 and CRP to be lower after nine weeks of BCT in female soldiers [25]. Such an outcome suggests that any exercise-related inflammatory processes that were evident here were quickly returned to baseline levels during the subsequent recovery period.

Recently, Auersperger and colleagues [14] investigated the effects of an eight week continuous or interval running program on hepcidin, inflammatory markers and iron status in females. These authors reported that serum hepcidin levels in both groups were significantly lower (compared to baseline) after the first three week period, as well as one week after completing a competitive race at the end of the study (10 or 21 km). Additionally, Ma et al. [26] reported that basal serum hepcidin and IL-6 gene expression were not significantly different between female distance runners and matched controls. The contradictory results of Auersperger et al. [14] and Ma et al. [26] to those of the current investigation may have been influenced by two factors: (a) their populations declining (or pre-existing poor) iron status during the training period, and (b) hormonal fluctuations in the menstrual cycle. Previously, these factors have both been raised as potential mechanisms that could attenuate hepcidin production (for review see [27]). For example, serum ferritin has recently been reported to dictate hepcidin activity in athletes [17]. Here, Peeling and colleagues [17] demonstrated that low serum ferritin levels (<30 $\mu g.L^{-1}$) were linked to the suppression of pre-exercise levels of hepcidin, and the magnitude of hepcidin response to an acute exercise stimulus. Additionally, concerns were raised for individuals with 'suboptimal' iron stores (serum ferritin 30–50 $\mu g.L^{-1}$), as the post-exercise hepcidin response in these individuals was still evident after 3 h of recovery, at a similar magnitude to those athletes presenting with more healthy iron stores. Considering that both the running and control groups in Ma et al. [26] presented with poor iron stores (at the time of biological sampling; serum ferritin of < 35 $ug.L^{-1}$), they would also be classified as Stage One Iron Deficient according to numerous published guidelines for athletes [2,28]. Consequently, these previous findings may only be relevant to populations displaying a poor iron status.

Karl et al. [25] also reported that serum hepcidin levels were unchanged in female soldiers who had performed a nine week BCT training program while receiving an iron fortified food bar (twice daily) or a placebo equivalent. However, when soldiers were regrouped according to their iron status (either Normal [NORM], Iron Deficient [ID] or Iron Deficient Anemic [IDA]), post-BCT basal hepcidin levels were significantly lower in IDA as compared to NORM, while the ID group showed similar decreases without reaching significance ($p = 0.06$). Most importantly, it should be highlighted that during the aforementioned investigations, basal hepcidin samples were obtained at the end of specific training phases [14,25] or at a single time point [26], without measuring any acute changes over the course of the training period. In our investigation, basal hepcidin levels were measured on five occasions (D1, D2, R3, D6, R7), in addition to 3 h post-exercise samples (D1, D2, D6) to highlight the acute hepcidin response. Additionally, this is the first investigation to explore if any benefits associated with iron metabolism might be present after completing a series of non-weight-bearing exercise (cycling) sessions as compared to weight-bearing activity (running) in active males.

Numerous exercise investigations have explored the hepcidin response acutely [3-9], showing that the hormone levels are significantly elevated 3 h post-exercise (as compared to baseline) after each exercise session. However, such a response was only recorded here on D1 of RTB, with moderate to large ES recorded for the majority of the other running and cycling sessions. Such findings may be linked to the accumulation of acute post-exercise increases in hepcidin (supported by moderate to large ES), which may be responsible for raising basal levels (as seen at R3 and R7). As such, elevated basal hepcidin activity may have reduced the magnitude by which hepcidin increases acutely, as a result of the exercise task. Despite this, it would appear that acute bouts of running (and to a lesser degree cycling) performed over a seven day period, may still have the ability to increase basal urinary hepcidin levels (e.g. D1 vs. R7).

In consideration of this finding, the accumulation of hepcidin levels over an extended training program might help to explain the high incidence of iron deficiency commonly observed amongst athletes. Such a proposition is supported by McClung et al. [16], where four days of military specific training followed by a three day cross-country ski march performed by male soldiers (~20 km/day, with 45 kg backpacks), caused an increase in serum IL-6 and hepcidin. This increase in hepcidin activity after their military training would be comparable to the significant hepcidin increases recorded at R7 (as compared to D1 in RTB). However, since training volume has been shown to influence hepcidin production [3], the findings of McClung and colleagues [16] are likely to be exacerbated in comparison to those presented here, possibly as a result of the greater training load undertaken. Furthermore, since the aforementioned investigations have only adopted weight-bearing activity [14,16,25], it is also possible that these results may be different under the influence of non-weight-bearing exercise. With this in mind, it is evident that basal hepcidin levels were likely higher at R7 as compared to D1 in the CTB. Therefore, it is possible that cycling training also has the potential to elevate basal hepcidin levels.

However, given the weight supported nature of the exercise task, it might be that exercise of an extended duration, and/or additional training sessions are required before a similar magnitude of response is recorded comparative to running-based training.

Finally, although the findings of this investigation are novel and important, a limitation of this study may be perceived from the measurement of hepcidin in the urine instead of serum. Previously, it has been demonstrated that urinary hepcidin measures were substantially lower than circulating serum levels [29]. As such, serum measurements are preferable to detect small changes in hepcidin levels. However, due to the nature of the current experimental design, involving numerous sampling time points and logistical requirements for each seven day period, urinary measurements were selected as it represented the most practical option for sample collection. Regardless, it is possible that if serum hepcidin measurements were performed here instead of urine (similar to [16]), the tendency for hepcidin levels to be higher at the end of RTB and CTB may have become stronger and more consistent.

Iron parameters

This investigation demonstrated that iron parameters (serum ferritin and iron, transferrin saturation) remained relatively stable over the course of RTB and CTB, possibly due to the relatively short duration of the experimental period (seven days), as compared to other investigations that obtained conflicting results [14,15,25].

Currently, numerous studies have highlighted the importance of maintaining optimal iron stores throughout a training program. However, a reduction in iron status over the course of an extended training period has been commonly reported [15,25,30]. McClung et al. [15] previously examined how iron parameters may be altered by BCT. These authors reported that markers of both iron storage (serum ferritin) and transport (transferrin saturation) had decreased post-BCT. In support of these findings, Di Santolo et al. [31] also suggested that athletes who performed ~11 h per week of training had reduced ferritin and transferrin saturation levels compared to sedentary controls. The discrepancy between our results and these investigations is potentially due to the shorter duration of the intervention employed here (five sessions over seven days) as compared to the substantially greater number of accumulated sessions over the two month period in other studies [15,25]. Considering that both hepcidin and iron parameters during CTB were not significantly different at R7 as compared to D1, perhaps the use of cycling (as opposed to running) may be better suited to iron deficient individuals, who are required to maintain fitness levels, while consuming iron supplements to replenish iron stores. Specifically, as hemolysis contributes towards iron loss [32], the use of non-weight bearing activity (such as cycling) to reduce hemolysis [13] may be beneficial.

Previously, Telford and colleagues [13], demonstrated significantly higher levels of hemolysis after completing an intensity matched running, as compared to cycling trial (1 h run or cycle at 75% VO_{2peak}). These results were attributed to the impact forces associated with footstrike that increased hemolysis, possibly having implications for exercise-induced iron loss in athletes [32]. Similar results were also reported by Sim et al. [7], where 10 well trained male triathletes performed four separate experimental sessions consisting of high (8 × 3 min intervals at 85% v or pVO_{2peak}, W:R 2:1) and low (40 min continuous exercise at 65% v or pVO_{2peak}) intensity running and cycling, with significant increases in hemolysis immediately post-exercise reported in all trials except for low intensity cycling. However, since the current investigation adopted both high and low intensity sessions during CTB (within a relatively short duration of seven days), any benefits associated with reduced hemolysis during this training period may not have been reflected by the serum iron parameters. To this end, it remains unknown if these findings may be altered over the course of an extended cycling program (e.g. >2 months).

Conclusion

In summary, these results suggest that basal urinary hepcidin levels may be significantly elevated after a series of acute running sessions (five sessions over seven days). However, such events may not be observed if an identical cycling program is adopted. Perhaps, more exercise sessions, or sessions of greater duration may be undertaken with cycling as an exercise medium, before a significant increase in basal hepcidin levels is recorded. Additionally, despite any variations in hepcidin, this did not appear to influence serum iron parameters in RTB and CTB. This study supports the idea that basal hepcidin levels may increase (due to an accumulation of acute exercise-induced responses) over the course of an extended training program; although it remains to be established if such a response may compromise an individual's ability to absorb and recycle iron, which may explain the high incidence of iron deficiency commonly reported in athletes.

Competing interests

The authors wish to declare that no competing interests existed as part of the preparation of this manuscript.

Authors' contributions

MS: Study concept and design, data collection and analysis, measurement of biological samples, manuscript preparation. BD: Study concept and design, data analysis and interpretation, manuscript preparation. GL: Study concept and design, data analysis and interpretation, manuscript preparation. DS: Study concept and design, measurement of hepcidin samples, manuscript preparation. HT: Study concept and design, measurement of hepcidin samples, manuscript preparation. EW: Study concept and design, measurement of hepcidin samples, manuscript preparation. DT: Study concept and design, data analysis and interpretation, manuscript preparation. PP: Study concept and design, measurement of biological samples, data analysis and interpretation, manuscript preparation. All authors read and approved the final manuscript.

Acknowledgements
Debbie Trinder is the recipient of a Senior Research Fellowship from the National Health and Medical Research Council of Australia (APP1020437).

Author details
[1]School of Sport Science, Exercise and Health, The University of Western Australia, Crawley, Western Australia, Australia. [2]Department of Laboratory Medicine, Laboratory of Genetic, Endocrine and Metabolic Disease, Radboud University Medical Centre, Nijmegen, The Netherlands. [3]School of Medicine and Pharmacology, The University of Western Australia, Fremantle Hospital, Fremantle, Western Australia, Australia. [4]Harry Perkins Institute for Medical Research, Nedlands, Western Australia, Australia.

References

1. Lukaski HC: **Vitamin and mineral status: effects on physical performance.** *Nutrition* 2004, **20**(7–8):632–644.
2. Peeling P, Dawson B, Goodman C, Landers G, Trinder D: **Athletic induced iron deficiency: new insights into the role of inflammation, cytokines and hormones.** *Eur J Appl Physiol* 2008, **103**(4):381–391.
3. Newlin MK, Williams S, McNamara T, Tjalsma H, Swinkels DW, Haymes EM: **The effects of acute exercise bouts on hepcidin in women.** *Int J Sport Nutr Exer Metab* 2012, **22**(2):79–88.
4. Peeling P, Dawson B, Goodman C, Landers G, Wiegerinck E, Swinkels D, Trinder D: **Training surface and intensity: inflammation, hemolysis, and hepcidin expression.** *Med Sci Sport Exer* 2009, **41**(5):1138–1145.
5. Peeling P, Dawson B, Goodman C, Landers G, Wiegerinck E, Swinkels D, Trinder D: **Cumulative effects of consecutive running sessions on hemolysis, inflammation and hepcidin activity.** *Eur J Appl Physiol* 2009, **106**(1):51–59.
6. Peeling P, Dawson B, Goodman C, Landers G, Wiegerinck E, Swinkels D, Trinder D: **Effects of exercise on hepcidin response and iron metabolism during recovery.** *Int J Sport Nutr Exer Metab* 2009, **19**(6):583–597.
7. Sim M, Dawson B, Landers G, Swinkels DW, Tjalsma H, Trinder D, Peeling P: **Effect of exercise modality and intensity on post-exercise interleukin-6 and hepcidin levels.** *Int J Sport Nutr Exer Metab* 2013, **23**(2):178–186.
8. Sim M, Dawson B, Landers G, Swinkels DW, Tjalsma H, Yeap BB, Trinder D, Peeling P: **Oral contraception does not alter typical post-exercise interleukin-6 and, hepcidin levels in females.** *J Science Med Sport* 2013. in press.
9. Sim M, Dawson B, Landers G, Wiegerinck ET, Swinkels DW, Townsend M-A, Trinder D, Peeling P: **The effects of carbohydrate ingestion during endurance running on post-exercise inflammation and hepcidin levels.** *Eur J Appl Physiol* 2012, **112**(5):1889–1898.
10. Nemeth E, Rivera S, Gabayan V, Keller C, Taudorf S, Pedersen BK, Ganz T: **IL-6 mediates hypoferremia of inflammation by inducing the synthesis of the iron regulatory hormone hepcidin.** *J Clin Invest* 2004, **113**(9):1271–1276.
11. Nemeth E, Tuttle MS, Powelson J, Vaughn MB, Donovan A, Ward DM, Ganz T, Kaplan J: **Hepcidin regulates cellular iron efflux by binding to ferroportin and inducing its internalization.** *Science* 2004, **306**(5704):2090–2093.
12. Troadec M-B, Laine F, Daniel V, Rochcongar P, Ropert M, Cabillic F, Perrin M, Morcet J, Loreal O, Olbina G, Westerman M, Nemeth E, Ganz T, Brissot P: **Daily regulation of serum and urinary hepcidin is not influenced by submaximal cycling exercise in humans with normal iron metabolism.** *Eur J Appl Physiol* 2009, **106**(3):435–443.
13. Telford RD, Sly GJ, Hahn AG, Cunningham RB, Bryant C, Smith JA: **Footstrike is the major cause of hemolysis during running.** *J Appl Physiol* 2003, **94**(1):38–42.
14. Auersperger I, Knap B, Jerin A, Blagus R, Lainscak M, Skitek M, Skof B: **The effects of 8 weeks of endurance running on hepcidin concentrations, inflammatory parameters, and iron status in female runners.** *Int J Sport Nutr Exer Metab* 2012, **22**(1):55–63.
15. McClung JP, Karl JP, Cable SJ, Williams KW, Young AJ, Lieberman HR: **Longitudinal decrements in iron status during military training in female soldiers.** *Brit J Nutr* 2009, **102**(4):605–609.
16. McClung JP, Martini S, Murphy NE, Montain SJ, Margolis LM, Thrane I, Spitz MG, Blatny J-M, Young AJ, Gundersen Y, Pasiakos SM: **Effects of a 7-day military training exercise on inflammatory biomarkers, serum hepcidin, and iron status.** *Nutr J* 2013, **12:**141.
17. Peeling P, Sim M, Badenhorst CE, Dawson B, Govus AD, Abbiss CR, Swinkels DW, Trinder D: **Iron status and the acute post-exercise hepcidin response in athletes.** *PLoS One* 2014. in press.
18. Nieman DC, Nehlsen-Cannarella SL, Fagoaga OR, Henson DA, Utter A, Davis JM, Williams F, Butterworth DE: **Influence of mode and carbohydrate on the cytokine response to heavy exertion.** *Med Sci Sport Exer* 1998, **30**(5):671–678.
19. Borg GA: **Psychophysical bases of perceived exertion.** *Med Sci Sport Exer* 1982, **14**:377–381.
20. Kroot JCC, Laarakkers CM, Geurts-Moespot A, Grebenchtchikov N, Pickkers P, Van Ede A, Peters HP, Van Dongen-Lases E, Wetzels JFM, Sweep FC, Tjalsma H, Swinkels DW: **Immunochemical and mass spectrometry-based serum hepcidin assays for a variety of iron metabolism disorders.** *Clin Chem* 2010, **56**(10):1570–1579.
21. Van Santen S, Van Dongen-Lases EC, De Vegt F, Laarakkers CM, Van Riel PL, Van Ede AE, Swinkels DW: **Hepcidin and hemoglobin content parameters in the diagnosis of iron deficiency in rheumatoid arthritis patients with anemia.** *Arthritis Rheum* 2011, **63**(12):3672–3680.
22. Swinkels DW, Girelli D, Laarakkers C, Kroot J, Campostrini N, Kemna E, Tjalsma H: **Advances in quantitative hepcidin measurements by time-of-flight mass spectrometry.** *PLoS One* 2008, **3:**e2706.
23. Calabro P, Chang DW, Willerson JT, Yeh ET: **Release of C-reactive protein in response to inflammatory cytokines by human adipocytes: linking obesity to vascular inflammation.** *J Am Coll Cardiol* 2005, **46**(6):1112–1113.
24. Moshage H, Roelofs H, Van Pelt J, Hazenberg B, Van Leeuwen M, Limburg P, Aarden L, Yap SH: **The effect of interleukin-1, interleukin-6 and its interrelationship on the synthesis of serum amyloid A and C-reactive protein in primary cultures of adult human hepatocytes.** *Biochem Bioph Res Co* 1988, **155**(1):112–117.
25. Karl JP, Lieberman HR, Cable SJ, Williams KW, Young AJ, McClung JP: **Randomized, double-blind, placebo-controlled trial of an iron-fortified food product in female soldiers during military training: relations between iron status, serum hepcidin, and inflammation.** *Am J Clin Nutr* 2010, **92**(1):93–100.
26. Ma X, Patterson KJ, Gieschen KM, Bodary PF: **Are serum hepcidin levels chronically elevated in collegiate female distance runners?** *Int J Sport Nutr Exer Metab* 2013. in press.
27. Sim M, Dawson B, Landers G, Trinder D, Peeling P: **Iron regulation in athletes: exploring the menstrual cycle and effects of different exercise modalities on hepcidin production.** *Int J Sport Nutr Exer Metab* 2013. in press.
28. Peeling P, Blee T, Goodman C, Dawson B, Claydon G, Beilby J, Prins A: **Effect of iron injections on aerobic-exercise performance of iron-depleted female athletes.** *Int J Sport Nutr Exer Metab* 2007, **17**(3):221–231.
29. Kroot JJC, Hendriks JCM, Laarakkers CMM, Klaver SM, Kemna E, Tjalsma H, Swinkels DW: **(Pre)analytical imprecision, between-subject variability, and daily variations in serum and urine hepcidin: Implications for clinical studies.** *Anal Biochem* 2009, **389**(2):124–129.
30. Schobersberger W, Tschann M, Hasibeder W, Steidl M, Herold M, Nachbauer W, Koller A: **Consequences of 6 weeks of strength training on red cell O_2 transport and iron status.** *Eur J Appl Physiol Occ Physiol* 1990, **60**(3):163–168.
31. Di Santolo M, Stel G, Banfi G, Gonano F, Cauci S: **Anemia and iron status in young fertile non-professional female athletes.** *Eur J Appl Physiol* 2008, **102**(6):703–709.
32. Reeder BJ, Wilson MT: **Hemoglobin and myoglobin associated oxidative stress: from molecular mechanisms to disease states.** *Curr Med Chem* 2005, **12**(23):2741–2751.

10

Effects of short-term ingestion of Russian Tarragon prior to creatine monohydrate supplementation on whole body and muscle creatine retention and anaerobic sprint capacity: a preliminary investigation

Jonathan M Oliver[1], Andrew R Jagim[2], Ivo Pischel[3], Ralf Jäger[4], Martin Purpura[4], Adam Sanchez[5], James Fluckey[6], Steven Riechman[7], Michael Greenwood[5], Katherine Kelly[5], Cynthia Meininger[8], Christopher Rasmussen[8] and Richard B Kreider[5*]

Abstract

Background: Extracts of Russian Tarragon (RT) have been reported to produce anti-hyperglycemic effects and influence plasma creatine (Cr) levels while supplementing with creatine monohydrate (CrM). The purpose of this preliminary study was to determine if short-term, low-dose aqueous RT extract ingestion prior to CrM supplementation influences whole body Cr retention, muscle Cr or measures of anaerobic sprint performance.

Methods: In a double-blind, randomized, and crossover manner; 10 recreationally trained males (20 ± 2 yrs; 179 ± 9 cm; 91.3 ± 34 kg) ingested 500 mg of aqueous RT extract (*Finzelberg, Andernach, Germany*) or 500 mg placebo 30-minutes prior to ingesting 5 g of CrM (*Creapure®, AlzChem AG, Germany*) twice per day for 5-days then repeated after a 6-week wash-out period. Urine was collected at baseline and during each of the 5-days of supplementation to determine urine Cr content. Whole body Cr retention was estimated from urine samples. Muscle biopsies were obtained for determination of muscle free Cr content. Participants also performed two 30-second Wingate anaerobic capacity tests prior to and following supplementation for determination of peak power (PP), mean power (MP), and total work (TW). Data were analysed by repeated measures MANOVA.

Results: Whole body daily Cr retention increased in both groups following supplementation (0.0 ± 0.0; 8.2 ± 1.4, 6.5 ± 2.4, 5.6 ± 3.2, 6.1 ± 2.6, 4.8 ± 3.2 g · d^{-1}; p = 0.001) with no differences observed between groups (p = 0.59). After 3 and 5-days of supplementation, respectively, both supplementation protocols demonstrated a significant increase in muscle free Cr content from baseline (4.8 ± 16.7, 15.5 ± 23.6 mmol · kg^{-1} DW, p = 0.01) with no significant differences observed between groups (p = 0.34). Absolute change in MP (9 ± 57, 35 ± 57 W; p = 0.031), percent change in MP (2.5 ± 10.5, 6.7 ± 10.4%; p = 0.026), absolute change in TW (275 ± 1,700, 1,031 ± 1,721 J; p = 0.032), and percent change in TW (2.5 ± 10.5, 6.6 ± 10.4%; p = 0.027) increased over time in both groups with no differences observed between groups.

Conclusions: Short-term CrM supplementation (10 g · d^{-1} for 5-days) significantly increased whole body Cr retention and muscle free Cr content. However, ingesting 500 mg of RT 30-min prior to CrM supplementation did not affect whole body Cr retention, muscle free Cr content, or anaerobic sprint capacity in comparison to ingesting CrM with a placebo.

Keywords: Creatine supplementation, Russian Tarragon, Anaerobic capacity, Muscle creatine

* Correspondence: rkreider@hlkn.tamu.edu
[5]Department of Health and Kinesiology, Exercise and Sport Nutrition Lab, Texas A&M University, College Station, TX 77843-4243, USA
Full list of author information is available at the end of the article

Introduction

Research has consistently shown that creatine (Cr) supplementation is an effective strategy to increase muscle Cr content by up to 10-40% [1-3] which can significantly improve anaerobic performance, increase training volume, and enhance training adaptations [4-9]. By following a typical loading dose of 5 g of Cr, 4 times per day (total 20 g daily); muscle Cr content can significantly increase in as little as 3 to 7 days [2]. It has been suggested that the uptake of Cr into muscle is heavily influenced by initial intramuscular Cr concentrations and the type as well as amount of Cr ingested [10]. In this regard, studies have suggested that individuals who start Cr supplementation with low muscle Cr and phosphocreatine (PCr) content are more responsive to Cr supplementation. However, there are other factors that may influence the extent to which Cr is transported into the muscle cells, such as concentrations of glucose and insulin.

The most common form of Cr found in dietary supplements, food products, and referred to in scientific literature is creatine monohydrate (CrM) [10]. Despite consistent findings demonstrating CrM to be effective at increasing muscle Cr content [1-3,10], manufacturers have sought to develop alternative forms to increase market share. Several researchers have investigated the effect of these various forms of Cr in terms of Cr retention, uptake into the muscle cell, and effects on performance [11-15], confirming CrM as the most effective formulation [10]. (For review of alternative forms see [10]) Previous research has also shown that the addition of certain nutrients to Cr may improve Cr retention [16-19]. For example, researchers have found that the co-ingestion of 5 g of CrM with 93 g of glucose significantly increased Cr retention by 60% compared to CrM alone after 5 days of 20 $g \cdot d^{-1}$ [17]. Similarly the addition of certain macronutrients have also been shown to improve Cr retention [18]. Steenge et al. [18] found that the addition of 96 g of carbohydrates and/or 47 g of carbohydrates with 50 g of protein to 20 g of CrM daily improved Cr retention by roughly 25% ($p < 0.05$) compared to 5 g carbohydrates. Results of the study suggest that higher insulin levels, in response to the additional macronutrients, may augment Cr uptake into the muscle.

While co-ingesting large amounts of carbohydrate and/or protein with Cr has been reported to augment muscle and/or whole body Cr retention, some athletes or recreationally active individuals may be interested in lower-calorie strategies to improve Cr uptake. Recently there has been an interest in the effects of combining Cr with additional ingredients to improve Cr uptake and retention. For example, Greenwood and associates [16] found that the co-ingestion of 1 g of D-pinitol (a plant extract with insulin-like properties) per day with CrM (20 g/d) for 3 days significantly improved Cr absorption and retention compared to CrM alone and a placebo. Ethanolic or aqueous extracts of Russian Tarragon (RT) (*artemisia dracunculus*) have been purported to have anti-hyperglycemic effects. Theoretically, co-ingestion of RT with Cr may help augment Cr uptake [20,21]. To support this theory, Jäger et al. [20] found that plasma Cr levels were reduced when RT was combined with CrM compared to CrM alone, suggesting an increase in Cr uptake. Therefore, the purpose of this study was to examine whether a low dose aqueous RT extract ingested 30 minutes prior to CrM intake during a 5-day loading phase significantly affected whole body Cr retention and/or anaerobic capacity in healthy, recreationally active males when compared to CrM ingestion alone.

Methods

Experimental design

The study was conducted in a double-blind, randomized, and crossover manner. The independent variable was RT extract supplementation. Dependent variables included intramuscular Cr concentration, whole body Cr retention, and anaerobic sprint performance capacity. Participants who qualified for the study participated in a familiarization session in which the study was explained following written consent. Participants were then randomly assigned to ingest 2 × 500 g of a placebo (P) or RT, 30-minutes prior to ingesting 5 g of CrM, twice a day for a 5-day period. Urine was collected at baseline and during each of the 5-days of supplementation to determine urine Cr content. At baseline and on days 3 and 5 of supplementation, participants returned to the lab for a muscle biopsy and a Wingate anaerobic capacity test. Urine was collected daily throughout the supplementation period for determination of whole-body Cr retention. Dietary intake was not controlled for but participants were asked to maintain normal dietary practices and record all food intake four days prior to the study and then replicate these practices prior to the next testing session. It has been reported that Cr stores return to baseline after approximately 30 days following cessation of supplementation [1]. To ensure a return to baseline levels, participants then completed a 6-week wash-out period prior to repeating the experiment following the alternate supplementation regimen.

Participants

A consort diagram is provided in Figure 1 outlining reasons for drop out and/or exclusion. Reasons for drop out included scheduling conflicts with no one reporting drop out due to supplementation protocol. Ten apparently healthy recreationally trained males (20 ± 2 yrs; 179 ± 9 cm; 91.3 ± 34 kg) with no self-reported recent history of Cr supplementation completed the entire study. Participants were not allowed to participate in this study if they had any metabolic disorder including known electrolyte

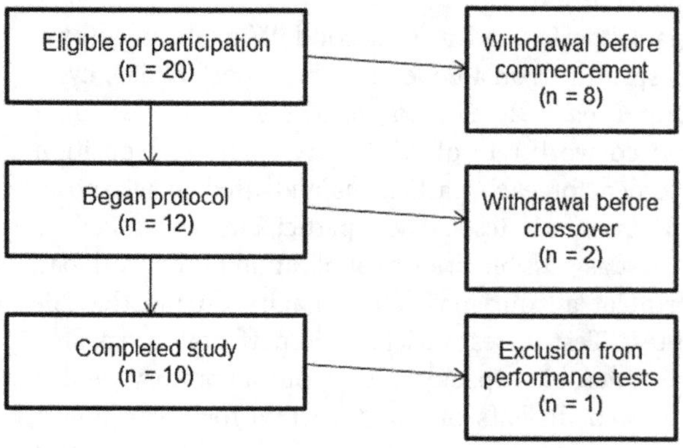

Figure 1 Consort diagram.

abnormalities; heart disease, arrhythmias, diabetes, thyroid disease, or hypogonadism; a history of hypertension, hepatorenal, musculoskeletal, autoimmune, or neurologic disease; if they were taking thyroid, anti-hyperlipidemic, hypoglycemic, anti-hypertensive, anti-inflammatory, or androgenic medications; or, if they had taken dietary supplements containing creatine within three months prior to the start of the study. Participants were recruited from the student population and from area fitness facilities. All participants responding to advertisement and met eligibility criteria were informed of the requirements of the study and invited to a familiarization session. Following explanation of the study procedures, participants signed an informed consent statement in compliance with the Human Subjects Guidelines of Texas A&M University and the American College of Sports Medicine. Participants then completed demographic, health history, and exercise history forms followed by performance of the Wingate anaerobic capacity test (WAnT), which served as familiarization for testing sessions. None of the participants reported training for a sport and/or recreational event during the time of the study. Participants were asked to maintain their normal recreational activities throughout the duration of the study.

Testing sessions

Following familiarization, participants were provided urine collection containers in order to collect 24 hour urine samples throughout the study. Participants reported daily to the laboratory to drop off urine samples and turn in their reported supplement side effects form as well as the requested supplement adherence questionnaire. Muscle biopsies and exercise testing occurred on days 0, 3, and 5. Participants were instructed to refrain from exercise for 48 hours and fast for 8-hours prior to testing sessions. Muscle biopsies were obtained on day 0, 3, and 5. Since this was a cross-over design, the same number of biopsies were obtained on the contralateral leg after the washout period; totaling 6 biopsies per participant. Following muscle biopsy procedures, participants performed two 30-second WAnT separated by 3 minutes.

Supplementation protocol

Participants were randomly assigned to ingest, in a double-blind and cross-over manner, capsules containing 500 mg of an aqueous extract of RT (*Finzelberg, Andernach, Germany*) or a placebo (P) (Luvos Heilerde) with CrM [*Creapure, AlzChem, Trostberg, Germany*]. The RT and P supplements were provided in capsules and two (2x) were consumed 30-minutes prior to ingesting 5 grams of CrM two times daily for 5 days. After a 6-week wash out period, participants repeated the experiment and consumed the alternate supplement capsules prior to CrM supplementation. Participants were instructed to ingest the supplements at 0800 and 2000 each day in order to standardize supplement intake/absorption for the 5 day period. Supplements were comprised of similar texture, taste, and appearance and placed in generic single serving packets for double-blind administration. The supplements were prepared for distribution by the supporting sponsors of this research endeavor. Supplementation compliance was monitored by having the participants return empty containers of the supplement at the end of each testing session. In addition, participant compliance was verified by collecting daily supplement adherence questionnaires when dropping off urine containers. Participants were then provided the supplement dosage for the next day.

Procedures

Muscle and urine samples

Following familiarization, participants were provided eight, 3 L urine collection containers in order to collect 24 hour urine samples for baseline (day 0) and day 1, 2, 3, 4, and 5. Participants were also requested to record the number of times they urinated each day. The 24 hour baseline urine sample time parameter was initiated at 0800 am the day before the supplementation protocol began. Participants were asked to refrigerate their urine samples during the 24 hour time period. Participants reported daily to the laboratory between 0700 and 0800 to drop off urine samples. Whole body creatine retention was estimated as the difference between orally ingested CrM (10 $g \cdot d^{-1}$) and the amount of Cr excreted daily in urine as previously described [22].

Muscle biopsies were obtained using a modified Bergstrom needle biopsy technique following standard procedures [23]. Percutaneous muscle biopsies (50–70 mg) were obtained from the middle portion of the vastus lateralis muscle at the midpoint between the patella and the greater trochanter of the femur at a depth between 1 and 2 cm into the muscle. For the remaining two biopsies, attempts were made to extract tissue from approximately the same location as the initial biopsy by using the pre-biopsy scar, depth markings on the needle, and successive incisions that were made approximately 2 cm proximal to the former site. The initial leg was chosen by the flip of a coin and the contralateral leg was used during the cross-over. After removal of adipose tissue, the muscle specimens were immediately frozen in liquid nitrogen and then stored at–80°C for later analysis. Three muscle samples were obtained (Days 0, 3, & 5) with the same number repeated during crossover on the contralateral leg for a total of six muscle biopsies.

Muscle tissue samples were prepared for spectrophotometric analysis for Cr using methods developed by Harris and colleagues [22,24,25]. Briefly, approximately 50–70 mg of muscle tissue was cut and transferred into a microfuge tube, followed by a dehydration process in a vacuum centrifuge (*Savant ISS110 SpeedVac Concentrator, Thermo Scientific, Milford, MA*) and centrifuged for 18–24 hours. Connective tissue was removed from the dried samples which were then grinded into a powder in a porcelain plate and placed into pre-weighed microfuge tubes. Muscle metabolites were extracted in a 0.5 M perchloric acid/ 1 mM EDTA solution on ice for 15 minutes, while periodically vortexing. Samples were then centrifuged at 7,000 rpm for 5 minutes. The supernatant was transferred into a pre-weighed microfuge tube and neutralized with 2.1 M KHCO3/0.3 M MOPS solution. The samples were then centrifuged again at 7,000 rpm for 5 minutes and the supernatant was removed and placed into microfuge tubes and frozen at–80°C.

Muscle extracts and urine samples were assayed for Cr in the presence of 50 mM imidazole buffer, pH 7.4; 5 mM magnesium chloride; 20 mM potassium chloride; 25 µM phosphoenolpyruvate; 200 µM ATP; 45 µM NADH; 1250 U/mL lactate dehydrogenase; 2000 U/mL pyruvate kinase. The assay was carried out in a standard fluorescence microplate reader using 10 µL of sample to 1 mL of reagent. The reactant solution was vortexed and read using a fluorometer (*Shimadzu RFMini 150, Japan*) with an excitation wavelength of 340 nm and an emission wavelength of 460 nm for baseline absorbance values. Five µL of CK (25 µ/mg) was added to 1 mL of the above buffer and stabilized using 1 mL of reagent. After 10 minutes the plate was read again for post-reaction absorbance values. Test to test reliability of duplicate muscle Cr assays was 0.01 ± 0.10 ($r = 0.81$) with a coefficient of variation of 2.62. Test to test reliability of duplicate of urine Cr assays was 0.01 ± 0.04 ($r = 0.99$) with a coefficient of variation of 1.13. We also assayed muscle and urine samples for PCr, but several values were out of normal ranges in both muscle and urine. Further, there was large variability in the values observed. This suggested lack of validity of this assay and therefore, these data were not reported.

Performance tests

Participants performed a 30-second Wingate anaerobic capacity sprint test on a Lode Excalibur Sport 925900 cycle ergometer (*Lode BV, Groningen, The Netherlands*) at a standardized work rate of 7.5 J/kg/rev. The seat position was recorded for each participant and used in all subsequent performance tests. Each participant was asked to pedal as fast as possible prior to application of the workload and sprint at all-out maximal capacity during the 30-second test. Test-to-test variability in performing repeated Wingate anaerobic capacity tests in our laboratory yielded correlation coefficients of $r = 0.98 \pm 15\%$ for mean power [12]. Participants practiced the anaerobic capacity test during the familiarization session to minimize learning effects. One participant opted out of performance testing due to a prior injury not resulting from participation in the study.

Side effect assessment

Participants were given daily questionnaires on how well they tolerated the supplement, how well they followed the supplement protocol, and if they experienced any medical problems/symptoms during the study. Compliance to the supplementation protocol was monitored daily as participants returned to the lab to hand in urine jugs and complete a daily questionnaire. After completing the compliance procedures, participants were given the required supplements and dosages for the following supplementation period.

Statistical analysis

All statistical analysis was performed using SPSS V.20 (*Chicago, IL*) software. Study data were analyzed by Multivariate Analysis of Variance (MANOVA) with repeated measures. Overall MANOVA effects were examined using the Wilks' Lambda time and group x time p-levels as well as MANOVA univariate ANOVA group effects. Greenhouse-Geisser univariate tests of within-subjects time and group × time effects and between-subjects univariate group effects were reported for each variable analyzed within the MANOVA model. The sum of daily-whole body Cr retention during the study was evaluated by a studentized t-test to determine any differences between groups. Data were considered statistically significant when the probability of type I error was 0.05 or less. If a significant group, treatment, and/or interaction alpha level was observed, Tukey's least significant differences (LSD) post-hoc analyses was performed to determine where significance was obtained.

Results

Urinary creatine excretion and retention

Table 1 presents daily urinary Cr excretion and whole-body Cr retention data. A significant time effect was observed

Table 1 Daily urinary creatine (Cr) excretion and retention

		Day							
Variable	**Group**	**0**	**1**	**2**	**3**	**4**	**5**		**p-level**
Urinary Cr Excreted(g·day^{-1})	P + CrM	0.3 ± 0.4	1.9 ± 1.60	3.5 ± 2.300	4.7 ± 3.3000	3.2 ± 2.800	5.0 ± 3.4000	Time	0.001
	RT + CrM	0.5 ± 0.6	1.7 ± 1.10	3.4 ± 2.700	4.2 ± 3.3000	4.6 ± 2.200	5.4 ± 3.2000	Group	0.801
	Combined	0.4 ± 0.5	1.8 ± 1.4*	3.5 ± 2.4*†	4.4 ± 3.2*†‡	3.9 ± 2.6*†	5.2 ± 3.2*†‡	GxT	0.59
Whole body Cr Retention(g·day^{-1})	P + CrM	0.0 ± 0.0	8.1 ± 1.60	6.5 ± 2.300	5.3 ± 3.3000	6.8 ± 2.800	5.0 ± 3.4000	Time	0.001
	RT + CrM	0.0 ± 0.0	8.3 ± 1.10	6.6 ± 2.700	5.8 ± 3.3000	5.4 ± 2.200	4.6 ± 3.2000	Group	0.82
	Combined	0.0 ± 0.0	8.2 ± 1.4*	6.5 ± 2.4*†	5.6 ± 3.2*†‡	6.1 ± 2.6*†	4.8 ± 3.2*†‡	GxT	0.59

(n = 10).
Values are means ± standard deviations. (n = 10) Greenhouse-Geisser time and group x time (G x T) interaction p-levels are reported with univariate group p-levels. *Significantly different than Day 0. †Significantly different than Day 1. ‡Significantly different than Day 2.

in both daily urinary Cr excretion (p = 0.001) and whole-body retention (p = 0.001), in which post hoc analysis demonstrated similar time effects throughout the supplementation protocol (Table 1). No significant differences were observed between groups (p = 0.82) in total whole-body Cr retention throughout the supplementation protocol, 31.7 ± 11.1 and 30.6 ± 9.9 grams for P + CrM and RT + CrM, respectively.

Muscle creatine analysis

Table 2 presents muscle free Cr content data. Sufficient muscle samples were obtained to measure baseline and subsequent creatine on all (n = 10) participants. A MANOVA was run on muscle Cr expressed in mmol · kg^{-1} DW, changes from baseline expressed in mmol · kg^{-1} DW and percent changes from baseline. An overall MANOVA time effect (Wilks' Lambda p = 0.03) was observed with no significant overall group × time interactions (Wilks' Lambda p = 0.34). MANOVA univariate analysis revealed significant time effects in muscle free Cr content expressed in absolute terms (p = 0.019), changes from baseline (p = 0.019), and percent changes from baseline (p = 0.006), in which post hoc analysis revealed a significant increase in muscle free Cr content by day 5. No significant differences were observed between groups.

Anaerobic capacity

Table 3 presents changes in peak power, mean power, and total work as observed during the 30-second WAnT. One participant did not participate in performance tests during crossover and thus all data were excluded for analysis (n = 9). No overall time or time x group effects were observed for peak power (Wilks' Lambda p = 0.40 and p = 0.52, respectively). An overall MANOVA time effect (Wilks' Lambda p = 0.025 and p = 0.025) was observed for mean power and total work, respectively, with no overall group x time interactions observed. MANOVA univariate analysis revealed significant time effects in mean power and total work. Post hoc analysis revealed significant increases in both mean power and total work by day 5. No significant differences were observed between groups.

Side effect assessment

For all participants who completed the study, supplement compliance was 100%. No side effects were reported for the duration of the study.

Table 2 Muscle free creatine (Cr) levels

Variable	**Group**	**0**	**Day 3**	**5**		**p-level**
Cr (mmol·kg^{-1} DW)	P + CrM	72.1 ± 26.0	81.2 ± 26.0	94.9 ± 40.5	Time	0.019
	RT + CrM	103.0 ± 21.1	103.2 ± 27.2	111.0 ± 19.0	Group	0.049
	Combined	87.5 ± 28.0	92.3 ± 28.2	102.9 ± 31.9*	GxT	0.34
Cr (Δ mmol·kg^{-1} DW)	P + CrM	0.0 ± 0.0	9.3 ± 14.3	22.8 ± 28.2	Time	0.019
	RT + CrM	0.0 ± 0.0	0.3 ± 18.4	8.1 ± 16.2	Group	0.097
		0.0 ± 0.0	4.8 ± 16.7	15.5 ± 23.6*	GxT	0.34
Cr (Δ%)	P + CrM	0.0 ± 0.0	21.1 ± 30.0	37.3 ± 41.7	Time	0.008
	RT + CrM	0.0 ± 0.0	0.7 ± 20.5	9.6 ± 18.1	Group	0.035
	Combined	0.0 ± 0.0	10.9 ± 27.1	23.5 ± 34.4*	GxT	0.13

(n = 10).
Values are means ± standard deviations. (n = 10) Δ represents change from baseline values. Data were analyzed by MANOVA with repeated measures. Greenhouse-Geisser time and group x time (G x T) interaction p-levels are reported with univariate group p-levels. *Significantly different than Day 0.

Table 3 Changes in peak power, mean power, and total work during Wingate

Variable	Group	0	Day 3	5		p-level
Peak power (W)	P + CrM	1,472 ± 451	1,435 ± 182	1,380 ± 244	Time	0.68
	RT + CrM	1,559 ± 213	1,565 ± 398	1,519 ± 339	Group	0.31
	Combined	1,515 ± 345	1,500 ± 307	1,450 ± 295	GxT	0.92
Mean power (W)	P + CrM	591 ± 94	599 ± 89	642 ± 8300	Time	0.031
	RT + CrM	590 ± 103	601 ± 78	608 ± 9600	Group	0.79
	Combined	591 ± 96	600 ± 81	625 ± 89*†	GxT	0.27
Total work (J)	P + CrM	17,742 ± 2,822	17,970 ± 2,663	19,264 ± 2,48200	Time	0.032
	RT + CrM	17,706 ± 3,098	18,029 ± 2,339	18,246 ± 2,88800	Group	0.79
	Combined	17,724 ± 2,875	17,999 ± 2,432	18,755 ± 2,664*†	GxT	0.27

(n = 9).
Values are means ± standard deviations. Δ represents change from baseline values. Data were analyzed by MANOVA with repeated measures. Greenhouse-Geisser time and group x time (G x T) interaction p-levels are reported with univariate group p-levels. *Significantly different than Day 0. †Significantly different than Day 3.

Discussion

Ethanolic and aqueous extracts of Russian Tarragon (RT) (*artemisia dracunculus*) have been purported to have anti-hyperglycemic effects [21,26,27]. A previous study found that ingesting this same dose of RT with CrM resulted in a greater reduction in plasma Cr levels suggesting greater uptake [20]. The purpose of this study was to examine whether a low dose aqueous RT extract ingested 30 minutes prior to CrM intake during a 5-day loading phase significantly affected whole body Cr retention and/or anaerobic capacity in healthy, recreationally active males when compared to CrM ingestion alone. Our preliminary findings indicate that ingesting 500 mg RT 30-min prior to CrM supplementation did not affect whole body Cr retention or muscle free Cr content during a short-period of CrM supplementation ($10\ g \cdot d^{-1}$ for 5-days) in comparison to ingesting a placebo prior to CrM supplementation. Further, results of this preliminary study indicate that ingesting 500 mg RT 30-min prior to CrM supplementation had no additive effects on anaerobic sprint capacity in comparison to ingesting CrM with a placebo.

While oral ingestion of CrM alone increases total muscle Cr content, the addition of other nutrients has been shown to enhance the absorption, thereby increasing muscle Cr content to a greater degree than CrM alone. Green et al. [17] demonstrated that ingesting 5 g CrM followed by 93 g simple carbohydrate (glucose and simple sugars) resulted in an increase in muscle Cr content compared to CrM alone. Later investigations have shown that a lesser amount of carbohydrate (35 g) with each dose of CrM may promote greater adaptations than CrM alone. Based on these findings, it has been hypothesized that Cr retention during supplementation may be mediated in part by the insulin pathway. In support of this hypothesis, Steenge et al. [28] demonstrated that insulin can enhance muscle Cr accumulation, but only when present at physiologically high or supraphysiological concentrations. While co-ingesting large amounts of carbohydrate and/or protein with Cr have been reported to promote muscle Cr retention, some athletes or recreationally active individuals may be interested in lower-calorie strategies to improve Cr uptake. Greenwood et al. [16] found that the co-ingestion of 1 g of D-Pinitol (a plant extract with insulin-like properties) per day with CrM (20 g/d) for 3 days significantly improved whole body Cr retention. While D-Pinitol provides a non-caloric substitute to other higher calorie nutrients, it is relatively expensive. Further, no other studies have demonstrated D-Pinitol to increase total muscle Cr.

Extracts of RT have been purported to have anti-hyperglycemic effects. The effect of RT on carbohydrate metabolism is most noted in animal models. For instance, Ribnicky et al. [27] showed the ethanolic extract of RT to reduce insulin concentrations by 33% compared to 48% and 52% for the antidiabetic drugs troglitzaone and metformin, respectively. Further, this same research group has shown ethanolic RT to significantly lower blood glucose concentrations by 20% in streptozotocin-induced diabetic mice, compared to control. However, the dosage in that study was significantly greater than the present study (500 mg/kg bodyweight). Further evidence of the anti-hyperglycemic effects of RT has been provided by Pischel et al. [29]. Using the same aqueous extract of RT and dosage used in the current study, Pischel et al. [29] reported lower blood glucose levels in both animals and humans (albeit non-statistically) following ingestion.

While the antidiabetic properties of RT are a relatively new discovery [30], current investigations are focusing on alterations in the insulin pathway. Given the purported role of insulin in enhanced muscle Cr accumulation, RT may serve as a means to augment Cr retention without the ingestion of carbohydrate and the resulting greater caloric intake. Jäger et al. [20] demonstrated a significant reduction in plasma Cr levels following ingestion of similar dose of RT followed by CrM compared with CrM alone. However, the current study suggests no additive effect of RT when combined with CrM on muscle Cr retention. Despite similar RT and CrM dosing strategy, 10 $g \cdot day^{-1}$ in current study compared to 60 $g \cdot kg$ bodyweight (just over 10 g using current participant average weight), measuring muscle Cr content demonstrated no additive effect of RT. It must be noted that despite there not being a statistically significant difference, the baseline muscle free Cr during the supplementation of RT and CrM appears to be slightly higher than CrM alone. There is no doubt large inter-individual differences in the change in Cr in muscle as evidenced by the work of Harris et al. [31] and Greenhaff et al. [2]. More importantly, Greenhaff et al. [2] demonstrated that any measureable effect on PCr resynthesis as a result of Cr ingestion was only observed in individuals demonstrating greater than a 20 $mmol \cdot kg^{-1}$ increase in TCr. Thus, the apparent higher baseline free Cr may have contributed to the current findings.

Despite finding no additive effect of RT, a novel aspect of the current study was the finding that ingesting as little as 5 g of CrM twice daily (i.e., 10 $g \cdot d^{-1}$) increased total muscle Cr content by 23.5 ± 34.5%. This dosing strategy was based on the previous study by Jäger et al. [20]. To the authors' knowledge, this is the first study to report significant increases in muscle Cr following low dose supplementation. This occurred despite being lower than dosage strategies used in previous studies (20 $g \cdot d^{-1}$ or 0.3 $g \cdot kg^{-1} \cdot bw^{-1}$) [5,9]. Harris et al. [31] were the first to demonstrate supplementation with 5 g CrM taken orally 4–6 times per day for two or more days resulted in a significant increase in muscle Cr content. The authors further noted the greatest change occurred in those individuals with low initial total Cr content. The increase in muscle Cr content observed in the current study is similar to values reported in the literature with higher loading doses (25 ± 3%) [2]. Further, we observed a significant improvement in both MP and TW by 2-7% following a lower dosing strategy suggesting that this level of Cr supplementation may be sufficient to affect anaerobic exercise capacity. This finding furthers the research in the area of the optimal loading phase dosing strategy to effectively increase muscle Cr stores.

In summary, the most important finding in this study were as little as 5 g CrM taken twice daily for 3–5 days increases total muscle Cr, whole body Cr retention, and improves MP and TW. However, results of this pilot study do not support contentions that ingesting 500 mg of RT prior to CrM supplementation enhances whole body Cr retention, muscle free Cr content, or provides an additive effect on anaerobic sprint capacity during a short-period of CrM supplementation. Additional research is needed with a larger sample size to examine: 1.) whether ingestion of greater amounts of RT prior to and/or in conjunction with CrM ingestion would affect Cr retention; 2.) whether ingestion of RT with CrM over longer periods of time would affect Cr retention; and, 3.) whether co-ingesting RT with CrM and carbohydrate may reduce the need for ingesting large amounts of carbohydrate with CrM in order to promote greater Cr retention.

Competing interests

Martin Bauer Group, Finzelberg GmbH & Co. KG. provided funding for this study through a research grant to Texas A&M University. All researchers involved independently collected, analyzed, and interpreted the results from this study and have no financial interests concerning the outcome of this investigation. RBK has received grants as Principal Investigator through institutions with which he has been affiliated to conduct exercise and nutrition related research, has served as a legal and scientific consultant, and currently serves as a scientific consultant for Woodbolt International (*Bryan, TX*). MP, IP, and RJ have been named as inventors on pending patents by the Martin Bauer Group. Remaining co-authors have no competing interests to declare. Data from this study have been presented at the International Society of Sports Nutrition Annual meeting and have not been submitted for publication to any other journals. Publication of these findings should not be viewed as endorsement by the investigators or their institutions of the nutrients investigated.

Authors' contributions

JMO served as the study coordinator, oversaw all testing, and assisted in data analysis and writing of the manuscript. ARJ assisted in data collection and statistical analysis. IP, RJ, and MP assisted in the experimental design, data analysis, and manuscript preparation. AS assisted with data collection JF and SR supervised the biopsy procedures. MG assisted in experimental design, data analysis, and manuscript preparation. KK supervised muscle assays and CM served as a collaborating scientist. CR served as lab coordinator and oversaw data collection and quality control of the study. RBK served as Principal Investigator and contributed to the design of the study, statistical analysis, manuscript preparation, and procurement of external funding. All authors read and approved the final manuscript.

Funding

Supported by the Martin Bauer Group, Finzelberg GmbH & Co. KG.

Author details

[1]Kinesiology Department, Texas Christian University, Fort Worth, TX 76129, USA. [2]Sport & Exercise Science Department, Gannon University, Erie, PA 16541, USA. [3]Phytolab GmbH & Co. KG, Vestenbergsgreuth, Germany. [4]Increnovo LLC, 2138 E Lafayette Pl, Milwaukee, WI 53202, USA. [5]Department of Health and Kinesiology, Exercise and Sport Nutrition Lab, Texas A&M University, College Station, TX 77843-4243, USA. [6]Department of Health and Kinesiology, Muscle Biology Laboratory, Texas A&M University, College Station, TX 77843-4243, USA. [7]Department of Health and Kinesiology, Human Countermeasures Laboratory, Texas A&M University, College Station, TX 77843-4243, USA. [8]Department of Systems Biology and Translational Medicine, Texas A&M Health Science Center, College Station, TX 77843-1114, USA.

References

1. Hultman E, Soderlund K, Timmons JA, Cederblad G, Greenhaff PL: **Muscle creatine loading in men.** *J Appl Physiol* 1996, **81**:232–237.
2. Greenhaff PL, Bodin K, Soderlund K, Hultman E: **Effect of oral creatine supplementation on skeletal muscle phosphocreatine resynthesis.** *Am J Physiol* 1994, **266**:E725–730.
3. Kreider RB, Ferreira M, Wilson M, Grindstaff P, Plisk S, Reinardy J, Cantler E, Almada AL: **Effects of creatine supplementation on body composition, strength, and sprint performance.** *Med Sci Sports Exerc* 1998, **30**:73–82.
4. Branch JD: **Effect of creatine supplementation on body composition and performance: a meta-analysis.** *Int J Sport Nutr Exerc Metab* 2003, **13**:198–226.
5. Buford TW, Kreider RB, Stout JR, Greenwood M, Campbell B, Spano M, Ziegenfuss T, Lopez H, Landis J, Antonio J: **International Society of Sports Nutrition position stand: creatine supplementation and exercise.** *J Int Soc Sports Nutr* 2007, **4**:6.

6. Clark JF: **Creatine and phosphocreatine: a review of their use in exercise and sport.** *J Athl Train* 1997, **32**:45–51.
7. Dempsey RL, Mazzone MF, Meurer LN: **Does oral creatine supplementation improve strength? A meta-analysis.** *J Fam Pract* 2002, **51**:945–951.
8. Kreider RB, Leutholtz BC, Katch FI, Katch VL: *Exercise and Sport Nutrition.* Santa Barbara, CA: Fitness Technologies Press; 2009.
9. Williams MH, Kreider R, Branch JD: *Creatine: The power supplement.* Human Kinetics Publishers; 1999.
10. Jager R, Purpura M, Shao A, Inoue T, Kreider RB: **Analysis of the efficacy, safety, and regulatory status of novel forms of creatine.** *Amino Acids* 2011, **40**:1369–1383.
11. Jager R, Metzger J, Lautmann K, Shushakov V, Purpura M, Geiss KR, Maassen N: **The effects of creatine pyruvate and creatine citrate on performance during high intensity exercise.** *J Int Soc Sports Nutr* 2008, **5**:4.
12. Jagim AR, Oliver JM, Sanchez A, Galvan E, Fluckey J, Riechman S, Greenwood M, Kelly K, Meininger C, Rasmussen C, Kreider RB: **A buffered form of creatine does not promote greater changes in muscle creatine content, body composition, or training adaptations than creatine monohydrate.** *J Int Soc Sports Nutr* 2012, **9**:43.
13. Kreider RB, Willoughby D, Greenwood M, Parise G, Payne E, Tarnopolsky M: *Effects of serum creatine supplementation on muscle creatine and phosphagen levels.* Online: J Exerc Physiol; 2003:6.
14. Greenwood M, Kreider R, Earnest C, Rasmussen C, Almada A: **Differences in creatine retention among three nutritional formulations of oral creatine supplements.** *Journal of Exercise Physiology Online* 2003, **6**:2.
15. Tallon MJ, Child R: **Kre-alkalyn® supplementation has no beneficial effect on creatine-to-creatinine conversion rates.** In *Book Kre-alkalyn® supplementation has no beneficial effect on creatine-to-creatinine conversion rates*; 2007.
16. Greenwood M, Kreider RB, Rasmussen C, Almada AL, Earnest CP: **D-Pinitol augments whole body creatine retention in man.** *J Exerc Physiol Online* 2001, **4**:41–47.
17. Green AL, Hultman E, Macdonald IA, Sewell DA, Greenhaff PL: **Carbohydrate ingestion augments skeletal muscle creatine accumulation during creatine supplementation in humans.** *Am J Physiol* 1996, **271**:E821–826.
18. Steenge GR, Simpson EJ, Greenhaff PL: **Protein- and carbohydrate-induced augmentation of whole body creatine retention in humans.** *J Appl Physiol* 2000, **89**:1165–1171.
19. Kreider RB: **Effects of creatine supplementation on performance and training adaptations.** *Mol Cell Biochem* 2003, **244**:89–94.
20. Jager R, Kendrick I, Purpura M, Harris R, Ribnicky, Pischel I: **The effect of Russian Tarragon (artemisia dracunculus L.) on the plasma creatine concentration with creatine monohydrate administration.** In *Book The effect of Russian Tarragon (artemisia dracunculus L.) on the plasma creatine concentration with creatine monohydrate administration*, Volume 5; 2008:4.
21. Wang ZQ, Ribnicky D, Zhang XH, Raskin I, Yu Y, Cefalu WT: **Bioactives of Artemisia dracunculus L enhance cellular insulin signaling in primary human skeletal muscle culture.** *Metabolism* 2008, **57**:S58–64.
22. Harris RC, Hultman E, Nordesjo LO: **Glycogen, glycolytic intermediates and high-energy phosphates determined in biopsy samples of musculus quadriceps femoris of man at rest. Methods and variance of values.** *Scand J Clin Lab Invest* 1974, **33**:109–120.
23. Evans WJ, Phinney SD, Young VR: **Suction applied to a muscle biopsy maximizes sample-size.** *Med Sci Sports Exerc* 1982, **14**:101–102.
24. Soderlund K, Hultman E: **Effects of delayed freezing on content of phosphagens in human skeletal muscle biopsy samples.** *J Appl Physiol* 1986, **61**:832–835.
25. Tarnopolsky MA, Parise G: **Direct measurement of high-energy phosphate compounds in patients with neuromuscular disease.** *Muscle Nerve* 1999, **22**:1228–1233.
26. Bloomer RJ, Canale I, Pischel I: **Effect of an aqueous Russian tarragon extract on glucose tolerance in response to an oral dextrose load in non-diabetic men.** *Nutr Diet Suppl* 2011, **3**:43–49.
27. Ribnicky DM, Poulev A, Watford M, Cefalu WT, Raskin I: **Antihyperglycemic activity of Tarralin, an athanolic extract of *Artemisia dracunculus L.*** *Phytomedicine* 2006, **13**:550–557.
28. Steenge GR, Lambourne J, Casey A, Macdonald IA, Greenhaff PL: **Stimulatory effect of insulin on creatine accumulation in human skeletal muscle.** *Am J Phys* 1998, **275**:E974–E979.
29. Pischel I, Burkard N, Kauschka M, Butterweck V, Bloomer RJ: **Potential application of Russian tarragon (artemisia dracunculus l.) in health and sports.** *Journal of International Society of Sports Nutrition* 2011, **8**:16.
30. Graf BL, Raskin I, Cefalu WT, Ribnicky DM: **Plate-derived therapeutics for the treatment of metabolic syndrome.** *Curr Opin Investig Drugs* 2010, **11**:1107–1115.
31. Harris RC, Soderlund K, Hultman E: **Elevation of creatine in resting and exercised muscle of normal subjects by creatine supplementation.** *Clin Sci (Lond)* 1992, **83**:367–374.

Effects of rehydration and food consumption on salivary flow, pH and buffering capacity in young adult volunteers during ergometer exercise

Mai Tanabe[1], Toshiyuki Takahashi[1*], Kazuhiro Shimoyama[2], Yukako Toyoshima[3] and Toshiaki Ueno[1]

Abstract

Background: The aim of this study was to investigate the influences of rehydration and food consumption on salivary flow, pH, and buffering capacity during bicycle ergometer exercise in participants.

Methods: Ten healthy volunteers exercised on a bicycle ergometer at 80% of their maximal heart rate. These sessions lasted for two periods of 20 min separated by 5-min rest intervals. Volunteers were subjected to one of the following conditions: (1) no water (mineral water) or food consumption, (2) only water for rehydration, (3) water and food consumption, (4) a sports drink only for rehydration, and (5) rehydration with a sports drink and food. Statistical significance was assessed using one-way analysis of variance and Dunnett's test ($p < 0.05$).

Results: The salivary pH decreased significantly during and after exercise in conditions 4 and 5. The salivary buffering capacity decreased significantly during exercise and/or after the exercise in conditions 1, 3, 4, and 5.

Conclusions: The results showed that salivary pH and buffering capacity decreased greatly depending on the combination of a sports drink and food.

Keywords: Saliva, Rehydration, Sports drink, Exercise, Oral care

Background

It was reported that the decayed, missing, and filled teeth index and the risk of tooth erosion in athletes is relatively high as compared with that of ordinary people [1-3]. The mouth should be functional and free from disease, facilitating good nutrition and physical wellbeing to achieve maximum sporting potential [2]. In general, dental caries and erosion seen in athletes are thought to be caused by dry mouth with exercise-induced rehydration, large consumption of sports drinks and foods, and poor brushing of teeth because of physical fatigue. Among them, the sensation of dry mouth and dehydration means a decrease in the salivary flow rate, which causes a decline in the irrigation function in the oral environment. Many studies have also shown that a decrease in salivary secretion causes a decline in oral sugar clearance capacity in patients with dry mouth symptoms. A previous study in our laboratory reported that treadmill and ergometer exercises induced decreases of both the salivary flow rate and the salivary buffering capacity [4-6]. Thus, a decrease of salivary secretion indicates an increase in the risk of dental caries and erosion [4,7,8]. In addition, in many studies regarding the risk of dental caries and erosion, salivary secretion, salivary pH, and salivary buffering capacity were used as the parameters. Hirose et al. indicated that significant positive correlations were noted between salivary flow rate and salivary pH, but positive correlations were not noted between salivary flow rate and salivary buffering capacity [9]. If the pH of saliva is <5.5, the critical pH of dental enamel, then the mineral of dental enamel tends to dissolve [10]. Therefore, using the salivary pH and salivary buffering capacity to discuss dental caries and erosion is important.

However, many athletes were observed drinking isotonic and/or soft drinks that contained high acid and/or sugar contents, which resulted in an increased risk of dental caries and erosion. Drinking water during exercise can prevent excessive dehydration and changes in electrolyte

* Correspondence: t.takahashi.spmd@tmd.ac.jp
[1]Department of Sports Medicine/Dentistry, Graduate School of Medical and Dental Sciences, Tokyo Medical and Dental University, Bunkyo-ku, Japan
Full list of author information is available at the end of the article

balance, and can maintain the salivary secretion function [11]. Peter et al. studied the effects of rehydration on performance following moderate dehydration, and found that constituents other than water, simple transportable monosaccharides and sodium, are important for maximal exercise performance and effective recovery associated with endurance exercise-induced dehydration [12].

Moreover, people commonly consume foods such as fruits and supplements during exercise. Studies have reported that salivary pH values immediately increase after food consumption [13]. However, the influence on the oral environment of exercise with water and nutritional support is unclear. In the present study, we investigated the influences of rehydration and food consumption on salivary flow, pH, and buffering capacity during bicycle ergometer exercise in healthy volunteer participants.

Methods

Experiments were performed on 10 healthy volunteers [4 females, mean ± standard deviation (SD) age, height, and weight: 20.5 ± 1.1 years, 160.5 ± 3.8 cm, and 55.7 ± 4.3 kg, respectively; 6 males, mean ± SD of age, height, and weight: 23.0 ± 3.1 years, 175.6 ± 7.47 cm, and 65.3 ± 4.3 kg, respectively]. The volunteers were fully dentate and had no oral disorders or braces. This study was approved by the Ethical Committee for Human Research of the Faculty of Dentistry, Tokyo Medical and Dental University, and the participants provided informed consent according to institutional guidelines.

The test was started at least 2 h after the last meal and at least 1 h after brushing the teeth [4-6]. The test exercise on the bicycle ergometer (Aerobike Ai, Combi Wellness Corporation, Tokyo, Japan) consisted of a warm-up of 5–10 min, a 20-min aerobic exercise at the test intensity determined to be 80% of the maximal heart rate, a warm-down exercise (1 min), 10-min rest, and repetition of the first warm-up/exercise cycle. The ergometer recorded the heart rate in real time from a sensor attached to the earlobe. The load of the pedal for exercise was automatically controlled by the ergometer at an intensity from level 1 to level 20, determined by the heart rate, and the pedal did not allow freewheeling.

Each volunteer tested the five conditions on different days in a random order. The fluid intake was at each participant's discretion during exercise, but the food intake was assigned in the resting period (jelly-type nutritional supplement) and just after the exercise (banana). The conditions were as follows: (1) no intake of fluid or food, (2) intake of mineral water, (3) intake of mineral water and food (jelly-type nutritional supplement and banana), (4) intake of sports drink, and (5) intake of sports drink and food.

We used mineral water (Evian, Danone Waters of Japan Co., Tokyo, Japan) and a sports drink (Aquarius, Coca-Cola & Co., Ltd., Tokyo, Japan) as the sources of the fluid intake. Aquarius is one of the major sports drink brands in Japan. We used a jelly-type nutritional supplement (Wider In Jerry, Morinaga & Co., Ltd., Tokyo, Japan) and bananas (mean weight 147.9 ± 18.0 g) as the sources of food.

Salivary production was stimulated by chewing a piece of unflavored paraffin wax for 3 min and 30 s. After 30 s of prestimulation, whole saliva samples were collected in a container for 3 min. The volume of the stimulated whole saliva samples was measured. Whole saliva samples were collected before, during, and after exercise. Salivary pH and buffering capacity were measured using a hand-held pH meter (Checkbuf™, Horiba Ltd., Tokyo, Japan) [4-6]. Calibration of the pH meter was done for each participant and each test with usage of dedicated standard pH-4.0 and pH-7.0 solutions. Salivary pH was directly measured from 0.25 ml of a saliva sample placed on the electrode sensor of the pH meter. To examine the salivary buffering capacity, 0.25 ml of dedicated lactic acid solution (pH 3.0) was dripped into the saliva sample on the electrode sensor. The pH meter was gently shaken for 20 s to mix the saliva sample and the lactic acid solution.

The statistical significance of the results was assessed using one-way analysis of variance and Dunnett's test. For all the statistical analyses, p-values of <0.05 were considered significant.

Results

In conditions 2 and 4, the mean quantities of the mineral water consumed were 642.4 ± 230.1 ml and 630.1 ± 188.7 ml, respectively. In conditions 3 and 5, those of the sports drink were 751.0 ± 152.9 ml and 714.0 ± 155.6 ml, respectively. No significant difference was present between the two groups.

Figure 1(a) shows the salivary flow rates. In condition 1, the salivary flow rate after exercise decreased by 40.3% compared with that before exercise ($p < 0.05$). In the other conditions, there was no significant difference in the salivary flow rate or its variations during the experiment.

Figure 1(b) shows the changes of salivary pH. In condition 4, salivary pH during and after exercise significantly decreased by 5.5% and 6.6%, respectively, compared with before exercise, and in condition 5, salivary pH during and after exercise significantly decreased by 4.6% and 4.3%, respectively, compared with before exercise. In condition 2, salivary pH during and after exercise did not decrease compared with that before exercise.

Figure 1(c) shows the changes of salivary buffering capacity. In condition 1, salivary buffering capacity during and after exercise significantly decreased by 5.6% and 7.2%, respectively, compared with before exercise. In condition 4, salivary buffering capacity during and after exercise significantly decreased by 9.8% and 9.3%, respectively, compared

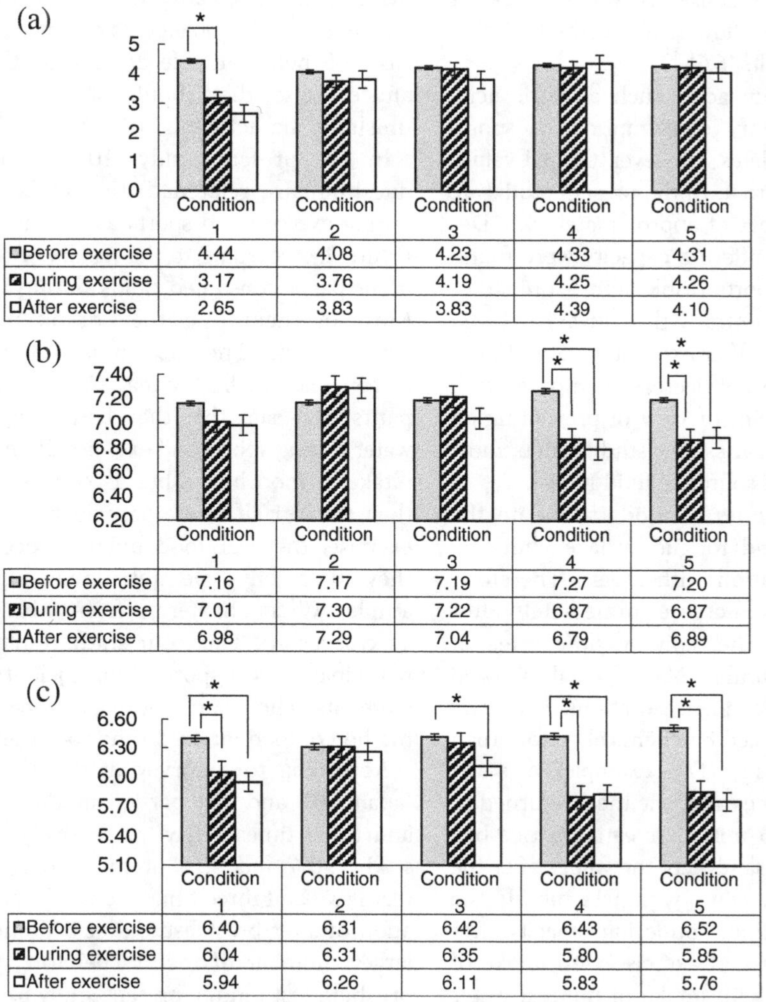

(a)

	Condition 1	Condition 2	Condition 3	Condition 4	Condition 5
Before exercise	4.44	4.08	4.23	4.33	4.31
During exercise	3.17	3.76	4.19	4.25	4.26
After exercise	2.65	3.83	3.83	4.39	4.10

(b)

	Condition 1	Condition 2	Condition 3	Condition 4	Condition 5
Before exercise	7.16	7.17	7.19	7.27	7.20
During exercise	7.01	7.30	7.22	6.87	6.87
After exercise	6.98	7.29	7.04	6.79	6.89

(c)

	Condition 1	Condition 2	Condition 3	Condition 4	Condition 5
Before exercise	6.40	6.31	6.42	6.43	6.52
During exercise	6.04	6.31	6.35	5.80	5.85
After exercise	5.94	6.26	6.11	5.83	5.76

Figure 1 Changes of salivary flow rate (a), salivary pH (b) and salivary buffering capacity (c). Numerical values in table are the means of 10 participants.

with before exercise. In condition 5, salivary buffering capacity during and after exercise significantly decreased by 10.3% and 11.7%, respectively, compared with before exercise. In condition 3, salivary buffering capacity after exercise significantly decreased by 4.8% compared with before exercise. In condition 2, salivary buffering capacity was almost constant throughout the experiment.

Discussion

The mean stimulated salivary flow rate induced by chewing was reported to be 1.6 ml/min [7]. In the present study, the mean salivary flow rate after exercise was 0.77 ml/min in condition 1. Salivary secretion is strongly affected by the neural control of the autonomic nervous system, which indirectly regulates the salivary flow rate. The salivary flow rate depends on the autonomic state [14]. Because an increase of sympathetic activation is caused by sports and exercise, active exercise was expected to decrease the salivary flow rate [15]. Comparing the salivary secretion function of mineral water and the sports drink, the sports drink had a stronger inhibitory action on salivary secretion than mineral water. The taste of the sports drink is thought to bring about a difference in the quantity of the fluid intake during sports and exercise [4]. The results of the present study indicate that adequate hydration during sports and exercise inhibited the decrease of the salivary secretion function and the risk of dental caries and erosion.

Carbonic acid is known to decrease blood pH, and salivary secretion always requires adequate supply of nutrients from the blood [16,17]. The change in salivary pH depends on the level of CO_2 in the blood [17]. With an increase in the blood CO_2 level, CO_2 is transferred from the blood to the saliva at a higher rate, with a subsequent decrease in salivary pH [14]. This function could explain the decrease in salivary pH during and after exercise compared with before exercise in condition 1. Nakano et al. studied the effects of exercise on salivary flow rate and buffering capacity, and found that exercise was a significant factor decreasing both salivary flow rate and the buffering capacity, in line with our results [5,6].

Many sports drinks contain acids such as citric acid, which increases the voluntary consumption of sports drinks, including that by athletes. However, the pH values of sports drinks vary from 3 to 4. In the present study, we used a sports drink with a pH of approximately 4.0. Decreases in salivary pH and buffering capacity were found in conditions 4 (intake of sports drink) and 5 (intake of sports drink and food). In contrast, the salivary pH and buffering capacity during and after exercise in condition 2 (intake of mineral water), did not decrease compared with before exercise. From the point of view of preventing an increase in the risk of dental caries, our study results show that mineral water is the best source of fluid intake.

Physical and chemical factors of foods stimulate the oral mucous membranes and tongue surface, inducing salivary secretion in association with meals. Therefore, salivary pH values generally increase immediately after meals [13]. In this study, the salivary flow rates in conditions 3 and 5 were similar. Nanba et al. showed that the salivary secretion-dependent variations in salivary pH values were more influenced by chemical factors than physical factors of food [13]. For example, a study reported that salivary pH values after the meal returned to the original values within 35 min after eating a rice ball [13]. However, after eating a sandwich, the values after the meal returned to the original values within 15 min. In the present study, the salivary pH and buffering capacity after exercise was lower in the case of exercise with intake of sports drink and food, than with intake of mineral water and food. With regard to the risk of dental caries and erosion, consumption of mineral water with food during sports and exercise is desirable in people who participate in exercise and/or competitions.

Nutrients such as glucose, proteins, amino acids, fat, fatty acids, minerals, electrolytes, and vitamins obtained from ingested food are essential for athletes' growth, development, and maturation [18]. Carbohydrate supplementation is effective in improving performance and deferring fatigue because glucose is the only source of energy for the brain [19]. Human sweat is known to contain minerals such as Na^+, Cl^-, and at least 25 other electrolytes and trace elements [20-22]. Consequently, supplements are necessary to maintain the appropriate distribution of electrolytes in the fluid compartment of the body [21,22]. Because K^+ has a relationship to muscle fatigue, K^+ supplementation to athletes during prolonged sports and exercise by administering nutritional supplements like bananas is considered necessary [23]. Moreover, they contain many nutrients such as water, protein, carbohydrates, Mg^{2+}, and K^+, the levels of which are three times as high in bananas as in apples [24]. Therefore, in order to maintain a proper amount of electrolytes, athletes should take nutritional supplements during sports and exercise. In case of being unable to taking them during sports and exercise, they should do as early as possible after finishing the activities.

In the present study, 10 participants answered a questionnaire related to the intake of fluids and food during exercise and sports as well as oral health behavior Figure 2. According to the results of the questionnaire, all participants consumed fluids during sports and exercise. Most of them said they drank mineral water or a sports drink. The next most common fluid was tea (green tea and barley tea). Approximately 30% participants who said that they had only tea and/or mineral water during sports and exercise did not consider the fluid intake as food intake but as consumption for quenching their thirst. Half of the participants answered that during exercise, they eat food often or occasionally, and that they liked jelly-type nutritional supplements (for example, Wider In Jerry, from Morinaga & Co., Ltd., Tokyo, Japan). Thus, our study results indicate that 70% participants used sports drinks, jelly-type nutritional supplements, chocolate, and/or rice balls as the preferred method of food intake during sports and exercise.

According to a survey of dental diseases in 2005 in Japan, 50% and 21% participants brushed their teeth two and three times a day, respectively [25]. In the present study, 70% and 30% of the participants brushed their teeth two and three times a day, respectively. The combination of after breakfast and at bedtime accounted for the largest number of them. Therefore, the daily frequency brushing teeth in the present study participants was above the national average. Although 70% participants used sports drinks and half of them nutritional supplements during sports and exercise, none brushed their teeth after snacking. The present study indicated that the risk of dental caries could increase as a result of the conditions of water and nutritional supplementation; therefore, we should pay more attention to oral health care.

There are many adjunctive devices for tooth brushing such as dental floss, interdental brushes, one-tuft brushes, tongue brushes, and toothpaste. Tooth brushing is not sufficient for plaque control, and daily dental flossing has been emphasized for plaque control of proximal surfaces [26]. The American Dental Association reported that up to 80% of plaque might be removed by dental flossing [27]. The present study results revealed that only 10% of the participants used dental floss every day, and indicated that dental flossing is not accepted as a common oral health behavior yet. In addition, the questionnaire survey results indicated that 60% participants had been taught how to brush their teeth, and that only 30% participants had been taught how to use dental floss. Thus, dentists and dental hygienists should help people understood the

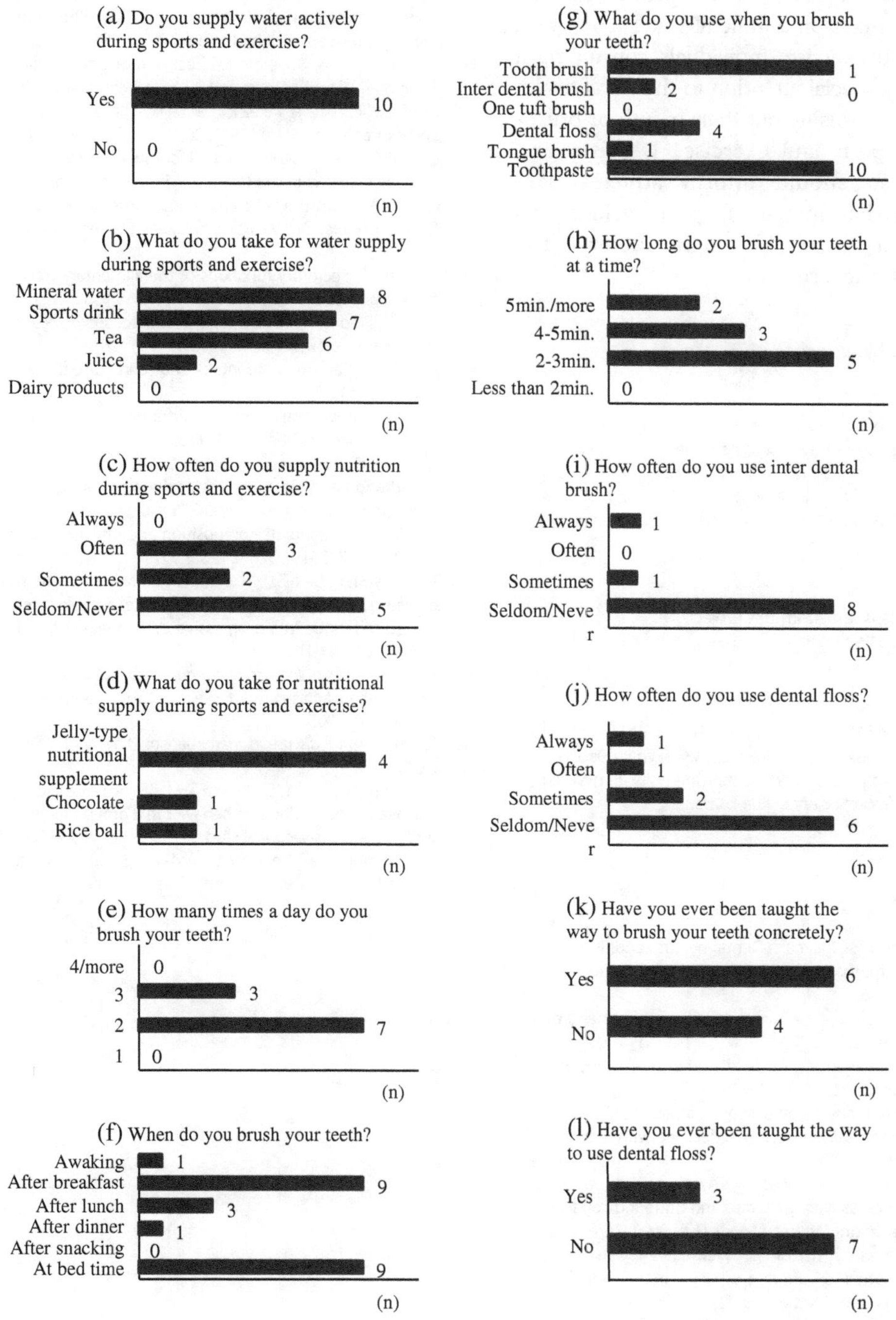

Figure 2 Questionnaire and frequency related to intake of fluids and food during exercise and sports, and oral health behavior. Histograms showing the number of responders to each of the questions.

importance of dental floss for tooth care and the proper way to use dental floss.

Conclusion

The present study's results indicated that adequate hydration during sports and exercise decreased salivary secretion and increased the risk of dental caries and erosion. However, during bicycle ergometer exercise, intake of sports drinks and foods were shown to significantly influence the oral circumstances, salivary pH, and buffering capacity, and increased the risk of dental caries and erosion. Therefore, from the point of view of the risks of dental caries and erosion, we advise that people who participate in exercise and competition should consume mineral water along with food during sports and exercise. Individuals consuming a sports drink should pay special attention to their oral health care by measures such as rinsing out their mouth or brushing their teeth after sports and exercise. Dentists and dental hygienists also should inform athletes, laypeople, and coaches that intake of sports drinks and food during sports and exercise might increase the risks of dental caries and erosion.

Competing interests

The authors declare that they have no competing interests.

Authors' contributions

MT participated in the design of the study, carried out the experiment and drafted the manuscript. TT performed the coordination and data analyses of the study, and helped to draft the manuscript. KS participated in the design of the study. YT participated in data arrangement. TU conceived of the study and participated in its design. All authors read and approved the final manuscript.

Acknowledgements

There has been no financial assistance with this project.
The authors would like thank all participants for their contribution to this study.

Author details

[1]Department of Sports Medicine/Dentistry, Graduate School of Medical and Dental Sciences, Tokyo Medical and Dental University, Bunkyo-ku, Japan. [2]Oral health care science, Tokyo Medical and Dental University, Bunkyo-ku, Japan. [3]Japanese Institute of Sports Science, Kita-ku, Japan.

References

1. Sumita Y, Yamanaka T, Ueno T, Ohyama T: **Dental health conditions of Japanese amateur rugby football players and their mouthguard uses.** *J Sports Dent* 2002, **5**(1):30–36.
2. Bryant S, McLaughlin K, Morgaine K, Drummond B: **Elite athletes and oral health.** *Int J Sports Med* 2011, **32:**720–724.
3. Sirimaharaj V, Brearley ML, Morgan MV: **Acidic diet and dental erosion among athletes.** *Aus Dent J* 2002, **47**(3):228–236.
4. Ueno T, Nakano S, Takahashi T, Abe K, Toyoshima Y, Tanabe M, Shimoyama K: **Effect of fluid replacement on salivary secretion declined with exercise load.** *J Sports Dent* 2012, **15**(2):53–60.
5. Yamamoto-Nakano S, Yamanaka T, Takahashi T, Toyoshima Y, Kawahara T, Ueno T: **Effect of exercise on salivary flow rate and buffering capacity in healthy female and male volunteers.** *Int J Sports Dent* 2009, **2:**25–32.
6. Yamamoto-Nakano S, Takahashi T, Toyoshima Y, Kawahara T, Ueno T: **Changes in salivary flow rate and buffering capacity after treadmill exercise of varied intensity and duration.** *Int J Sports Dent* 2010, **3:**37–45.
7. Heintze U, Birkhed D, Bjorn H: **Secretion rate and buffer effect of resting and stimulated whole saliva as a function of age and sex.** *Swed Dent J* 1983, **7:**227–238.
8. Moritsuka M, Kitasako Y, Burrow MF: **The pH change after HCL titration into resting and stimulated saliva for a buffering capacity test.** *Aus Dent J* 2006, **51**(2):170–174.
9. Hirose M, Fukuda A, Yahata S, Matsumoto D, Igarashi S: **Individual variations in salivary buffer capacity measured by Checkbuff and relationship among salivary flow rate, pH, buffer capacity, phosphate ion, and protein concentrations in saliva.** *J Dent Hlth* 2006, **56:**220–227.
10. Colin D: **What is the critical pH and why does a tooth dissolve in acid?** *J Can Dent Assoc* 2003, **69**(11):722–724.
11. Sawka MN, Burke LM, Eichner ER, Maughan RJ, Stachenfeld NS: **American college of sports medicine. Position stand on exercise and fluid replacement.** *Med Sci Sports Exerc* 2007, **39:**377–390.
12. Peter GS, Robert W, Chithan K, Sidney JS: **Comparative effects of selected non-caffeinated rehydration sports drinks on short-term performance following moderate dehydration.** *J Int Soc Sports Nutr* 2010, **7:**28.
13. Nanba R, Itaya A, Norimoto E: **Effect of foods on salivary pH.** *Bulletin of Faculty of Education Okayama University* 1988, **77**(1):11–21.
14. Chicharo JL, Lucia A, Perez M, Vaquero AF, Urena R: **Saliva composition and exercise.** *Sports Med* 1998, **26**(1):17–27.
15. Elena P, George PN: **Saliva as a tool for monitoring steroid, peptide and immune markaers in sport and exercise science.** *J Sci Med Sport* 2011, **10:**1016.
16. Guyton AC: **Transport of oxygen and carbon dioxide in blood and tissue fluids.** In *Textbook of medical physiology*, 11th ed. Philadelphia: WB Saunders Company; 2006.
17. Guyton AC: **Secretory functions of the alimentary tract.** In *Textbook of medical physiology*, 11th ed. Philadelphia: WB Saunders Company; 2006.
18. Allan JR, Fred LA: **Nutrition for the athlete.** *Sports medicine. A Subsidiary of Harcount Jovanovich* 1989:141–159.
19. Kovacs MS: **Carbohydrate intake and tennis, are there benefits.** *Br J Sports Med* 2006, **40:**el3.
20. Clarkson PM: **Minerals, exercise performance and supplementation in athletes.** *J Sport Sci* 1991, **9:**91–116.
21. Armstrong LE, Hubbard RW, Szlyk PC, Matthew WT, Sils IV: **Voluntary dehydration and electrilyte losses during prolonged exercise in the heat.** *Aviat Space Environ Med* 1985, **56:**765–770.
22. Costill DL: **Sweating, its composition and effects on body fluids.** *Ann NY Acad Sci* 1977, **301:**160–174.
23. Matthew ST, Robert GM, Troy B, Melanie M, Kyle L: **The relationship between blood potassium, blood lactate, and electromyography signals related to fatigue in a progressive cycling exercise test.** *Electromyogr Kinesiol* 2011, **21**(1):25–32.
24. *Standard tables of food composition in Japan fifth revised and enlarged edition.* Japan: Ministry of Education, Culture, Sports, Science and Technology; 2005.
25. *Survey of dental disease in Japan.* Japan: Ministry of Health, Labor and Welfare; 2005.
26. Hossain N, Masaumeh E, Maryam T, Mana HA, Keiwan K: **Major differences in oral health knowledge and behavior in a group of Iranian pre-university students; a cross-sectional study.** *J Oral Sci* 2011, **53:**177–184.
27. Council on Dental Therapeutics: *Accepted Dental Therapeutics, 40th ed. Section III.* Chicago, USA: American Dental Association; 1984.

12

Low-intensity and moderate exercise training improves autonomic nervous system activity imbalanced by postnatal early overfeeding in rats

Wilson Rinaldi[1], Rodrigo Mello Gomes[2], Dionízia Xavier Scomparin[3], Sabrina Grassiolli[3], Tatiane Aparecida Ribeiro[4], Gabriel Sergio Fabricio[1], Luiz Felipe Barella[4], Audrei Pavanello[4], Amanda Bianchi Trombini[4], Paulo Cezar de Freitas Mathias[4] and Júlio Cezar de Oliveira[4*]

Abstract

Background: Postnatal early overfeeding and physical inactivity are serious risk factors for obesity. Physical activity enhances energy expenditure and consumes fat stocks, thereby decreasing body weight (bw). This study aimed to examine whether low-intensity and moderate exercise training in different post-weaning stages of life is capable of modulating the autonomic nervous system (ANS) activity and inhibiting perinatal overfeeding-induced obesity in rats.

Methods: The obesity-promoting regimen was begun two days after birth when the litter size was adjusted to 3 pups (small litter, SL) or to 9 pups (normal litter, NL). The rats were organized into exercised groups as follows: from weaning until 90-day-old, from weaning until 50-day-old, or from 60- until 90-days-old. All experimental procedures were performed just one day after the exercise training protocol.

Results: The SL-no-exercised (SL-N-EXE) group exhibited excess weight and increased fat accumulation. We also observed fasting hyperglycemia and glucose intolerance in these rats. In addition, the SL-N-EXE group exhibited an increase in the vagus nerve firing rate, whereas the firing of the greater splanchnic nerve was not altered. Independent of the timing of exercise and the age of the rats, exercise training was able to significantly blocks obesity onset in the SL rats; even SL animals whose exercise training was stopped at the end of puberty, exhibited resistance to obesity progression. Fasting glycemia was maintained normal in all SL rats that underwent the exercise training, independent of the period. These results demonstrate that moderate exercise, regardless of the time of onset, is capable on improve the vagus nerves imbalanced tonus and blocks the onset of early overfeeding-induced obesity.

Conclusions: Low-intensity and moderate exercise training can promote the maintenance of glucose homeostasis, reduces the large fat pad stores associated to improvement of the ANS activity in adult rats that were obesity-programmed by early overfeeding.

Keywords: Moderate exercise training, Overfeeding-induced obesity, Autonomic nervous system, Parasympathetic nervous system, Glucose homeostasis

Background

Obesity has reached epidemic proportions in many of the developed countries of the world. This phenomenon is frequently ascribed to the combination of excess food consumption and decreased physical activity [1]. The habits acquired in childhood have a major impact on adult life, and in most cases, determine the state of health during adulthood, particularly with respect to metabolic and endocrine disturbances. Extensive findings indicate that metabolic programming occurs in humans, and this metabolic programming is correlated with the increased risk of adverse health effects, such as diabetes, hypertension and cardiovascular disease [2-4]. Animal studies demonstrate that nutritional programming during the early periods of postnatal life has numerous long-term growth consequences [5-9]. The intrauterine

* Correspondence: biojborges@gmail.com
[4]Department of Biotechnology, Genetics and Cell Biology, State University of Maringá, Maringá, PR, Brazil
Full list of author information is available at the end of the article

and lactation phases of life are crucial periods in brain growth and development processes; it is during these stages that critical events of cell migration and differentiation occur [10,11]. Nutritional insults, by either low or overfeeding, on these stages may be responsible for the changes in the hypothalamic pathways involved in metabolic balance and energy homeostasis [12,13]. As reported, early overfeed-programmed obese rats exhibit disrupted neuronal firing in the central nervous regulation of body weight (bw) [14].

Several maternal environmental insult conditions have been linked to obesity in both human and rodent offspring, which, in turn, has been shown to affect neural development. Interestingly, both maternal caloric deprivation and maternal overfeeding can leads to metabolic syndrome in offspring [15,16]. Overfeeding and obesity are often accompanied by alterations in both sympathetic and parasympathetic autonomic function. Several lines of evidence support the hypothesis that derangements in the autonomic nervous system (ANS) play an important role in the development of obesity [17,18]. As reported, other different models of obesity display imbalanced function of the ANS [19,20]. The sympathetic and parasympathetic nervous systems are critical in the coordination of the catabolic and anabolic responses, respectively. In response to physical activity, glucose uptake is increased in the adipose and skeletal muscle cells; which happens regardless of insulin action [21,22].

The major metabolic changes induced by exercise training are caused by the enhancement of sympathetic tonus. Adrenodemedullated rats that were submitted to swimming training showed low fat mobilization; where was showed that the long-term exercise training led to the mobilization of fat, and the fat gains in these adrenodemedullated rats were more consistent [23]. Thus, it is important to keep in mind that the exercise training may increase the basal metabolism to promote further increases in fat store consumption, even at rest. As previously reported by our group, the low-intensity and moderate swimming training was able to attenuate obesity onset induced by monosodium L-glutamate (MSG) in mice. However, the benefits of this protocol were observed only in cases where exercise was started early, soon after weaning [24].

Rat's litter size reduction provokes overfeeding behavior in suckling pups, which induces a high chow intake post-weaning and subsequent obesity. The early overfeeding model of obesity is interesting because the development of obesity in childhood and adolescence is highly correlated with the onset of the metabolic syndrome in adulthood [25,26]. In the present study, we aimed to evaluate the effects of low-intensity and moderate exercise training applied during different post-weaning development stages on modulating the ANS activity and its role on blocks the obesity progression in rats that were early overfeed.

Materials

Ethical approval

All experiments were undertaken according to the norms established by the Brazilian Association for Animal Experimentation (COBEA) and were previously approved by the Ethics Committee in Animal Research of the State University of Maringá (protocol number 084/2009).

Animals and obesity induction

Sets of 3 female and 1 male Wistar rats, 70 days old, were mated. After 1 week, the pregnant rats were separated. On the 2nd day of life, the size of the normal litters (NL) was set to 9 pups; while the small litter (SL) size was set to 3 pups. After weaning (21st day), males were selected, and all females were discharged. Young male rats from the NL and SL groups were randomly chosen for exercise. Animals received water and a commercial diet (Nuvital®; Curitiba/PR, Brazil) *ad libitum*. During all protocol stages, the animals were placed in an environmentally controlled room (23 ± 3°C; 12 hour light/dark photocycle (07:00–19:00 h).

Exercise training protocol

Rats from the NL exercised (NL-EXE) and SL exercised (SL-EXE) groups were trained on an animal treadmill (model ET-2000 Insight®; Ribeirão Preto/SP, Brazil). Three trained groups were established: exercise beginning after weaning in 21-day-old rats and ending at 90-day-old (EXE_{21-90}); exercise beginning at weaning and stopped at 50-day-old (EXE_{21-50}); and exercise beginning at 60 days old and ending at 90 days old ($EXE60_{60-90}$). Another group of NL and SL rats did not exercise at all (N-EXE). Running protocols, including running speeds and times, were set to induce moderate-intensity exercise training, promoting a 50-70% total oxygen uptake (VO_{2max}) for each animal, independent of age. The running protocols used have been described previously [27,28] with some modifications. The anaerobic threshold of the rats is approximately 20 $m.min^{-1}$ and was used to delimit the maximal velocity reached in the training program. This protocol was intended to guarantee the same aerobic exercise intensity across all ages as the animals grew.

Adaptation period of exercise protocol

Exercise sessions lasted 10 min on the first day of the adaptation period, and the rats were run at a velocity of $10\ m \times min^{-1}$. The sessions were increased to 20 min at $12\ m \times min^{-1}$ for the subsequent sessions. The rats in the group exercised from days 21–90 had an adaptation time of two weeks, and the rats in the 21–50 day group and the 60–90 day group had an adaption time of one week, as previously reported [27]. The running sessions were performed in the afternoon. The rats that did not adapt were eliminated.

Training period

In the EXE_{21-90} groups, the initial training speed was 12 m × min^{-1} for 20 min and was increased to 20 m × min^{-1} for 60 min over ten weeks (Figure 1A). The initial speed of the EXE_{21-50} and EXE_{60-90} groups was 12 m × min^{-1} for 20 min and was increased to 20 m × min^{-1} for 50 min over four weeks (Figure 1B). The variation of the training period time and velocity was adjusted for each protocol and their specific sessions.

Food intake

After weaning, rats from all groups were weighed, and food intake was determined every week by non-ingested chow. Food intake was calculated for each animal as chow consumed divided by bw. The total area under the curve (AUC) of food consumption throughout experimental protocol was calculated.

Intravenous glucose tolerance test (ivGTT)

At 91-day-old, rats from all groups underwent a surgery for the silicone cannula implantation into the right jugular vein, as previously described [29]. At 24 h after the surgery, and after to be fasted overnight (12 h; 7:00 PM to 7:00 AM) the rats received a glucose infusion (1 g/kg bw) by a cannula implanted in the right jugular vein. Blood samples were collected in heparinized syringes at 0 (before glucose administration), 5, 15, 30 and 45 min after the glucose administration. Plasma samples were stored at −20°C for determination of glucose concentrations by the glucose oxidase method (Gold Aanlisa®; Belo Horizonte/MG, Brazil). The AUC of glycemia throughout the ivGTT was calculated.

Autonomic nerves activity assessment

At 91-day-old, a batch of rats from all of the experimental groups, after to be fasted overnight was subsequently anesthetized with thiopental (45 mg/kg bw). As previously described [29], surgical longitudinal incisions were made on the anterior cervical region. Under the dissection microscope, the nerve bundle of the left superior branch of the upper vagus nerve was severed from the carotid artery close to the trachea. The nerve trunk was pulled with a fine cotton line, and a pair of recording silver electrodes (0.6 mm diameter), similar to a hook, were placed under the nerve. The nerve was covered with silicone oil to prevent dehydration. The electrode was connected to an electronic device (Bio-Amplificator, Insight®; Riberão Preto/SP, Brazil), which amplified the electrical signals up to 10,000 times, and the low and high frequencies, 1–80 kHz, were filtered. The neural signal output was acquired by an Insight interface (Insight®; Riberão Preto/SP, Brazil), viewed online and stored by a personal computer running software developed by Insight (Bio-Amplificator, Insight®; Riberão Preto/SP, Brazil). During all data acquisition, the animals were placed in a Faraday cage to avoid any electromagnetic interference. Nerve activity was analyzed as the number of spikes during 5 sec. After stabilization of the signal for 2 min, 20 record frames of 15 sec from each animal were randomly chosen for spike counting. The average number of spikes was used as the nerve firing rate for each rat.

The branch of the sympathetic nerve from the lumbar plexus that innervates the retroperitoneal white fat tissue,

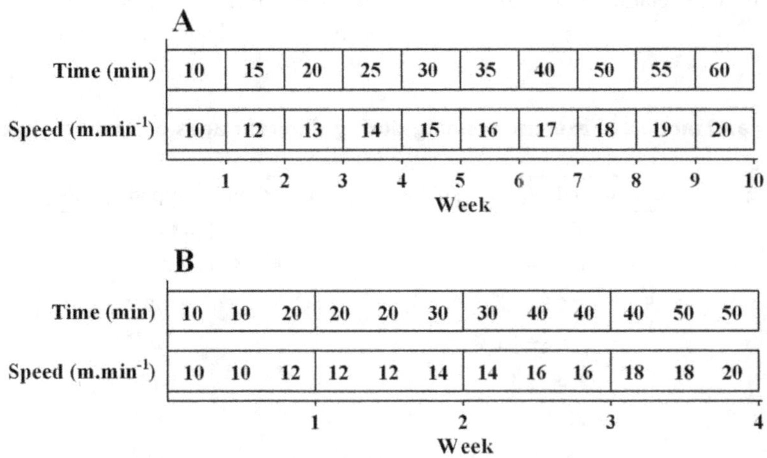

Figure 1 Schematical figure depicting the treadmill exercise training protocol. The time sessions, speed and duration depict the intensity of exercise training throughout the period in which exercise training protocol was performed. Exercise training protocol applied from 21- until 90-days-old **(A)**; and applied from 21- until 50-days-old or from 60- until 90-days-old **(B)**.

which may be called the greater splanchnic nerve, was dissected from another batch of anesthetized rats from all experimental groups, as described above. The electrode was placed under the greater splanchnic nerve, close to the retroperitoneal area. Firing rates from the nerve were obtained as described for the vagus nerve.

Obesity assessment

After all experimental procedure, as described above, both exercised and no-exercised rats were anaesthetized by an intraperitoneal injection of pentobarbital sodium (thiopental 45 mg/kg bw) and killed by cervical dislocation. The retroperitoneal fat pads were removed and weighed. The fat mass of this tissue was used as a simple reliable estimation of total body fat in normal and obese rodents.

Statistical analysis

The results are expressed as the mean ± SEM. Data were submitted to variance analysis (one-way ANOVA). In the case of analyses with a significant F, the differences between the means were evaluated by Tukey's test. Probability values less than .05 ($p < .05$) were considered statistically significant. Tests were performed using GraphPad Prism version 5.0 for Windows (GraphPad Software Inc., San Diego/CA, USA).

Results

Biometric parameters

As shown in Table 1, the SL-N-EXE group exhibited larger bw (10%) when compared to the NL-N-EXE group ($p < .01$). In the NL-EXE$_{21-90}$ group, exercise reduced the bw by 13% compared to the NL-N-EXE group ($p < .05$). No differences were observed among the NL-N-EXE, NL-EXE$_{21-50}$ and NL-EXE$_{60-90}$ groups. In contrast, the SL-EXE$_{21-90}$, SL-EXE$_{21-50}$ and SL-EXE$_{60-90}$ groups exhibited bw reductions around of 10%, in relation to the SL-N-EXE ($p < .05$).

As showed in Table 1, the retroperitoneal fat pad content was larger in the SL-N-EXE group (88%) compared to the NL-N-EXE group ($p < .01$). Moderate exercise training reduced the retroperitoneal fat pad in the NL-EXE$_{21-90}$ group by 25% ($p < .05$), whereas no differences were observed among the NL-N-EXE, NL-EXE$_{21-50}$ and NL-EXE$_{60-90}$ groups. In all of the SL-EXE groups (21–90, 21–50 and 60–90), moderate exercise training reduced the weight of the retroperitoneal fat pads (35%, 27% and 41%, respectively) in relation to those of the SL-N-EXE group ($p < .05$).

Food intake

The AUC of food intake exhibited significant differences between the NL-N-EXE and the SL-N-EXE groups ($p < .05$; Table 1). Exercise training did not change food intake in either group (NL-EXE and SL-EXE), independent of the period in which exercise protocol was applied (21–90, 21–50 or 60–90).

Glycemic homeostasis

When compared with the NL-N-EXE group, the fasting blood glucose levels were reduced by 34% in the SL-N-EXE group ($p < .05$; Table 1). Exercise altered fasting plasma glucose concentrations independent of the period in which protocol was applied, decreasing levels by 18%, 14% and 20% in the SL-EXE$_{21-90}$, SL-EXE$_{21-50}$ and SL-EXE$_{60-90}$ groups, respectively, when compared to the SL-N-EXE group ($p < .05$; Table 1). Exercise did not change fasting blood glucose levels in the NL-EXE groups compared to NL-N-EXE group (Table 1).

Throughout the ivGTT, the SL-N-EXE group exhibited plasma glucose levels higher than those of the NL-N-EXE group (Figure 2A). As shown by the AUC (inset of the Figure 2A), postnatal early overfeeding in rats increased glycemia by 54% during the ivGTT when compared to the NL-N-EXE group ($p < .05$). No significant difference was observed between the NL-N-EXE and

Table 1 Effect of low-intensity and moderate exercise training during different ages on fasting glycemia and biometric parameters

		Body weight (g)	AUC food intake (g/100 g of bw)	Retroperitoneal fat pad (g/100 g bw)	Glycemia (mg/dL)
N-EXE	**NL**	386.7 ± 4.2	179.0 ± 5.1	0.88 ± 0.02	81.8 ± 3.0
	SL	423.1 ± 6.4**	205.0 ± 4.2**	1.66 ± 0.03**	109.4 ± 2.2**
EXE$_{21-90}$	**NL**	334.5 ± 4.4*	180.5 ± 3.2	0.66 ± 0.02*	83.4 ± 2.1
	SL	384.6 ± 5.0#	204.8 ± 1.3	1.07 ± 0.02#	89.5 ± 2.9#
EXE$_{21-50}$	**NL**	395.8 ± 4.9	193.3 ± 3.2	0.76 ± 0.04	78.2 ± 1.9
	SL	385.3 ± 10.1#	206.5 ± 1.5	1.21 ± 0.04#	94.2 ± 3.4#
EXE$_{60-90}$	**NL**	387.7 ± 3.9	185.0 ± 5.7	0.73 ± 0.04	86.2 ± 3.2
	SL	380.2 ± 9.6#	209.8 ± 4.7	0.97 ± 0.02#	87.2 ± 1.5#

All values are expressed as the mean ± SEM of 10–16 rats from each experimental group. *$p < .05$ and **$p < .01$ v.s. NL-N-EXE; #$p < .05$ v.s. SL-N-EXE; by one-way ANOVA followed by the Tukey's test.

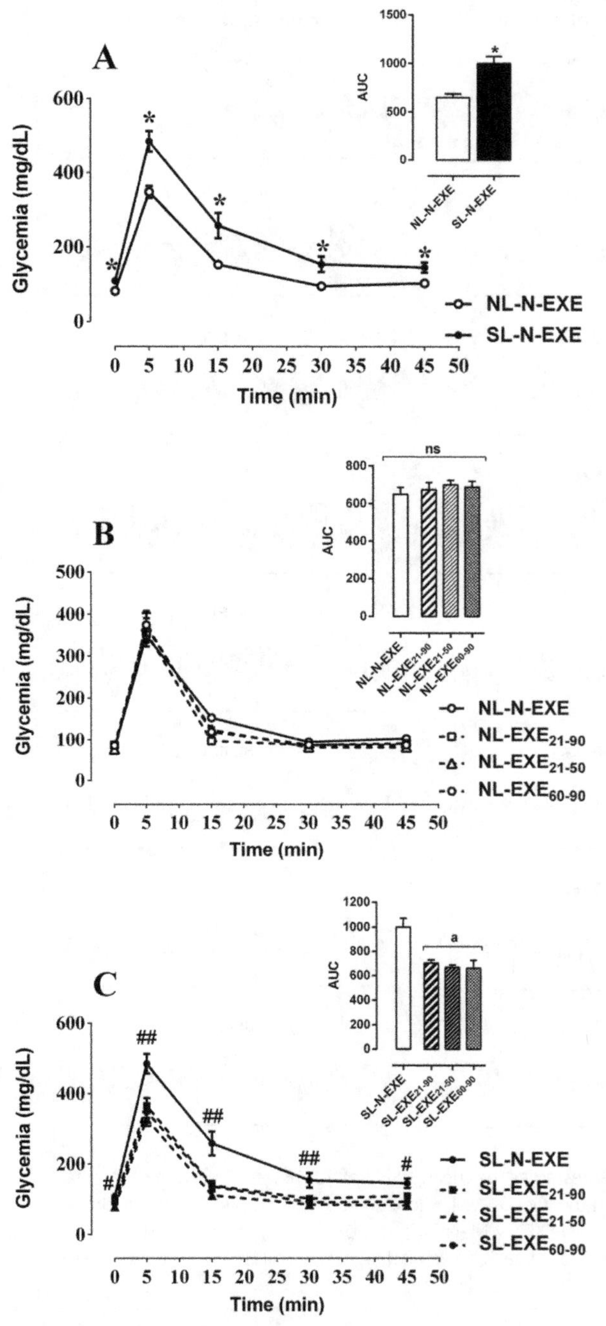

Figure 2 Intravenous glucose tolerance test (ivGTT). All values are expressed as the mean ± SEM of 12–15 rats for each experimental group. **(A)** NL-N-EXE versus SL-N-EXE; **(B)** NL-N-EXE versus all NL-EXE groups and **(C)** SL-N-EXE versus all SL-EXE groups. Symbols on the lines as well as letters on the bars represents the statistical difference by one-way ANOVA followed by Tukey's test among groups. *p < .01 for NL-N-EXE v.s. SL-N-EXE, (Figure 2**A**); ##p < .01, #p < .05 for each one of SL-EXE group v.s. SL-N-EXE, (Figure 2**C**). The upper panel of each figure represents the area under the curve of glycemia during the ivGTT. (ns) Represents no statistical difference in the Figure 2**B** and **(A)** represents SL-N-EXE group in the Figure 2**C**.

NL-EXE groups (Figure 2B). However, the exercise training was able on improves the glucose intolerance of the SL rats. As showed in the inset of the Figure 2C, the SL-EXE (SL-EXE$_{21-90}$, SL-EXE$_{21-50}$ and SL-EXE$_{60-90}$) groups exhibited lower plasma glucose levels in relation to the NL-N-EXE group, which were similar to those of the NL-N-EXE rats.

Autonomic nervous activity

The SL-N-EXE group exhibited a 31% increase in the vagus nerve firing rate when compared to the NL-N-EXE group ($p < .05$; Figure 3A). While the low-intensity and moderate exercise training did not cause any significant modifications in the number of vagus nerve spikes in the NL rats (NL-EXE$_{21-90}$, NL-EXE$_{21-50}$ and NL-EXE$_{60-90}$ groups); a significant decrease in vagus nerve electrical activity was observed in the SL rats (SL-EXE$_{21-90}$, SL-EXE$_{21-50}$ and SL-EXE$_{60-90}$ groups) when compared to their respective no-exercised groups ($p < .01$; Figure 3A).

The sympathetic activity is showed in the Figure 3B, demonstrating that low-intensity and moderate exercise training increases the triggering rate of the greater splanchnic nerve by two-fold in both the NL and SL rats compared to their respective no-exercised groups ($p < .05$). No change was observed in the number of greater splanchnic nerve spikes in the SL-N-EXE rats when compared to the NL-N-EXE rats (Figure 3B). The representative records of each nerve discharge, which illustrate the data for each experimental group, are given in the Figure 3C.

Discussion

As expected, a reduction in litter size during the suckling phase induced obesity in adult rats, as indicated by increased bw and increased fat tissue accumulation. Confirming data reporting that this experimental model of obesity is caused by the overfeeding behavior of young rats during lactation [30], this metabolic imprinting model displays glucose intolerance, insulin resistance, hyperphagia among others important metabolic disturbances [6,31].

The afferent vagus projects from the periphery to the nucleus of the solitary tract in the brainstem, a brain region situated in the dorsal vagal complex that functions as a port of entry for visceral information to the brain. Interestingly, the incoming peripheral signals about glucose levels can be modified by central glucose-sensing neurons at nearly every level of the central nervous system [32], and populations of neurons in the ventromedial and lateral hypothalamus are reported to increase their firing rates in response to the application of glucose [33].

The balance of the ANS is important to maintain constant glycemia. Overall, the parasympathetic stimulates insulin secretion, whereas the sympathetic inhibits it, which can produces decreases and increases in glycemia that are dependent on the glucose demand of cells,

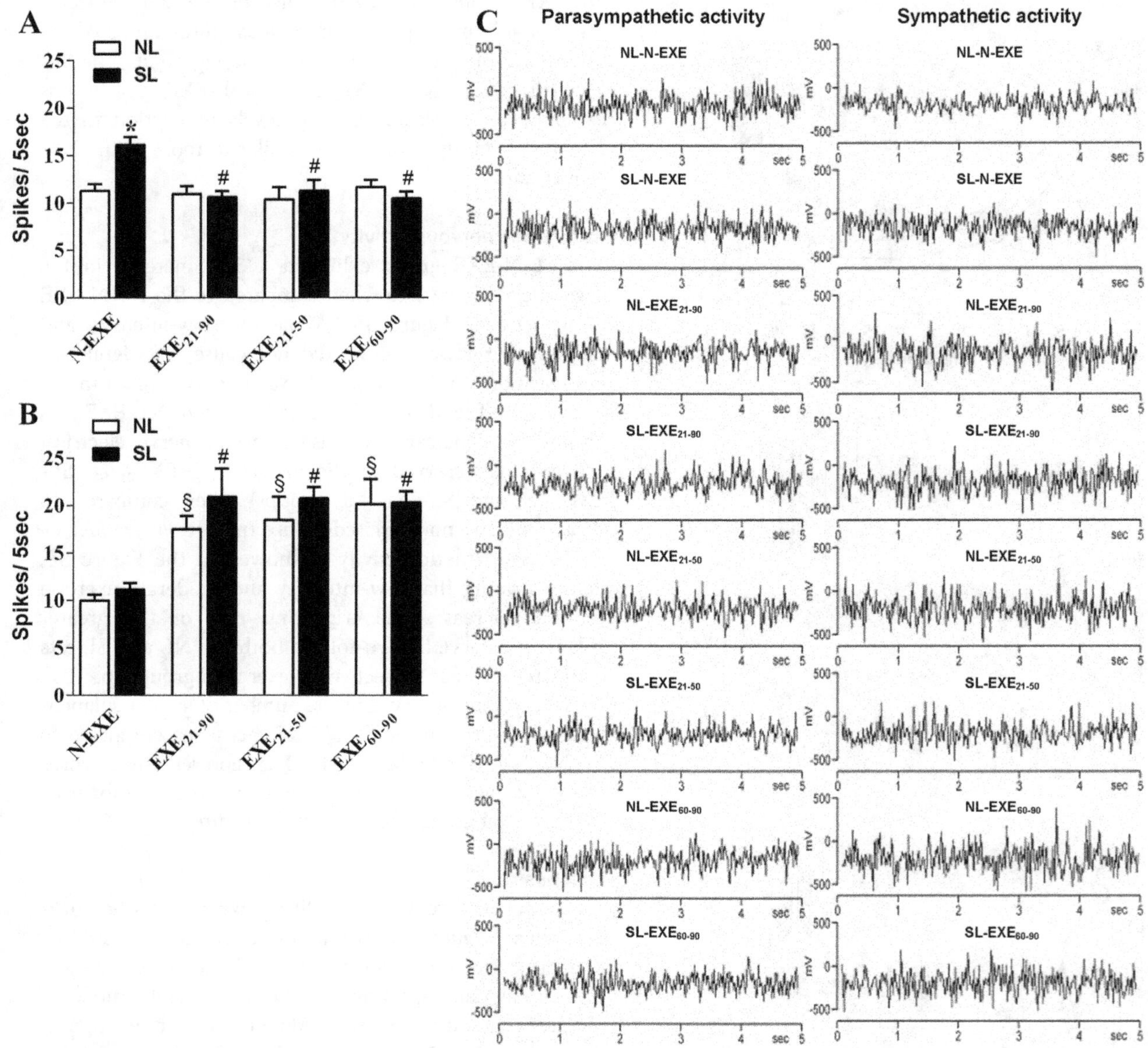

Figure 3 Electrical activity of the autonomic nervous system. All values are expressed as the mean ± SEM of 10–18 rats of each experimental group. The vagus **(A)** and greater splanchnic nerve **(B)** electrical activity. Symbols on the lines as well as letters on the bars represents the statistical difference by one-way ANOVA followed by Tukey's test among groups. *$p < .01$ for SL-N-EXE v.s. NL-N-EXE; $^{\#}p < .01$ for each one of SL-EXE group v.s. SL-N-EXE; $^{\S}p < .05$ for each one of NL-EXE group v.s. NL-N-EXE. Representative records of each nerve discharge, which illustrate the data for each experimental group, are given in the Figure 3**C**.

skeletal muscles and fat tissue. The data of the current research reveal, for the first time, that higher vagal nerve activity is observed in obese rats induced by early overfeeding. Our group also observed this feature in other different model of obesity [19,20,27,34], in all of these obesity model high fasting insulinemia and insulin resistance were observed. The method used in the present work cannot discriminate afferent from efferent signals; however, the firing rates from control rats are very similar to those reported by other authors [35,36]. Increased activation of the parasympathetic branch and/or reduced outflow of the sympathetic branch have been suggested to be responsible, at least in part, for the insulin oversecretion. Thus, in the current work we suggest that autonomic dysfunction could be indirectly responsible by the large fat pad accumulation in the SL rats, through the insulin lipogenesis action.

The most important find in the present work, is the observation that ANS may be modulated by the low-intensity and moderated exercise training, even in rats ran until puberty, and rats that start to run at begin of adulthood that includes later stages of developmental plasticity. Interestingly, using the swimming training protocol at the same periods of life that were used in the present work, we showed that MSG-obese mice displayed the metabolic ameliorations, however it was more prominent in mice that began to swim at weaning and stopped to do it at the end of puberty or at 90-day-old. Swimming training protocol did not improve the metabolic changes in mice swam between 60- and 90-day-old, like as is observed in early stages of life [24]. In agreement with, it has been demonstrated that exercise applied immediately after weaning is able to improve the cognitive ability of rats and it is correlated with high neuronal density in the neurons of the hippocampal area [37,38]. Concerning, in previous studies we reported that the puberty is one important phase of life in which metabolic changes can happen similar to those occur early in perinatal phases [19,20], which can be an important window to either malprogramming or deprogramming the metabolism.

It is known that physical exercise is a potent attenuator of obesity, activating energy expenditure, promoting lipolysis and increasing the consumption of fatty acids by peripheral tissues to reduce body fat deposits [39-41]. The peripheral metabolic adaptations promoted by physical exercise are activated by the hypothalamic neural pathways involved in the regulation of the sympathetic nervous system [40]. Our data demonstrate that physical exercise was able to improve the imbalanced parasympathetic activity of SL-obese rats, which was observed to be closely associated with reduction on the fat pad deposition in these obese rats. Interestingly, beyond high vagus nerve tonus no difference was observed in sympathetic activity of these overfeeding rats. On the same line the improvement of vagus nerve tonus was able in ameliorate the disrupted glucose homeostasis and fat pad stores, independent of the time exercise training protocol had begun.

In previous studies, using the same exercise training protocol applied throughout life, we showed that obese rats induced by high-fat diet restores the imbalanced autonomic function beyond other metabolic dysfunctions [27]. Similar results were obtained in rats fed hypercaloric diets that ran voluntarily [39].

Although our study to be a phenomenological study, our data are suggestive that autonomic changes are modulating the increased energy expenditure, the mobilization of fat stores, and the reduction in bw. The current work demonstrates that low-intensity and moderate exercise training is able to improve the glycemia, either in early- or late-exercised rats similar to NL rats. Even SL rats whose exercise training was stopped at the end of puberty, and SL rats that began to be trained at begin of adulthood, exhibited improvement of all metabolic impairment observed in the no-exercised SL-obese rats. These metabolic changes are acquired due to early training, especially during perinatal and puberty, because the brain is still forming, which could be also happen at begin of adulthood. Therefore, any stimulation of the abnormal nervous system activity, especially the ANS, contributes to a body spender phenotype.

In fact, to making a parallel with human condition, a body of data in the present work could suggest that a continual moderate walks and/or slow running, since moderate and low-intensity aerobic training, might help obese young children to reach a well health condition by preventing fat pad stores accumulation, heart diseases and/or type 2 diabetes. However, it is need to have caution regarding to make some paradigms between the exercise training in rats and in human. On this line, the necessity to have more experimental and epidemiological data, to do more precise recommendation about that exercise training to children is very important.

Conclusion

These results demonstrate that low-intensity and moderate exercise training, independent of period that begin or stop improves the vagus nerves activity in adult-obese rats early programmed by overfeeding during suckling phase; and this exercise protocol provokes increased activity of the greater splanchnic nerve in both lean and SL-obese rats. Thus, the body of data in the current study highlights that low-intensity and moderate exercise training, independent of the age it could to be applied, can be one important no pharmacological tool against the metabolic syndrome problems that threat the human health around the word, specially childhood obesity, once it is a great risk factor to adulthood metabolic syndrome.

Regarding this point, more clinical and/or experimental studies should be performed to better explain the molecular pathways involved on interaction of exercise training on the ANS action. Given that, it could be one essential pharmacological target greatly important to improve health problem around the world.

Abbreviations

AUC: Area under the curve; ANS: Autonomic nervous system; bw: Body weight; ivGTT: Intravenous glucose tolerance test; MSG: Monosodium L-glutamate; NL: Normal litter; NL-N-EXE: Normal litter no-exercised; NL-EXE: Normal litter exercised; NL-EXE_{21-90}: Normal litter exercised from 21- to 90-days-old; NL-EXE_{21-90}: Normal litter exercised from 21- to 50-days-old; NL-EXE_{60-90}: Normal litter exercised from 21- to 90-days-old; SL: Small litter; SL-N-EXE: Small litter no-exercised; SL-EXE_{21-90}: Small litter exercised from 21- to 90-days-old; SL-EXE_{21-90}: Normal litter exercised from 21- to 50-days-old; SL-EXE_{60-90}: Normal litter exercised from 21- to 90-days-old; VO_{2max}.: Maximal voluve of oxygen uptake.

Competing interests

The authors declare that they have no competing interests.

Author's contributions

WR, RMG, DXS, ABT and GSF designed the study and acquired the data; SG, AP, LFB and TAR interpreted and analysed the data; PCFM and JCde O drafted and wrote the manuscript; JCde O, TAR, LFB and PCFM revised intellectual and critically the manuscript. All of the authors approve the final version of the manuscript.

Acknowledgements
This work was supported by the Brazilian research agencies: Conselho Nacional de Desenvolvimento Científico e Tecnológico – CNPq; Coordenação de Aperfeiçoamento de Pessoal de Nível Superior – CAPES; and Fundação Araucária. We are also grateful to National Starch Company.

Author details
[1]Department of Physical Education, State University of Maringá, Maringá, PR, Brazil. [2]Department of Physiological Sciences, State University of Maringá, Maringá, PR, Brazil. [3]Department of General Biology, State University of Ponta Grossa, Ponta Grossa, PR, Brazil. [4]Department of Biotechnology, Genetics and Cell Biology, State University of Maringá, Maringá, PR, Brazil.

References

1. Novak CM, Levine JA: **Central neural and endocrine mechanisms of non-exercise activity thermogenesis and their potential impact on obesity.** *J Neuroendocrinol* 2007, **19:**923–940.
2. Armitage JA, Poston L, Taylor PD: **Developmental origins of obesity and the metabolic syndrome: the role of maternal obesity.** *Front Horm Res* 2008, **36:**73–84.
3. Hales CN, Barker DJ: **The thrifty phenotype hypothesis.** *Br Med Bull* 2001, **60:**5–20.
4. Breton C: **The hypothalamus-adipose axis is a key target of developmental programming by maternal nutritional manipulation.** *J Endocrinol* 2013, **216:**R19–R31.
5. Ooshima T, Yoshida T, Hamada S: **Detection of caries-inducing microorganisms in hyposalivated rats without infection of mutans streptococci.** *Microbiol Immunol* 1994, **38:**39–45.
6. Aessopos A, Tsironi M, Andreopoulos A, Farmakis D: **Heart disease in thalassemia intermedia.** *Hemoglobin* 2009, **33**(Suppl 1):S170–S176.
7. Yoshida T, Sakane N, Umekawa T, Yoshioka K, Kondo M, Wakabayashi Y: **Usefulness of mazindol in combined diet therapy consisting of a low-calorie diet and Optifast in severely obese women.** *Int J Clin Pharmacol Res* 1994, **14:**125–132.
8. Soeters MR, Lammers NM, Dubbelhuis PF, Ackermans M, Jonkers-Schuitema CF, Fliers E, Sauerwein HP, Aerts JM, Serlie MJ: **Intermittent fasting does not affect whole-body glucose, lipid, or protein metabolism.** *Am J Clin Nutr* 2009, **90:**1244–1251.
9. Erickson AR, Enzenauer RJ, Bray VJ, West SG: **Musculoskeletal complaints in persian gulf war veterans.** *J Clin Rheumatol* 1998, **4:**181–185.
10. Markakis EA: **Development of the neuroendocrine hypothalamus.** *Front Neuroendocrinol* 2002, **23:**257–291.
11. Morgane PJ, Mokler DJ, Galler JR: **Effects of prenatal protein malnutrition on the hippocampal formation.** *Neurosci Biobehav Rev* 2002, **26:**471–483.
12. Plagemann A, Harder T, Rake A, Waas T, Melchior K, Ziska T, Rohde W, Dorner G: **Observations on the orexigenic hypothalamic neuropeptide Y-system in neonatally overfed weanling rats.** *J Neuroendocrinol* 1999, **11:**541–546.
13. Plagemann A, Harder T, Rake A, Melchior K, Rohde W, Dorner G: **Hypothalamic nuclei are malformed in weanling offspring of low protein malnourished rat dams.** *J Nutr* 2000, **130:**2582–2589.
14. Davidowa H, Plagemann A: **Different responses of ventromedial hypothalamic neurons to leptin in normal and early postnatally overfed rats.** *Neurosci Lett* 2000, **293:**21–24.
15. Velkoska E, Morris MJ, Burns P, Weisinger RS: **Leptin reduces food intake but does not alter weight regain following food deprivation in the rat.** *Int J Obes Relat Metab Disord* 2003, **27:**48–54.
16. Vickers MH, Gluckman PD, Coveny AH, Hofman PL, Cutfield WS, Gertler A, Breier BH, Harris M: **Neonatal leptin treatment reverses developmental programming.** *Endocrinology* 2005, **146:**4211–4216.
17. Inoue S, Nagase H, Satoh S, Saito M, Egawa M, Tanaka K, Takamura Y: **Role of the efferent and afferent vagus nerve in the development of ventromedial hypothalamic (VMH) obesity.** *Brain Res Bull* 1991, **27:**511–515.
18. Lee HC, Curry DL, Stern JS: **Tonic sympathetic nervous system inhibition of insulin secretion is diminished in obese Zucker rats.** *Obes Res* 1993, **1:**371–376.
19. Barella LF, de Oliveira JC, Branco RC, Camargo RL, Gomes RM, Mendes FC, Miranda RA, Gravena C, Torrezan R, Grassiolli S, de Freitas Mathias PC: **Early exposure to a high-fat diet has more drastic consequences on metabolism compared with exposure during adulthood in rats.** *Horm Metab Res* 2012, **44:**458–464.
20. de Oliveira JC, Lisboa PC, de Moura EG, Barella LF, Miranda RA, Malta A, Franco CC, Ribeiro TA, Torrezan R, Gravena C, Mathias PC: **Poor pubertal protein nutrition disturbs glucose-induced insulin secretion process in pancreatic islets and programs rats in adulthood to increase fat accumulation.** *J Endocrinol* 2013, **216:**195–206.
21. Purev E, Giordano A, Soprano DR, Soprano KJ: **Interaction of PP2A catalytic subunit with Rb2/p130 is required for all-trans retinoic acid suppression of ovarian carcinoma cell growth.** *J Cell Physiol* 2006, **206:**495–502.
22. Wente W, Brenner MB, Zitzer H, Gromada J, Efanov AM: **Activation of liver X receptors and retinoid X receptors induces growth arrest and apoptosis in insulin-secretion cells.** *Endocrinology* 2007, **148**(4):1843–1849. doi:10.1210/en.2006-1247.
23. Oyama K, Minami K, Ishizaki K, Fuse M, Miki T, Seino S: **Spontaneous recovery from hyperglycemia by regeneration of pancreatic beta-cells in Kir6.2G132S transgenic mice.** *Diabetes* 2006, **55:**1930–1938.
24. Scomparin DX, Grassiolli S, Marcal AC, Gravena C, Andreazzi AE, Mathias PC: **Swim training applied at early age is critical to adrenal medulla catecholamine content and to attenuate monosodium L-glutamate-obesity onset in mice.** *Life Sci* 2006, **79:**2151–2156.
25. Sawaya A, Benoit JP, Benita S: **Binding mechanism of doxorubicin in ion-exchange albumin microcapsules.** *J Pharm Sci* 1987, **76:**475–480.
26. Chen M, Gavrilova O, Zhao WQ, Nguyen A, Lorenzo J, Shen L, Nackers L, Pack S, Jou W, Weinstein LS: **Increased glucose tolerance and reduced adiposity in the absence of fasting hypoglycemia in mice with liver-specific Gs alpha deficiency.** *J Clin Invest* 2005, **115:**3217–3227.
27. Gomes RM, Tofolo LP, Rinaldi W, Scomparin DX, Grassiolli S, Barella LF, de Oliveira JC, Branco RC, Agostinho AR, da Silva Ribeiro TA, Gravena C, Mathias PC: **Moderate Exercise Restores Pancreatic Beta-Cell Function and Autonomic Nervous System Activity in Obese Rats Induced by High-Fat Diet.** *Cell Physiol Biochem* 2013, **32:**310–321.
28. Negrao CE, Moreira ED, Santos MC, Farah VM, Krieger EM: **Vagal function impairment after exercise training.** *J Appl Physiol* 1992, **72:**1749–1753.
29. de Oliveira JC, Scomparin DX, Andreazzi AE, Branco RC, Martins AG, Gravena C, Grassiolli S, Rinaldi W, Barbosa FB, Mathias PC: **Metabolic imprinting by maternal protein malnourishment impairs vagal activity in adult rats.** *J Neuroendocrinol* 2011, **23:**148–157.
30. Leithauser M, Kahl C, Aepinus C, Prall F, Maruschke M, Riemer H, Wolff D, Jost K, Hilgendorf I, Freund M, Junghanss C: **Invasive zygomycosis in patients with graft-versus-host disease after allogeneic stem cell transplantation.** *Transpl Infect Dis* 2010, **12:**251–257.
31. Fehr M, Templeton A, Cogliatti S, Aebersold F, Egli F, Gillessen S, Cathomas R: **Primary manifestation of small lymphocytic lymphoma in the prostate.** *Onkologie* 2009, **32:**586–588.
32. D'Agostino MA, Conaghan PG, Naredo E, Aegerter P, Iagnocco A, Freeston JE, Filippucci E, Moller I, Pineda C, Joshua F, Backhaus M, Keen HI, Kaeley G, Ziswiler HR, Schmidt WA, Balint PV, Bruyn GA, Jousse-Joulin S, Kane D, Moller I, Szkudlarek M, Terslev L, Wakefield RJ: **The OMERACT ultrasound task force – Advances and priorities.** *J Rheumatol* 2009, **36:**1829–1832.
33. Hallemans A, Aerts P: **Effects of visual deprivation on intra-limb coordination during walking in children and adults.** *Exp Brain Res* 2009, **198:**95–106.
34. Scomparin DX, Gomes RM, Grassiolli S, Rinaldi W, Martins AG, de Oliveira JC, Gravena C, de Freitas Mathias PC: **Autonomic activity and glycemic homeostasis are maintained by precocious and low intensity training exercises in MSG-programmed obese mice.** *Endocrine* 2009, **36:**510–517.
35. Gennarelli G, Rovei V, Novi RF, Holte J, Bongioanni F, Revelli A, Pacini G, Cavallo-Perin P, Massobrio M: **Preserved insulin sensitivity and {beta}-cell activity, but decreased glucose effectiveness in normal-weight women with the polycystic ovary syndrome.** *J Clin Endocrinol Metab* 2005, **90:**3381–3386.
36. Okada K, Fujii Y, Uema K, Yoshimoto T, Nakatsu T, Yoshida T, Hasegawa T: **Pseudosarcomatous myofibroblastic tumor of the urinary bladder with massive intraperitoneal hemorrhage in a child.** *Acta Paediatr Jpn* 1998, **40:**470–473.
37. Uysal N, Tugyan K, Kayatekin BM, Acikgoz O, Bagriyanik HA, Gonenc S, Ozdemir D, Aksu I, Topcu A, Semin I: **The effects of regular aerobic**

exercise in adolescent period on hippocampal neuron density, apoptosis and spatial memory. *Neurosci Lett* 2005, **383:**241–245.

38. Neeper SA, Gomez-Pinilla F, Choi J, Cotman CW: **Physical activity increases mRNA for brain-derived neurotrophic factor and nerve growth factor in rat brain.** *Brain Res* 1996, **726:**49–56.
39. Kumazaki T, Sakano T, Yoshida T, Hamada K, Sumida H, Teranishi Y, Nishiyama M, Mitsui Y: **Enhanced expression of mitochondrial genes in senescent endothelial cells and fibroblasts.** *Mech Ageing Dev* 1998, **101:**91–99.
40. Nakamura S, Kuroda T, Sugai T, Ono S, Yoshida T, Akasaka I, Nakashima F, Sasou S: **The first reported case of intestinal spirochaetosis in Japan.** *Pathol Int* 1998, **48:**58–62.
41. Chauvatcharin S, Siripatana C, Seki T, Takagi M, Yoshida T: **Metabolism analysis and on-line physiological state diagnosis of acetone-butanol fermentation.** *Biotechnol Bioeng* 1998, **58:**561–571.

13

Quercetin intake with exercise modulates lipoprotein metabolism and reduces atherosclerosis plaque formation

Mahdi Garelnabi*, Halleh Mahini and Thomas Wilson

Abstract

The pathogenesis of atherosclerosis, the major cause of cardiovascular diseases (CVD), is multifactorial and therefore its treatment approaches and the ability to regress the plaque are complicated. Data from research on animal models and clinical studies have indicated that moderate daily exercise can alleviate the risk for the development of atherosclerotic plaques, while the same has not been true for the supplementation of antioxidants.

Study objectives: We proposed that mice supplemented with quercetin, a class of flavonoids known to have antioxidant and anti-inflammatory properties, will have profound effects on the pathophysiology of atherosclerosis when combined with exercise.

Study design: Forty C57BL6 LDLr −/− mice were divided into four groups (n = 10): control untreated (NN); control group supplemented with 100 μg/day of quercetin (NQ); exercise group (EN); and exercise group supplemented with 100 μg/day of quercetin (EQ). All animals were fed atherogenic diet. The exercise groups were run on a treadmill for 30 minutes, 15 m/min for 5 days/week for 30 days. After 30 day animals were sacrificed and tissues were harvested.

Results and conclusion: Mice supplemented with quercetin during exercise sessions had 78% atherosclerotic plaque reduction compared to control mice and 40% less atherosclerotic plaque formation compared to control group supplemented with quercetin. The manifestation of the combination of quercetin supplementation with exercise was more evident in the pro-reverse cholesterol transport genes, indicating a plausible mechanism for their combined beneficial effect.

Keywords: Lipoproteins, Quercetin, Flavonoids, Inflammation, Exercise

Introduction

Atherosclerosis is a chronic disease of the large arteries and is a major cause of heart disease, stroke, and death in westernized societies. The etiology of cardiovascular disease (CVD) is complex and multifactorial, however there is substantial evidence [1,2] that oxidative stress [3] and inflammation [4] play an important role in the initiation and progression of the disease. Oxidative modification of low density lipoprotein (LDL) is believed to turn the otherwise native lipoprotein into an antigenic molecule that attracts monocytes turned macrophages to the vascular wall with a subsequent triggering of a complex immune response mediated by inflammatory modulators [5-7]. Recent insights into the pathogenesis of atherosclerosis underscore the importance of chronic inflammation in both the initiation and progression of the disease [8-11].

Exercise which induces a severe oxidative stress resulting in the depletion of plasma and tissue antioxidants has been shown to be an important deterrent of CVD [12-14]. This paradigm is supported by a large number of experimental animal studies and by epidemiological investigations. Over the past 5 decades, numerous scientific reports have examined the relationships between physical activity, physical fitness, and cardiovascular health [15-18]. Studies from our previous work have indicated that exercise induced the reverse cholesterol transport in mice that were exercised on a treadmill [19]. Others have reported that mice fed a high fat diet had increased numbers of macrophage clusters in adipose tissue [20], which were reduced by exercise training compared to sedentary

* Correspondence: Mahdi_Garelnabi@uml.edu
Department of Clinical Laboratory and Nutritional Sciences, University of Massachusetts, 3 Solomont Way, Suite 4 01854, Lowell, MA, USA

mice. The sedentary mice also had higher levels of tumor necrosis factor α (TNF-α) mRNA, increased numbers of CD11c inflammatory macrophages and CD8 T cells [20]. Recently published study by Wen *et. al.* [21] reported that treadmill exercise training modulated hepatic cholesterol metabolism and circulating PCSK9 concentration in high-fat-fed mice.

Studies that combined antioxidants with exercise have also shown conflicting outcomes. Early study by Ramachandran et. al., [22] have showed that exercise reduced preexisting atherosclerotic lesions in LDL receptor knockout (−/−) mice, and that the addition of vitamin E supplementation to exercising did not reduce atherosclerotic lesion formation significantly when compared to untreated exercised mice [22]. Moreover, vitamin E supplementation was found to counteract the beneficial effects of exercise by preventing the induction of aortic catalase activity and endothelial NO synthase expression [23]. Flavonoids are a class of naturally occurring compounds widely present in fruits, vegetables and beverages derived from plants that have known antioxidant activity [24,25]. One such flavonoid, quercetin, has been shown to be an effective free-radical scavenger that inhibits lipoprotein oxidation [24]. Recent studies have also suggested that quercetin possesses anti-inflammatory properties as well as antioxidant activity. As an antioxidant and anti-inflammatory, quercetin appears to alleviate oxidative stress via diverse pathways, including NF-κB dependent mechanism [25], decrease activity of JAK3 [26], and/or by blocking the activation of pro-inflammatory/oxidative stress mediator signal transduction [27]. Quercetin has also been shown to prevent the accumulation of fat in the liver of mice fed a high fat diet [28] and to lower blood lipids in people with dyslipidemia [29]. Chang *et. al.* [30] have demonstrated that quercetin promotes cholesterol efflux from macrophages on a concentration-dependent manner through ATP-binding cassette transporter (ABCA-1) mediated mechanisms. It appears from these studies that the combination of exercise and quercetin supplementation may produce greater cardiovascular benefits than exercise alone. We propose that quercetin supplementation will have a profound effect on the pathophysiology of atherosclerosis when combined with exercise and that this action will be attributed to the inhibition of lipid oxidation, lowering of arterial lipid deposition and decreased development of plaque.

Materials and methods

Animals, diets, and exercise

All animal studies were performed in agreement with Public Health Service policy on use of laboratory animals, and in conformity with the Guide for the Care and Use of Laboratory Animals published by the US National Institutes of Health. The animal use protocol was approved by the Institutional Animal Care and Use Committee of the University of Massachusetts Lowell. All animals were fed an atherogenic diet containing 1.5% cholesterol as part of a 42% Fat Kcal Diet without antioxidants (Cat: TD.110489; Harlan Laboratories, Madison, WI).

Forty 4-week-old male LDLr$^{-/-}$mice on C57BL/6 J background (B6.129S7-Ldlr^{tm1Her}/J strain) were obtained from Jackson Laboratory (Bar Harbor, ME). Mice were divided into four groups (10 mice each): control mice (NN) left untreated; control mice supplemented with quercetin (NQ); exercise group (EN); and exercise group supplemented with quercetin (EQ). Animals groups supplemented with quercetin were orally fed 100 μg/day, 5 days per week for 30 days 15 min prior to exercise. The quercetin solution was prepared in water with 1% sodium lauryl sulfate (SLS). Although the solution is very stable however; was gently mixed before pipetting to ensure correct dosage concentration. Pipette was used to deliver the correct amount; mouse was held upright until it swallowed the fluid. The exercise groups were run on a treadmill (Columbus Instruments, Columbus, OH) for 30 minutes at 15 meters/min, 5 days/week for 30 days.

Materials

Quercetin was purchased from Cayman Chemicals (Ann Arbor, MI), with all other chemicals and reagents being purchased from Sigma-Aldrich Chemical Co. (St. Louis, MO). Gene expression reagents were obtained from Bio-Rad (Hercules, CA). Primers were designed and purchased along with TRIzol® from Life Technologies (Carlsbad, CA).

Methods

Initially animals were acclimatized to the housing facility and the use of the treadmill instrument prior to starting the actual protocol. After 30 days of treatment the animals were fasted overnight (>12 hours), sacrificed with 100% CO_2 exposure, and blood was collected via cardiac puncture. The plasma was collected after centrifugation at 4°C at 3000 rpm for 20 min and frozen at −80°C until assayed. The aorta and liver were perfused with cold phosphate buffered saline (PBS) prior to being harvested. All tissues were instantaneously frozen in liquid nitrogen following collection and stored at −80°C until assayed.

Assessment of atherosclerotic lesions

At the completion of the livers perfusion and tissue collection the aorta was kept wet with cold PBS through the dissection process which was performed under a stereomicroscope from the iliac bifurcation up to the heart, including the beginning of the brachiocephalic, carotid, and subclavian arteries. Pictures of the aorta were obtained using a digital camera. Lesion area size was quantified using Image J software [31]. The lesion area was marked on the pictures under direct microscopic observation and quantified.

Quantitative real-time PCR (qPCR)

Liver RNA was extracted using TRIzol according to the manufacturer's protocol and the quantity was measured by Qubit (Life Technologies, Carlsbad, CA). cDNA was generated from 10–100 ng of total RNA and 1/20th of the sample was taken for qPCR. cDNA synthesis and qPCRs were performed with SYBR GreenER Two-Step qRT-PCR Kit according to the manufacturer's protocol. qPCR was run in 20 μL of reaction mixture in sealed 96-well plates with iScriptTM Reverse Transcription Supermix and SsoFastTM EvaGreen® Supermix on an RTPCR MyiQTM2 system (Bio-Rad; Hercules, CA). Threshold cycle (CT) was determined by Bio-Rad iQ5 v.2.1 software. The melting curve and efficiency were assessed for all primer pairs. The level of mRNA was calculated using glyceraldehyde 3-phosphate dehydrogenase (GAPDH) as an internal control gene. Data are expressed as fold induction of mRNA level in one group compared to another.

Enzyme-Linked Immunosorbent Assay (ELISA)

Plasma TNF-α, monocyte chemoattractant protein (MCP)-1, and interleukin (IL)-17α levels were determined according to manufacturer protocols by ELISA kits purchased from BioLegend (San Diego, CA).

Statistical analysis

All data are presented as mean ± SD. Statistical significance for differences in lesion areas were evaluated using Student's *t*-test. Statistical significance for relative gene expression was evaluated using one-way ANOVA with Tukey post-hoc test using 95% confidence intervals. Differences were considered significant at P <0.05.

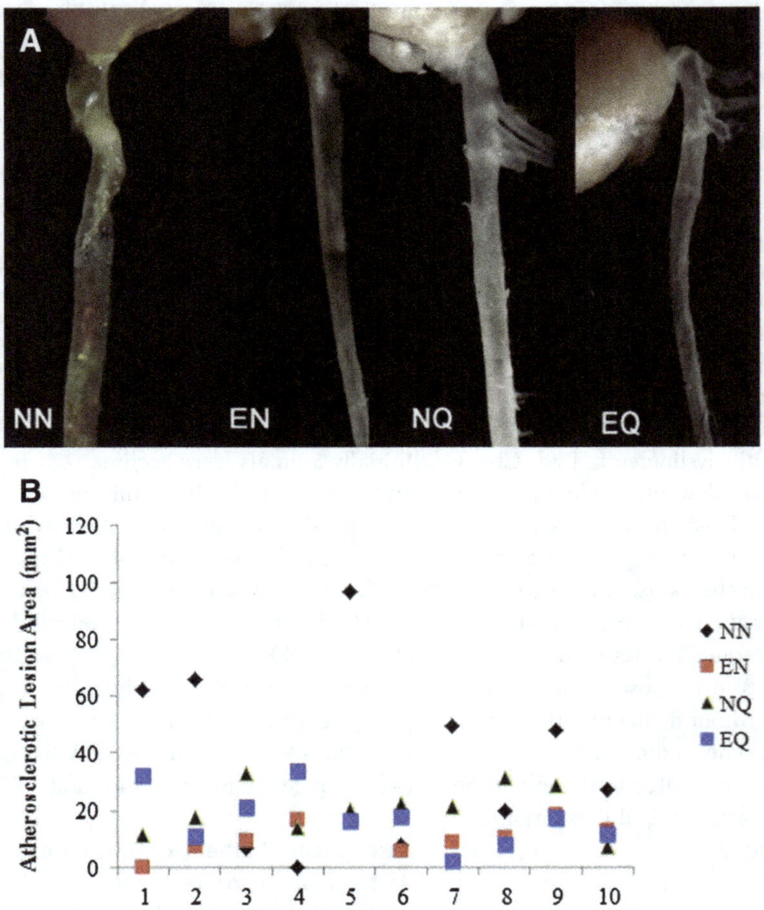

Figure 1 Effect of quercetin and exercise on atherosclerotic lesion development. A: Images of the atherosclerotic lesions in aortas. Atherosclerotic lesions in aortas of LDLr–/–mice fed a high-fat diet. NN: Control group; mice on atherogenic diet without quercetin and exercise treatment; EN: Mice on atherogenic diet and exercise without quercetin supplementation; NQ: Mice on atherogenic diet and quercetin supplementation; EQ: Mice on atherogenic diet, exercise and quercetin supplementation. Massive formation of atherosclerotic plaque can be seen on control and relatively less lesion formation on the other groups. **B**: Lesions areas dot plot representation in the 4 groups. EN: Mice on atherogenic diet and exercise without quercetin intake NQ: Mice on atherogenic diet and quercetin intake. EQ: Mice on atherogenic diet and exercise and quercetin intake. Compared to NN mice; the aorta lesion areas in EN, NQ and EQ showed significant decreases of 79%, 64% and 70% respectively (P < 0.05).

Results

All mice completed the study, tolerated the supplemented quercetin amount; there was no differences in the amount of consumed food between the groups or the physical appearance of the mice as a result of the quercetin intake. There was, however, a significant reduction in body weight in the EQ mice after 30 days of treatment compared to baseline (data not shown). The weight reduction appears to have resulted from the combination of the exercise and quercetin intake; however the mechanism for this weight loss is not very clear.

Atherosclerotic lesion

Atherosclerotic plaque formation in selected mice from all groups is shown in Figure 1A. The average lesion areas for the groups were: 56.04 mm^2, 11.84 mm^2, 19.95 mm^2 and 16.63 mm^2 for NN, EN, NQ, and EQ respectively, revealing a decrease of 79% ($P < 0.01$); 64% ($P < 0.05$) and 70% ($P < 0.05$) between each group, respectively, and the NN (Figure 1B).

Plasma cytokines

The plasma concentrations of IL-17, MCP-1 and TNF-α measured by ELISA are shown in (Figure 2A,B and C). The average plasma concentrations for TNF-α were: 473.1 pg/mL, 534.4 pg/mL, 534 pg/mL and 502.3 pg/mL for the NN EN, NQ, and EQ groups respectively, depicting a significant increase ($P < 0.05$) in TNF-α level among the EN and NQ groups compared to the NN group.

On the other hand, plasma MCP-1 concentrations decreased among the EQ, EN, and NQ groups compared to the NN. The greatest decrease was observed in the EQ group (54.7%). The average plasma levels were: 2529.37 pg/mL, 2021.81 pg/mL, 1996.81 pg/mL, and 1384.69 pg/mL for the NN, EN, NQ, and EQ groups respectively.

The average plasma concentrations of IL-17 were 8775.0 pg/mL, 8646.6 pg/mL, 8460.6 pg/mL, and 10,053.1 pg/mL for the NN EN, NQ, and EQ groups respectively; showing an increase trend in the EQ group compared to the NN group but not significantly.

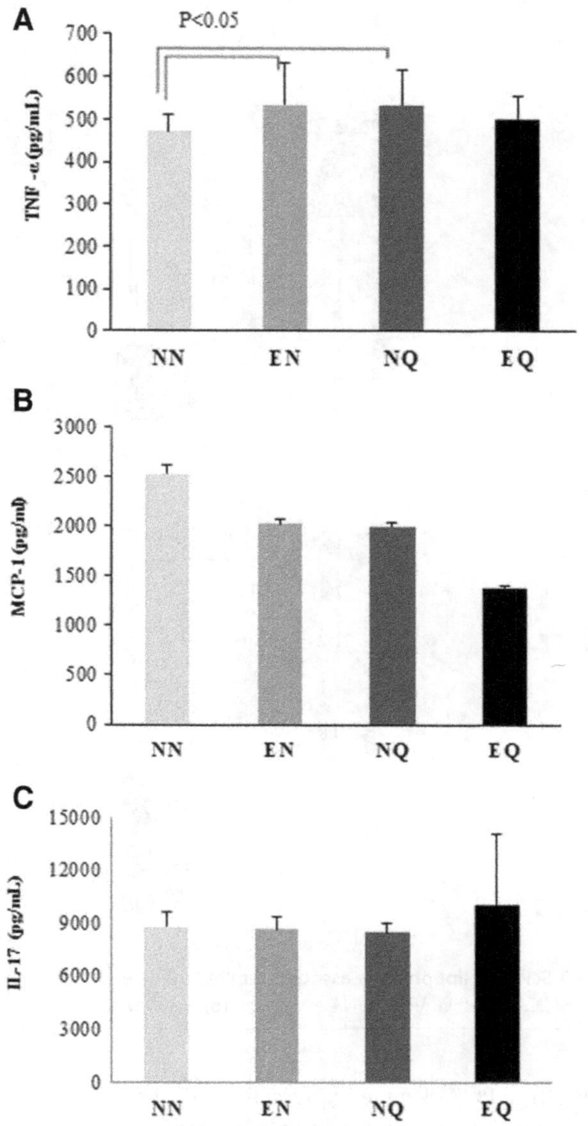

Figure 2 Effect of quercetin intake and exercise on selected plasma biomarkers. Plasma levels of TNF-α, MCP-1 and IL-17α. The figure shows average plasma levels of TNF-α **(A)**, MCP-1 **(B)** and IL-17 **(C)** . TNF-α levels significantly increased in the EN and NQ mice compared to NN group. However no significant changes were noticed between the groups MCP-1 and IL-17 levels.

Gene expressions in mouse liver

The mice in the EQ group showed a significant down regulation of apolipoprotein (APO)A-1 gene expression levels compared to NN (Figure 3A). However, the decrease in APOA-1 gene expression in the NQ and EN groups was not significantly different from the NN (Figure 3A). The APOA-1 gene expression level in the EQ group was also significantly lower ($P < 0.001$) compared to the EN group (Figure 3A). APOA-5 gene expression showed similar trends with all treatment groups having down regulated gene expression compared to the NN group. However, only the decrease in the EQ group was significant ($P < 0.001$) compared to the NN (Figure 3B). Interestingly, APOA-5 gene expression levels were significantly higher in the EQ compared to the NQ group as well (Figure 3B). Ironically, gene expressions for APOA-4, ABCA-1, and peroxisome proliferator-activated receptor (PPAR)-α followed a contrasting trend to what was observed with the APOA-1 and APOA-5. ABCA-1 gene expression was significantly ($P < 0.001$) up regulated in the EQ group compared to NN group (Figure 3B). Furthermore, the EQ group showed a significant ($P < 0.05$) ABCA-1 gene induction compared to the NQ group

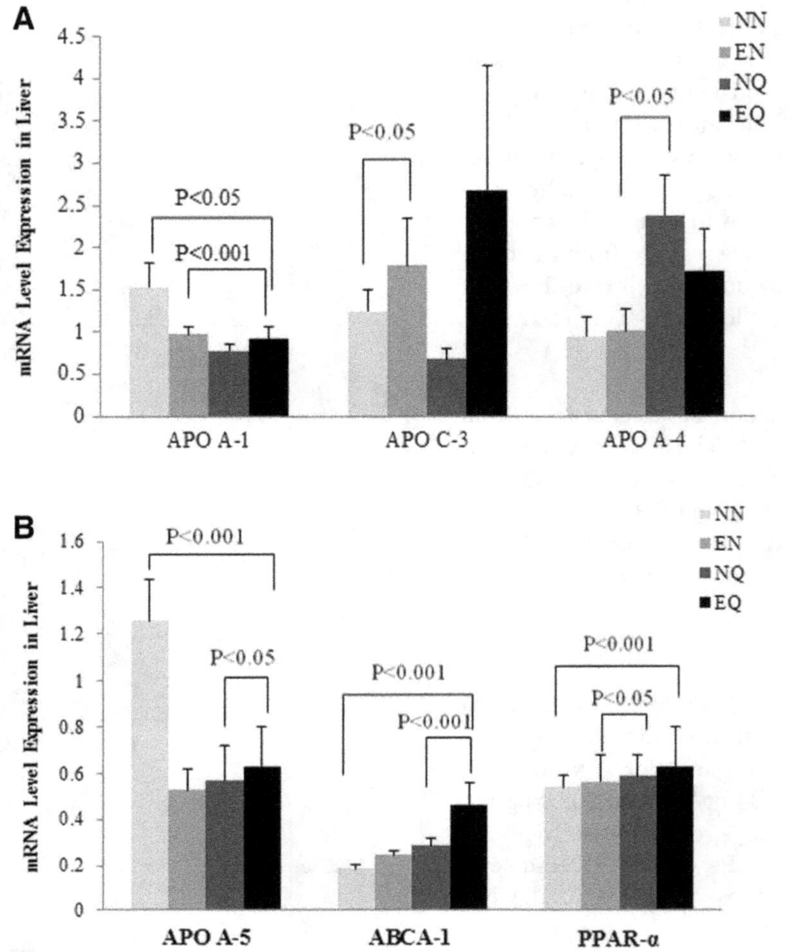

Figure 3 Selected lipoproteins associated mRNA gene expression levels. Levels of APOA-1, APOC3, APOA-4 mRNA expressions **(A)** and APOA-5, ABCA-1 and PPAR-α mRNA expression **(B)** are shown in these figures.

(Figure 3B). APOA-4 gene expression was also up regulated among all treatment groups compared to the NN group, however, only the difference between the EN and NQ groups was significant ($P < 0.05$) (Figure 3A). PPAR-α gene expression levels were also increased in all treatment groups compared to the NN group (Figure 3B). The EQ was shown to have the most significant induction ($P < 0.001$) compared to the NN group (Figure 3B). APOC-3 gene expression was up regulated with exercise, with the differences between NE group and NN group being significant ($P < 0.05$) (Figure 3A). A similar trend was observed between the EQ group and NQ group but not significantly (Figure 3A), which may suggest that quercetin and exercise down regulate APOC-3.

The liver gene expression for the inflammatory, oxidative stress markers and transcription factors; signal transducer and activator of transcript (STAT)3, paraoxonase/arylesterase (PON)1, nuclear factor kappa-light-chain-enhancer of activated B cells (NF-κB), and suppressor of cytokine signaling (SOCS)1 showed varied responses. While exercise appears to down regulate STAT3 gene expression; it up regulated PON1 gene expression with no effect for the quercetin supplementation compared to the NN group (Figure 4A). SOCS1 was influenced by the exercise depicting up regulation in the exercise groups compared to the NN group but none of these changes was significant (Figure 4B). NF-κB gene expression levels varied, however, the EQ group had a significant ($P < 0.05$) induction compared to the EN group (Figure 4B).

Discussion

Considerable attention has been given to polyphenols, such as quercetin, due to their anti-inflammatory and antioxidant properties [27-30]. Several mechanisms have been described and attributed to the anti-atherogenic effects of exercise and quercetin. It is commonly accepted that moderate exercise is an important component of a healthy lifestyle that helps to prevent or delay the onset of coronary artery disease [15-18]. These beneficial effects are lost when subjects become sedentary. Exercise

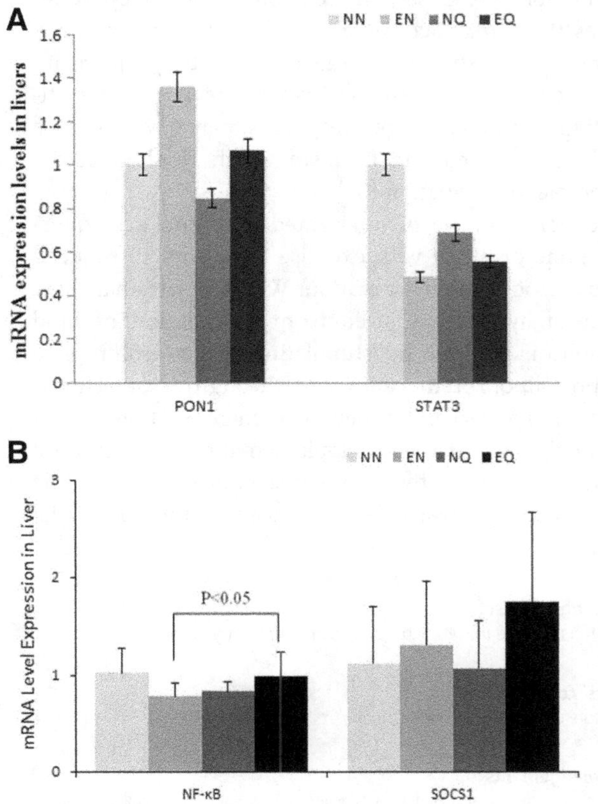

Figure 4 Selected inflammation and oxidative stress associated gene expression levels. Average relative level of mRNA expression for STAT3, and PON1 **(A)**. (The differences between the levels of PON1 and STAT3 in the various groups were not significant). **(B)** Average of relative level of mRNA of NF-κB and SOCS1expression (no significant differences between the groups), up regulation of NF-κB among the EQ is significant.

intensity and duration are also critical determinants of the cardiovascular beneficial effects [32,33]. A wide range of mechanisms have been described for the beneficial effects of exercise; including: enhancing serum HDL levels; up regulation of PON1 and SRB1; inducing anti-inflammatory cytokines; and up regulation of the antioxidant enzymes contributing towards their ability to counteract the oxidative stress that is generated during exercise [34-36]. Quercetin on the other hand has been shown to act through various mechanisms mainly linked to reducing the inflammation and oxidative stress levels which are responsible for the atherosclerotic pathogenesis. Earlier studies have shown that quercetin significantly inhibit in vitro LDL oxidation, and also protects macrophages from oxidized low-density lipoprotein-induced apoptosis [37,38]. Quercetin has also been reported to inhibit the progression of atherosclerosis via up-regulating the expression of PON1 [18]; indicating a possible cholesterol reverse transportation mechanism.

Studies combining antioxidants with exercise are not new; our previous work has extensively studied the possible role of the intake of antioxidant vitamins, such as vitamin E during exercise on cardiovascular health in humans and mouse models. However, the current study is unique in a way, it has combined quercetin supplementation with exercise to examine their anti-atherogenic roles. To our knowledge this has not been explored previously. The C57BL LDLr−/− mouse model has been commonly used for the rapid development of the atherogenic diet-induced atherosclerotic plaque. One of the major findings in the current study is the atherosclerotic reduction in the three groups of mice on exercise alone, exercise with quercetin supplementation, and quercetin supplementation alone. The current quercetin dosage was selected since mice have been previously shown to tolerate and respond to this concentration (28). Exercise is well known to help reduce plaque formation [22]; however, earlier work by Parthasarathy's group did not find significant reduction in the aortic plaque formation in exercising LDL receptor-deficient mice supplemented with vitamin E [23]. Moreover, it appears that vitamin E offset the beneficial effects of exercise by preventing the induction of aortic catalase activity and endothelial NO synthase expression [23]. The duration of this study was 30 days, which was sufficient to allow fatty streaks and plaque development to resemble early atherosclerosis development. We also chosen low intensity exercise regimen to provide the opportunity to study the effect of the combination of quercetin with low intensity exercise on the plaque formation. In the current study, we observed a 64-79% reduction in plaque formation in all treatment groups compared to control. Exercise alone greatly reduced plaque formation. Conversely quercetin supplementation alone and with exercise resulted in similar reductions of plaque formation. This outcome suggests a strong anti-athrogenic role for quercetin supplementation.

To further investigate the mechanisms that may have contributed to the reduced plaque formation, we measured plasma lipids, selected cytokines, and we assessed certain genes expression in mouse livers. Interestingly there were no significant changes in the plasma lipids profiles (data not shown). There was a slight increase in the plasma TNF-α levels in the treated groups compared to control, however, the changes between the group on the quercetin supplementation alone and the control was the only difference in TNF-α that was significant. It is not clear why this difference was observed considering the known anti-inflammatory role for quercetin. Plasma MCP-1 levels on the other hand slightly decreased with exercise or quercetin supplementation alone greatly decreased with the combination of the exercise and quercetin supplementation. MCP-1 is critical for the initiation and development of atherosclerotic lesions. It is known to participate in the progression of atherosclerosis, by promoting direct migration of inflammatory cells to the vascular wall. MCP-1 has also been detected in atherosclerotic lesions using specific antibodies [35]. It appears quercetin supplementation alone or combined with exercise has potent anti-MCP-1 effects. Plasma IL-17α levels decreased with exercise or quercetin supplementation alone and slightly increased with the combination of the two. IL-17α plays an important pro-inflammatory role in atherosclerotic plaque development. Interestingly plasma IL-17α levels were decreased with exercise or quercetin intake but not with the combination. Interleukin 17 acts as a potent mediator by increasing chemokine production in various tissues to recruit monocytes and neutrophils to the site of inflammation, its involvement in inducing and mediating pro-inflammatory responses is well understood. It is not clear if the combination of exercise and quercetin will mediate IL 17 levels as indicated by this result.

The gene expression data shown in this study for lipoprotein is differentiated. The discrepancy between the treatment and the control groups for the APOA-1, APOC-3, and APOA-5 genes cannot be explained. However, on other lipoprotein metabolism associated genes, specifically, ABCA-1, PPAR-α, and APOA-4 did show significant up regulation among the treatment groups compared to the control, indicating that quercetin supplementation alone or with exercise may modulate the reverse cholesterol transport genes. Recent reports have shown that quercetin does modulate lipid reduction. Earlier studies by us and others [19] have shown that exercise promotes plasma lipid reductions. PON1 gene expression was up regulated among exercise groups compared to the control. This data goes along the ABCA-1 data suggesting a reverse transportation mechanism which may be responsible for the decreased plaque formation. The changes in NF-κB regulations among all treatment groups compared to the control indicate a possible reduced plaque formation mechanism mediated by NF-κB. Previous studies have pointed to NF-κB as potentially one of the most important pro-inflammatory pathways in atherosclerosis [36]. NF-κB is known to be activated in smooth muscle cells, macrophages, and endothelial cells in atherosclerotic lesions. In this study its gene induction levels appears to be at the intersection of the acute inflammatory response accompanying the acute atherosclerotic plaque formation. SOCS1 and STAT3 demonstrated varied responses to exercise and quercetin supplementation between the various groups. While STAT3 gene expression levels appear down regulated in the treatment groups compared to the control, SOCS1 was up regulated in these groups compared to the control, although none of these changes were significant. SOCS-1 is known to potently restrict transduction of various inflammatory signals and, thereby modulate T-cell development. STAT3 activation by selected cytokines such IL-6 is known to preferentially induce pro-inflammatory responses, whereas other sets of cytokines such as IL-10 may activate STAT3 and promote an anti-inflammatory response. In the current study, quercetin supplementation and exercise, which are known for stimulating anti-inflammatory responses, may have activated STAT3 by a specific mechanism which resulted in decreased plaque formation [39].

In conclusion, we demonstrated that intake of quercetin alone or along with exercise will result in reduced atherosclerotic plaque formation. We speculate that these changes may have resulted from modulation of lipid metabolism, possibly by stimulating cholesterol reverse transport lipoprotein genes and through a set of anti-inflammatory cytokine genes. The manifestation of the combination of quercetin supplementation with exercise was more evident in the pro-reverse cholesterol transport genes indicating a plausible mechanism for their beneficial effect.

Competing interests
The authors declare that they have no competing interests.

Authors' contributions
All authors read and approved the final manuscript.

Acknowledgements
This study was supported by the University of Massachusetts, Lowell: Advancing Research, Scholarship and Creative Work Seed Grant 2011.

References
1. Hansson GK, Robertson AK, Söderberg-Nauclér C: **Inflammation and atherosclerosis.** *Annu Rev Pathol* 2006, **1**:297–329.
2. Wool GD, Reardon CA: **The influence of acute phase proteins on murine atherosclerosis.** *Curr Drug Targets* 2007, **8**(11):1203–1214.
3. Garelnabi M: **Emerging evidences from the contribution of the traditional and new risk factors to the atherosclerosis pathogenesis.** *J Med Sci* 2010, **10**:153–161.
4. Parthasarathy S, Litvinov D, Selvarajan K, Garelnabi M: **Lipid peroxidation and decomposition–conflicting roles in plaque vulnerability and stability.** *Biochim Biophys Acta* 2008, **1781**(5):221–231.
5. Tobias PS, Curtiss LK: **Toll-like receptors in atherosclerosis.** *Biochem Soc Trans* 2007, **35**(Pt 6):1453–1455.
6. Litvinov D, Mahini H, Garelnabi M: **Antioxidant and anti-inflammatory role of paraoxonase 1: implication in arteriosclerosis diseases.** *N Am J Med Sci* 2012, **4**(11):523–532.
7. Ohashi K, Ouchi N, Matsuzawa Y: **Anti-inflammatory and anti-atherogenic properties of adiponectin.** *Biochimie* 2012, **94**(10):2137–2142.
8. Paccou J, Brazier M, Mentaverri R, Kamel S, Fardellone P, Massy ZA: **Vascular calcification in rheumatoid arthritis: prevalence, pathophysiological aspects and potential targets.** *Atherosclerosis* 2012, **224**(2):283–290.
9. Ansell BJ: **Targeting the anti-inflammatory effects of high-density lipoprotein.** *Am J Cardio* 2007, **100**(11 A):n3–n9.
10. Parthasarathy S, Raghavamenon A, Garelnabi MO, Santanam N: **Oxidized low-density lipoprotein.** *Methods Mol Biol* 2010, **610**:403–417.
11. Rosenson RS, Stafforini DM: **Modulation of oxidative stress, inflammation, and atherosclerosis by lipoprotein-associated phospholipase A2.** *J Lipid Res* 2012, **53**(9):1767–1782.
12. Dietz P, Hoffmann S, Lachtermann E, Simon P: **Influence of exclusive resistance training on body composition and cardiovascular risk factors in overweight or obese children: a systematic review.** *Obes Facts* 2012, **5**(4):546–560.

13. Leung FP, Yung LM, Laher I, Yao X, Chen ZY, Huang Y: **Exercise, vascular wall and cardiovascular diseases: an update (Part 1).** *Sports Med* 2008, **38**(12):1009–1024.
14. Heckman GA, McKelvie RS: **Cardiovascular aging and exercise in healthy older adults.** *Clin J Sport Med* 2008, **18**(6):479–485.
15. Garelnabi M, Veledar E, White-Welkley J, Santanam N, Abramson J, Weintraub W, Parthasarathy S: **Vitamin E differentially affects short term exercise induced changes in oxidative stress, lipids, and inflammatory markers.** *Nutr Metab Cardiovasc Dis* 2012, **22**(10):907–913.
16. Garelnabi M, Veledar E, Abramson J, White-Welkley J, Santanam N, Weintraub W, Parthasarathy S: **Physical inactivity and cardiovascular risk: baseline observations from men and premenopausal women.** *J Clin Lab Anal* 2010, **24**(2):100–105.
17. Siebel AL, Carey AL, Kingwell BA: **Can exercise training rescue the adverse cardiometabolic effects of low birth weight and prematurity?** *Clin Exp Pharmacol Physiol* 2012, **39**(11):944–957.
18. Fernandes-Silva MM, Carvalho VO, Guimarães GV, Bacal F, Bocchi EA: **Physical exercise and microRNAs: new frontiers in heart failure.** *Arq Bras Cardiol* 2012, **98**(5):459–466.
19. Wei C, Penumetcha M, Santanam N, Liu YG, Garelnabi M, Parthasarathy S: **Exercise might favor reverse cholesterol transport and lipoprotein clearance: potential mechanism for its anti-atherosclerotic effects.** *Biochim Biophys Acta* 2005, **1723**(1–3):124–127.
20. Cesar L, Vasallo Suarez S, Adi J, Adi N, Vazquez-Padron R, Yu H, Ma Q, Goldschmidt-Clermont PJ, Agatston A, Kurlansky P, Webster KA: **An essential role for diet in exercise-mediated protection against dyslipidemia, inflammation and atherosclerosis in ApoE−/− mice.** *PLoS One* 2011, **6**(2):e17263.
21. Wen S, Jadhav KS, Williamson DL, Rideout TC: **Treadmill exercise training modulates hepatic cholesterol metabolism and circulating PCSK9 concentration in high-Fat-Fed mice.** *J Lipids* 2013, **2013**:908048. doi:10.1155/2013/908048. Epub 2013 Jun 19, PubMed PMID: 23862065.
22. Ramachandran S, Penumetcha M, Merchant NK, Santanam N, Rong R, Parthasarathy S: **Exercise reduces preexisting atherosclerotic lesions in LDL receptor knockout mice.** *Atherosclerosis* 2005, **178**(1):33–38.
23. Meilhac O, Ramachandran S, Chiang K, Santanam N, Parthasarathy S: **Role of arterial wall antioxidant defense in beneficial effects of exercise on atherosclerosis in mice.** *Arterioscler Thromb Vasc Biol* 2001, **21**(10):1681–1688.
24. Yang T, Luo F, Shen Y, An J, Li X, Liu X, Ying B, Liao Z, Dong J, Guo L, Wang T, Xu D, Chen L, Wen F: **Quercetin attenuates airway inflammation and mucus production induced by cigarette smoke in rats.** *Int Immunopharmacol* 2012, **13**(1):73–81.
25. Boly R, Gras T, Lamkami T, Guissou P, Serteyn D, Kiss R, Dubois J: **Quercetin inhibits a large panel of kinases implicated in cancer cell biology.** *Int J Oncol* 2011, **38**(3):833–842.
26. Wang G, Wang JJ, Chen XL, Du SM, Li DS, Pei ZJ, Lan H, Wu LB: **The JAK2/STAT3 and mitochondrial pathways are essential for quercetin nanoliposome-induced C6 glioma cell death.** *Cell Death Dis* 2013, **4**:e746. doi:10.1038/cddis.2013.242. PubMed PMID: 23907460.
27. Michaud-Levesque J, Bousquet-Gagnon N, Béliveau R: **Quercetin abrogates IL-6/STAT3 signaling and inhibits glioblastoma cell line growth and migration.** *Exp Cell Res* 2012, **318**(8):925–935.
28. Song Y, Liu J, Zhang F, Zhang J, Shi T, Zeng Z: **Antioxidant effect of quercetin against acute spinal cord injury in rats and its correlation with the p38MAPK/iNOS signaling pathway.** *Life Sci* 2013, **92**(24–26):1215–1221.
29. Jung CH, Cho I, Ahn J, Jeon TI, Ha TY: **Quercetin reduces high-fat diet-induced fat accumulation in the liver by regulating lipid metabolism genes.** *Phytother Res* 2013, **27**(1):139–143.
30. Chang YC, Lee TS, Chiang AN: **Quercetin enhances ABCA1 expression and cholesterol efflux through a p38-dependent pathway in macrophages.** *J Lipid Res* 2012, **53**(9):1840–1850.
31. Litvinov D, Selvarajan K, Garelnabi M, Brophy L, Parthasarathy S: **Anti-atherosclerotic actions of azelaic acid, an end product of linoleic acid peroxidation, in mice.** *Atherosclerosis* 2010, **209**(2):449–454.
32. Thijssen DH, Cable NT, Green DJ: **Impact of exercise training on arterial wall thickness in humans.** *Clin Sci (Lond)* 2012, **122**(7):311–322.
33. Rankin AJ, Rankin AC, MacIntyre P, Hillis WS: **Walk or run? Is high-intensity exercise more effective than moderate-intensity exercise at reducing cardiovascular risk?** *Scott Med J* 2012, **57**(2):99–102.
34. Bowles DK, Laughlin MH: **Mechanism of beneficial effects of physical activity on atherosclerosis and coronary heart disease.** *J Appl Physiol* 2011, **111**(1):308–310.
35. Namiki M, Kawashima S, Yamashita T, Ozaki M, Hirase T, Ishida T, Inoue N, Hirata K, Matsukawa A, Morishita R, Kaneda Y, Yokoyama M: **Local overexpression of monocyte chemoattractant protein-1 at vessel wall induces infiltration of macrophages and formation of atherosclerotic lesion: synergism with hypercholesterolemia.** *Arterioscler Thromb Vasc Biol* 2002, **22**(1):115–120.
36. Bereta J, Cohen MC, Bereta M: **Stimulatory effect of ouabain on VCAM-1 and iNOS expression in murine endothelial cells: involvement of NF-kappa B.** *FEBS Lett* 1995, **377**(1):21–25.
37. Naderi GA, Asgary S, Sarraf-Zadegan N, Shirvany H: **Anti-oxidant effect of flavonoids on the susceptibility of LDL oxidation.** *Mol Cell Biochem* 2003, **246**(1–2):193–196.
38. Yao S, Sang H, Song G, Yang N, Liu Q, Zhang Y, Jiao P, Zong C, Qin S: **Quercetin protects macrophages from oxidized low-density lipoprotein-induced apoptosis by inhibiting the endoplasmic reticulum stress-C/EBP homologous protein pathway.** *Exp Biol Med (Maywood)* 2012, **237**(7):822–831.
39. Suzuki M, Yamamoto M, Sugimoto A, Nakamura S, Motoda R, Orita K: **Delta-4 expression on a stromal cell line is augmented by interleukin-6 via STAT3 activation.** *Exp Hematol* 2006, **34**(9):1143–1150.

High-intensity interval training and β-hydroxy-β-methylbutyric free acid improves aerobic power and metabolic thresholds

Edward H Robinson IV[1,2†], Jeffrey R Stout[1,2*†], Amelia A Miramonti[1,2†], David H Fukuda[1,2†], Ran Wang[1,2†], Jeremy R Townsend[1,2†], Gerald T Mangine[1,2†], Maren S Fragala[1,2†] and Jay R Hoffman[1,2†]

Abstract

Background: Previous research combining Calcium β-hydroxy-β-methylbutyrate (CaHMB) and running high-intensity interval training (HIIT) have shown positive effects on aerobic performance measures. The purpose of this study was to examine the effect of β-hydroxy-β-methylbutyric free acid (HMBFA) and cycle ergometry HIIT on maximal oxygen consumption (VO_2peak), ventilatory threshold (VT), respiratory compensation point (RCP) and time to exhaustion (T_{max}) in college-aged men and women.

Methods: Thirty-four healthy men and women (Age: 22.7 ± 3.1 yrs ; VO2peak: 39.3 ± 5.0 ml · kg^{-1} · min^{-1}) volunteered to participate in this double-blind, placebo-controlled design study. All participants completed a series of tests prior to and following treatment. A peak oxygen consumption test was performed on a cycle ergometer to assess VO_2peak, T_{max}, VT, and RCP. Twenty-six participants were randomly assigned into either a placebo (PLA-HIIT) or 3 g per day of HMBFA (BetaTor™) (HMBFA-HIIT) group. Eight participants served as controls (CTL). Participants in the HIIT groups completed 12 HIIT (80-120% maximal workload) exercise sessions consisting of 5–6 bouts of a 2:1 minute cycling work to rest ratio protocol over a four-week period. Body composition was measured with dual energy x-ray absorptiometry (DEXA). Outcomes were assessed by ANCOVA with posttest means adjusted for pretest differences.

Results: The HMBFA-HIIT intervention showed significant ($p < 0.05$) gains in VO_2peak, and VT, versus the CTL and PLA-HIIT group. Both PLA-HIIT and HMBFA-HIIT treatment groups demonstrated significant ($p < 0.05$) improvement over CTL for T_{max}, and RCP with no significant difference between the treatment groups. There were no significant differences observed for any measures of body composition. An independent-samples t-test confirmed that there were no significant differences between the training volumes for the PLA-HIIT and HMBFA-HIIT groups.

Conclusions: Our findings support the use of HIIT in combination with HMBFA to improve aerobic fitness in college age men and women. These data suggest that the addition of HMBFA supplementation may result in greater changes in VO_2peak and VT than HIIT alone.

Study registration: The study was registered on ClinicalTrials.gov (ID NCT01941368).

Keywords: High-intensity interval training, β-Hydroxy-β-Methylbutyric free acid, Aerobic, Endurance, VO_2peak, Respiratory compensation point, Ventilatory threshold

* Correspondence: jeffrey.stout@ucf.edu
†Equal contributors
[1]Institute of Exercise Physiology & Wellness, University of Central Florida, 4000, Orlando, FL 32816, USA
[2]College of Education & Human Performance, 12494 University Boulevard, Orlando, FL 32816, USA

Background

High-intensity interval training (HIIT) has become a popular training modality in competitive athletes, recreationally-trained individuals, and clinical populations [1]. HIIT consists of repeated bouts of short to moderate duration exercise completed at intensities greater than the anaerobic threshold, interspersed with brief periods of low intensity or passive rest. The salient features of HIIT over constant rate aerobic training (CRT) are shorter training periods and the reported improvements of both oxidative and glycolytic energy systems [1,2].

Physiological adaptations associated with HIIT include improved metabolic efficiency [3,4] related to a more efficient skeletal muscle substrate utilization, and improved respiratory control sensitivity resulting from increased mitochondrial density [5]. Helgerud et al. [6] reported that an eight-week running HIIT program improved VO_2max and time to exhaustion (TTE) more than CRT in moderately trained males. Further, Smith et al. [7] reported a 7% to 10% increase in VO_2peak and ventilatory threshold (VT) values after only 3 weeks of HIIT on a cycle ergometer using college age males. HIIT, therefore, is a time-efficient exercise strategy that has shown consistent positive results following relatively short duration training programs.

The branched-chain amino acid, leucine, has shown to be the key contributor for muscle protein synthesis and may play a role as a substrate during this process [8]. As such, dietary supplementation of leucine and its metabolites has been demonstrated to provide anabolic or anti-catabolic effects on lean body mass during training or periods of energy imbalance [9-11]. Ingestion of one of these metabolites, β-hydroxy-β-methylbutyrate in the free acid form (HMBFA), has been suggested to provide similar benefits to those of leucine with regard to muscle protein synthesis [12]. Additional investigation with CaHMB and resistance training in humans has shown improvement in muscle mass and strength in both younger and older subjects [13-16]. Recently, scientists have suggested CaHMB may enhance the benefits of intense aerobic training by attenuating skeletal muscle damage and accelerating recovery between training bouts. In support, Knitter et al. [17] examined the effect of three grams of CaHMB or placebo per day in trained endurance athletes for six weeks. Following the training and supplementation period, blood markers of muscle damage, creatine phosphokinase (CPK) and lactate dehydrogenase (LDH), were measured in response to a 20-km race. Following the race, LDH and CPK levels were 10.5% and 17% lower in the CaHMB supplemented group, respectively compared to the placebo group. These results [17] suggest that CaHMB supplementation may attenuate some of the muscle damage often observed with endurance training, possibly reducing the incidence of overtraining and allowing for greater training adaptations.

Ingestion of CaHMB during an aerobic training program appears to provide additional benefits. Vukovich and Dreifort [18] examined the effect of 3 grams of CaHMB or placebo per day for 14 days in elite cyclists while average training volume was 300 miles per week. In response to only the CaHMB condition, the cyclists demonstrated a significant increase in peak oxygen consumption rate (VO_2peak) and an increase in the onset of blood lactate accumulation during a graded exercise test. Those investigators suggested that changes in maximal and submaximal performance following CaHMB supplementation may have been related to both the attenuation of protein breakdown and the augmentation of mitochondrial protein synthesis resulting in greater oxidative energy capacity. In further support, Lamboley et al. [19] examined the effect of 5 weeks of CaHMB supplementation and HIIT in physically-active college students. They measured changes in VO_2max, VT and respiratory compensation point (RCP) during a graded exercise test at baseline and post training. The HIIT running program was performed 3 times per week on a treadmill (1% grade) and participants supplemented with 3 grams per day of CaHMB or placebo. The results of the investigation demonstrated significant increases in VO_2max, VT and RCP in both treatment groups from the HIIT; however, the CaHMB group resulted in a 19% to 45% greater increase in all metabolic variables. The investigators' suggested that CaHMB may have attenuated the muscle damage often observed from running and might have accelerated recovery between training bouts. Further, CaHMB supplementation may have enhanced the training stimulus of HIIT on VT and RCP by increasing mitochondrial biogenesis, thus improving oxidative energy capacity and efficiency [13,18,19].

It appears that HMBFA supplementation is most effective during muscle damaging exercise [20]. Lamboley et al. [19] indicated that they specifically selected running to induce delayed onset muscle soreness, a non-invasive indicator of muscle damage. However, to date, no one has examined the effect of HMBFA supplementation while undergoing a HIIT program on a cycle ergometer. If muscle damage is needed to observe the potential benefits of HMBFA supplementation, then HIIT training on a cycle ergometer, which produces much less muscle damage [21] than running, may provide no additional benefit. Therefore, the purpose of this study was to examine the effects of chronic (4-weeks) HMBFA supplementation in combination with cycle ergometry HIIT on endurance performance measures in active college age men and women.

Methods

Participants

For inclusion in the study, all males were required to have a VO_2peak greater than 35 $ml \cdot kg^{-1} \cdot min^{-1}$ and all female participants greater than 30 ml·kg^{-1}·min^{-1}. After initial testing, forty recreationally-active individuals (men = 21, women = 19) between the ages of 18 and 35 were recruited to participate in this study. Three female and two male participants were removed due to health reasons not associated with the study. One female participant was removed after a family emergency. Therefore, data for 19 men and 15 women (Table 1) were included in the final analysis. All participants completed a questionnaire to assess ability to participate in physical activity and to ascertain any prior supplementation regime. Individuals self-reported to be free of musculoskeletal injury as determined by a physical activity readiness questionnaire (PAR-Q). Following an explanation of all procedures, risks and benefits, each participant provided his/her informed consent to participate in the study.

A minimum sample size of n = 8 per group was determined using previously published data [19] and the formula derived by Gravettier and Wallnau [22] to achieve a statistical power (1-β) of 0.80. Therefore, with an expectation of subject dropout, a final sample size of n = 15 in each experimental group and n = 10 in the control group were recruited. The study was registered on ClinicalTrials.gov (ID NCT01941368).

Research design

A double-blind, placebo-controlled design, stratified for gender, was used to examine the effects of HMBFA and HIIT training on measures of metabolic performance. Each participant was required to visit the Human Performance Laboratory on four separate occasions for pre- and post- testing, with each testing session occurring on nonconsecutive days. The same testing protocols were repeated at the beginning and end of the 4-week training period. On the first testing day, anthropometric measures of participants were collected (Table 1). Each participant then performed a graded exercise test to determine peak oxygen consumption (VO_2peak), time to exhaustion (T_{max}), respiratory compensation point (RCP), and ventilatory threshold (VT). The peak wattage achieved during this test was used to establish individual training intensity. On the second day of testing, a baseline blood draw was performed to measure serum HMB, and total lean soft tissue (TLST) and body fat percentage (BF) were assessed using dual energy x-ray absorptiometry (DEXA) (Prodigy™; Lunar Corporation, Madison, WI, USA).

After baseline testing, the participants were randomly assigned to one of three groups: a control group (CTL), a placebo with HIIT group (PLA-HIIT) or HMBFA with HIIT group (HMBFA-HIIT). Of the 40 subjects that were recruited for this study, 10 subjects were assigned to CTL and 15 to each of the training groups (PLA-HIIT or HMBFA-HIIT).

Exercise protocol

Participants in the PLA-HIIT and HMBFA-HIIT groups participated in 4-weeks of high-intensity interval training with three sessions per week—with at least one day between each training session—on a calibrated, electronically-braked cycle ergometer (Lode Corival 400, Groningen, the Netherlands). The exercise training program consisted of alternating training sessions of sub-maximal and supra-maximal workloads (Figure 1). Each participant's training load was determined as a percentage of the peak power output (P_{peak}) from the graded exercise test. Individuals began each training session with a 5-minute warm up at a self-selected wattage, followed by an exercise protocol of five 2-minute exercise bouts at a predetermined percentage of their power output at VO_2peak. Between each exercise bout, the participant had 1 minute of complete rest. In the event that there was an inability to complete the entire 2-min exercise bout, the participant completed the 1-min rest period and attempted subsequent bouts. Total time completed and power output was recorded for each exercise session to calculate total training volume (Power output (Watts) × Total time = Training Volume). Participants assigned to CTL were asked to continue their normal activity pattern for 4 weeks before returning to undergo post-testing.

Supplementation

The HMBFA supplement consisted of 1 gram of β-hydroxy-β-methylbutyrate in the free acid form (BetaTor™, Metabolic Technologies Inc, Ames, IA), reverse osmosis water, de-bittering agent, orange flavor, stevia

Table 1 Participant descriptive statistics

Variable	Control (n = 8)	PLA-HIIT (n = 13)	HMBFA-HIIT (n = 13)	p-value
Age (y)	21.0 ± 2.4	23.6 ± 3.7	22.9 ± 2.4	0.166
Height (cm)	171.4 ± 5.7	172.6 ± 12.2	173.0 ± 9.2	0.939
Body mass (kg)	76.3 ± 12.8	74.9 ± 16.6	72.4 ± 9.9	0.793
% Body fat	22.4 ± 8.1	19.7 ± 8.6	24.8 ± 8.1	0.301
Training volume (kJ)	N/A	1437.0 ± 309.6	1456.8 ± 378.6	0.313

Values are presented as means ± SD. HIIT, high-intensity interval training. HMBFA, β-hydroxy-β-methylbutyrate in the free acid form (BetaTor™, Metabolic Technologies Inc, Ames, IA), PLA, placebo.

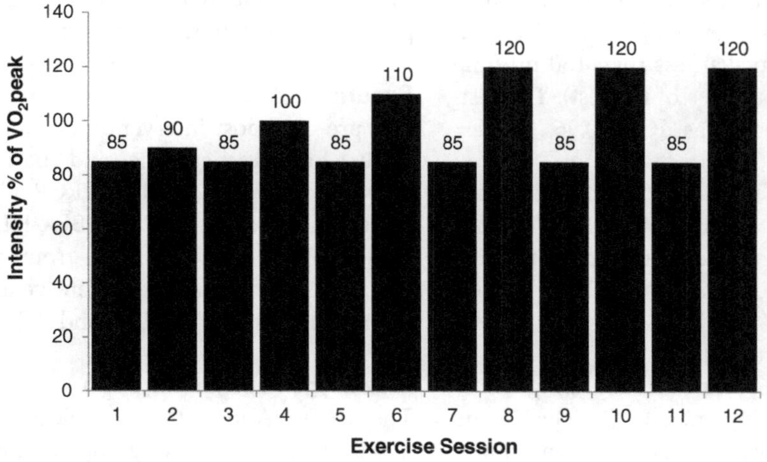

Figure 1 Exercise training intensity protocol.

extract, and potassium carbonate. Each serving of placebo contained 1 gram of polydextrose that was equivalent to β-hydroxy-β-methylbutyrate in the free acid, citric acid, corn syrup, stevia extract, de-bittering agent, and orange flavoring. Identical in appearance and taste, the HMBFA and PL treatments were produced and supplied by Metabolic Technologies Inc. (Ames, IA). Prior to the first training session, subjects were randomly assigned to receive either 3 g per day of HMBFA or a placebo divided equally into three servings, given 30 minutes prior to exercise and again 1 hour later and then a final 1 g dose 3 hours post exercise on training days. To ensure compliance, investigators watched as the subjects consumed the supplement prior to and immediately after each exercise session. On the non-training days, subjects were instructed to consume one packet with three separate meals throughout the day. Empty packets were presented to the investigators upon returning to the laboratory following non-training days.

Blood measurements and HMB analysis

During testing days, resting blood samples were drawn following a 15-min equilibration period. These blood samples were obtained from an antecubital arm vein using a 20-gauge disposable needle equipped with a Vacutainer® tube holder (Becton Dickinson, Franklin Lakes, NJ) containing K_2EDTA. Each participant's blood samples were obtained at the same time of day during each testing session. The blood was centrifuged at 3,000 × g for 15 min along and the resulting plasma was placed into s 1.8-mL microcentrifuge tube and frozen at −80°C for later analysis.

Plasma HMB concentrations were analyzed by gas chromatography–mass spectrometry which was performed by Metabolic Technologies Inc. in a blinded fashion using methods previously described by Nissen et al. [23].

Dietary analysis

Prior to training, participants were asked to complete a 3-day food log, to establish macronutrient content and average leucine intake. This diet was considered the participant's standard diet and they were asked to maintain a similar regimen throughout the duration of the study. These data were entered into a software program (Food Works 13, The Nutrition Company; Long Valley, NJ) which provided calculation for daily leucine intake (g) and total calories (kcal).

Determination of VO_2peak, VT, and RCP

An incremental test to volitional exhaustion was performed on an electronically-braked cycle ergometer (Lode Excalibur Sport; Groningen, The Netherlands) to determine VO_2peak and the P_{peak} in watts (W) at VO_2peak. Prior to testing, each participant was fitted with a Polar Heart Watch system to record the participants' heart rate (Polar Electro Inc., Lake Success, NY). Following the procedures described by Bergstrom et al. [24], participants were instructed to maintain a pedaling cadence of 70–75 revolutions per minute (RPM) at an initial workload of 75 W. The workload increased 25 W every two minutes until he or she was unable to maintain a cadence above 70 RPM for ~10s despite verbal encouragement, or volitional fatigue. Prior to each graded exercise test, open-circuit spirometry (TrueOne 2400® Metabolic Measurement System, Parvo Medics, Inc., Sandy, UT) was calibrated with room air and gases of known concentration, which was used to estimate VO_2peak ($ml{\cdot}kg^{-1}{\cdot}min^{-1}$) by sampling and analyzing breath-by-breath expired gases. Oxygen (O_2), carbon dioxide (CO_2), ventilation (V_E), and respiratory exchange ratio (RER)—were monitored continuously and expressed as 30-second averages [25]. VO_2peak was determined to be the highest 30-s VO_2 value during the test and coincided with at least two of the following three criteria: (a) 90% of age-predicted maximum heart rate; (b) respiratory exchange ratio > 1.1; and/or (c) a plateau of oxygen uptake (less than 150 mL/min increase in VO_2 during the last 60 s of the test). The test-retest reliability for VO_2peak was ICC = 0.96 (SEM = 1.4 ml·kg·min^{-1}).

Ventilatory threshold (VT) and RCP were determined by common methods for determining gas exchange thresholds [26-29]. The VT was determined by plotting and determining the point of increase in the V_E/VO_2 versus VO_2 curve as the V_E/VCO_2 versus VO_2 curve remained constant or decreased [24,26]. The RCP as described by Beaver et al. [26] was identified using the V-Slope method by plotting the V_E versus VCO_2. The VT and RCP were reported as the corresponding VO_2 and power output in watts (PVT and PRCP). The test-retest reliability for VT and RCP was ICC = 0.97 (SEM 0.1 ml·kg·min^{-1}) and 0.87 (SEM 0.2 ml·kg·min^{-1}), respectively.

Anthropometric measures

Body composition was estimated from a scan by DEXA (GE Medical Systems Lunar, Madison, WI, USA; software version 13.60.033) performed by a state licensed x-ray technician. Participants were positioned supine in the center of the platform and were scanned using the default scan mode for total body scanning. Measures for total lean soft tissue (LSTM) and fat mass were calculated by the system software (Encore 2011, software version 13.60.033). Body composition was analyzed using estimated body fat percentage (%BF) and total lean soft tissue mass (LSTM). The test-retest reliability for LSTM and% BF was ICC = 0.99 (SEM 0.4 kg) and 0.99 (SEM 0.8%BF), respectively.

Statistical analyses

Statistical software (IBM SPSS Statistics for Windows, Version 21.0; Armonk, NY: IBM Corp) was used to perform all statistical analysis. Separate one-way analyses of covariance (ANCOVA) were used to analyze all dependent performance and metabolic variable data based on the recommendations of Huck and McLean [30]. The independent variable, group, included 3 levels: PLA-HIIT, HMBFA-HIIT, and CTL. The pretest and posttest values were used as the covariate and dependent variable, respectively. When appropriate, LSD post hoc pairwise comparisons were used to examine the differences among the groups. For effect size, the partial eta squared statistic was calculated, and according to Green et al. [31], 0.01, 0.06, and 0.14 were interpreted as small, medium, and large effect sizes, respectively. Two-way ANOVA (Time × treatment) was used to examine changes in plasma HMB concentration between PLA-HIIT and HMBFA-HIIT. Independent-samples t-tests' were performed to compare total training volume, total energy and leucine intake for the PLA-HIIT and HMBFA-HIIT groups. An alpha of $p < 0.05$ was established a priori.

Results

The pre- and post-intervention mean and standard deviations for all metabolic and performance measures (VO_2peak, P_{peak}, T_{max}, RCP, PRCP, VT, and PVT) for all groups (CTL, PLA-HIIT, HMBFA-HIIT) are provided in Table 2. Table 3 provides the group mean and standard deviations for pre- to post-intervention body composition measures (BW, LSTM, and BF).

Peak oxygen uptake (VO_2peak)

The ANCOVA indicated a significant difference ($p = 0.003$, $\eta^2 = 0.322$) among the group means for the posttest VO_2peak values after adjusting for pre-test differences (Figure 2). The strength of the association (i.e., effect size, η^2) indicated that the treatment groups (CTL, PLA-HIIT, HMBFA-HIIT) accounted for 32% of the variance of the post-test VO_2peak values, holding constant the pre-test VO_2peak scores. The LSD pairwise comparisons indicated that the increase in VO_2peak from pre- to post-testing was greater for the HMBFA-HIIT group than for the CTL ($p = 0.001$) and the PLA-HIIT groups ($p = 0.032$), however, no differences were found between PLA-HIIT and CTL groups ($p = 0.09$). The group means (±SEM) for the post-test VO_2peak values, adjusted for initial differences in pre-test scores, are shown in Figure 2.

Peak power (P_{peak})

The ANCOVA indicated a significant difference ($p = 0.013$, $\eta^2 = 0.251$) among the group means for the post-test P_{peak} values after adjusting for pre-test differences (Figure 3). The strength of the association (i.e., effect size, η^2) indicated that the treatment groups (CTL, PLA-HIIT, HMBFA-HIIT) accounted for 25% of the variance of the post-test P_{peak} values, holding constant the pre-test P_{peak} scores. The LSD pairwise comparisons indicated that the increase in P_{peak} from pre- to post-testing was greater for the HMBFA-HIIT ($p = 0.04$) and PLA-HIIT ($p = 0.018$) groups than for the CTL group, however, no differences were found between HMBFA-HIIT and PLA-HIIT groups ($p = 0.51$). The group means (±SEM) for the post-test P_{peak} values, adjusted for initial differences in pre-test scores, are shown in Figure 3.

Time to exhaustion (T_{max})

The ANCOVA indicated a significant difference ($p = 0.002$, $\eta^2 = 0.35$) among the group means for the post-test T_{max} values after adjusting for pre-test differences (Figure 4). The strength of the association (i.e., effect size, η^2) indicated that the treatment groups (CTL, PLA-HIIT, HMBFA-HIIT) accounted for 35% of the variance of

Table 2 Metabolic and performance measures for pre- and post-supplementation

	Control ($n = 8$)		PLA-HIIT ($n = 13$)		HMBFA-HIIT ($n = 13$)	
Measure	**Pretest**	**Posttest**	**Pretest**	**Posttest**	**Pretest**	**Posttest**
VO_2peak (ml · kg^{-1} · min^{-1})	39.1 ± 4.5	38.9 ± 4.0	38.9 ± 3.4	40.3 ± 2.6	39.8 ± 6.7	42.7 ± 5.1
P_{peak} (W)	218.8 ± 41.7	215.6 ± 32.6	221.2 ± 46.6	236.5 ± 48.5	226.9 ± 56.3	246.2 ± 54.8
T_{max} (min)	12.5 ± 2.9	12.2 ± 2.3	13.0 ± 3.8	14.2 ± 3.7	13.6 ± 4.7	14.9 ± 4.5
RCP (ml · kg^{-1} · min^{-1})	30.5 ± 5.0	28.7 ± 2.7	29.3 ± 3.1	31.9 ± 2.2	32.2 ± 4.2	33.7 ± 3.8
PRCP (W)	175.3 ± 38.8	167.0 ± 24.8	168.4 ± 36.0	185.0 ± 33.5	182.6 ± 33.6	196.5 ± 35.1
VT (ml · kg^{-1} · min^{-1})	27.7 ± 3.3	27.2 ± 2.7	28.6 ± 3.1	29.0 ± 4.1	27.8 ± 4.8	31.7 ± 3.7
PVT (W)	156.3 ± 17.7	153.1 ± 28.2	159.6 ± 40.2	169.2 ± 37.0	161.5 ± 39.02	184.6 ± 37.6

Values are means ± SD. HIIT, high-intensity interval training; HMBFA, β-hydroxy-β-methylbutyrate in the free acid form (BetaTor™, Metabolic Technologies Inc, Ames, IA); PLA, placebo; VO_2peak, peak oxygen uptake; P_{peak}, peak power achieved; Tmax, time to exhaustion during graded exercise test; RCP, respiratory-compensation point; VT, ventilatory threshold.

the post-test T_{max} values, holding constant the pre-test T_{max} scores. The LSD pairwise comparisons indicated that the increase in T_{max} from pre- to post-testing was greater for the HMBFA-HIIT ($p = 0.001$) and PLA-HIIT ($p = 0.002$) groups than for the CTL group, however, no differences were found between HMBFA-HIIT and PLA-HIIT groups ($p = 0.62$). The group means (±SEM) for the post-test T_{max} values, adjusted for initial differences in pretest scores, are shown in Figure 4.

Respiratory Compensation Point (RCP)

The ANCOVA indicated a significant difference ($p < 0.001$, $\eta^2 = 0.436$) among the group means for the posttest RCP values after adjusting for pre-test differences (Figure 5). The strength of the association (i.e., effect size, η^2) indicated that the treatment groups (CTL, PLA-HIIT, HMBFA-HIIT) accounted for 44% of the variance of the post-test RCP values, holding constant the pre-test RCP scores. The LSD pairwise comparisons indicated that the increase in RCP from pre- to post-testing was greater for the HMBFA-HIIT ($p < 0.001$) and PLA-HIIT ($p < 0.001$) groups than for the CTL group, however, no differences were found between HMBFA-HIIT and PLA-HIIT groups ($p = 0.77$). The group means (±SEM) for the posttest RCP values, adjusted for initial differences in pretest scores, are shown in Figure 5.

Power at Respiratory Compensation Point (PRCP)

The ANCOVA indicated a significant difference ($p = 0.001$, $\eta2 = 0.375$) among the group means for the posttest PRCP values after adjusting for pre-test differences (Table 2, Figure 6). The strength of the association (i.e., effect size, η^2) indicated that the treatment groups (CTL, PLA-HIIT, HMBFA-HIIT) accounted for 38% of the variance of the post-test PRCP values, holding constant the pre-test PRCP scores. The LSD pairwise comparisons indicated that the increase in PRCP from pre- to post-testing was greater for the HMBFA-HIIT ($p < 0.001$) and PLA-HIIT ($p < 0.001$) groups than for the CTL group, however, no differences were found between HMBFA-HIIT and PLA-HIIT groups ($p = 0.97$). The group means (±SEM) for the posttest PRCP values, adjusted for initial differences in pretest scores, are shown in Figure 6.

Ventilatory Threshold (VT)

The ANCOVA indicated a significant difference ($p = 0.016$, $\eta2 = 0.24$) among the group means for the post-test VT values after adjusting for pre-test differences (Figure 7). The strength of the association (i.e., effect size, η^2) indicated that the treatment groups (CTL, PLA-HIIT, HMBFA-HIIT) accounted for 24% of the variance of the posttest VT values, holding constant the pre-test VT scores. The LSD pairwise comparisons indicated that the increase in VT from pre- to post-testing was

Table 3 Body composition measures for pre- and post-supplementation

	Control ($n = 8$)		PLA-HIIT ($n = 13$)		HMBFA-HIIT ($n = 13$)	
Measure	**Pretest**	**Posttest**	**Pretest**	**Posttest**	**Pretest**	**Posttest**
Body weight (kg)	76.3 ± 12.8	75.5 ± 12.7	74.9 ± 16.6	75.2 ± 16.3	72.4 ± 9.9	72.5 ± 10.0
Lean soft tissue mass (kg)	56.5 ± 11.7	56.4 ± 10.7	58.4 ± 16.6	58.6 ± 16.6	52.2 ± 10.9	52.2 ± 10.9
Total body fat mass (kg)	15.9 ± 7.0	14.3 ± 8.4	13.3 ± 4.8	13.2 ± 4.6	16.9 ± 5.3	17.0 ± 5.4
Body fat %	22.4 ± 8.1	22.0 ± 2.8	19.7 ± 8.6	19.5 ± 8.4	24.8 ± 8.1	24.6 ± 7.7

Values are means ± SD. HIIT, high-intensity interval training; HMBFA, β-hydroxy-β-methylbutyrate in the free acid form (BetaTor™, Metabolic Technologies Inc, Ames, IA); PLA, placebo.

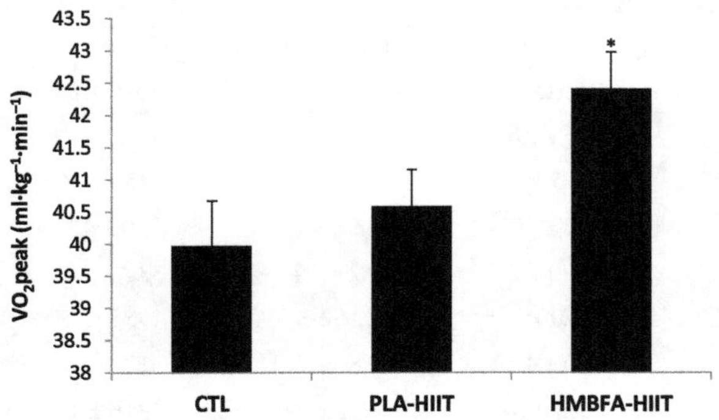

Figure 2 VO_2peak obtained during graded exercise test. Mean values (+SEM) for posttest VO_2peak scores adjusted for the initial differences in pretest VO_2peak (covariate; adjusted pretest mean = 39.3). *HMBFA-HIIT significantly greater than PLA-HIIT ($p = 0.032$) and CTL ($p = 0.001$).

greater for the HMBFA-HIIT group than for the CTL ($p = 0.012$) and the PLA-HIIT groups ($p = 0.017$), however, no differences were found between PLA-HIIT and CTL groups ($p = 0.6$). The group means (±SEM) for the posttest VT values, adjusted for initial differences in pretest scores, are shown in Figure 7.

Power at Ventilatory Threshold (PVT)

The ANCOVA indicated a significant difference ($p = 0.009$, $\eta^2 = 0.267$) among the group means for the post-test PVT values after adjusting for pre-test differences (Figure 8). The strength of the association (i.e., effect size, η^2) indicated that the treatment groups (CTL, PLA-HIIT, HMBFA-HIIT) accounted for 27% of the variance of the post-test PVT values, holding constant the pre-test PVT scores. The LSD pairwise comparisons indicated that the increase in PVT from pre- to post-testing was greater for the HMBFA-HIIT group than for the CTL ($p = 0.004$) and the PLA-HIIT groups ($p = 0.027$), however, no differences were found between PLA-HIIT and CTL groups ($p = 0.277$). The group means (±SEM) for the posttest PVT values, adjusted for initial differences in pretest scores, are shown in Figure 8.

Body composition

The ANCOVA indicated no significant difference for body mass ($p = 0.31$, $\eta^2 = 0.074$) percent body fat ($p = 0.88$, $\eta^2 = 0.009$), and lean soft tissue mass ($p = 0.247$, $\eta^2 = 0.089$) between the groups (Table 3).

Training volume

There was no significant difference ($p = 0.31$) between training volumes for PLA-HIIT (1437.0 ± 309.6 kJ) and HMBFA-HIIT (1456.8 ± 378.6 kJ).

Dietary analysis

There was no significant difference for daily energy intake ($p = 0.159$; PLA-HIIT, 2398.7 ± 619 Kcal; HMBFA-HIIT, 2011 ± 620 Kcal) or leucine intake ($p = 0.561$; PLA-HIIT, 3.3 ± 1.7 g; HMBFA-HIIT, 3.9 ± 2.1 g) between the two treatment groups.

Supplementation compliance and plasma HMBFA concentrations

Placebo or HMBFA intake was recorded on individual intake logs, which were returned to the laboratory and monitored and resulted in 99% compliance. In addition, there was a significant interaction (F = 5.9, p = 0.02) for blood plasma HMBFA concentrations. The HMBFA-HIIT group increased by 2.6 ± 2.1 $nmol{\cdot}ml^{-1}$ with little change in the PLA-HIIT group (0.1 ± 0.9 $nmol{\cdot}ml^{-1}$), further supporting compliance in the treatment group.

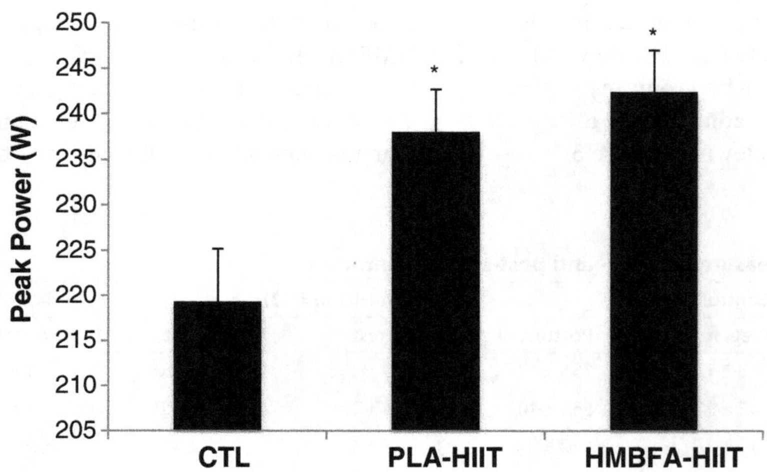

Figure 3 Peak power (P_{peak}) obtained during graded exercise test. Mean values (+SEM) for posttest P_{peak} scores adjusted for the initial differences in pretest P_{peak} (covariate; adjusted pretest mean = 222.79). *Indicates significantly different than CTL (PLA-HIIT, p = 0.018; HMBFA-HIIT, $p = 0.04$).

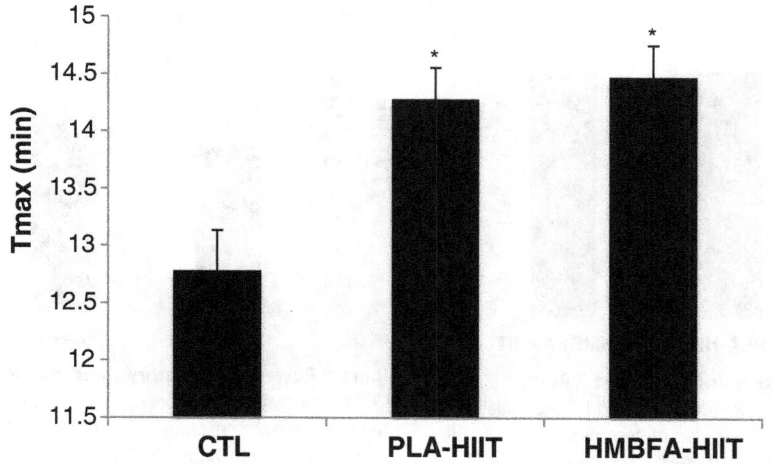

Figure 4 Time to exhaustion (T_{max}) for the graded exercise test. Mean values (+SEM) for posttest T_{max} scores adjusted for the initial differences in pretest T_{max} (covariate; adjusted pretest mean = 13.11). *Indicates significantly different than CTL (PLA-HIIT, p = 0.002; HMBFA-HIIT, $p = 0.001$).

Discussion

To the best of our knowledge, this is the first study to examine the effects of the free-acid form of β-hydroxy-β-methylbutyrate (HMB) supplementation and high-intensity interval training (HIIT) using a cycle ergometer on metabolic and performance measures in young men and women. The primary findings support the use of HIIT in combination HMBFA as a training method to improve aerobic fitness. Furthermore, the results of the current study suggest that HMBFA supplementation significantly improved the benefits of the 4-week HIIT program on VO2peak, VT and PVT aerobic and metabolic measures when compared to HIIT alone.

The HIIT protocol used in the current study (Figure 1) resulted in a 4 to 11% increase in aerobic performance measures (VO_2peak, P_{peak}, T_{max}; Table 2). This is consistent with Smith et al. [7] who reported a 7% to 11% increase in VO_2peak and T_{max} after 3 weeks of HIIT using a similar protocol. In agreement, several other studies have reported 7 to 10% increases in VO_2peak using HIIT protocols in college-aged participants [6,32,33]. Although previous studies utilizing this method of HIIT utilized a 5-day per week training routine, Jourkesh et al. [34] also reported a significant increase in T_{max} after 3 weeks of periodized HIIT and a significant increase in VO_2peak after 6 weeks with training 3 times per week.

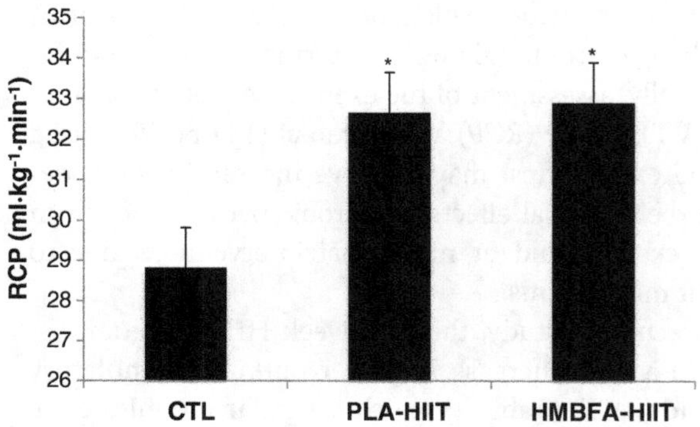

Figure 5 Respiratory compensation point (RCP). Mean values (+SEM) for posttest RCP scores adjusted for the initial differences in pretest RCP (covariate; adjusted pretest mean = 30.69). *Indicates significantly different than CTL (PLA-HIIT, p < 0.001; HMBFA-HIIT, p < 0.001).

In the current investigation, the addition of HMBFA ingestion with HIIT significantly (7.3%) increased VO_2peak (Table 2, Figure 2) greater than training alone. The present results are in agreement with Lamboley et al. [19] who reported a 15% increase in VO_2max after 5 weeks of a running HIIT program while supplementing with 3 grams per day of calcium β-hydroxy-β-methylbutyrate (CaHMB) in college age men and women. In contrast, previous studies, which involved supplementation of CaHMB while endurance training, found no increase in VO_2peak with 2 to 6 weeks of supplementation [17,18]. In a cross-over design, Vukovich and Dreifort [18], examined the effect of CaHMB supplementation in endurance-trained cyclists, and reported no significant increase in VO_2peak in these highly trained athletes, however, there was a significant increase (3.6%) in the time to reach VO_2peak (T_{max}). The increase in T_{max} observed by Vukovich and Dreifort [18], was smaller than our observed 8% increase in younger untrained men and women (Table 2). The discrepancy between our study and the previous endurance training studies [18] examining CaHMB could be due to the training experience of the participants used in the investigation. It has been suggested that active men and women who are unaccustomed to HIIT may benefit more from

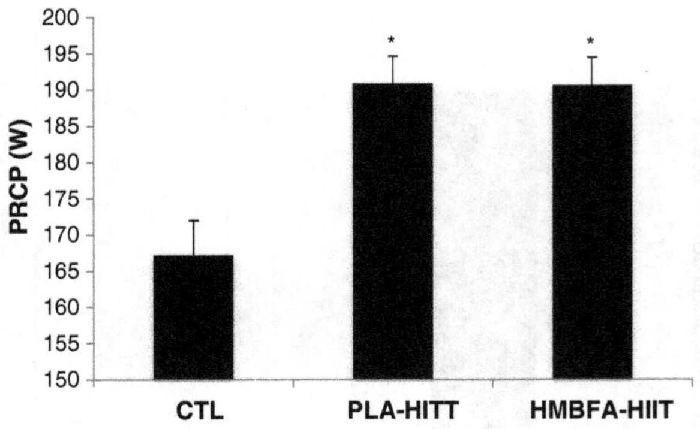

Figure 6 Power at respiratory compensation point (PRCP). Mean values (+SEM) for posttest PRCP scores adjusted for the initial differences in pretest PRCP (covariate; adjusted pretest mean = 175.43). *Indicates significantly different than CTL (PLA-HIIT, p = 0.001; HMBFA-HIIT, p = 0.001).

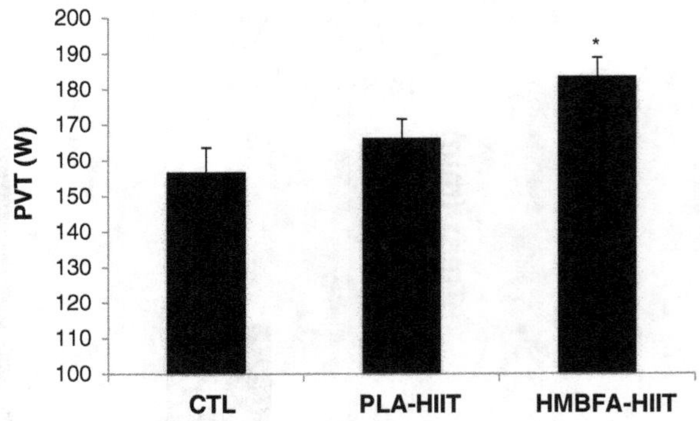

Figure 8 Power at ventilatory threshold (PVT). Mean values (+SEM) for posttest PVT scores adjusted for the initial differences in pretest PVT (covariate; adjusted pretest mean = 160.29). *HMBFA-HIIT significantly greater than PLA-HIIT ($p = 0.027$) and CTL ($p = 0.004$).

CaHMB supplementation than trained athletes who are accustomed to HIIT [19]. The participants in the current study were unfamiliar with HIIT, which may explain why our results were similar to Lamboley et al. [19] and not Vukovich et al. [18] who used trained endurance athletes. However, Knitter et al. [17] also examined individuals unaccustomed to HIIT, but reported no additive effect of HMB supplement on endurance performance measures. Therefore, training status and previous experience with HIIT could have influenced the current results while explaining differences from previous investigations.

The differences reported by Lamboley et al. [19] and our findings versus other studies may be due to the fact that individualized HIIT programs were developed based on each participant's baseline fitness level and monitored throughout the 28 days of training, while it was unclear what endurance program was used in other studies [18]. Therefore, the difference in results by Knitter [17] and Vukovich et al. [18] in comparison to Lamboley et al. [19] and our data may be related to an insufficient training stimulus that was unable to stimulate physiological adaptation [13,20,35].

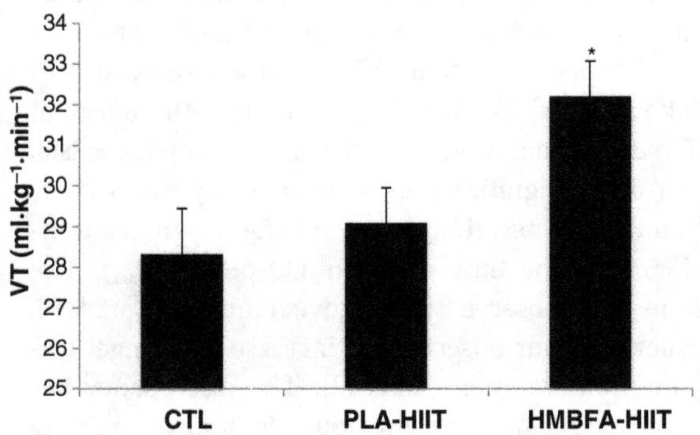

Figure 7 Ventilatory Threshold (VT). Mean values (+SEM) for posttest VT scores adjusted for the initial differences in pretest VT (covariate; adjusted pretest mean = 28.68). *HMBFA-HIIT significantly greater than PLA-HIIT ($p = 0.017$) and CTL ($p = 0.012$).

Fatigue threshold measures, such as VT, RCP, and onset of blood lactate accumulation (OBLA), have been used as non-invasive measures of health and performance, and in the evaluation of the efficacy of endurance training and/or nutritional supplementation [19,36,37]. Further, the measurement of specific fatigue thresholds during a graded exercise test, like VT and RCP, may be useful for demarcating the heavy or severe exercise intensity domains, respectively [24]. For example, VT has been associated with the minimum exercise intensity that results in excessive CO_2 production from the bicarbonate buffering of hydrogen ions [38,39], while exercise above RCP has been associated with the severe intensity domain which leads to excessive minute ventilation resulting from hyperkalemia [24,40]. The measurement of fatigue thresholds (VT, RCP), therefore, may provide possible mechanistic explanation for aerobic performance changes from training or nutritional interventions. Additionally, assessment of the exercise intensity domains, heavy (VT), severe (RCP) and maximal ($\dot{V}O_2$peak), during a graded exercise test may improve the sensitivity of detecting the potential effects on aerobic performance from various exercise and or nutritional interventions due to different mechanisms.

In the current study, the four-week HIIT program resulted in a 6.3% increase in power output at ventilatory threshold (PVT) (Table 2) which is similar to Smith et al. [7] who reported a ~9% increase using a comparable three-week HIIT cycling protocol in untrained college aged men. In addition, our study demonstrated an 8.6% increase in RCP which was very similar to the changes reported by Lamboley et al. [19] of an 8.5% increase from 5 weeks of HIIT on a treadmill. Our data, along with Smith et al. [7] and Lamboley et al. [19], support previous studies that demonstrate HIIT consistently improves metabolic threshold measures [6,41,42].

The addition of HMBFA to the four weeks of HIIT (HMB-HIIT) resulted in a ~14% increase in VT which was significantly greater than HIIT alone (Table 2, Figure 7). However, there was no difference between HMBFA-HIIT and PLA-HIIT groups for changes in RCP (Table 2, Figure 5). While our changes in VT are similar to values reported by Lamboley et al. [19], they described no significant difference between CaHMB-HIIT and PLA-HIIT groups. However, Lamboley et al. [19] reported significantly greater changes in RCP for CaHMB-HIIT compared to PLA-HIIT, whereas the current investigation resulted in similar changes between groups. Furthermore, Vukovich and Dreifort [18] reported a 9.1% increase in OBLA after two weeks of CaHMB supplementation in elite cyclists. Previous researchers have used OBLA as a method to identify the crossover point between moderate to heavy exercise intensities denoted by blood lactate concentrations greater than 4 $mmol{\cdot}L^{-1}$ during an incremental exercise test [43]. With previous evidence supporting OBLA and VT as fatigue thresholds representing similar exercise domains, the increases in exercise intensity at OBLA (+9.1%) reported by Vukovich and Dreifort [18] and the increase in VT (+14%) observed in our study (Table 2) may reflect similar physiological adaptations. Our results, along with Vukovich and Dreifort [18] and Lamboley et al. [19], suggest that HMBFA may augment the beneficial effects of HIIT on aerobic performance by increasing fatigue threshold measures that reflect the physiological response to moderate and/or severe intensity exercise.

The physiological changes observed in aerobic performance from HIIT have been shown to improve $\dot{V}O_2$peak, muscle buffering capacity, and whole body fat oxidation [1,44,45]. Further, the improved aerobic power associated with HIIT has been linked to an up-regulation of glycolytic enzymes, as well as, increased mitochondrial density and blood flow [46,47]. HMBFA supplementation may improve HIIT training by up-regulating fatty acid oxidation, adenosine monophosphate kinase (AMPK), Sirt1, and Sirt3 activity in muscle cells [48,49]. Sirt1, Sirt3, and AMPK have been shown to augment mitochondrial biogenesis, lipolysis, energy metabolism and the reactive oxygen defense system [50,51]. Additionally, Pinheiro et al. [49] reported that 28 days of CaHMB administration in male Wistar rats resulted in significantly increased intramuscular ATP and glycogen content. While speculative, HMBFA supplementation may have enhanced the effects of HIIT by improving mitochondrial biogenesis, fat oxidation, and metabolism. However, more research is needed to support these proposed mechanisms in humans.

Conclusions

In conclusion, our findings support the use of HIIT in combination with HMBFA as an effective training stimulus for improving aerobic performance. In addition, the use of HMBFA supplementation, in combination with HIIT, appeared to result in greater changes in $\dot{V}O_2$peak, PVT and VT than HIIT alone. While more research is needed, the current investigation suggests that in this sample of college age men and women, the use of HMBFA supplementation may enhance the benefits of HIIT on aerobic performance measures.

Competing interests

The authors declare that they have no competing interests.

Authors' contributions

All authors contributed equally to this work. All authors have read and approved the final manuscript.

Authors' information

The authors responsible for this work are members of the Institute of Exercise Physiology and Wellness at the University of Central Florida. All authors are faculty and graduate students in the College of Education and Human Performance.

Acknowledgements

This study was funded by a grant from Metabolic Technologies Inc., Ames Iowa.

References

1. Laursen PB, Jenkins DG: **The scientific basis for high-intensity interval training.** *Sports Med* 2002, **32**(1):53–73.
2. Perry CGR, Heigenhauser GJF, Bonen A, Spriet LL: **High-intensity aerobic interval training increases fat and carbohydrate metabolic capacities in human skeletal muscle.** *Appl Physiol Nutr Metab* 2008, **33**(6):1112–1123.
3. Laursen PB, Shing CM, Peake JM, Coombes JS, Jenkins DG: **Influence of high-intensity interval training on adaptations in well-trained cyclists.** *J Strength Cond Res* 2005, **19**(3):527–533.
4. Jenkins DG, Quigley BM: **The influence of high-intensity exercise training on the Wlim-Tlim relationship.** *Med Sci Sports Exerc* 1993, **25**(2):275–282.
5. Jacobs RA, Boushel R, Wright-Paradis C, Calbet JA, Robach P, Gnaiger E, Lundby C: **Mitochondrial function in human skeletal muscle following high-altitude exposure.** *Exp Physiol* 2013, **98**(1):245–255.
6. Helgerud J, Hoydal K, Wang E, Karlsen T, Berg P, Bjerkaas M, Simonsen T, Helgesen C, Hjorth N, Bach R: **Aerobic High-Intensity Intervals Improve VO2max More Than Moderate Training.** *Med Sci Sports Exerc* 2007, **39**(4):665.
7. Smith AE, Walter AA, Graef JL, Kendall KL, Moon JR, Lockwood CM, Fukuda DH, Beck TW, Cramer JT, Stout JR: **Effects of β-alanine supplementation and high-intensity interval training on endurance performance and body composition in men; a double-blind trial.** *J Int Soc Sports Nutr* 2009, **6**(1):1–9.
8. Churchward-Venne TA, Breen L, Di Donato DM, Hector AJ, Mitchell CJ, Moore DR, Stellingwerff T, Breuille D, Offord EA, Baker SK, Phillips SM: **Leucine supplementation of a low-protein mixed macronutrient beverage enhances myofibrillar protein synthesis in young men: a double-blind, randomized trial.** *Am J Clin Nutr* 2014, **99**(2):276–286.
9. Norton LE, Layman DK: **Leucine regulates translation initiation of protein synthesis in skeletal muscle after exercise.** *J Nutr* 2006, **136**(2):533S–537S.
10. Katsanos CS, Kobayashi H, Sheffield-Moore M, Aarsland A, Wolfe RR: **A high proportion of leucine is required for optimal stimulation of the rate of muscle protein synthesis by essential amino acids in the elderly.** *Am J Physiol Endocrinol Metab* 2006, **291**(2):E381–E387.

11. Carbone JW, McClung JP, Pasiakos SM: **Skeletal muscle responses to negative energy balance: effects of dietary protein.** *Adv Nutr* 2012, **3**(2):119–126.
12. Wilkinson DJ, Hossain T, Hill DS, Phillips BE, Crossland H, Williams J, Loughna P, Churchward-Venne TA, Breen L, Phillips SM: **Effects of leucine and its metabolite β-hydroxy-β-methylbutyrate on human skeletal muscle protein metabolism.** *J Physiol Lond* 2013, **591**(11):2911–2923.
13. Wilson GJ, Wilson JM, Manninen AH: **Effects of beta-hydroxy-beta-methylbutyrate (HMB) on exercise performance and body composition across varying levels of age, sex, and training experience: a review.** *Nutr Metab (Lond)* 2008, **5**:1.
14. Stout JR, Smith-Ryan AE, Fukuda DH, Kendall KL, Moon JR, Hoffman JR, Wilson JM, Oliver JS, Mustad VA: **Effect of calcium β-hydroxy-β-methylbutyrate (CaHMB) with and without resistance training in men and women 65 yrs: A randomized, double-blind pilot trial.** *Exp Gerontol* 2013, **48**(11):1303–1310.
15. Nissen S, Sharp R, Ray M, Rathmacher JA, Rice D, Fuller JC Jr, Connelly AS, Abumrad N: **Effect of leucine metabolite β-hydroxy-β-methylbutyrate on muscle metabolism during resistance-exercise training.** *J Appl Physiol (1985)* 1996, **81**(5):2095–2104.
16. Flakoll P, Sharp R, Baier S, Levenhagen D, Carr C, Nissen S: **Effect of β-hydroxy-β-methylbutyrate, arginine, and lysine supplementation on strength, functionality, body composition, and protein metabolism in elderly women.** *Nutrition* 2004, **20**(5):445.
17. Knitter A, Panton L, Rathmacher J, Petersen A, Sharp R: **Effects of β-hydroxy-β-methylbutyrate on muscle damage after a prolonged run.** *J Appl Physiol* 2000, **89**(4):1340–1344.
18. Vukovich MD, Dreifort GD: **Effect of [beta]-Hydroxy-[beta]-Methylbutyrate on the Onset of Blood Lactate Accumulation and VO2peak in Endurance-Trained Cyclists.** *J Strength Cond Res* 2001, **15**(4):491–497.
19. Lamboley CR, Royer D, Dionne IJ: **Effects of beta-hydroxy-beta-methylbutyrate on aerobic-performance components and body composition in college students.** *Int J Sport Nutr Exerc Metab* 2007, **17**(1):56–69.
20. Wilson JM, Lowery RP, Joy JM, Walters JA, Baier SM, Fuller JC, Stout JR, Norton LE, Sikorski EM, Wilson S: **β-Hydroxy-β-methylbutyrate free acid reduces markers of exercise-induced muscle damage and improves recovery in resistance-trained men.** *Br J Nutr* 2013, **1**(1):1–7.
21. Koller A, Mair J, Schobersberger W, Wohlfarter T, Haid C, Mayr M, Villiger B, Frey W, Puschendorf B: **Effects of prolonged strenuous endurance exercise on plasma myosin heavy chain fragments and other muscular proteins. Cycling vs running.** *J Sports Med Phys Fitness* 1998, **38**(1):10–17.
22. Gravettier FJ, Wallnau LB: *Statistics for the Behavioral Sciences.* St. Paul, MN: West Publishing Co.; 1996.
23. Nissen S, Van Koevering M, Webb D: **Analysis of β-hydroxy-β-methylbutyrate in plasma by gas chromatography and mass spectrometry.** *Anal Biochem* 1990, **188**(1):17–19.
24. Bergstrom HC, Housh TJ, Zuniga JM, Traylor DA, Camic CL, Lewis RW Jr, Schmidt RJ, Johnson GO: **The Relationships Among Critical Power Determined From a 3-Min All-Out Test, Respiratory Compensation Point, Gas Exchange Threshold, and Ventilatory Threshold.** *Res Q Exerc Sport* 2013, **84**(2):232–238.
25. Day JR, Rossiter HB, Coats EM, Skasick A, Whipp BJ: **The maximally attainable VO2 during exercise in humans: the peak vs. maximum issue.** *J Appl Physiol (1985)* 2003, **95**(5):1901–1907.
26. Beaver WL, Wasserman K, Whipp BJ: **A new method for detecting anaerobic threshold by gas exchange.** *J Appl Physiol (1985)* 1986, **60**(6):2020–2027.
27. Gaskill SE, Ruby BC, Walker AJ, Sanchez OA, Serfass RC, Leon AS: **Validity and reliability of combining three methods to determine ventilatory threshold.** *Med Sci Sports Exerc* 2001, **33**(11):1841–1848.
28. Wasserman K, Whipp B, Koyal S, Beaver W: **Anaerobic threshold and respiratory gas exchange during exercise.** *J Appl Physiol* 1973, **35**(2):236–243.
29. Caiozzo VJ, Davis JA, Ellis JF, Azus JL, Vandagriff R, Prietto C, McMaster W: **A comparison of gas exchange indices used to detect the anaerobic threshold.** *J Appl Physiol* 1982, **53**(5):1184–1189.
30. Huck SW, McLean RA: **Using a repeated measures ANOVA to analyze the data from a pretest-posttest design: A potentially confusing task.** *Psychol Bull* 1975, **82**(4):511.
31. Green S, Salkind N, Akey T: **Methods for controlling type I error across multiple hypothesis tests.** In *Using SPSS for Windows: Analysing and Understanding Data.* 2nd edition. New Jersey: Prentice-Hall; 2000:395–396.
32. Duffield R, Edge J, Bishop D: **Effects of high-intensity interval training on the response during severe exercise.** *J Sci Med Sport* 2006, **9**(3):249–255.
33. Talanian JL, Galloway SD, Heigenhauser GJ, Bonen A, Spriet LL: **Two weeks of high-intensity aerobic interval training increases the capacity for fat oxidation during exercise in women.** *J Appl Physiol* 2007, **102**(4):1439–1447.
34. Jourkesh M, Ahmaidi S, Keikha B, Sadri I, Ojagi A: **Effects of six weeks sodium bicarbonate supplementation and high-intensity interval training on endurance performance and body composition.** *Ann Biol Res* 2011, **2**(2):403–404. 413.
35. Zanchi N, Gerlinger-Romero F, Guimarães-Ferreira L, de Siqueira Filho M, Felitti V, Lira F, Seelaender M, Lancha A: **HMB supplementation: clinical and athletic performance-related effects and mechanisms of action.** *Amino Acids* 2011, **40**(4):1015–1025.
36. Stout J, Cramer J, Zoeller R, Torok D, Costa P, Hoffman J, Harris R, O'kroy J: **Effects of β-alanine supplementation on the onset of neuromuscular fatigue and ventilatory threshold in women.** *Amino Acids* 2007, **32**(3):381–386.
37. Zoeller R, Stout J, O'kroy J, Torok D, Mielke M: **Effects of 28 days of beta-alanine and creatine monohydrate supplementation on aerobic power, ventilatory and lactate thresholds, and time to exhaustion.** *Amino Acids* 2007, **33**(3):505–510.
38. Gaesser GA, Poole DC: **The slow component of oxygen uptake kinetics in humans.** *Exerc Sport Sci Rev* 1996, **24**(1):35–70.
39. Wasserman K, Beaver WL, Whipp BJ: **Gas exchange theory and the lactic acidosis (anaerobic) threshold.** *Circulation* 1990, **81**(1 Suppl):II14–II30.
40. Paterson DJ, Friedland JS, Bascom DA, Clement ID, Cunningham DA, Painter R, Robbins PA: **Changes in arterial K + and ventilation during exercise in normal subjects and subjects with McArdle's syndrome.** *J Physiol* 1990, **429**:339–348.
41. Berger NJ, Campbell IT, Wilkerson DP, Jones AM: **Influence of acute plasma volume expansion on VO2 kinetics, VO2 peak, and performance during high-intensity cycle exercise.** *J Appl Physiol (1985)* 2006, **101**(3):707–714.
42. Eddy DO, Sparks KL, Adelizi DA: **The effects of continuous and interval training in women and men.** *Eur J Appl Physiol Occup Physiol* 1977, **37**(2):83–92.
43. Heck H, Mader A, Hess G, Mucke S, Muller R, Hollmann W: **Justification of the 4-mmol/l lactate threshold.** *Int J Sports Med* 1985, **6**(3):117–130.
44. Edge J, Bishop D, Goodman C: **The effects of training intensity on muscle buffer capacity in females.** *Eur J Appl Physiol* 2006, **96**(1):97–105.
45. Weston SB, Zhou S, Weatherby RP, Robertson SJ: **Does exogenous coenzyme Q10 affect aerobic capacity in endurance athletes?** *Int J Sport Nutr* 1997, **7**(3):197.
46. Henriksson J: **Effects of physical training on the metabolism of skeletal muscle.** *Diabetes Care* 1992, **15**(11):1701–1711.
47. Krustrup P, Söderlund K, Mohr M, Bangsbo J: **The slow component of oxygen uptake during intense, sub-maximal exercise in man is associated with additional fibre recruitment.** *Pflugers Arch* 2004, **447**(6):855–866.
48. Bruckbauer A, Zemel MB, Thorpe T, Akula MR, Stuckey AC, Osborne D, Martin EB, Kennel S, Wall JS: **Synergistic effects of leucine and resveratrol on insulin sensitivity and fat metabolism in adipocytes and mice.** *Nutr Metab (Lond)* 2012, **9**(1):77.
49. Pinheiro C, Gerlinger-Romero F, Guimarães-Ferreira L, Souza-Jr A, Vitzel K, Nachbar R, Nunes M, Curi R: **Metabolic and functional effects of beta-hydroxy-beta-methylbutyrate (HMB) supplementation in skeletal muscle.** *Eur J Appl Physiol* 2012, **112**(7):2531–2537.
50. Verdin E, Hirschey MD, Finley LW, Haigis MC: **Sirtuin regulation of mitochondria: energy production, apoptosis, and signaling.** *Trends Biochem Sci* 2010, **35**(12):669–675.
51. Hardie DG, Sakamoto K: **AMPK: a key sensor of fuel and energy status in skeletal muscle.** *Physiology (Bethesda)* 2006, **21**(1):48–60.

15

Do glucose containing beverages play a role in thermoregulation, thermal sensation, and mood state?

Yongsuk Seo[1*], Corey A Peacock[2], John Gunstad[3], Keith J Burns[1], Brandon S Pollock[1] and Ellen L Glickman[1]

Abstract

Introduction: Dehydration limits the appropriate delivery of oxygen and substrates to the working muscle. Further, the brain's ability to function may also be compromised whereby thermal sensation and mood state may be altered.

Purpose: The purpose of the present investigation was to compare the thermoregulatory, perceptual, and negative mood state profile in glucose (GLU) vs. non-glucose beverage (NON-GLU) condition.

Methods: Ten healthy men volunteered and were counterbalanced either a GLU or NON-GLU containing beverage on separate mornings. In each condition, they were exposed to 37°C, 50% relative humidity (RH) for baseline, exercise, rehydration, and recovery periods. The exercise period elicited the desired level of dehydration (mean of 2.6 ± 0.3% body weight losses). Upon completion of the protracted exercise, participants were administered either a GLU or NON-GLU containing electrolyte based sports drink ad libitum for 30 min, followed by a recovery period of 15 min in 37°C, 50% RH. Rectal (Tre) and mean skin temperatures (Tsk) were continuously monitored. Gagge (TS) and heated thermal sensation (HTS), profile of mood state (POMS) were measure at the end of each period.

Results: During recovery after rehydration, Tre was not significantly different between conditions (GLU vs. NON-GLU) (37.4 ± 0.8 vs. 37.0 ± 1.2°C); Tsk was also not affected by rehydration in both conditions (36.0 ± 0.5 vs. 36.0 ± 0.6°C) and, TS and HTS did not differ between conditions (0.9 ± 1.3 vs.1.3 ± 0.7) and (1.0 ± 0.8 vs.0.8 ± 0.3). Total mood disturbance (TMD) score for the POMS was utilized for overall negative mood state and demonstrated a main effect for time ($p < 0.05$). TMD during recovery was decreased compared to before hydration in both conditions.

Conclusion: The non-glucose containing beverage maintained plasma volume and was effective at maintaining body temperature homeostasis in a similar fashion compared to the glucose containing beverage. Furthermore, negative mood state was not different between the two conditions. The non-glucose beverages can serve a valuable role in the exercise environment depending upon the sport, the ambient temperature, the individual, duration of the exercise, the age and training states of the individual.

Introduction

Exercise in hot environments can cause a reduction in plasma volume due in part to the thermoregulation via sweating, which can decrease the blood supply to the muscle tissue. If fluid loss continues and is not replaced with water and electrolytes, body fluid distribution will then limit the appropriate delivery of oxygen and substrate to the working muscle [1]. Furthermore, heat exposure, hyperthermia, and dehydration affect the brain's ability to function normally and can adversely impact cognitive performance whereby thermal sensation and mood state may be altered.

While much is known regarding the physiology of dehydration, the psychological effects are less clear due in part to inconsistent data in the experimental literature. Dehydration and other adverse physiological stressors have been shown to have a negative impact on mood state [2,3]. Such mood changes can then impact cognitive function [4,5].

Exercise can also impact blood glucose levels, as the body requires the use of glucose to fuel physical activity [6].

* Correspondence: yseo@kent.edu
[1]Exercise and Environmental Physiology Laboratory, Kent State University, Kent, OH, USA
Full list of author information is available at the end of the article

Strenuous, prolonged exercise can result in hypoglycemia, as the blood's level of glucose may become lower because it is utilized to allow for continued physical activity. Reduced levels of glucose may exhibit as physical symptoms including shakiness, hunger, nervousness, sweating, dizziness, confusion, visual disturbance, and weakness [7]. Reduced blood sugar and the subsequent symptoms have been observed across a variety of populations following strenuous exercise, including both professional and amateur athletes [8-10]. Existing literature also indicates glucose does not directly affect hydration status. A study by Hargreaves and colleagues reported that after 40 minutes of exercise in the heat, continuous administration of glucose did not alter plasma volume or hydration status [11]. These results may be attributes to experimental methodologies, such as timing of fluid replacement and environmental conditions (i.e., temperature and exercise duration), both of which can impact fluid homeostasis.

Additionally, it has been accepted by the American College of Sports Medicine that it is appropriate to consume a drink that is comprised of glucose and electrolytes to combat the loss of these ingredients during exercise and the stressor of heat [12]. Many sport beverages contain glucose and additional nutritional components, specifically electrolytes (i.e., sodium, potassium, vitamin B12, etc.) which element(s) benefitted cognitive function relative to water. Therefore, rehydration with comparable beverages, with the exception of carbohydrate content, would allow for more accurate examination of between-condition differences.

The purpose of the current investigation is to examine the effects of a fluid replacement drink that contains electrolytes, glucose and calories versus a fluid replacement drink containing solely electrolytes (GLU), non-digestible artificial sweeteners, and zero calories (NON-GLU) on rectal temperature, skin temperature, and mood state after protracted exercise in 37°C for 90 minutes. It was hypothesized that a GLU containing drink will elicit improved mood state during recovery after prolonged exercise in the heat compared to a NON-GLU beverage. The findings increase our knowledge and safety for exercise in the heat and the role of glucose on mental and physiological processes during rehydration.

Methods

Subjects

Ten males (22 ± 2 yrs, 181.4 ± 6.6 cm, 88.4 ± 10.4 kg) volunteered to take part in the current investigation and reported to the laboratory on three occasions (preliminary, GLU, NON-GLU). Through completion of a medical history screening, subjects were excluded with the presence or history of medical, neurological, developmental, or psychiatric disorders or a history of heat illness. The sample consisted of males, as exercise intensity and duration could be confounded with a co-ed sample (i.e., males vs. females may require a different level of exercise to produce the level of dehydration desired) [13-15]. Further, only Caucasian males were utilized, as non-whites and female have demonstrated differences in thermoregulation [16,17]. The study protocol was approved by the Institutional Review Board at Kent State University. All subjects provided written informed consent before participating.

Measurements

Rectal temperature (Tre) was measured by a thermistor inserted 13 cm into the rectum (ER400-12, Respiratory Diagnostic Products, Irvine, CA). Skin thermistors (Model 409B, Yellow Springs, OH) were used to measure skin temperature at the following sites: chest, triceps, forearm, thigh, and calf [18]. Rectal, skin and air temperatures were collected by an interface (iNet-100HC, Omega Engineering, Stamford, CT). Mean skin temperature (Tsk) was calculated using the formula supported in the current literature [18]: Tsk = (0.22 × calf temperature) + (0.28 × thigh temperature) + (0.28 × chest temperature) + (0.14 × forearm temperature) + (0.08 × triceps temperature).

Participants' metabolic rate (VO_2) was assessed via Parvo metabolic measurement system (Parvo Metabolic Cart, Sandy, Utah), which analyzed expired air samples via an indirect automated open circuit system to determine oxygen consumption.

The Profile of Mood State-Short Form (POMS-SF) is a 37 item, condensed version of the original Profile of Mood State questionnaire which preserves the six measures of mood disturbance. The questionnaire consists of a five-point Likert scale, with mood-related items that provide answers ranging from 0 (not at all) to 4 (extremely) to answer the question, "how are you feeling right now?". The POMS-SF yields six subscales including fatigue-inertia, vigor-activity, tension-anxiety, depression-dejection, anger-hostility, and confusion-bewilderment.

The thermal sensation was measured using the Gagge thermal sensation scale (TS) [19] and heated thermal sensation (HTS) [20], both of which are valid and reliable measures of subjective whole body thermal sensation. Participants were asked to quantify their thermal sensation utilizing these scales.

Procedures

During the initial visit, in order to determine cardiovascular fitness and capacity, resting and peak blood pressure, resting and peak heart rate (HR), and peak oxygen uptake (VO_2max) data were collected. The graded exercise test (GXT) was conducted on an electronically braked cycle ergometer (Lode, Quinton Excalibur, Netherlands). The expired air was analyzed for oxygen and carbon dioxide concentration using an automated open circuit system to determine maximal oxygen consumption (VO_2max). Following completion of the VO_2max test and health history questionnaire, those participants deemed eligible for participation were then scheduled for two additional counterbalanced (GLU and NON-GLU) testing sessions. All experiments were conducted in the morning hours following an overnight fast. Each counterbalanced experimental trial (GLU vs. NON-GLU), lasted approximately 180 minutes (Figure 1). Prior to the experimental trials, participants were provided a standardized breakfast (a bagel and a banana) and water (500 ml) intake to minimize possible confounds. During each experimental trial (GLU vs. NON-GLU), a baseline measure of Tre, Tsk, VO_2, profile of mood state, thermal sensation [19] and Heated thermal sensation [20] were collected in an environmentally-controlled room set at 37°C and 50% RH. Participants were then asked to exercise on a cycle ergometer in the climatically controlled chamber, inducing an average dehydration of 2.6 ± 0.3% of their initial body weight. In order to assess the individuals percentage of body weight lost, they were asked during this period to exercise for 25-minute intervals, with interspersed 5 minutes rest periods to measure weight loss. Cycling intensity was set to 50% of the participants VO_2max. Prior to the completion of every exercise bout, during minutes 22–25, data was collected for thermal sensation, metabolic rate, Tre, and Tsk. The individuals were then weighed during the 5 minute rest period.

These 25-minute exercise blocks and 5-minute assessment blocks were continued until desired level of dehydration of loss of 2.6% of body weight or a maximum of 4 exercise bouts (total of 100 minutes of exercise) were achieved.

Immediately following the last exercise protocol, and still in the 37°C chamber, participants were assessed for TS, VO_2, Tsk, POMS and Tre. Following these assessments, participants received a fluid replacement drink consisting of GLU or NON-GLU. They were permitted to drink ad-libitum for 30-minutes to allow for adequate re-hydration. The quantity consumed by each participant was recorded.

Tre, Tsk, VO_2, POMS, and thermal sensation data were recorded for 30 minutes after the rehydration period.

Statistical analyses

Using SPSS 17.0, two-way repeated measures analyses of variance (condition and time) were performed for Tre, Tsk, VO_2, POMS, TS, and HTS. The level of significance was set a priori at $p \leq 0.05$ and to examine the main effects of time; the dehydrated state (immediately post last exercise bout) and most rehydrated (immediately post rehydration bout) and condition (GLU vs. NON-GLU). If a significant interaction was found, post-hoc paired sample t-tests were utilized. The POMS was administrated four total times per trial. However, the main goal of this study was on the post-rehydration recovery mood state.

Results

The amount of fluid consumed during the rehydration periods was not statistically different from one another (*p = 0.997*) with an average of 987.5 ± 197.3 ml consumed via the GLU replacement drink and 990.0 ± 224.1 ml consumed via the NON-GLU replacement drink. Therefore, any difference in physiological measures detected between conditions is not a result of differing amounts of re-hydration drinks consumed.

Baseline measures of the Baseline measures of Tre, Tsk, VO_2, POMS, TS, and HTS and were assessed within 10 minutes upon entering an environmentally controlled chamber set 37°C. Baseline physiological measurements were similar between conditions. In particular, Tre (37.3 ± 0.3 vs. 37.0 ± 0.5°C) and Tsk (34.7 ± 1.4 vs. 35.1 ± 0.5°C), Glucose level (115.3 ± 19.6 vs. 127.1 ± 23.1 ml/dl), and VO_2 (4.9 ± 1.3 vs. 5.5 ± 2.7 ml/kg/min) were not different

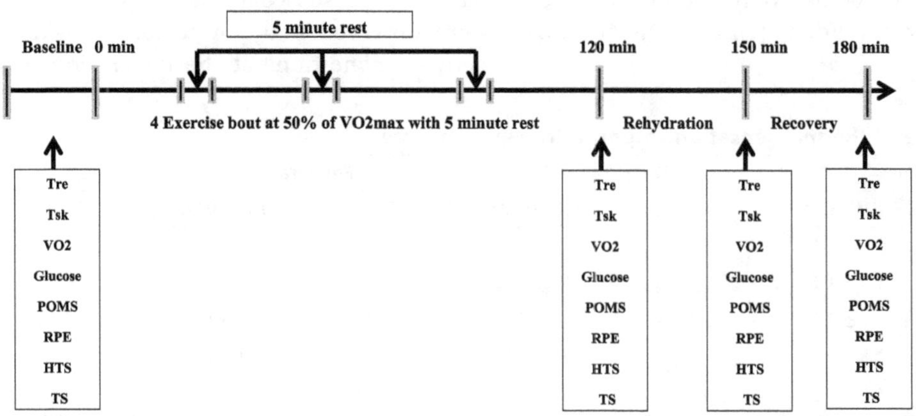

Figure 1 The experimental procedure and time line.

between GLU and NON-GLU, respectively. In addition, baseline POMS TMD (−2.8 ± 11.1 vs. -4.3 ± 8.5), TS (1.5 ± 0.7 vs. 1.5 ± 0.7), and HTS (1.4 ± 1.4 vs. 0.9 ± 0.5) were not different between two conditions, respectively. After dehydration (2.6% of body weight loss) Tre and Tsk were elevated in both conditions (Table 1). However, there were no significant differences in Tre and Tsk between conditions. Despite the elevated body temperature, metabolic rate did not increase compared to baseline and no difference was found between two conditions. The blood glucose was decreased compared to baseline but there was no significant difference observed between groups. These data showed that upon completion of the exercise bout both conditions were equally dehydrated and in similar physiologic states. POMS TMD at dehydration increased compared to baseline values, but no difference was exhibited between conditions.

Upon completion of the rehydration period, there was no significant difference between conditions for Tre and Tsk. Expectedly, metabolic rate was different between conditions after rehydration. An average the VO_2 of 4.9 ± 1.1 ml/kg/min observed in the glucose electrolyte containing beverage and the average VO_2 4.3 ± 1.2 ml/kg/min observed in the non-glucose electrolyte containing beverage ($p = 0.007$). In addition, blood glucose levels in GLU condition statistically greater compared to NON-GLU fluid replacement drink were ($p = 0.000$). However, in both thermal scales, there is no significantly different between two conditions.

Following the recovery period, there was no significant difference between the two conditions on Tre, Tsk, and both thermal scale. However, oxygen consumption was significantly higher in GLU condition compared to NON-GLU condition. Furthermore, blood glucose level remained higher in GLU condition compare to NON-GLU condition ($p = 0.009$). The change in POMS TMD demonstrated no main effect for condition ($p = 0.554$), time ($p = 0.273$), and time by condition interaction ($p = 0.053$). Analyses of paired sample t-test showed that POMS TMD was decreased compared to before rehydration. However, did not differ between conditions (GLU vs. NON-GLU) (Figure 2).

Discussion

The purpose of this study was to quantify changes in mood state during and following intake of fluid in hot ambient condition. The results of this study elucidate the need for fluid during exercise in the heat; however, the fluid does not need to contain high glucose or calories to maintain homeostasis.

With the amount of calories that individuals consumes daily, and the amount of ergogenic aids marketed for post-exercise rehydration the data presented is noteworthy. For the most part, investigators believe a high caloric type of beverage is the optimal hydration beverage during prolonged exercise in the heat and the subsequent recovery process. Results from the current study contradict this theory. Although, glucose is utilized during strenuous exercise, it is the loss of electrolytes via sweat that contributes mostly to the hypohydration of athletes [21]. As indicated by the statistical analyses provided, there were no differences in amount of liquid consumed after the strenuous exercise bout in the heat between the GLU and NON-GLU conditions. Additionally, rectal and skin temperature also demonstrated that there are no significant differences between conditions. This provides support that the main mechanism of controlling body temperature is not mediated by glucose, simply due to the consumption of liquid and electrolytes. However, significant differences were indicated between the conditions in subsequently metabolic rate. The VO_2 is directly associated with the full-calorie drink (i.e., ≈ 220 calories/ 960 ml). VO_2 is significantly higher due to the thermic effect of feeding, whereas the higher blood glucose is attributed to the sugar (56 g of sugar/960 ml) in the full-calorie drink, or, ≈ 220 calories. These two variables being significantly higher will to lead to an inhibition of fat metabolism. Inhibiting fat metabolism is detrimental reducing body fat and consequently is one of the many factors that contribute to obesity [22].

Additionally, the increased metabolic rate observed in the full-caloric condition could have an impact on exercise recovery and subsequent exercise bouts. No differences were observed between rectal and skin temperature between conditions at the conclusion of the post re-

Table 1 Physiological and thermal sensation response to heat exposure

	Baseline		Dehydration		Rehydration		Recovery	
	GLU	NON-GLU	GLU	NON-GLU	GLU	NON-GLU	GLU	NON-GLU
Tre	37.3 ± 0.3	37.0 ± 0.5	37.8 ± 1.2	37.9 ± 0.5	37.7 ± 0.8	37.7 ± 0.5	37.4 ± 0.8	37.0 ± 1.2
Tsk	35.2 ± 0.5	37.0 ± 0.5	36.5 ± 0.5	36.0 ± 1.2	35.0 ± 0.6	36.5 ± 0.6	36.0 ± 0.5	36.0 ± 0.6
VO_2	4.9 ± 1.3	5.5 ± 2.7	4.9 ± 1.5	4.4 ± 0.8	4.9 ± 1.1*	4.2 ± 0.7	5.5 ± 1.0*	4.3 ± 1.2
TS	1.5 ± 0.7	1.5 ± 0.7	2 ± 1.0	1.8 ± 0.9	1.3 ± 0.8	0.9 ± 0.6	0.9 ± 1.3	1.3 ± 0.7
HTS	1.4 ± 1.4	0.9 ± 0.5	2.9 ± 2.5	1.7 ± 1.4	1.4 ± 1.2	0.9 ± 1.2	1.0 ± 0.8	0.8 ± 0.3

Data are Mean ±SD. *denotes significant difference from NON-GLU condition at same time ($p < 0.05$).
Rectal temperature (Tre), mean skin temperature (Tsk), metabolic rate (VO_2), Gagge (TS) and heated thermal sensation (HTS).

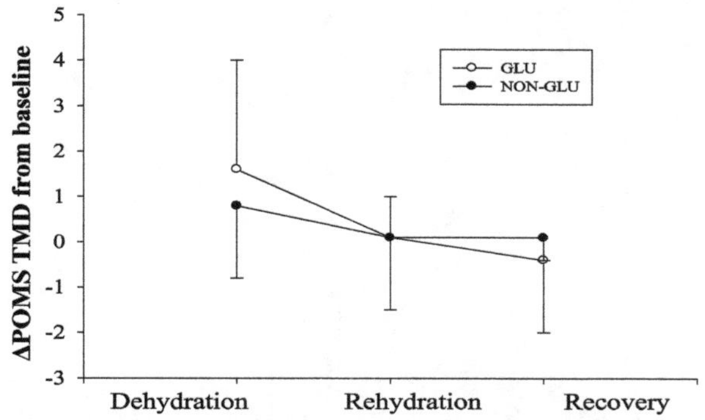

Figure 2 Delta POMS-SF total score with higher scores indicative of greater mood-related symptoms and thus poorer mood.

hydration period indicating a similar level of recovery and thermal homeostasis were achieved between the differing fluid replacement drinks. However, due to the thermic effect of food and the energy needed for the active process of carbohydrate absorption and subsequent breakdown and utilization the increased metabolic rate observed in the full-calorie condition may have an impact on long term exercise recovery [22]. Instead of the recovery and rebuilding of muscle damaged during the exercise bouts, the body is using additional energy and physiologic processes to aid in the digestion of the glucose absorbed. Further investigation is needed to determine the long term recovery and exercise performance between a full calorie and eucaloric fluid replacement drink.

The eucaloric drink was equally effective in maintaining temperature homeostasis, thus rejecting the hypothesis of the researchers. Although no significant differences were detected between the volume of fluid replacement drink consumed, subjects did drink slightly more of the eucaloric beverage. This small increased consumption of the eucaloric beverage in the 30-min period post exercise may support evidence that the high glucose containing beverages are less palatable than non-glucose containing beverages. Davis and colleagues reported that subjects after exercise in heat drank less of a high glucose drink due to the onset of nausea [23]. More research is needed in this area to provide further evidence of the palatability of glucose containing beverages. Furthermore, since the sodium is present in the NON-GLU drink it was equally effective in maintaining plasma volume more so than a water alone beverage [21].

Some limitations could be identified in the present study. Dehydration state was confirmed by weight loss and change of Tre (0.7°C). However, it would be beneficial to include other assessments of hydration status such as urine specific gravity or plasma osmolality. Although urine specific gravity or plasma osmolality are widely used to determine dehydration status in research and clinical setting [24], these techniques were not used during this study. Thus, we were not able to directly determine the effect of dehydration state on mood state. Other limitations include studying only the physically active young population and testing a single aspect of mood state. Hence, a wide range of subjects (e.g., women and older population) and additional measurements of mood state will be needed for future experiments.

Conclusion

The non-glucose containing beverage maintained plasma volume and was effective at maintaining body temperature homeostasis in a similar fashion compared to the glucose containing beverage. Furthermore, negative mood state was not different between the two conditions. The non-glucose beverages can serve a valuable role in the exercise environment depending upon the sport, the ambient temperature, the individual, duration of the exercise, the age and training states of the individual.

Competing interests

The authors declare that they have no competing interests.

Authors' contributions

All authors contributed equally to this manuscript. All authors have read and approved the final manuscript.

Author details

[1]Exercise and Environmental Physiology Laboratory, Kent State University, Kent, OH, USA. [2]Nova Southeastern University, Fort Lauderdale, FL, USA. [3]Departments of Psychology, Kent State University, Kent, OH, USA.

References

1. Sawka MN, Montain SJ: **Fluid and electrolyte supplementation for exercise heat stress.** *Am J Clin Nutr* 2000, **72:**564S–572S.
2. D'Anci KE, Vibhakar A, Kanter JH, Mahoney CR, Taylor HA: **Voluntary dehydration and cognitive performance in trained college athletes.** *Percept Mot Skills* 2009, **109**(1):251–269.
3. Choma CW, Sforzo GA, Keller BA: **Impact of rapid weight loss on cognitive function in collegiate wrestlers.** *Med Sci Sports Eexerc* 1998, **30**(5):746–749.
4. Herrmann LL, Le Masurier M, Ebmeier KP: **White matter hyperintensities in late life depression: a systematic review.** *J Neurol Neurosurg Psychiatry* 2008, **79**(6):619–624.
5. Nebes RD, Pollock BG, Houck PR, Butters MA, Mulsant BH, Zmuda MD, Reynolds CF 3rd: **Persistence of cognitive impairment in geriatric patients following antidepressant treatment: a randomized, double-blind clinical trial with nortriptyline and paroxetine.** *J Psychiatr Res* 2003, **37**(2):99–108.
6. McMahon SK, Ferreira LD, Ratnam N, Davey RJ, Youngs LM, Davis EA, Fournier PA, Jones TW: **Glucose requirements to maintain euglycemia after moderate-intensity afternoon exercise in adolescents with type 1 diabetes are increased in a biphasic manner.** *J Clin Endocrinol Metab* 2007, **92**(3):963–968.
7. Cryer PE: **Symptoms of hypoglycemia, thresholds for their occurrence, and hypoglycemia unawareness.** *Endocrinol Metab Clin North Am* 1999, **29**(3):495–500. v-vi.
8. Billat VL, Demarle A, Slawinski J, Paiva M, Koralsztein JP: **Physical and training characteristics of top-class marathon runners.** *Med Sci Sports Exerc* 2001, **33**(12):2089–2097.
9. di Prampero PE, Atchou G, Bruckner JC, Moia C: **The energetics of endurance running.** *Eur J Appl Physiol Occup Physiol* 1986, **55**(3):259–266.
10. Rapoport BI: **Metabolic factors limiting performance in marathon runners.** *PLoS Comput Biol* 2010, **6**(10):1–13.

11. Hargreaves M, Angus D, Howlett K, Conus NM, Febbraio M: **Effect of heat stress on glucose kinetics during exercise.** *J Appl Physiol* 1996, **81**(4):1594–1597.
12. American College of Sports M, Sawka MN, Burke LM, Eichner ER, Maughan RJ, Montain SJ, Stachenfeld NS: **American College of Sports Medicine position stand. Exercise and fluid replacement.** *Med Sci Sports Exerc* 2007, **39**(2):377–390.
13. Bar-Or O: **Effects of age and gender on sweating pattern during exercise.** *Int J Sports Med* 1998, **19**(Suppl 2):S106–S107.
14. Kelley GA, Lowing L, Kelley K: **Gender differences in the aerobic fitness levels of young African-American adults.** *J Natl Med Assoc* 1999, **91**(7):384–388.
15. Mehnert P, Brode P, Griefahn B: **Gender-related difference in sweat loss and its impact on exposure limits to heat stress.** *Int J Ind Ergonom* 2002, **29**(6):343–351.
16. Kaciuba-Uscilko H, Grucza R: **Gender differences in thermoregulation.** *Curr Opin Clin Nutr Metab Care* 2001, **4**(6):533–536.
17. Hessemer V, Bruck K: **Influence of menstrual-cycle on shivering, skin blood-flow, and sweating responses measured at night.** *J Appl Physiol* 1985, **59**(6):1902–1910.
18. Toner MM, Sawka MN, Foley ME, Pandolf KB: **Effects of body mass and morphology on thermal responses in water.** *J Appl Physiol* 1986, **60**(2):521–525.
19. Gagge AP, Stolwijk JAJ, Hardy JD: **Comfort and thermal sensations and associated physiological responses at various ambient temperatures.** *Environ Res* 1967, **1**(1):1–20.
20. Glickman EL, Peacock C, Gunstad J, Kakos L, Burns KJ, Pollock B, Feeback M, Seo Y: **A thermal perception scale for use during rest and exercise in 37°C ambient air [abstract].** *Med Sci Sports Exerc* 2013, **45**(5):S70.
21. Armstrong LE: *Exertional Heat Illnesses.* Champaign, IL: Human Kinetics; 2003.
22. Brooks GA, Fahey TD, Baldwin KM: *Exercise Physiology: Human Bioenergetics and Its Applications with PowerWeb Bind-in Card.* New York, NY: McGraw-Hill Higher Education; 2004.
23. Davis JM, Burgess WA, Slentz CA, Bartoli WP, Pate RR: **Effects of ingesting 6% and 12% glucose/electrolyte beverages during prolonged intermittent cycling in the heat.** *Eur J Appl Physiol Occup Physiol* 1988, **57**(5):563–569.
24. Armstrong LE: **Assessing hydration status: the elusive gold standard.** *J Am Coll Nutr* 2007, **26**(Suppl 5):575S–584S.

16

Effect of carbohydrate mouth rinsing on multiple sprint performance

James L Dorling and Conrad P Earnest*

Abstract

Background: Research suggests that carbohydrate mouth rinsing (CMR) improves endurance performance; yet, little is known regarding the effect of CMR on multiple sprint efforts. As many sports involve multiple sprinting efforts, followed by periods of recovery, the aim of our current study was to investigate the influence of CMR on multiple sprint performance.

Methods: We recruited eight active males (Age; 22 ± 1 y; 75.0 ± 8.8 kg; estimated $VO2_{max}$ 52.0 ± 3.0 ml/kg/min) to participate in a randomly assigned, double-blind, counterbalanced study administering a CMR (6.4% Maltodextrin) or similarly flavoured placebo solution. Primary outcomes for our study included: (a) time for three repeated sprint ability tests (RSA) and (b) the Loughborough Intermittent Shuttle Test (LIST). Time was expressed in seconds (sec). Secondary outcomes included ratings of perceived exertion (RPE) and blood glucose concentration. Tertiary outcomes included two psychological assessments designed to determine perceived activation (i.e., arousal) and pleasure-displeasure after each section of the LIST. We analysed our data using a two-way analysis of variance (ANOVA) for repeated measures, a Bonferroni adjusted *post hoc* t-test to determine significant differences in treatment, and a liberal 90% confidence interval between treatment conditions. Effect sizes were calculated between trials and interpreted as ≤ 0.2 trivial, > 0.2 small, > 0.6 moderate, > 1.2 large, > 2 very large and > 4 extremely large. Data are means ± SD. Overall statistical significance was set as $P < 0.05$; yet, modified accordingly when Bonferroni adjustments were made.

Results: Overall, we observed no significant difference in average (3.46 ± 0.2 vs. 3.44 ± 0.17; P = 0.11) or fastest time (3.38 ± 0.2 vs. 3.37 ± 0.2; P = 0.39) in the RSA test for the placebo vs. CMR conditions, respectively. Similar findings were also noted for the placebo vs. CMR, respectively, during the LIST test (3.52 ± 0.2 vs. 3.54 ± 0.2 sec; P = 0.63). Despite a significantly higher within group RPE during the 3rd and 4th sections of the LIST (< 0.05), no between group differences were otherwise noted. No differences were noted for blood glucose concentrations throughout the testing protocol. Lastly, from a psychological perspective, we observed no differences in pleasure-displeasure or perceived activation.

Conclusions: The results of our current study suggest that CMR does not improve exercise performance, RPE or perceived pleasure-displeasure during high intensity activity requiring repeated, intermittent, sprint efforts.

Background

It is well established that carbohydrate (CHO) ingestion improves prolonged (> 2 hours) steady-state [1] and intermittent endurance performance [2]. The proposed mechanisms for this ergogenic effect include a sparing of endogenous glycogen stores, an enhanced oxidation of exogenous CHO and the maintenance of high CHO oxidation rates during the later stages of exercise [3]. The ingestion of CHO before and during high intensity exercise over shorter durations (~ 1 hour) has also been found to enhance performance [4]. However, under these conditions, CHO ingestion exerts no influence on exogenous glucose uptake and total CHO oxidation [4]. To explain these findings, some authors hypothesize that CHO ingestion facilitates ergogenesis via the central nervous system, mediated by receptors in the oral cavity [5].

To investigate this theory, Carter et al. [5] examined the influence of mouth rinsing a CHO drink solution on time trial performance in nine cyclists. Interestingly, when compared to a placebo solution, mouth rinsing with a CHO solution resulted in a 2.9% improvement in

* Correspondence: cpe22@bath.ac.uk
Department for Health, Sport, Health and Exercise Science, University of Bath, Eastwood 22-23 3.4, Bath BA2 7AY, UK

performance [5]. Subsequent research has further demonstrated that carbohydrate mouth rinsing (CMR) enhances endurance performance during cycling [6] and running [7]. While others have reported contrary findings [8], research examining different exercise modes has indicated that CMR has no influence on maximal 30 sec sprint performance [9] or maximal strength [10].

Although the precise ergogenic mechanisms of CMR are not fully understood, Gant et al. [11] reported that mouth rinsing both sweet and non-sweet CHO enhanced motor evoked potentials to fresh and fatigued muscle by 9 and 30%, respectively. Other studies also suggest that CMR stimulates receptors in the mouth, which activate neural pathways to lower the perceptions of effort and improve subjective experiences during exercise [5]. Chambers et al. [6] provided support for this notion by demonstrating that CMR activates areas of the brain associated with reward and motivation using functional MRI.

Collectively, these findings raise the possibility that CMR may improve performance during multiple sprint exercise. To our knowledge, only one study has examined the influence of CMR on multiple sprint performance on a cycle ergometer [12]. Interestingly, Beaven and colleagues reported that CMR enhanced initial sprint performance, but also resulted in a greater performance decrement over their repeated sprint protocol [12]. Despite these findings, there is no published literature that has examined CMR during running activities which simulates multiple sprint sports. As such, further research would be useful to investigate whether CMR can provide an ergogenic benefit during a field test that replicates field-based team games. Furthermore, as previous research suggests an increased perception of exercise intensity may hinder performance during field-based team games [13], investigation of the influence of CMR on subjective experiences during multiple sprint exercise is required. The primary aim of our current study was to examine the effect of CMR on multiple sprint performance during a field-based exercise protocol. Secondary and tertiary aims included assessments regarding CMR on subjective experiences during multiple sprint exercise.

Methods

Participants

Eight physically active males (Age; 22 ± 1 y; 75.0 ± 8.8 kg; estimated $VO2_{max}$ 52.0 ± 3.0 ml/kg/min) volunteered to take part in the study. Seven of the participants habitually participated in field-based multiple sprint sport such as football (i.e., soccer) and rugby, while the other was a recreationally active runner. After participants were briefed about the nature of the study, they provided written informed consent. The exclusion criteria included usage of creatine supplements in the 12 weeks prior to the study, due to its influence on multiple sprint performance [14]. The ethics committee for the Department of Health at the University of Bath approved, which was according to the Declaration of Helsinki. We have presented a schematic representation of the experimental conditions is presented in Figure 1.

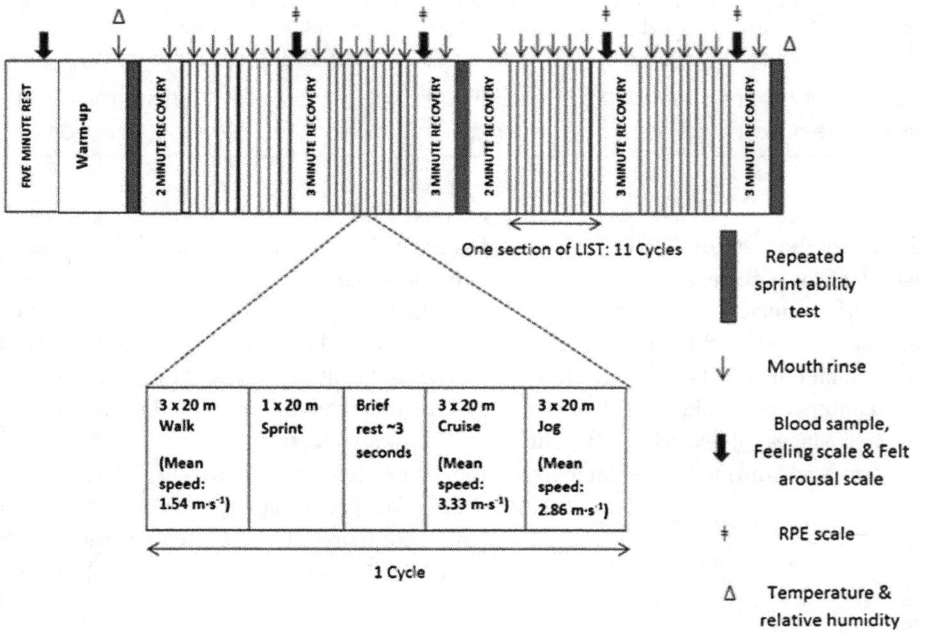

Figure 1 Schematic representation of the time line of study procedures.

Preliminary measures and test familiarization

Five days prior to the first experimental trial, participants reported to an indoor sprints track for preliminary measurements including the participant's height and body mass. During this visit each participant completed a progressive multistage shuttle run test, which estimated maximal oxygen uptake [15]. Following this, each participant completed one 15 min section of the Loughborough Intermittent Shuttle Test (LIST) and one repeated sprint ability (RSA) test in order to familiarize themselves with the experimental tests. At the completion of this visit, participants were familiarized with the psychological scales used in this study.

Experimental trials

During each experimental condition, participants completed two trials consisting of a CMR and placebo (PLA) supplement administered in a randomized, counterbalanced order. To maintain blinding to the investigators and participants, all treatments were pre-labelled and subsequently dispersed by a non-affiliated researcher not participating in this trial. Experimental trials were conducted 7-9 days apart and at the same time of day. In the 24 h preceding the first experimental trial, participants were asked to record their diet and then replicate it before the second trial. Participants were also asked to refrain from strenuous exercise and to abstain from caffeine and alcohol ingestion in the 24 h before each trial. On the day of the experimental trial, participants were asked to ingest 568 ml of water to maintain euhydration, and arrive in a fasted condition.

On the morning of each trial, participants presented at an indoor sprint track to perform a standardized warm up (10-min), which consisted of jogging, cruising, sprinting, dynamic stretching and the RSA protocol. This RSA was used as part of the warm-up and not as a measurement test. Temperature and relative humidity were recorded (Testo, Hampshire, UK) at the start and at the end of each experimental trial to check for changes in environmental conditions. Following the warm-up period, participants initiated the testing phase of the trial by performing the RSA test, followed by a 2-min recovery. Participants then completed the LIST [16].

The LIST was comprised of 15-min sections of intermittent shuttle running over a 20-m distance. Each section of the LIST consisted of 11 cycles of a set running protocol. One cycle was comprised of three 20-m walks (mean speed: 1.54 $m \cdot s^{-1}$), one 20 metre sprint, ~ 3 sec of rest, three 20 metre cruises (mean speed: 3.33 $m \cdot s^{-1}$) and three 20 metre jogs (mean speed: 2.86 $m \cdot s^{-1}$). Following each section, there was a 3-min recovery period. Appropriate speeds for the walk, cruise and jog shuttles of the LIST were dictated by audible signals from a prerecorded disc. On completion of the 3-min recovery of the second and fourth section of the LIST, participants completed the RSA test, followed by 2-min recovery period (Figure 1). Throughout the experimental protocol, every attempt was made to ensure that the participants were not distracted. No interaction or encouragement occurred between the investigator and the participants, except for mouth rinse administration.

Carbohydrate solutions

The CHO solution was a 6.4% maltodextrin solution, containing 64 g of maltodextrin (HighFive, Bardon, England) per 1000 ml of water. Maltodextrin was used because it is a non-sweet and colourless [5]. The PLA solution was water. To make solutions indistinguishable both treatments contained a non-calorific artificial sweetener consisting of sucralose (FlavDrops, MyProtein, Norwich, England). Each rinse solution was provided as a 25-ml bolus in a preweighed plastic cup. Participants were instructed to swirl all of the solution in their mouth for ~ 5 sec, before expectorating the solution back into the cup. Participants rinsed a solution 30 sec prior to each section of the LIST and each RSA test. Participants were also instructed to rinse a solution during the first 20 metre shuttle of the second, fourth, sixth, eighth and tenth cycles of each LIST section. In total, this equated to 27 rinses and 675 ml of solution being rinsed and expectorated during each trial (Figure 1). On completion of the study, participants were asked whether they could distinguish which solution contained CHO.

Repeated sprint ability test and sprint measures

All 20 m sprints from the RSA test and the LIST were recorded using infrared timing gates (Smartspeed, Fusion Sport, Australia) and were commenced from a standing position 0.5 m from the first start gate. Individual sprint times of all 44 sprints of the LIST were recorded and the mean sprint time from each section was calculated.

The RSA test was comprised of four straight-line 20 m sprints, separated by 20 sec of active recovery. During the active recovery, participants were given verbal encouragement to jog back to the start line within ~ 10-12 sec. On return to the start line, participants were instructed to prepare for the next sprint. Following a three second countdown, participants were given the 'go' command, which instructed them to initiate the sprint. A hand-held stopwatch was used to monitor recovery time. From each RSA test, the fastest and mean 20 m sprint times were recorded. During the RSA test of the warm-up, sprint times were recorded and within-subject coefficient of variation was derived from six participants. The coefficient of variation for both the fastest time and mean time was 1.2%.

Blood sampling and analysis

Blood glucose was measured to examine any potential metabolic effects of CMR. A capillary blood sample was taken at baseline and during each 3 min recovery period of the LIST. Blood samples were obtained in EDTA prepared tubes (Microvette 5000, Sarstedt, Leicestershire) and placed in ice. Following completion of the trial, blood samples were analysed in duplicate using an automated analyser (YSI 2300 Stat Plus, YSI, Yellow Springs, Ohio). The coefficient of variation for 10 replicates for blood glucose was 3.2%.

Psychological scales

As a tertiary measure we performed a series of psychological inventory throughout the trial to assess the effects of CMR on the participant's subjective experiences. The perceived activation scale (FAS) was used to assess the participant's perceived arousal [17]. The FAS is a six-point measure ranging from 1 (*low arousal*) to 6 (*high arousal*). Backhouse et al. [18] reported the FAS as a valid measure when examining supplementation interventions. The feeling scale (FS) was used to measure the dimension of pleasure-displeasure [19]. The FS is an 11 point scale which ranges from -5 to +5. Anchors are placed at 0 (*neutral*) and at odd integers, ranging from +5 (*very good*) to -5 (*very bad*) [20]. The FS and FAS were administered at rest and immediately after each section of the LIST (Figure 1). The participant's ratings of perceived exertion (RPE) were obtained using the Ratings of Perceived Exertion Scale [21]. The Ratings of Perceived Exertion Scale was administered immediately following each section of the LIST (Figure 1).

Statistical analysis

Data were analysed using a two-way repeated measures ANOVA. If sphericity was violated, a Greenhouse-Geisser correction was applied for epsilon < 0.75, while the Huynh-Feldt correction was utilised for less severe asphericity (> 0.75). A Bonferroni adjusted *post hoc* test was used to locate variance, where significant statistical effects occurred.

Magnitude-based inferences were calculated for sprint measures to examine whether the differences between the CMR and PLA trials were meaningful [22]. Using a function of the *P*-value, *F*-value and degrees of freedom generated by an ANOVA, the effect of the intervention was expressed as 90% confidence intervals and likelihoods of whether the true effect indicated a positive, negative or trivial change in performance [22]. Cohen's effect size [23] was calculated between trials for the three sprint measures: RSA test mean times, RSA test fastest times and the mean sprint times of the LIST. Effect sizes were interpreted as ≤ 0.2 trivial, > 0.2 small, > 0.6 moderate, > 1.2 large, > 2 very large and > 4 extremely large [24].

An effect was deemed unclear if the confidence intervals spanned both positive and negative thresholds for the smallest worthwhile effect, i.e., the effect could be beneficial or detrimental [22]. The smallest worthwhile change in sprint time was assumed to be 0.8% of the mean time for each sprint measure [25]. All results are means ± standard deviation (SD) or 90% confidence intervals when appropriate. Statistical significance was set as $P < 0.05$.

Results

Repeated sprint ability and Loughborough intermittent shuttle tests

Throughout the testing protocol we observed no between trials for temperature (PLA, 21.9 ± 0.9°C; CHO, 22.0 ± 1.0°C; $P = 0.84$) or relative humidity (PLA, 60 ± 2%; CHO, 59 ± 3%; $P = 0.43$). With regard to the RSA, we observed a modest trend for the fastest sprint time of the RSA to increase throughout the trial as a whole; however, there was no main statistical effect for time ($P = 0.07$), treatment, or the time-by-treatment interaction effect ($P = 0.56$; Figure 2). The fastest sprint times of the RSA test were not significantly between treatment conditions for the CMR (3.37 ± 0.2) and PLA trial (3.38 ± 0.2 sec, $P = 0.39$). There were also no significant main effects of trial (PLA, 3.46 ± 0.19 sec; CHO, 3.44 ± 0.17 sec; $P = 0.49$), time ($P = 0.11$) and no interaction effect ($P = 0.56$) for mean RSA test time (Figure 2B). Although fastest sprint times of the RSA test tended to improve during the second trial ($P = 0.09$), there were no significant order effects for the three sprint measures ($P > 0.05$).

Despite a significant effect of time ($P = 0.001$), showing an increase in sprint time throughout the LIST, there was no main effect of the treatment condition for the mean sprint times of the LIST (PLA, 3.52 ± 0.2 sec; CHO, 3.54 ± 0.2 sec; $P = 0.63$) and no interaction effect ($P = 0.42$; Figure 3). Finally, we observed no significant difference in blood glucose concentrations between trials (PLA, 4.90 ± 0.4 $mmol \cdot l^{-1}$; CHO, 4.90 ± 0.6 $mmol \cdot l^{-1}$; $P = 0.78$) and at no time point was blood glucose different (Figure 3). We deemed the effect sizes for all sprint measures as trivial ((≤ 0.2); Table 1). With regards to magnitude-based inferences, 90% confidence intervals overlapped the 0.8% smallest worthwhile effect for all sprint measures (Table 1).

Psychological scales

We observed no significant effects of time on perceived pleasure-displeasure (FS; $P = 0.033$), but no differences were found between trials and no interaction effect was evident ($P = 0.55$; Table 2). We also observed no difference in perceived activation (FAS) between PLA and CHO trials (2.4 ± 1.2 vs. 2.5 ± 1.2, respectively; $P = 0.28$) and no effect of time ($P = 0.25$; Table 2). There was no main effect of trial on RPE (PLA, 13 ± 2; CHO, 14 ± 2; $P = 0.84$) or interaction effect. There was, however, a main effect of time on RPE ($P = 0.001$), with *post-hoc* tests revealing that RPE was greater following the third ($P < 0.02$) and fourth sections ($P < 0.02$) of the LIST, when compared to the first (Table 2).

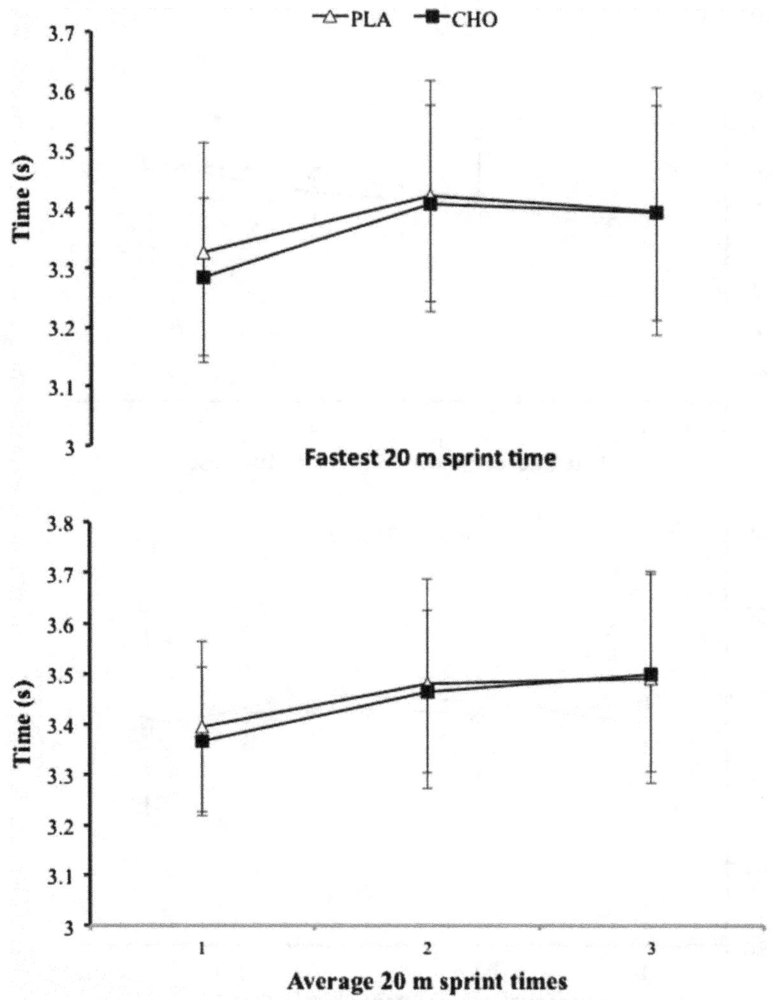

Figure 2 Data (mean ± SD) represent the fastest 20 m sprint time (top panel), and average 20 m sprint times (lower panel) for the RSA tests each experimental trial.

Discussion

The primary aim of the current study was to investigate the influence of CMR on multiple sprint performance. Primary measures included actual sprint times; while secondary measures examined RPE, blood glucose concentrations and psychological constructs of perceived activation and pleasure-displeasure. Our primary findings demonstrate that CMR does not improve intermittent high-intensity exercise performance as measured via the RSA and LIST. We also found that CMR had no effect on three subjective indices associated with exercise performance. Direct comparisons with the current literature are difficult as we are unaware of any published studies examining the influence of CMR during field-based multiple sprint performance. Nevertheless, the findings are broadly in line with those of Chong et al. [9] who reported trivial effect sizes of 0.01 - 0.14 for peak and mean power measures while examining the effect of CMR on sprint performance on a cycle ergometer. At odds with the current study's findings, Beaven et al. [12] reported that CMR enhanced initial sprint performance during repeated cycle sprint exercise, but did not maintain power over multiple sprints. The precise reasons for this discrepancy are unknown but may be due to the increased demand of the protocol used in the current study. Indeed, as the current protocol, including the warm up, was used to simulate field-based team game activity, the increased number of sprints may have led to other overruling factors that caused fatigue to accrue. Specifically, other mechanisms of fatigue seen during team-game sport such as alterations in intramuscular phosphates and the reduction in phosphocreatine may have negated any ergogenic influence of the CMR [26,27]. Though this notion requires further research, it is supported by Jeukendrup and Chambers [28] who suggested that the mechanisms, which cause fatigue during intense activity, may nullify any performance enhancing effects of CMR.

Many studies which report an ergogenic benefit while using CMR postulate that the presence of CHO in the

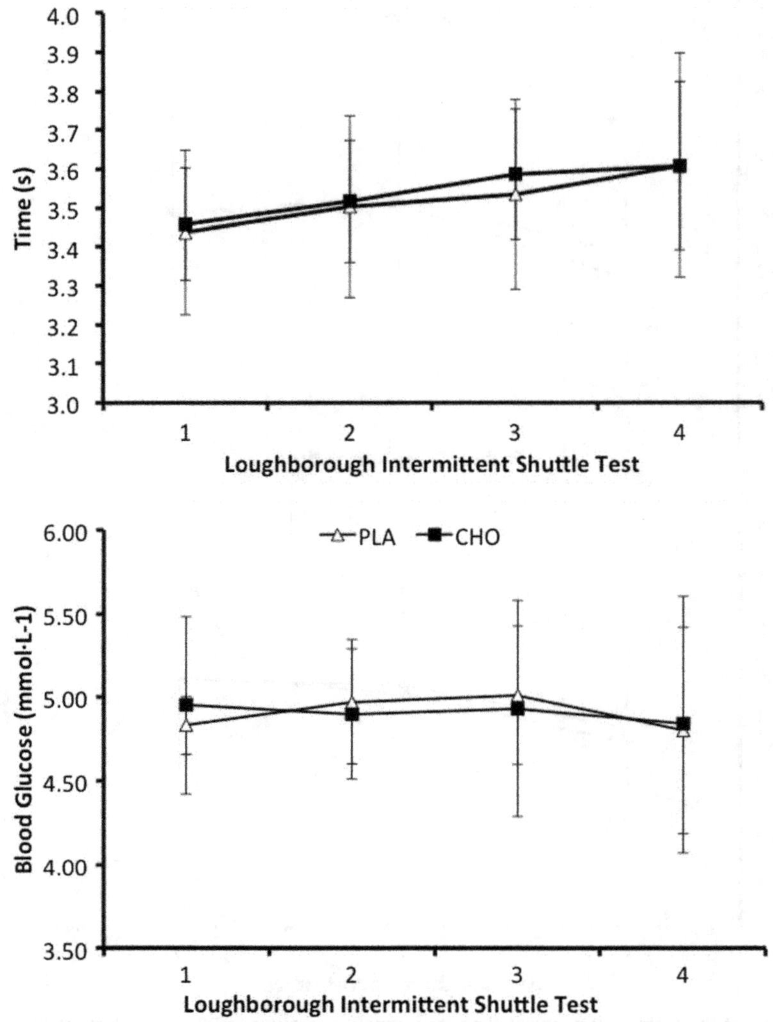

Figure 3 **Data (mean ± SD) represent time (upper panel) and respective blood glucose concentrations (lower panel) observed during the LIST test.**

oral cavity triggers receptor cells in the mouth, which stimulate reward centres in the brain such as the orbitofrontal cortex and the ventral striatum [6]. In turn, this stimulus may lower perceptions of effort and/or improve motor output without an increase in perceived exertion [5]. In the current study, mouth rinsing CHO elicited no reductions in RPE or any evident dissociations between motor output (sprint times) and RPE. This is at odds with studies that report CMR augments exercise intensity for a given RPE score [5] and decreases RPE for a given absolute work rate [29]. Although further research is warranted to fully elucidate this difference, the results from the current study may suggest that CMR is incapable of reducing perceived exercise intensity during multiple sprint exercise. Of course,

Table 1 Absolute and standardized differences (effect size) between trials for sprint measures during the RSA and LIST tests

	Absolute difference	Effect size	Percentage difference (90% confidence intervals)	Practical interpretation
RSA average sprint time (s)	0.016 (↑)	0.09	0.5 (± 3.2)	Unclear
RSA fastest sprint time (s)	0.018 (↑)	0.10	0.8 (± 3.7)	Unclear
LIST average sprint time (s)	0.022 (↓)	0.10	0.3 (± 2.4)	Unclear

Percentage change with 90% confidence intervals and practical interpretations of magnitude-based inferences are also shown.
Note: Absolute differences are differences in mean. Upward (↑) and downward (↓) arrows represent whether the absolute difference is an improvement or decrement in performance when mouth rinsing CHO. Practical interpretations were considered unclear if 90% confidence intervals overlapped the smallest worthwhile change (0.8%).

Table 2 Scores for the FAS, FS and RPE during the CMR and PLA trials

		Time point				
Scale	**Trial**	**Baseline**	**Section 1**	**Section 2**	**Section 3**	**Section 4**
FS	CHO	1.1 ± 1.4	−0.3 ± 1.0	−0.8 ± 1.2	−1.1 ± 1.1	−0.9 ± 2.5
	PLA	1.4 ± 1.2	−0.1 ± 0.8	0.0 ± 0.5	−0.5 ± 0.9	0.0 ± 1.2
FAS	CHO	2.3 ± 0.5	2.6 ± 1.4	2.4 ± 1.3	2.5 ± 1.5	2.6 ± 1.2
	PLA	2.0 ± 0.8	2.6 ± 1.3	2.3 ± 1.2	2.4 ± 1.5	2.8 ± 1.4
RPE (6-20)	CHO	n/a	13 ± 1	13 ± 1	14 ± 2*	15 ± 2*
	PLA	n/a	12 ± 1	13 ± 1	14 ± 1*	14 ± 2*

* Significant within (i.e., time) effect noted for each group different to Section 1 ($P < 0.05$). No between group differences are otherwise noted. Data are mean ± SD.

as the oral sensing of CHO may be just one of a large number of physiological and psychological inputs which modify RPE during multiple sprint activity [30], any reduction in perceived exertion due to CMR is perhaps negligible.

Further to the effects on perceived intensity, it has been proposed that CMR may improve the subjective evaluation of 'how one feels' during exercise [7]. The current study administered the FAS and FS to assess feelings of perceived activation and pleasure-displeasure, respectively. Results from the current study suggest that CMR was unable to improve perceptions of pleasure and activation. In contrast, Rollo et al. [7] reported that CMR increased feelings of pleasure during the first five minutes of a 30 min running procedure. Discrepancies between these findings are likely to be due to the different demands of the exercise protocols. Specifically, the aim of Rollo and colleagues protocol was to sustain a pace, which denoted a rating of 15 on the RPE scale [7], while the current study required participants to perform the sprints of the LIST and RSA tests. Perhaps, as optimal performance in the current study required participants to perform maximally during the sprints, the overriding motivation to perform well may have negated any small changes in the feelings of pleasure-displeasure and activation induced by the presence of CHO in the oral cavity [30]. In addition, any central changes caused by CMR may be evident for multiple sprint activity of 60 min or greater in duration. Though further research is required to confirm this notion, it may be supported by Backhouse et al. [18] who reported that CHO ingestion only improves perceived activation between 60 and 90 min of the LIST protocol.

Hypothetically, Carter et al. [5] suggest that CMR results in a cephalic rise in insulin and blood glucose, which improves performance by facilitating glucose uptake into the muscle. Contrary to this postulation, our current study indicates that CMR exerts no effect on blood glucose during multiple sprint exercise. This agrees with previous literature reporting that CMR has no influence on blood glucose concentrations during endurance exercise [31]. Although we did not measure peripheral changes in metabolism in our current study, our results support to the notion that CMR exerts little or no metabolic changes.

Despite the relatively small sample size of our study, we are confident in our findings. A major strength of our current study is that it represents a fairly "real world" testing scenario synonymous with sport as the LIST correlates well with soccer and hockey performance [16,32]. Overall, we used a randomized, crossover treatment assignment to CMR and placebo conditions, whereby participants in our study served as their own controls.

The results of our RSA test coefficient of variations for fastest and mean sprint time (1.2%) were similar to other studies using RSA tests [33] and LIST [16]. The trivial effect sizes between trials questions whether there is any ergogenic influence of CMR on multiple sprint performance. We also observed very low coefficients of variation between testing each testing condition (*all*, < 2.0%). Thus, our study was additionally robust owing to the small variance that we observed between testing conditions, which ultimately attest to the reliability of our study protocol. Finally, though it is more common to use 95% confidence intervals, our use of fairly broad confidence intervals (90%) to detect magnitude of effect based inferences revealed that the influence of CMR on sprint times of the RSA test and LIST were unclear as suggested Batterham and Hopkins [22]. An additional strength of our study was ability to control temperature and relative humidity during testing conditions as environmental factors have been found to influence sprint performance [34].

In spite of these strengths, the current study has limitations. First, there was no procedure used to ascertain whether any CHO or fluid was ingested, such as measuring the expectorant to equate mouth rinse "ingestion" with expulsion. Though the blood glucose concentrations were similar between trials, there was insufficient time in the testing facility to reweigh each expectorated solution to establish absolutely whether any CHO or fluid was inadvertently ingested. Second, due to size and homogeneity of the sample studied, we are unable to generalize our results to other populations. Third, one criticism of our study is that we tested participants in a fasted state, which is at odds with training and competition. However, Lane et al (2013) have shown that CMR in the fasted state improves performance more so than a fed state [35]. Therefore, our results are not likely confounded by a fed vs. fasted treatment condition.

Finally, though the LIST is designed to be a field test emulating soccer performance, it does not adequately account for various time points during a match. Therefore, it may be worthwhile to assess CMR under more match appropriate time conditions such as at the beginning, half way point (~ 45 min) and ~90 min) of exercise.

Conclusions

On the whole, results from our current study suggest that CMR exerts no influence on multiple sprint performance during a field-based test designed to simulate team game sports. Though our results suggest that CMR is an ineffective ergogenic aid during field-based activity, further confirmatory study is required to examine CMR during time periods more applicable to team game sports and to investigate CMR following a period of preload.

Competing interests

The authors declare that they have no competing interests.

Authors' contributions

JD was the primary investigator for the current study and largely responsible for its inception, design and performance. CE was the supervising teacher for Mr. D final year, undergraduate, thesis project and provided advice during the design and carrying out of the study, as well as the statistical procedures involved in the study analysis. Both parties contributed equally to the writing and presentation of this manuscript. Both authors read and approved the final manuscript.

Acknowledgements

The authors would like to thank the University of Bath for internally funding this project and the use of the indoor track facility at the University of Bath Sports Training Village for testing. Additionally, the authors would like to thank the participants for their time and commitment to the project.

References

1. Tsintzas OK, Williams C, Wilson W, Burrin J: **Influence of carbohydrate supplementation early in exercise on endurance running capacity.** *Med Sci Sports Exer* 1996, **28:**1373–1379.
2. Nicholas CW, Williams C, Lakomy HKA, Phillips G, Nowitz A: **Influence of ingesting a carbohydrate-electrolyte on endurance capacity during intermittent, high-intensity shuttle running.** *J Sports Sci* 1995, **13:**283–290. 1987, 162:156-159.
3. Jeukendrup AE: **Carbohydrate intake during exercise and performance.** *Nutr* 2004, **20:**669–677.
4. Jeukendrup AE, Brouns F, Wagenmakers AJM, Saris WHM: **Carbohydrate-electrolyte feedings improve 1 h time trial cycling performance.** *Int J Sports Med* 1997, **18:**125–129.
5. Carter JM, Jeukendrup AE, Mann CH, Jones DA: **The effect of glucose infusion on glucose kinetics during a 1-h time trial.** *Med Sci Sports Exer* 2004, **36:**1543–1550.
6. Chambers ES, Bridge MW, Jones DA: **Carbohydrate sensing in the human mouth: effects on exercise performance and brain activity.** *J Physiol* 2009, **587:**1779–1794.
7. Rollo I, Williams C, Gant N, Nute M: **The influence of carbohydrate mouth rinse on self-selected speeds during a 30-min treadmill run.** *Int J Sports Nutr Exer Metab* 2008, **18:**585–600.
8. Rollo I, Williams C, Nevill M: **Influence of ingesting versus mouth rinsing a carbohydrate solution during a 1-h run.** *Med Sci Sports Exer* 2011, **43:**468–475.
9. Chong E, Guelfi K, Fournier P: **Effect of a carbohydrate mouth rinse on maximal sprint performance in competitive male cyclists.** *J Sci Med Sport* 2011, **14:**162–167.
10. Painelli V, Roschel H, Gualano B, Del-Favero S, Benatti F, Ugrinowitsch C, Tricoli V, Lancha A: **The effect of carbohydrate mouth rinse on maximal strength and strength endurance.** *Eur J Appl Physiol* 2011, **111:**2381–2386.
11. Gant N, Stinear CM, Byblow WD: **Carbohydrate in the mouth immediately facilitates motor output.** *Brain Res* 2010, **1350:**151–158.
12. Beaven CM, Maulder P, Pooley A, Kilduff L, Cook C: **Effects of caffeine and carbohydrate mouth rinses on repeated sprint performance.** *Appl Physiol Nutr Metab* 2013, **38:**633–637.
13. Knicker AJ, Renshaw I, Oldham ARH, Cairns SP: **Interactive processes link the multiple symptoms of fatigue in sport competition.** *Sports Med* 2011, **41:**307–328.
14. Mujika I, Padilla S, Ibanez J, Izquierdo M, Gorostiaga E: **Creatine supplementation and sprint performance in soccer players.** *Med Sci Sports Exer* 2000, **32:**518–525.
15. Ramsbottom R, Brewer J, Williams C: **A progressive shuttle run test to estimate maximal oxygen uptake.** *Br J Sports Med* 1988, **22:**141–144.
16. Nicholas CW, Nuttall FE, Williams C: **The Loughborough intermittent shuttle test: a field test that simulates the activity pattern of soccer.** *J Sports Sci* 2000, **18:**97–104.
17. Svek S, Murgatroyd S: **Metamotivational dominance – a multimethod validation of reversal theory constructs.** *J Person Soc Psch* 1985, **48:**107–116.
18. Backhouse SH, Ali A, Biddle SJH, Williams C: **Carbohydrate ingestion during prolonged high-intensity intermittent exercise: impact on affect and perceived exertion.** *Scand J Med Sci Sport* 2007, **17:**605–610.
19. Hardy CJ, Rejeski WJ: **Not what, but how one feels – the measurement of affect during exercise.** *J Sport Exer Psych* 1989, **11:**304–317.
20. Ekkekakis P, Backhouse SH, Gray C, Lind E: **Walking is popular among adults but is it pleasant? A framework for clarifying the link between walking and affect as illustrated in two studies.** *Psych Sport Exer* 2008, **9:**246–264.
21. Borg GAV: **Psyhophysical bases of perceived exertion.** *Med Sci Sports Exer* 1982, **14:**377–381.
22. Batterham AM, Hopkins WG: **Making meaningful inferences about magnitudes.** *Int J Sports Physiol Perform* 2006, **1:**50–57.
23. Cohen J: **A power primer.** *Psychological Bull* 1992, **112:**155–159.
24. Hopkins WG: **How to interpret changes in athletic performance test.** *Sportscience* 2004, **8:**1–7.
25. Paton CD, Hopkins WG, Vollebregt L: **Little effect of caffeine ingestion on repeated sprints in team-sport athletes.** *Med Sci Sports Exer* 2001, **33:**822–825.
26. Reilly T, Drust B, Clarke N: **Muscle fatigue during football match-play.** *Sports Med* 2008, **38:**357–367.
27. Bogdanis GC, Nevill ME, Boobis LH, Lakomy HKA: **Contribution of phosphocreatine and aerobic metabolism to energy supply during repeated sprint exercise.** *J Appl Physiol* 1996, **80:**876–884.
28. Jeukendrup AE, Chambers ES: **Oral carbohydrate sensing and exercise performance.** *Current Opinion Clin Nutr Metab Care* 2010, **13:**447–451.
29. Fares EJM, Kayser B: **Carbohydrate mouth rinse effects on exercise capacity in pre- and postprandial states.** *J Nutr Metab* 2011, **ID:**385962.
30. Rollo I, Williams C: **Effect of mouth-rinsing carbohydrate solutions on endurance performance.** *Sports Med* 2011, **41:**449–461.
31. Rollo I, Cole M, Miller R, Williams C: **Influence of mouth rinsing a carbohydrate solution on 1-h running performance.** *Med Sci Sports Exer* 2010, **42:**798–804.
32. Sunderland C, Nevill M: **High-intensity intermittent running and field hockey skill performance in the heat.** *J Sports Sci* 2005, **23:**531–540.
33. Glaister M, Howatson G, Pattinson JR, McInnes G: **The reliability and validity of fatigue measures during multiple-sprint work: an issue revisited.** *J Strength Cond Res* 2008, **22:**1597–1601.
34. Gray SR, De Vito G, Nimmo MA, Farina D, Ferguson RA: **Skeletal muscle ATP turnover and muscle fiber conduction velocity are elevated at higher muscle temperatures during maximal power output development in humans.** *Am J Physiol Regulat Inter Com Physiol* 2006, **290:**R376–R382.
35. Lane SC, Bird SR, Burke LM, Hawley JA: **Effect of a carbohydrate mouth rinse on simulated cycling time-trial performance commenced in a fed or fasted state.** *Appl Physiol Nutr Metab* 2013, **38**(2):134–139.

17

Acute versus chronic supplementation of sodium citrate on 200 m performance in adolescent swimmers

Colin Russell[1], Efthymios Papadopoulos[1], Yasmeen Mezil[1], Greg D Wells[2], Michael J Plyley[1], Mathew Greenway[3] and Panagiota Klentrou[1*]

Abstract

Background: A double-blinded, placebo-controlled, cross-over design was used to investigate whether two different sodium citrate dihydrate (Na-CIT) supplementation protocols improve 200 m swimming performance in adolescent swimmers.

Methods: Ten, male swimmers (14.9 ± 0.4 years of age; 63.5 ± 4 kg) performed four 200 m time trials with the following treatments: acute (ACU) supplementation (0.5 g kg^{-1} administered 120 min pre-trial), acute placebo (PLC-A), chronic (CHR) supplementation (0.1 g·kg^{-1} for three days and 0.3 g kg^{-1} on the forth day 120 min pre-trial), and chronic placebo (PLC-C). The order of the trials was randomized, with at least a six-day wash-out period between trials. Blood samples were collected by finger prick pre-ingestion, 100 min post-ingestion, and 3 min post-trial. Performance time, rate of perceived exertion, pH, base excess, bicarbonate and lactate concentration were measured.

Results: Post-ingestion bicarbonate and base excess were higher ($P < 0.05$) in both the ACU and CHR trials compared to placebo showing adequate pre-exercise alkalosis. However, performance time, rate of perceived exertion as well as post-trial pH and lactate concentration were not significantly different between trials. Further analysis revealed that five swimmers, identified as responders, improved their performance time by 1.03% ($P < 0.05$) and attained higher post-trial lactate concentrations in the ACU versus PLC-A trial ($P < 0.05$). They also had significantly higher post-trial lactate concentrations compared to the non-responders in the ACU and CHR trials.

Conclusions: Acute supplementation of Na-CIT prior to 200 m swimming performance led to a modest time improvement and higher blood lactate concentrations in only half of the swimmers while the chronic Na-CIT supplementation did not provide any ergogenic effect in this group of adolescent swimmers.

Trial registration: Clinicaltrials.gov NCT01835912.

Keywords: Ergogenic aid, Buffer, Alkalization, Responders, Blood lactate, Bicarbonate

Introduction

Alkalizing agents have been used in high performance sports as a strategy to postpone the onset of fatigue during high intensity exercise by slowing the decline in muscle and blood pH [1,2]. Studies have confirmed that increasing the extracellular pH, via an alkalizer, promotes the efflux of lactate and H^+ from the active muscles [1,3-5]. Therefore, artificially inducing alkalosis prior to anaerobic exercise may reduce intracellular acidosis and increase the time to fatigue [6,7]

The process known as "bicarbonate loading", in which sodium bicarbonate is ingested pre-performance, is a popular method of blood alkalization among athletes [6,8]. According to a recent meta-analysis by Carr et al. [8], sodium bicarbonate enhances performance by 1.7% (±2.0%) for a 60 sec maximal effort, with a dose of 0.3 g kg^{-1} of body mass being the optimal dose. However, the gastrointestinal (GI) acceptance profile of

* Correspondence: nklentrou@brocku.ca
[1]Department of Kinesiology, Faculty of Applied Health Sciences, Brock University, 500 Glenridge Av., St. Catharines, Ontario L2S 3A1, Canada
Full list of author information is available at the end of the article

sodium bicarbonate is narrow and 10% of humans cannot adequately tolerate the doses needed to elicit an ergogenic effect [6,9]. Thus, ingesting sodium bicarbonate in high enough doses to induce an adequate modification of the acid–base balance during exercise can be detrimental to performance [6,9,10]. Sodium citrate (Na-CIT) is another alkalizing agent that has been studied in sports over a broad array of doses, times and distances but the results on its ergogenic effect have been inconclusive [2-4,10-14]. Indeed, the meta-analysis by Carr et al. [8] reported an unclear effect on performance (0.0 ± 1.3%) for a 60 sec maximal effort, with a dose of 0.5 g kg^{-1}. Due to this uncertainty, in combination with its lower commercial availability, Na-CIT has not been used as an alternative to sodium bicarbonate although it has a higher GI tolerance [2,5,6]. Na-CIT can enter the sarcolemma through a recently discovered plasma membrane citrate transporter [15], providing new evidence to support its potential effect on performance.

Competitive swimming is an ideal model for studying the effectiveness of alkalizing agents due to its high reliance on anaerobic metabolism. Events range in duration from 22 sec (50 m freestyle) to 15 min (1500 m freestyle) with the highest blood lactate concentrations found in the 200 m (~2 min) events. Typical post-race blood lactate concentrations for these events are 6.4, 9.1, and 14.0 mmol/L in the 1500 m, 50 m, and 200 m events, respectively [16]. Furthermore, swimmers often compete in several events within a 30–90 min time frame during any given session. Swimmers must also contend with restrictions placed on their breathing frequency during intense exercise as a result a unique interaction between muscle physiology, technique, and ventilation. Exercise hyperpnoea is limited during high intensity swimming because turning or lifting the head to breathe may jeopardize execution of proper stroke technique [17,18]. Indeed, swimming requires that the athlete sustain a high rate of energy expenditure and the suspension of breathing for approximately 20 - 30% of a race [19]. Given these limitations and the physiological consequences, it is likely that anaerobic metabolism is a significant contributor to metabolic power in competitive swimming, and may also be a primary determinant of fatigue and limitations in performance [7].

Another reason why competitive swimming is an appropriate model for studying the effectiveness of alkalizing agents is that swimmers are often young when they reach elite level competition; among the swimming medalists in the 2012 Olympics ($n = 78$), twenty-five were under 21 and eight were under 18 years old. This creates a highly competitive environment, where 80% of elite adolescent athletes are using supplements and other non-doping strategies to improve performance [20]. It is, therefore, surprising that there is such a lack of research on the effectiveness of such ergogenic aids in this population [20], especially when acid base regulation in adolescents may be significantly different than that of adults.

The overall purpose of this study was to evaluate the ergogenic effect of two Na-CIT supplementation protocols, previously used in adults, in adolescent swimmers. Specifically, the types of Na-CIT supplementation protocols that have been previously applied include an acute (single) dose and a chronic (multi-day) dose prior to performance. During the acute delivery mode participants take one single dose (0.3 - 0.6 g· kg^{-1} body mass Na-CIT) 60 to 180 min before the start of competition [2-4,11,13] while a chronic dose (0.3 g· kg^{-1} body mass Na-CIT) is given for a number of days prior to performance [21]. Chronic dosing of alkalizing agents was first employed by McNaughton et al. [22] using sodium bicarbonate in an effort to elicit an ergogenic effect while minimizing GI upset, which often occurs with acute dosing protocols. Based on these studies, a double-blinded, placebo controlled, cross-over design was used to investigate the effects of an acute versus a chronic Na-CIT supplementation protocol on 200 m swimming performance and acid–base parameters in male, adolescent swimmers.

Methods

Participants

Sample size was calculated using pre- and post-trial blood lactate concentrations from a published 5 km run trial in adults, an 80% power, and a 0.05 level of significance; this resulted in a minimum sample size of 8 [13]. Thus, ten, well trained, male, adolescent swimmers (14.9 ± 0.4 years of age; 63.5 ± 4.0 kg), were recruited from competitive swimming clubs in Ontario, Canada to participate in the current study. All participants had at least 3 years experience in competitive swimming and had achieved regional, provincial and/or national level qualifications. Informed consent was obtained from all participants and their parents. The study procedures were approved by the Health Canada Natural Health Products Directorate and the Brock University Research Ethics Board.

Experimental design

The current study used a randomized, double-blinded, placebo controlled, cross-over design. All participants performed four swimming trials under four treatment conditions determined by the amount of, and time over which, Na-CIT dihydrate [$(HCOONa)_2 \cdot 2(H_2O)$] was ingested. Specifically, all participants randomly performed the following 4 trials; two experimental: 1) acute (ACU), 2) chronic (CHR), and 2 placebo: 3) acute placebo (PLC-A), and 4) chronic placebo (PLC-C). Each Na-CIT supplementation trial was separated by at least a six-day washout period. The order of trials was randomly assigned to each participant by a computerized random number generator.

The study was conducted during the mid-season training period (March-April) in a 4-week window without competition in order to minimize fluctuations in training volume and tapering effects. During this period, the swimmers trained 14–19 hours/week including 12–16 hours of swimming sets and 0–5 hours of weight training. Their training consisted of: a) seven to nine variant-load swimming sessions per week of medium to high-intensity, and b) two to three constant-load weight training sessions per week. The participants were instructed to maintain their individual training programs. Additionally, they were advised to refrain from any high-intensity exercise and to continue their nutritional habits between the four swimming trials.

Supplementation protocol

Sodium Citrate (Victoria Compounding Pharmacy) was delivered in solution with 500 mL of flavored water (Crystal Light Pink Lemonade); the placebo consisted of similarly flavored water (Crystal Light Pink Lemonade). Ten adult volunteers tested multiple flavors (Strawberry-Banana-Orange, Lemon-Lime, and Pink Lemonade), with and without Na-CIT, to find an optimal masking flavor in an effort to maintain blinded supplementation. Volunteers were blinded to which samples contained Na-CIT. After sampling and revealing which drinks contained Na-CIT, the volunteers chose the Pink Lemonade as the best masking flavor for the supplementation protocols.

According to McNaughton [4], the optimal ACU dose of Na-CIT was 0.5 g kg^{-1}; therefore, the ACU trial involved taking 0.5 g kg^{-1} of Na-CIT in solution with 500 mL of flavored water consumed 120 min prior to performance according to the timing protocol described by Oopik et al. [13]. The CHR dose involved taking 0.1 g kg^{-1} of Na-CIT three times per day for three days, and on the fourth day, a final dose of 0.3 g kg^{-1} was consumed 120 min prior to performance as previously done in adult athletes [21]. The PLC-A and PLC-C involved 500 mL of flavored water taken with the same frequency and timing as their corresponding experimental trial. The doses and the ingestion time frame of 120 min pre-trial were chosen to match previously published protocols using Na-CIT supplementation [13,23]. It is recognized that there are different ingestion times suggested in the literature, anywhere from 60 to 120 min pre-performance [6,22]. However, since all previous studies are in adult athletes and this is the first exploratory pediatric study the decision was to start with the time frame previously used for Na-CIT [13,21].

The placebo and Na-CIT bottles were coded by an independent researcher, and the key was used only at the time of data analysis by the primary investigator. Swimmers were simply asked anecdotally if they knew which solution they were ingesting and if they were experiencing any GI discomfort throughout each trial. In all cases, swimmers did not know which solution they were ingesting and no GI discomfort was reported during the study.

Swimming trials

The 200 m swimming trials were conducted in a short-course (25 m) pool. Participants swam a 200 m event of their preferred stroke at maximal effort. The choice of stroke was given to increase participant motivation and provide real life data. For each swimmer, the same stroke was used for all four trials (backstroke n = 1, breaststroke n = 2, freestyle n = 6, individual medley n = 1). The breaststrokers and three freestylers (n = 5) were National age group qualifiers, the backstroker and 2 freestylers were provincial qualifiers (n = 3), and the rest were regional qualifiers (n = 2). All swimmers wore the same, regular competition apparel across the four trials. Warm-up and warm-down procedures were based solely on each swimmer's typical competition routine. Every trial was done during the same time of the day (5:00–6:00 pm) in order to minimize diurnal and daily variations. The 200 m swim began with a dive from the blocks with a typical competition signal by the same starter. Performance times and rates of perceived exertion (RPE) were recorded at the end of each trial. Performance times were recorded with a manual stopwatch by the same investigator.

Blood sampling and analysis

Blood was collected pre-ingestion, 100 min post-ingestion (20 min pre-trial), and 3 min post-trial. The post-trial collection time was chosen based on previous research suggesting that blood lactate reaches its highest concentrations between 3–5 min post-exercise [16,24-26]. A mixed blood sample was collected by finger prick and analyzed immediately using an automated lactate analyzer (Arkray Lactate Pro LT-1710) to determine blood lactate concentrations. Using the same finger prick, ~95 μL blood was collected into a plain capillary tube and immediately analyzed for base excess (BE), bicarbonate, pH, and PCO_2 using an i-STAT 1 analyzer (Abbott Point of Care). The blood collection was consistently done by the same researcher for each analyzer and for all trials.

Statistical analysis

Sample size was calculated using pre- and post-trial blood lactate concentrations from a published 5 km run trial in adults, an 80% power, and a 0.05 level of significance; this resulted in a sample size of 8 [13]. The Statistical Package for Social Sciences (SPSS Inc., Version 19.0) was used for all data analyses, and statistical significance was accepted at $P < 0.05$. Descriptive data are presented as mean ± SEM.

Repeated measures ANOVA analysis was used to compare performance time and blood lactate concentrations among trials, and RPE to establish equal effort among all trials. Due to missing data points, BE, bicarbonate, pH, and PCO_2 were analyzed for differences between trials using an ANOVA and the assumption of equal sample sizes was not satisfied. This was accounted for in simple comparisons using a Gabriel's *post-hoc*. In addition, the time effects within trials for all physiological variables were analyzed using repeated measures ANOVA.

Further analysis was conducted within two sub-groups: "responders" and "non-responders", in which the athletes were "barred" on the basis of performance differences. Participants were classified as responders if they had a performance improvement greater than 0.4% in the ACU versus the PLC-A trial. This is considered a significant competitive improvement estimated by analyzing the magnitude of the improvement needed for a swimmer ranked in the Top 10 in the World to medal in the Olympics [27,28]. Of the ten swimmers, five were identified as responders. Anthropometric data were compared between responders and non-responders for differences in age and body mass using an independent sample T-test. Due to the small sample size, the responders' group did not satisfy the assumptions of normality for time and lactate concentrations, and therefore, were analyzed with a non-parametric Wilcoxon Signed Ranks test. Lactate concentrations of responders and non-responders were compared using a Mann–Whitney U test.

Results

There were no differences in performance times between the PLC-A and PLC-C trials (143.5 ± 4.7 and 143.5 ± 5.4 sec, respectively), indicating that the young swimmers were able to accurately reproduce their performance. When comparing the PLC-A versus the ACU trial, the PLC-C versus the CHR trial, and the ACU versus the CHR trial for all swimmers, no significant differences were found. Furthermore, RPE was not statistically different across all trials, confirming that the perception of effort was unaffected by any perception (or absence of) in regards to the nature of the supplement.

The five swimmers, identified as responders, improved their performance times by 1.03% ($P < 0.05$) in the ACU compared to the PLC-A trial (Figure 1). This improvement was statistically significant and more than the set minimum improvement of 0.4%. However, even after applying the 0.4% minimum improvement requirement there were no significant performance differences in the CHR compared to the PLC-C trial. In addition, no significant ergogenic or ergolytic effect was found in the non-responders. Although statistically non-significant, the five swimmers classified as responders were older and had a higher body mass and BMI than the non-responders (Table 1).

As expected, blood lactate concentrations were significantly increased from post-ingestion to post-trial ($P < 0.05$), across all trials. The responders had significantly higher blood lactate concentrations in the ACU compared to the PLC-A trial ($P < 0.05$), but this was not the case when comparing the CHR versus the PLC-C trial. Furthermore, responders had significantly higher post-trial blood lactate concentrations than non-responders in both the ACU ($P < 0.05$) and the CHR trials ($P < 0.05$) (Figure 2).

The analysis of the time effects for BE and bicarbonate showed similar results (Figures 3 and 4). The post-ingestion values were significantly higher than the basal

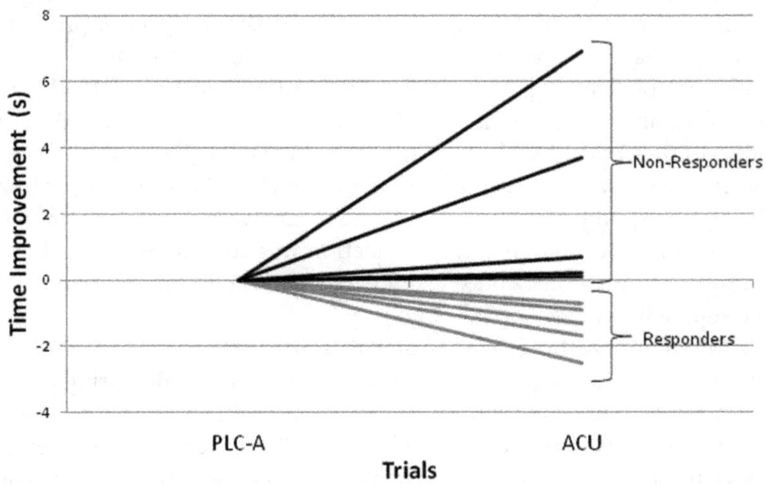

Figure 1 Absolute change in performance time for the responders (n = 5) and non-responders (n = 5) comparing acute (ACU) versus acute placebo (PLC-A) supplementation trials. Performance was significantly different in the ACU versus PLC-A ($P < 0.05$). Each *line* represents a different swimmer.

Table 1 Physical characteristics (mean ± SEM) of both the 5 responders and 5 non-responders

	Age (yrs)	Body mass (kg)	Height (cm)	BMI (kg/m^2)
All	14.9 ± 0.4	63.5 ± 4.0	168.6 ± 8.3	21.0 ± 0.6
Responders (n = 5)	15.4 ± 0.5	67.4 ± 4.1	172.2 ± 4.7	22.1 ± 1.1
Non-Responders (n = 5)	14.4 ± 0.4	59.3 ± 3.8	163.7 ± 2.2	19.8 ± 0.6

($P < 0.05$) and post-trial values ($P < 0.05$). Upon further analysis, the post-ingestion values in the ACU and the CHR trials were found to be significantly higher than the basal ($P < 0.05$) and post-trial values ($P < 0.05$). As expected, pH significantly decreased from post-ingestion to post trial ($P < 0.05$); however, pH only slightly increased ($P = 0.07$) from basal to post-ingestion in the ACU trial (Figure 5). Furthermore, PCO_2 significantly decreased from post-ingestion to post-trial ($P < 0.05$).

The between group comparisons indicated that basal BE (Figure 3) was significantly higher in the CHR trial versus the ACU trial ($P < 0.05$). Post-ingestion BE was significantly higher in the ACU versus the PLC-A trial ($P < 0.05$), and in the CHR versus the PLC-C trial ($P < 0.05$), suggesting a significant pre-exercise alkalosis in both ACU and CHR trials. However, there were no post-trial differences in BE between the Na-CIT supplementation trials and their corresponding placebo (Figure 3). As expected, post-ingestion bicarbonate concentrations were significantly different in both the ACU ($P < 0.05$) and CHR ($P < 0.05$) treatment conditions compared to their corresponding placebo (Figure 4). There was also a small, non-significant difference in the post-ingestion pH ($P = 0.06$) between the ACU and the PLC-A trial (Figure 5). However, there were no post-trial differences in bicarbonate concentration between the Na-CIT supplementation trials and their corresponding placebo. Similarly, PCO_2 values were not significantly different between conditions.

Discussion

This is the first study to investigate the potential ergogenic effects of Na-CIT in adolescent athletes. Ten, well-trained, adolescent swimmers performed four 200 m time trials at maximal effort, using two different Na-CIT supplementation protocols: ACU and CHR each with a corresponding placebo (PLC-A and PLC-C). The main finding was that acute supplementation of Na-CIT provided adequate pre-exercise alkalosis but did not result in an improved 200 m swimming performance or higher post-trial blood lactate concentrations in all young swimmers. This is also the first study to apply a chronic Na-CIT supplementation regimen in an effort to improve performance while minimizing GI discomfort. Indeed, the swimmers were regularly asked throughout the study if any GI discomfort occurred and none was reported. However, in our sample of adolescent swimmers, the chronic supplementation of Na-CIT did not have an effect on performance despite its significant pre-exercise alkalosis effect.

With all 10 swimmers included in the analysis, the 200 m performance times did not appear to improve with either the ACU or the CHR supplementation. Na-CIT is postulated to work predominantly as an alkalizing agent; however, more study is needed on its intracellular effects. Lactate facilitation out of working muscle is increased under alkalotic conditions compared to placebo [5]. However, post-trial lactate concentrations were also not statistically different between trials. The literature is predominantly in agreement; lactate concentrations are significantly higher post-trial with Na-CIT ingestion compared to control or placebo [4,11-14], even when performance outcomes were not improved with supplementation

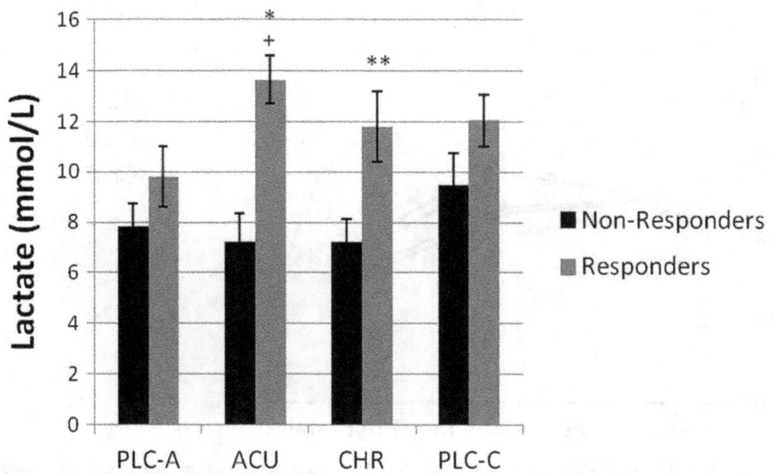

Figure 2 Post-trial lactate concentrations (mmol/L) of responders and non-responders. [a]Significantly different ($P < 0.05$) from acute placebo trial (PLC-A). [b]Significantly different ($P < 0.05$) from non-responders in the acute (ACU) trial. [c]Significantly different ($P < 0.05$) from non-responders in the chronic (CHR) trial. Values are Mean ± SEM.

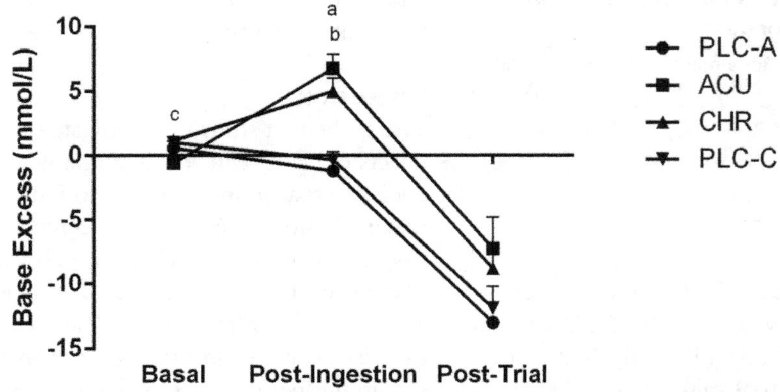

Figure 3 Base excess (BE) (mmol/L) at basal, post-ingestion, and post-trial time points for the acute placebo (PLC-A), acute (ACU), chronic (CHR) and chronic placebo (PLC-C) trials. [a]Significant difference during post-ingestion ($P < 0.05$) between ACU and PLC-A. [b]Significant difference during post-ingestion ($P < 0.05$) between CHR and PLC-C. [c]Significant difference during basal ($P < 0.05$) between CHR and ACU. Significant time effects ($P < 0.05$) basal to post-ingestion in ACU and PLC-C. Significant time effects ($P < 0.05$) post-ingestion to post-trial in ACU, CHR, and PLC-C. Values are Mean ± SEM.

[2,3,29]. Therefore, a higher lactate concentration post-trial, with Na-CIT ingestion, was expected.

It is well established that energy production through anaerobic glycolysis during high-intensity exercise is lower in children than adults [30,31]. This difference has been explained by several mechanisms including reduced activity of PFK [32-35], lower activity of lactate dehydrogenase [32-35], limited ability to recruit and use type IIb motor units [34,36], and a greater reliance on aerobic oxidative enzymes [30,32,34]. Furthermore, this difference may be the reason for the smaller intramuscular pH change and lower lactate concentration found in children and adolescents after maximal exercise compared to adults [31-34,37].

Given these age related metabolic differences we further investigated the potential to find participants that responded to Na-CIT at a greater magnitude than others. Therefore, the data were analyzed for responders and non-responders. Responders were chosen if they had greater than 0.4% improvement, which corresponds to a significant competitive improvement [27,28], in the ACU versus PLC-A trials. Interestingly, the responders (n = 5) were characterized with a higher mean age and body size compared to non-responders, and had a 1.03% mean performance improvement, which was greater than expected and statistically significant, in the ACU but not in the CHR trial. The acid–base response was favorable post-ingestion amongst the responders. Similarly, post-trial lactate concentrations were significantly higher in the ACU trial as compared to its placebo, but not in the CHR trial. When compared to non-responders, responders had higher post-trial lactate concentrations in both the

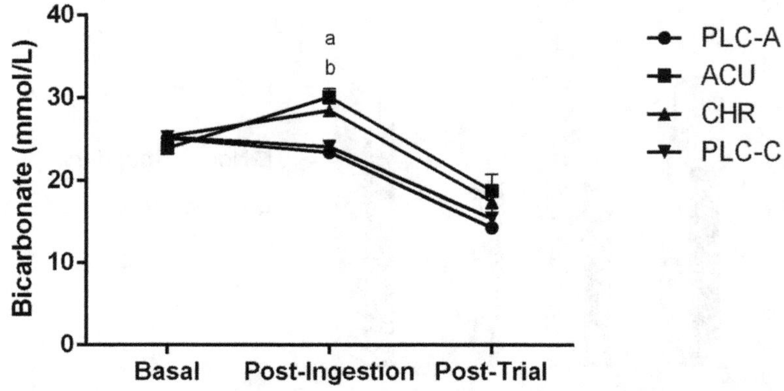

Figure 4 Bicarbonate concentration (mmol/L) at basal, post-ingestion, and post-trial time points for the acute placebo (PLC-A), acute (ACU), chronic (CHR) and chronic placebo (PLC-C) trials. [a]Significant difference during post-ingestion ($P < 0.05$) between ACU and PLC-A. [b]Significant difference during post-ingestion ($P < 0.05$) between CHR and PLC-C. Significant time effects ($P < 0.05$) basal to post-ingestion in ACU and PLC-C. Significant time effects ($P < 0.05$) post-ingestion to post-trial in ACU, CHR, and PLC-C. Values are Mean ± SEM.

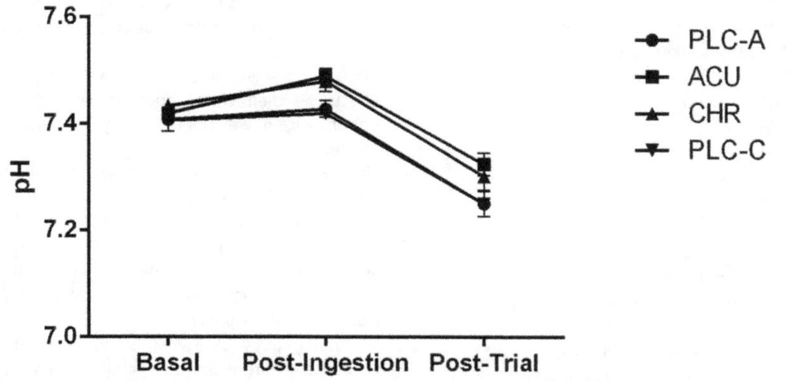

Figure 5 Blood pH at basal, post-ingestion, and post-trial time points for the acute placebo (PLC-A), acute (ACU), chronic (CHR) and chronic placebo (PLC-C) trials. Significant time effects ($P < 0.05$) from basal to post-ingestion. Trend to significance ($P = 0.06$) during post-ingestion between ACU and PLC-A. Values are Mean ± SEM.

ACU and CHR trials. In fact, Na-CIT did not induce any ergogenic or ergolytic effect in non-responders, and they did not attain typical blood lactate concentrations after the 200 m time trials, as was observed for the responders. Therefore, those who developed higher post-trial lactate levels benefited from the acute supplementation. These findings show a more active anaerobic metabolism amongst the group of responders, which is supported by the pre-mentioned age related differences. Indeed the responders were older as a group. Furthermore, responders had greater BMI indicating a difference in body composition. It is, therefore, possible that the responders had more muscle mass potentially enhancing their use of Na-CIT, and subsequently their anaerobic metabolism.

The effect on both swimming performance and plasma alkalization was dependent on the supplementation protocol. The acute supplementation benefited the performance of the responders; however, the chronic supplementation did not lead to significant improvement or increase lactate concentration. The CHR protocol was enacted to incrementally increase plasma BE over a longer time period to allow similar blood alkalization with a smaller dose at the basal time point. The rationale behind the chronic dosing supplementation was to minimize the potential for performance inhibiting GI upset. Perhaps the CHR pre-trial dose was insufficient to elicit performance enhancement, even with the chronic dosing protocol over the previous three days. Another factor could be the time between the last chronic dose and the pre-trial dose of Na-CIT. Optimally, the pre-trial dose would have been the morning after the last chronic dose; however, the swims were performed after school, in the late afternoon. Further experimentation with the timing of the last chronic dose and the pre-trial dose may be necessary to find an optimal protocol, should one exist

Sample size was a limitation of this study as is for most studies focused on athletic enhancement of specific age groups. Considering the post-study analysis of responders and non-responders, the absence of maturation data of the participants was a limitation based on the conclusions of this study. Differences in training volume may also be a limitation to studies attempting multi-day trials over a period of time. In addition, although allowing swimmers to warm-up and race using their preferred routine and stroke was chosen to improve motivation and real-life application it is possible that the discrepancies in the warm-up routines between swimmers and the different strokes swam could have added some noise into the data that cannot be controlled. Therefore, the study cannot answer whether the degree of the observed effect (or lack thereof) was mediated, at least in part, due to the different swimming strokes and warm-up routines.

Conclusions

This double-blinded, placebo controlled, cross-over trial of Na-CIT supplementation did not show a significant ergogenic effect in all adolescent swimmers. Specifically, acute supplementation of Na-CIT provided sufficient pre-exercise alkalosis (as shown by the higher BE and bicarbonate) for performance improvement in 200 m time trials in only half of the young swimmers, who were older and had higher body mass. Post-trial blood lactate concentrations were also higher for this group. However, the chronic supplementation protocol was not significantly advantageous for either responders or non-responders though it did provide a significantly increased BE and bicarbonate concentration post-ingestion. Adequate timing of the CHR dosing before the trial day may have been a factor in the lead up to the basal time measurement.

Abbreviations
ACU: Acute; PLC-A: Acute placebo; BE: Base excess; CHR: Chronic; PLC-C: Chronic placebo; GI: Gastrointestinal; RPE: Rate of perceived exertion; Na-CIT: Sodium citrate.

Competing interests
There is no conflict of interest in this study.

Authors' contributions
CR conceived of the study and carried out data acquisition, analysis, interpretation, and was the principal writer for the manuscript. EP participated in data acquisition and was a manuscript reviewer. YM participated in data acquisition and was a manuscript reviewer. GW conceived of the study and was a manuscript reviewer/reviser. MP carried out data interpretation and was a manuscript reviewer/reviser. MG was the medical advisor and was a manuscript reviewer/reviser. PK was the research supervisor for the study and was involved in its conception. PK also assisted in the statistical analysis and interpretation of the results, and was the senior manuscript writer/reviser. All authors read and approved the final manuscript.

Acknowledgements
The authors would like to thank the Canadian Sport Institute Ontario for their support of this study, and Izabella Ludwa her assistance in the data collection. A special thanks goes to the swimmers, parents, and coaches for their time and effort.

Author details
[1]Department of Kinesiology, Faculty of Applied Health Sciences, Brock University, 500 Glenridge Av., St. Catharines, Ontario L2S 3A1, Canada. [2]Faculty of Kinesiology and Physical Education, University of Toronto, 55 Harbord St., Toronto, Ontario M5S 2W6, Canada. [3]Michael G. DeGroote School of Medicine, McMaster University, 500 Glenridge Av., St. Catharines, Ontario L2S 3A1, Canada.

References
1. Katz A, Costill DL, King DS, Hargreaves M, Fink WJ: **Maximal exercise tolerance after induced alkalosis.** *Int J Sports Med* 1984, **5**(2):107–110.
2. Kowalchuk JM, Maltais SA, Yamaji K, Hughson RL: **The effect of citrate loading on exercise performance, acid-base balance and metabolism.** *Eur J Appl Physiol Occup Physiol* 1989, **58**(8):858–864.
3. Ibanez J, Pullinen T, Gorostiaga E, Postigo A, Mero A: **Blood lactate and ammonia in short-term anaerobic work following induced alkalosis.** *J Sports Med Phys Fitness* 1995, **35**(3):187–193.
4. McNaughton LR: **Sodium citrate and anaerobic performance: implications of dosage.** *Eur J Appl Physiol Occup Physiol* 1990, **61**(5–6):392–397.
5. Robergs R, Hutchinson K, Hendee S, Madden S, Siegler J: **Influence of pre-exercise acidosis and alkalosis on the kinetics of acid-base recovery following intense exercise.** *Int J Sport Nutr Exerc Metab* 2005, **15**(1):59–74.
6. McNaughton LR, Siegler J, Midgley A: **Ergogenic effects of sodium bicarbonate.** *Curr Sports Med Rep* 2008, **7**(4):230–236.
7. Noakes TD: **Physiological models to understand exercise fatigue and the adaptations that predict or enhance athletic performance.** *Scand J Med Sci Sports* 2000, **10**(3):123–145.
8. Carr AJ, Hopkins WG, Gore CJ: **Effects of acute alkalosis and acidosis on performance: a meta-analysis.** *Sports Med* 2011, **41**(10):801–814.
9. Requena B, Zabala M, Padial P, Feriche B: **Sodium bicarbonate and sodium citrate: ergogenic aids?** *J Strength Cond Res* 2005, **19**(1):213–224.
10. Schabort EJ, Wilson G, Noakes TD: **Dose-related elevations in venous pH with citrate ingestion do not alter 40-km cycling time-trial performance.** *Eur J Appl Physiol* 2000, **83**(4–5):320–327.
11. Linossier MT, Dormois D, Bregere P, Geyssant A, Denis C: **Effect of sodium citrate on performance and metabolism of human skeletal muscle during supramaximal cycling exercise.** *Eur J Appl Physiol Occup Physiol* 1997, **76**(1):48–54.
12. McNaughton L, Cedaro R: **Sodium citrate ingestion and its effects on maximal anaerobic exercise of different durations.** *Eur J Appl Physiol Occup Physiol* 1992, **64**(1):36–41.
13. Oopik V, Saaremets I, Medijainen L, Karelson K, Janson T, Timpmann S: **Effects of sodium citrate ingestion before exercise on endurance performance in well trained college runners.** *Br J Sports Med* 2003, **37**(6):485–489.
14. Shave R, Whyte G, Siemann A, Doggart L: **The effects of sodium citrate ingestion on 3,000-meter time-trial performance.** *J Strength Cond Res* 2001, **15**(2):230–234.
15. Sun J, Aluvila S, Kotaria R, Mayor JA, Walters DE, Kaplan RS: **Mitochondrial and plasma membrane citrate transporters: discovery of selective inhibitors and application to structure/function analysis.** *Mol Cell Pharmacol* 2010, **2**(3):101–110.
16. Vescovi JD, Falenchuk O, Wells GD: **Blood lactate concentration and clearance in elite swimmers during competition.** *Int J Sports Physiol Perform* 2011, **6**(1):106–117.
17. Wells GD, Norris SR: **Assessment of physiological capacities of elite athletes & respiratory limitations to exercise performance.** *Paediatr Respir Rev* 2009, **10**(3):91–98.
18. Wells GD, Plyley M, Thomas S, Goodman L, Duffin J: **Effects of concurrent inspiratory and expiratory muscle training on respiratory and exercise performance in competitive swimmers.** *Eur J Appl Physiol* 2005, **94**(5–6):527–540.
19. Craig A Jr: **Breath holding during the turn in competitive swimming.** *Med Sci Sports Exerc* 1986, **18**(4):402–407.
20. Braun H, Koehler K, Geyer H, Kleiner J, Mester J, Schanzer W: **Dietary supplement use among elite young german athletes.** *International Journal of Sport Nutrition and Exercise Metabolism* 2009, **19**(1):97–109.
21. Zochowski T, Sporer B, Sleivert G: **The effect of acute vs. chronic sodium citrate ingestion on 200m time trial swimming performance [abstract].** *Med Sci Sports Exerc* 2009, **41**(5):223–224. Supplement 1 (May 2009).
22. McNaughton L, Back K, Palmer G, Strange N: **Effects of chronic bicarbonate ingestion on the performance of high intensity work.** *European Journal of Applied Ahysiology* 1999, **80**:333–336.
23. Potteiger JA, Webster MJ, Nickel GL, Haub MD, Palmer RJ: **The effects of buffer ingestion on metabolic factors related to distance running performance.** *Eur J Appl Physiol Occup Physiol* 1996, **72**(4):365–371.
24. Bangsbo J, Graham T, Johansen L, Saltin B: **Muscle lactate metabolism in recovery from intense exhaustive exercise: impact of light exercise.** *J Appl Physiol* 1994, **77**(4):1890–1895.
25. Fournier M, Ricci J, Taylor AW, Ferguson RJ, Montpetit RR, Chaitman BR: **Skeletal muscle adaptation in adolescent boys: Sprint and endurance training and detraining.** *Med Sci Sports Exerc* 1982, **14**(6):453–456.
26. Rimaud D, Messonnier L, Castells J, Devillard X, Calmels P: **Effects of compression stockings during exercise and recovery on blood lactate kinetics.** *Eur J Appl Physiol* 2010, **110**(2):425–433.
27. Pyne D, Trewin C, Hopkins W: **Progression and variability of competitive performance of olympic swimmers.** *J Sports Sci* 2004, **22**(7):613–620.
28. Trewin CB, Hopkins WG, Pyne DB: **Relationship between world-ranking and olympic performance of swimmers.** *J Sports Sci* 2004, **22**(4):339–345.
29. Oopik V, Saaremets I, Timpmann S, Medijainen L, Karelson K: **Effects of acute ingestion of sodium citrate on metabolism and 5-km running performance: a field study.** *Can J Appl Physiol* 2004, **29**(6):691–703.
30. Boisseau N, Delamarche P: **Metabolic and hormonal responses to exercise in children and adolescents.** *Sports Med* 2000, **30**(6):405–422.
31. Ratel S, Duche P, Hennegrave A, Van Praagh E, Bedu M: **Acid-base balance during repeated cycling sprints in boys and men.** *J Appl Physiol* 2002, **92**(2):479–485.
32. Beneke R, Hutler M, Jung M, Leithauser RM: **Modeling the blood lactate kinetics at maximal short-term exercise conditions in children, adolescents, and adults.** *J Appl Physiol* 2005, **99**(2):499–504.
33. Eriksson BO, Gollnick PD, Saltin B: **Muscle metabolism and enzyme activities after training in boys 11–13 years old.** *Acta Physiol Scand* 1973, **87**(4):485–497.
34. Falk B, Dotan R: **Child-adult differences in the recovery from high-intensity exercise.** *Exerc Sport Sci Rev* 2006, **34**(3):107–112.
35. Feriche Fernandez-Castanys B, Delgado-Fernandez M, Alvarez GJ: **The effect of sodium citrate intake on anaerobic performance in normoxia and**

after sudden ascent to a moderate altitude. *J Sports Med Phys Fitness* 2002, **42**(2):179–185.
36. Dotan R, Mitchell C, Cohen R, Klentrou P, Gabriel D, Falk B: **Child-adult differences in muscle activation–a review.** *Pediatr Exerc Sci* 2012, **24**(1):2–21.
37. Dotan R, Ohana S, Bediz C, Falk B: **Blood lactate disappearance dynamics in boys and men following exercise of similar and dissimilar peak-lactate concentrations.** *J Pediatr Endocrinol Metab* 2003, **16**(3):419–429.

18

Menstrual cycle phase and carbohydrate ingestion alter immune response following endurance exercise and high intensity time trial performance test under hot conditions

Hideki Hashimoto[1,2*], Toshimichi Ishijima[1,3], Harumi Hayashida[1,4], Katsuhiko Suzuki[1] and Mitsuru Higuchi[1]

Abstract

Background: Sex hormones are known to regulate some responses during exercise. Evaluation of the differences in exercise response with regard to menstrual cycle will help understand the menstrual cycle phase specific adaptations to exercise and athletic performance.

Methods: We investigated the effects of menstrual cycle phase and carbohydrate (CHO) ingestion on immune response during endurance exercise at 30°C. Six healthy women completed 4 trials comprising 90 min of cycling at 50% peak aerobic power ($\dot{V}O_{2peak}$) and a high intensity time trial performance test (POST). They ingested a placebo- or CHO-containing beverage during the trials, which were performed during both the follicular and luteal phases of the menstrual cycle. In all trials, thermoregulatory, cardiorespiratory, and immune responses were measured during exercise and after POST.

Results: Although the thermoregulatory responses differed between the menstrual cycle phases, the cardiorespiratory responses were not different. After placebo ingestion, leukocyte concentration (cells/μL) at POST (15.9×10^3) in the luteal phase was significantly higher than that in the follicular phase (12.9×10^3). The rise in leukocyte concentration was attenuated upon CHO ingestion, and the difference between menstrual cycle phases disappeared. A significant positive correlation was found between leukocyte concentration and serum free fatty acid concentrations. Interleukin-6, calprotectin, and myeloperoxidase concentrations significantly increased at POST in all trials, but no significant differences were observed between menstrual cycle phase or beverage type. Concentrations of other cytokines did not change during exercise in any of the 4 trials. Menstrual cycle phase and beverage type had no significant effect on the POST outcome. Thus, differences in leukocyte mobilization between menstrual cycle phases could result from the effect of sex hormones on substrate utilization.

Conclusions: The menstrual cycle affected circulating leukocyte concentrations during endurance exercise with POST when a placebo was ingested. Therefore, we recommend ingesting CHO beverages to attenuate immune disturbances, especially in the luteal phase, even though they are unlikely to enhance test performance.

Keywords: Prolonged exercise, Leukocytes, Cytokines, Carbohydrate

* Correspondence: hideki.hashimoto@asahiinryo.co.jp
[1]Faculty of Sport Sciences, Waseda University, Saitama, Japan
[2]Products Research & Development Laboratory, Asashi Soft Drinks Co., Ltd, Ibaraki, Japan
Full list of author information is available at the end of the article

Background

With an increase in the number of women participating in sports for recreation, health, fitness, weight management, social interaction, competition, and/or personal accomplishment, the influence of menstrual cycle phase on physiologic response to exercise has received much attention, not only for athletes but also women in general. Sex hormones are known to regulate substrate utilization [1], muscle fatigue [2], temperature regulation [3], and endocrine response [4] during exercise. Evaluation of the differences in exercise response with regard to menstrual cycle phase will help understand the menstrual cycle phase–specific adaptations to exercise and athletic performance.

A number of studies involving male subjects have reported that exercise causes disturbances in circulating leukocyte concentrations and function and that these effects are dependent on the intensity of exercise and the associated release of stress hormones [5]. Furthermore, body temperature has been shown to affect leukocyte mobilization, cytokines, and markers of neutrophil activation during and after exercise in men. Thus, greater systemic mobilization was observed in a hot environment [6,7].

In women with a normal menstrual cycle, core temperature (Tc) rises by 0.3°–0.5°C in the luteal phase compared to the follicular phase [8]. Therefore, we hypothesized that a stressful condition (higher Tc and cardiorespiratory strain) in the luteal phase would affect immune response to prolonged exercise. Although several studies have reported the effect of exercise on immune response, very few have investigated the effect of menstrual cycle phase. One study reported that menstrual cycle phase did not significantly affect immune cell response (leukocytes, monocytes, neutrophils, and lymphocytes) after 90 min of cycling at 65% maximal aerobic power [9], However, there was no information on Tc during exercise, and it appeared that the concentration of progesterone, which is involved in body temperature regulation, was too low in the luteal phase.

Several studies have investigated the effect of menstrual cycle phase on endurance exercise performance, but consistent results have not been obtained [10,11]. One study showed that endurance performance was significantly decreased during the luteal phase compared with the follicular phase in a hot and humid condition (32°C, 60% relative humidity), even though there was no difference between menstrual cycle phases in a temperate condition (20°C, 45% relative humidity) [12]. One characteristic of that study was to set a strict progesterone concentration (>5.1 ng/mL) as the criterion threshold for definition of the luteal phase.

A number of previous studies involving male subjects reported that CHO ingestion during exercise could suppress the mobilization of leukocytes into the circulation [13-15] and secretion of cytokines [13,15-18]. Ingestion of CHO during prolonged exercise, maintains blood glucose concentration, lessens hypothalamic-pituitary-adrenal activation and diminishes the perturbation of circulating leukocyte concentration and function [19-21].

It is known that ovarian hormones can exert metabolic actions affecting substrate utilization. For example, administration of estradiol and progesterone in rats has been reported to decrease gluconeogenesis from alanine and to increase hepatic storage [22], and variations in plasma ovarian hormones concentrations have been shown to alter gluconeogenesis [23]. Furthermore, animal studies show that larger lipid, and lower CHO, utilization occurs during exercise when estrogen and progesterone, are elevated [24,25]. Exercise substrate utilization in women throughout menstrual cycle has generally been characterized by the measurement of respiratory exchange rate (RER). Although discrepancies occur when studying RER in women at rest or during exercise, some data shows the significant difference between the menstrual cycle phases. Furthermore, previous research shows decrease of blood glucose concentration in luteal phase compared to follicular phase during prolonged exercise [26]. This low blood glucose concentration in the luteal phase may have a different impact on immune response between menstrual phases during prolonged exercise.

The first purpose of our study was to examine the effect of menstrual cycle phase on immune response to exercise in a hot condition, with a progesterone concentration threshold for luteal phase verification. To our knowledge, the interaction between exercise in a hot condition and menstrual cycle phase with progesterone limitation on immune response has not been systematically studied because the exercise conditions in previous studies were not defined. The second purpose of our study was to investigate the effect of CHO ingestion on immune response. We hypothesized that menstrual cycle may affect immune responses and that CHO ingestion attenuates these effects.

Materials and methods

Subjects

Six healthy young women volunteered to take part in this study. All subjects maintained a regular menstrual cycle and were not taking any oral contraceptives before testing. Their mean characteristics were as follows: age, 23 (SD, 2.6) years; weight, 48.7 (SD, 6.1) kg; height, 156.2 (SD, 2.4) cm; and peak aerobic power ($\dot{V}O_{2peak}$), 39.5 (SD, 5.3) mL/kg/min. Four subjects had not performed regular physical activities for the previous 3 years, whereas two other subjects performed regular physical activities (e.g. swimming).

Experimental design

This study comprised 4 separate experimental trials. Subjects exercised in the condition (30 [SD, 2]°C and 50 [SD, 5]% relative humidity) during follicular and luteal phases of their menstrual cycle. During the exercise, subjects either consumed a CHO beverage containing 3.8% CHO (2.1% glucose and 1.7% fructose) or a placebo sweetened with an artificial sweetener (sucralose and acesulfame potassium) that tasted like the CHO beverage. We used a hypotonic CHO beverage (osmolality 195 mOsm/kg), which was reported to attenuate some inflammatory responses to exercise [27]. The components and ingredients of both beverages were otherwise identical. The composition of both beverages was as follows: protein and fat, 0 g/100 mL; sodium, 26 mg/100 mL; potassium, 6 mg/100 mL; calcium, 1 mg/100 mL;, and magnesium, 1 mg/100 mL. Both beverages had the same flavor and color (slightly cloudy) and were served to subjects in a transparent plastic cup. Thus, subjects were blinded as to which beverage they were consuming. Subjects were asked to ingest 300 mL of either beverage 30 min before exercise and another 107 mL every 15 min during the 90-min exercise (7 times), so that the total intake was 1,050 mL per participant. The amount and timing of intake were determined according to the position stands of the American College of Sports Medicine [28]. This study was approved by the Human Research Ethics Committee of the Faculty of Sport Sciences of Waseda University for the use of human subjects in accordance with the Declaration of Helsinki. Prior to participation, each subject provided her informed consent.

Preliminary testing

To estimate menstrual cycle phase, all subjects recorded their oral temperature upon waking every day for at least 2 months and the day of menstruation for 3 months before commencement of the trial. Additionally, blood samples taken before commencement of the exercise were analyzed for estradiol and progesterone concentrations to determine the menstrual phase.

($\dot{V}O_{2peak}$) was measured using a maximal graded exercise test with an electromagnetically braked cycle ergometer (Combi RS-232; Combi, Tokyo, Japan). The initial workload was 0 W for 4 min (warming up) and was increased by 30 W every 3 min thereafter, starting at 40 W, until subjects could no longer maintain the required pedaling frequency (70 rpm). Heart rate (HR) was monitored by electrocardiography (Cardiosuper 2E32; Sanei-Sokki, Yamagata, Japan) throughout the exercise. During the progressive exercise test, the expired gas of subjects was collected, and the rates of oxygen consumption ($\dot{V}O_2$) and carbon dioxide production $\dot{V}CO_2$ were measured and averaged over 30-s intervals using an automated breath-by-breath gas analyzer (Minato AE300; Minato Medical Science, Osaka, Japan). $\dot{V}O_{2peak}$ was defined as the highest 30-s value. At the end of each workload stage, subjects were asked to indicate the rating of perceived exertion (RPE) by using the Borg Scale [29].

Experimental trials

All subjects completed four separate experimental trials, with each trial occurring at a specific time during the menstrual cycle, previously determined for each subject by her basal body temperature. For the 2 CHO and 2 placebo trials, 1 trial each occurred in the follicular phase (FC and FA, respectively), and 1 trial each in the luteal phase (LC and LA, respectively). To avoid a confounding phase and beverage effect with trial order, subjects were randomly assigned trial orders, with 3 subjects commencing in the follicular phase and 3 in the luteal phase. Each experimental trial was performed on a separate day at least 1 week apart. Subjects were asked to only drink water after 21:00 h on the day before the experimental trial, and they ate a standardized breakfast (protein, 12.4 g; fat, 5.5 g; CHO, 75.7 g; and total energy, 395 kcal) at 06:00 h, i.e. 6–7 h before each trial. Thereafter, foods and beverages, except for water, were not allowed.

In all 4 trials, subjects cycled at 50% $\dot{V}O_{2peak}$ (60 [SD, 12.2] W) for 90 min in a hot condition (30 [SD, 2]°C and 50 [SD, 5]% relative humidity) and completed POST. The workload corresponding to 50% $\dot{V}O_{2peak}$ was determined from the graded exercise test by interpolation from the line of the best fit describing the relationship between power output and $\dot{V}O_2$. During endurance sports competitions, such as marathons, many participants attempt sprints in the final stage of the race. Therefore, in order to simulate an actual competition, our experimental protocol comprised of 2 parts: 90 min of cycling exercise at moderate intensity and a timed performance test. This study composed of a prolonged exercise and performance test under hot condition by untrained subjects. We set exercise intensity at 50% $\dot{V}O_{2peak}$, which was lower than the 65% $\dot{V}O_{2max}$ and room temperature condition set in the previous study [9] because we thought that the 65% $\dot{V}O_{2max}$ intensity under hot condition would be too strenuous for untrained subjects. To measure rectal temperature during the exercise, subjects self-inserted a rectal probe (401 J; Nikkeiso-YSI Co. Ltd., Musashino, Japan) 10 cm past the anal sphincter. During exercise, minute ventilation ($\dot{V}E$), expired gas concentration, HR, and rectal temperature were measured for 3 min at the 4-min (warm-up), 15-min, 30-min, 45-min, 60-min, 75-min, and 90-min time points. Subjects were asked to indicate their overall RPE, RPE-cardiovascular, and RPE-legs to identify specific locations of perceived exertion at every 15-min time point from the warm-up to the end of the 90-min cycling exercise.

Following the 90-min exercise, subjects completed POST that lasted approximately 10 min in the same condition. Subjects were required to complete a set amount of work (52.4 [SD, 8.6] kJ) as fast as possible. The total amount of work to be performed was calculated using the following formula [30]: Total work (J) = 0.65 Wpeak × 600. Wpeak (134.4 [SD, 22] W) was the maximal workload capacity determined in preliminary testing and 600 was the duration in seconds (equivalent to 10 min). The ergometer was connected to a computer that calculated and displayed the total amount of work performed. Subjects received only information on the percentage of work performed relative to the set amount of work from the examiner. A familiarization trial was also completed before commencement to allow subjects to familiarize themselves with the protocol and laboratory setting.

Blood sampling and analysis

Venous blood samples were collected by venipuncture from an antecubital vein before exercise (PRE); at the 30-min, 60-min, and 90-min time points during the exercise; and at POST. Blood samples were collected into serum separation tubes or vacutainers containing ethylenediaminetetraacetic acid (EDTA). A fraction of whole blood was used to measure hemoglobin, hematocrit, and full blood cell count. Serum separation tubes were left to allow blood to clot at room temperature for 30 min, while vacutainers containing EDTA for plasma separation were immediately centrifuged at 1,000 × *g* for 10 min. Serum and plasma were then removed and stored at −80°C for future analysis. Serum free fatty acid and plasma glucose concentrations, leukocyte concentrations, hemoglobin, and hematocrit were analyzed by BML, Inc. (Tokyo, Japan). Commercial enzyme-linked immunosorbent assay (ELISA) kits were used to measure plasma concentrations of the cytokines interleukin (IL)-1β, IL-1 receptor antagonist (IL-1ra), IL-6, tumor necrosis factor (TNF)-α (R&D Systems, Minneapolis, MN), IL-8, IL-10, and IL-12p40 (Becton Dickinson Bioscience, San Diego, CA), and the neutrophil activation markers myeloperoxidase (MPO) and calprotectin (HyCult Biotechnology, Uden, the Netherlands). ELISA measurements were performed according to the instructions for each ELISA kit using a microplate reader (VERSAmax; Molecular Devices, Sunnyvale, CA). Plasma concentrations of all these variables were adjusted for changes in plasma volume [31].

Statistical analysis

All data were checked for normal distribution using the Kolmogorov-Smirnov statistic. Data for rectal temperature, HR, VE, RER, blood glucose, serum free fatty acid, leukocyte concentrations, and performance test result were normally distributed. Data for serum sex hormones, IL-8, IL-12p40, and MPO concentrations were normally distributed after log transformation. Data for serum IL-1β, IL-1ra, IL-6, IL-10, calprotectin, and TNF-α concentrations were not normally distributed. Normally distributed data (sex hormones and POST result were analyzed using a 2 × 2 factor (menstrual cycle phase × beverage) repeated analysis of variance (ANOVA). For other normally distributed data (rectal temperature, HR, and RER), a 4 × 8 factor (trial × time) repeated ANOVA was used to determine trial effects, time effects, and trial × time interactions. For other normally distributed data (blood glucose, free fatty acid, leukocyte concentrations, IL-8, IL-12p40, and MPO), a 4 × 5 factor (trial × time) repeated ANOVA was used to determine trial effects, time effects, and trial × time interactions. When significant trial effects, time effects, or trial × time interactions were evident, Bonferroni posthoc multiple comparisons were used. Data for serum IL-1β, IL-1ra, IL-6, IL-10, calprotectin, and TNF-α were analyzed using nonparametric Friedman's ANOVA on ranks test to determine time effects. Kruskal-Wallis' one-way ANOVA was used to assess differences between trials at specific time points. Data were analyzed using SPSS version 19 for Windows (IBM Corporation, Armonk, NY) with the threshold for statistical significance set at $P = 0.05$. Relationships between dependent variables and leukocyte concentration were assessed with Pearson product correlations. The level of statistical significance was set at $P < 0.05$.

Results

Hormones

Table 1 shows the serum estradiol and progesterone concentrations of all subjects. Menstrual cycle phase × beverage did not affect serum estradiol and progesterone concentrations. A main effect of menstrual cycle phase ($P < 0.01$), but not of the beverage, on both hormones was observed. Serum estradiol and progesterone concentrations were significantly higher in the luteal phase than in the follicular phase [32]. We used the progesterone concentration limit 5.1 ng/mL for luteal phase verification according to previous studies [12,33].

Physiologic response

Rectal temperature data during exercise is shown in Figure 1.

The results show that menstrual cycle phase and beverage type had significant effect on rectal temperature during exercise ($P < 0.05$). Although there was a significant difference within a trial, there was no significant difference between the trials. Rectal temperature was significantly increased over time during exercise ($P < 0.01$).

Table 1 Resting hormone concentration of subjects before each trial

Subject	FA		LA		FC		LC	
	[E] (pg/mL)	[P] (ng/mL)	[E] (pg/mL)	[P] (ng/mL)	[E] (pg/mL)	[P] (ng/mL)	[E] (pg/mL)	[P] (ng/mL)
1	33.4	0.2	171.4	18.9	163.7	0.3	321.3	15.7
2	34.8	0.2	125.5	10.4	42.7	0.1	98.5	7.4
3	30.8	0.4	94.0	6.0	39.4	0.2	68.3	5.7
4	47.3	0.1	108.9	6.4	83.8	1.4	171.0	14.9
5	50.6	0.2	201.4	13.2	98.0	0.2	327.4	19.9
6	201.0	0.4	151.2	25.6	44.0	0.4	102.1	9.1
mean	66.3	0.3	142.1	13.4	78.6	0.4	181.4	12.1
SD	66.5	0.1	40.4	7.0	48.3	0.4	115.7	5.1

Abbreviations: *FA* follicular phase placebo trial, *LA* luteal phase placebo trial, *FC* follicular phase carbohydrate trial, *LC* luteal phase carbohydrate trial. *[E]*, estradiol concentration, *[P]* progesterone concentration.

Table 2 shows cardiorespiratory measures. The results show that menstrual cycle and beverage type had no significant effect on HR, $\dot{V}E$, and RER. However HR and $\dot{V}E$ significantly increased to over time during exercise ($P < 0.01$). RER significantly changed over time during exercise ($P < 0.01$). Furthermore, there was no significant effect of menstrual cycle phase or beverage type on RPE data (data not shown).

The total amount of CHO consumed in the CHO trials (FC and LC) was 40 g. Plasma glucose and free fatty acid data are shown in Figure 2.

There was no trial × time interaction with respect to change in glucose; however, there was a main effect in trial ($P < 0.05$) and time ($P < 0.01$). Blood glucose at 90 min in the LA was significantly lower than that in the LC ($P < 0.05$), and a lower trend compared with that in the FC ($P < 0.068$).

There was a trial × time interaction ($P < 0.05$), a main effect in time ($P < 0.01$), and a trend in trial ($P = 0.082$) in serum free fatty acid. The concentration at POST in the LA was significantly higher compared with that in the FC ($P < 0.01$).

Immune response

Leukocyte concentration data are shown in Figure 3.

There was a trial × time interaction ($P < 0.01$), and a main effect in trial ($P < 0.01$) and time in leukocyte concentration ($P < 0.01$). Leukocyte concentration at 90 min in the LA was significantly higher than that in the FC ($P < 0.01$), and that at POST in the LA were significantly higher than those in the FA ($P < 0.05$), LC ($P < 0.01$), and FC ($P < 0.01$). Leukocyte concentrations at 90 min in the LA was higher than those in the FA ($P = 0.073$) and LC ($P = 0.098$). Moreover, leukocyte concentrations at POST

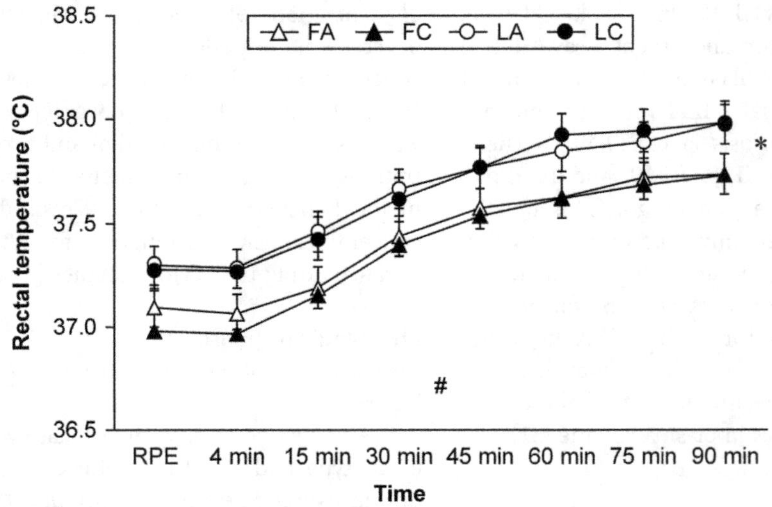

Figure 1 Rectal temperature during cycling exercise. Data are mean ± SEM (n = 6). *Significant repeated-measures ANOVA main effect difference between the trials ($P < 0.05$). #Significant repeated-measures ANOVA main effect in time ($P < 0.01$). Abbreviations: FA, follicular phase placebo trial; FC, follicular phase carbohydrate trial; LA, luteal phase placebo trial; LC, luteal phase carbohydrate trial; PRE, before exercise.

Table 2 Cardiorespiratory measures during 90 min exercise

	Trial	4 min	15 min	30 min	45 min	60 min	75 min	90 min
HR (beat/min)	FA	80 ± 50	131 ± 11	138 ± 12	140 ± 12	145 ± 12	149 ± 15	154 ± 15
	FC	83 ± 12	134 ± 14	143 ± 17	145 ± 20	148 ± 19	153 ± 21	156 ± 21
	LA	82 ± 40	137 ± 90	142 ± 11	149 ± 13	148 ± 18	154 ± 13	156 ± 17
	LC	91 ± 16	141 ± 12	149 ± 12	150 ± 12	153 ± 15	154 ± 14	156 ± 14
$\dot{V}E$ (L/min)	FA	11.1 ± 1.3	28.4 ± 2.4	29.6 ± 3.4	28.4 ± 4.5	29.8 ± 3.8	29.5 ± 3.3	29.8 ± 3.0
	FC	10.9 ± 1.0	28.7 ± 2.6	29.5 ± 2.3	28.9 ± 3.1	28.6 ± 2.3	30.0 ± 3.3	30.6 ± 3.5
	LA	10.9 ± 2.6	28.9 ± 1.9	30.1 ± 2.4	30.2 ± 4.0	31.0 ± 4.3	32.5 ± 4.9	33.2 ± 6.1
	LC	12.1 ± 1.0	29.1 ± 5.4	30.4 ± 3.4	30.5 ± 4.3	30.4 ± 4.5	30.7 ± 4.5	31.9 ± 4.8
RER	FA	0.81 ± 0.04	0.88 ± 0.03	0.88 ± 0.03	0.83 ± 0.05	0.84 ± 0.04	0.82 ± 0.04	0.80 ± 0.04
	FC	0.83 ± 0.08	0.89 ± 0.04	0.87 ± 0.04	0.83 ± 0.04	0.82 ± 0.04	0.82 ± 0.04	0.81 ± 0.04
	LA	0.84 ± 0.05	0.90 ± 0.07	0.89 ± 0.06	0.86 ± 0.08	0.85 ± 0.06	0.85 ± 0.07	0.84 ± 0.08
	LC	0.85 ± 0.11	0.89 ± 0.06	0.88 ± 0.05	0.86 ± 0.04	0.85 ± 0.05	0.84 ± 0.05	0.84 ± 0.05

Dates are shown as mean ± SD. *Abbreviations*: *FA* follicular phase placebo trial, *FC* follicular phase carbohydrate trial, *IL* interleukin, *LA* luteal phase placebo trial, *LC* luteal phase carbohydrate trial, *HR* heart rate, $\dot{V}E$ minute ventilation, *RER* respiratory exchange rate.

in the FA were significantly higher than those in the FC ($P < 0.01$). Pearson's correlation coefficient between serum free fatty acid concentration and leukocyte concentration was determined, and a significant positive correlation was found ($r = 0.661$, $P < 0.001$).Serum cytokine concentration data are shown in Table 3.

Serum IL-6 concentrations were significantly higher at 90 min ($P < 0.05$) and POST ($P < 0.01$) from PRE in 3 trials (FA, LA, and LC). Moreover, the concentrations at POST in these 3 trials were significantly higher ($P < 0.01$) than those at 30 min. In the FC trial, the concentration at POST was significantly higher compared with that at PRE and 30 min. However, there were no significant differences between the trials at any time point. Serum MPO concentrations were highest at POST in all trials. There was a main effect in time ($P < 0.01$), but no trial × time interaction or main effect in trial. Serum calprotectin concentrations were significantly higher ($P < 0.01$) at POST from PRE in all 4 trials. The concentrations at POST in the FC ($P < 0.05$), LA ($P < 0.01$), and LC ($P < 0.05$) were higher than those at 30 min. Moreover, the concentrations at 90 min in the FC ($P < 0.01$), LA ($P < 0.01$), and LC ($P < 0.05$) were significantly higher than those at PRE.

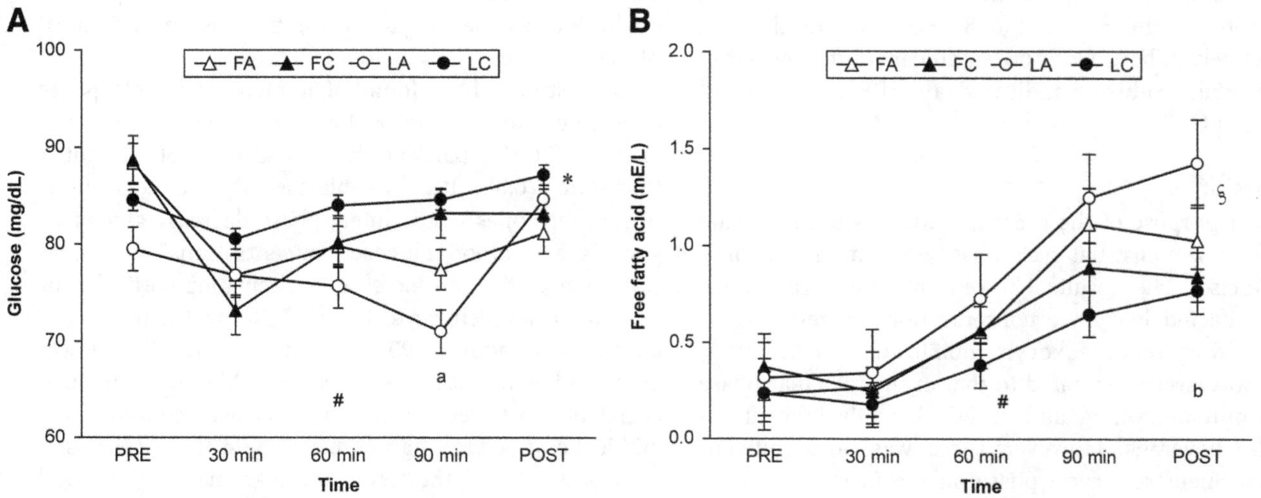

Figure 2 Blood glucose (A) and serum free fatty acid (B) concentrations. Data are mean ± SEM. *Significant repeated-measures ANOVA main effect difference between the trials ($P < 0.05$). #Significant repeated-measures ANOVA main effect in time ($P < 0.01$). [a]Significantly different between LA and LC ($P < 0.05$) §Significant repeated-measures ANOVA interaction between trial and time ($P < 0.05$). [b]Significantly different between LA and FC ($P < 0.01$). Abbreviations: FA, follicular phase placebo trial; FC, follicular phase carbohydrate trial; LA, luteal phase placebo trial; LC, luteal phase carbohydrate trial; PRE, before exercise; POST, high intensity time trial performance test.

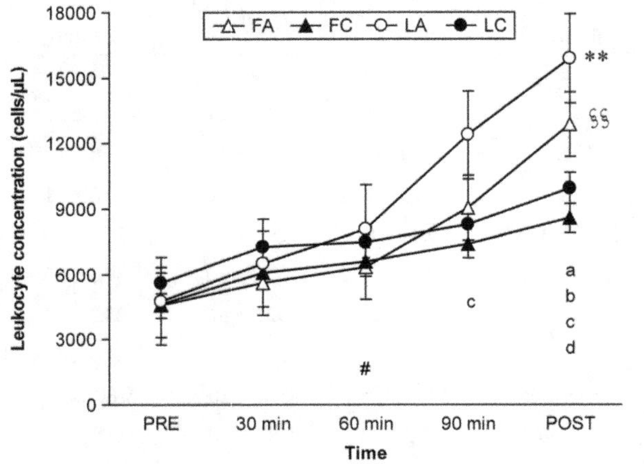

Figure 3 Leukocyte concentration during exercise and after performance test. Data are mean ± SEM. **Significant repeated-measures ANOVA a trial × time interaction ($P < 0.01$). §§Significant repeated-measures ANOVA main effect difference between the trials ($P < 0.01$). #Significant repeated-measures ANOVA main effect difference in time ($P < 0.01$). [a]Significantly different between LA and FA ($P < 0.05$). [b]Significantly different between LA and LC ($P < 0.01$). [c]Significantly different between LA and FC ($P < 0.01$). [d]Significantly different between FA and FC ($P < 0.01$). Abbreviations: FA, follicular phase placebo trial; FC, follicular phase carbohydrate trial; LA, luteal phase placebo trial; LC, luteal phase carbohydrate trial; PRE, before exercise; POST, high intensity time trial performance test.

Serum IL-1β, IL-1ra, IL-8, IL-10, IL-12p40, and TNF-α concentrations remained unchanged following the exercise in all 4 trials, and no significant differences were observed between trials.

Performance test

The mean time (s) required to complete POST was 675 (SD, 163) in the FA, 681 (SD, 147) in the LA, 692 (SD, 156) in the FC, and 678 (SD, 180) in the LC, respectively. There were no significant differences between trials. Subjects indicated an RPE of 20 for all trials at POST.

Discussion

The first purpose of the present study was to investigate the effect of menstrual cycle phase on immune response to exercise. The results showed that menstrual cycle phase affected leukocyte concentrations in response to prolonged exercise; leukocyte mobilization in the luteal phase was larger compared to that in the follicular phase at 90 min of cycling and at POST while ingesting a placebo beverage. However, there was no significant effect of menstrual cycle phase on serum cytokine concentrations. Thus, these results partially supported our hypothesis.

The second purpose of this study was to investigate whether CHO ingestion has an effect on immune response to prolonged exercise. The results showed that ingesting a CHO beverage attenuated leukocyte mobilization and eliminated the differences between menstrual cycle phases observed in the placebo beverage trials. However, there was no effect of CHO ingestion on serum cytokine concentrations, which partially supported our hypothesis.

A previous study showed that there was no significant difference in total leukocyte concentration between menstrual cycle phases after 90 min of cycling exercise [9]. The reason for the conflicting results between the previous and present study may be difference in the range of progesterone concentrations (10.3 [SD, 8.3] nmol/L) in the luteal phase. This range indicates that most subjects had a lower progesterone concentration than the 16 nmol/L limit, which may have weakened the effect of progesterone on body temperature [12]. However, the correlation between Tc and immune response could not be determined because no information on Tc was available in the previous study.

It is well known that there is a substantial increase in leukocyte concentration (mainly neutrophils) during endurance exercise, and this increase depends on the intensity and duration of exercise [34]. It has been shown that the elevation of neutrophils is due to several hormones (e.g., epinephrine, cortisol, growth hormone, and prolactin) that are known to have immunomodulatory effects [35]. We hypothesized that higher Tc and potentially increased cardiorespiratory strain in the luteal phase would result in a disturbance in immune response. However, the results of this study showed that there were no significant differences in cardiorespiratory responses between menstrual cycle phases even though thermoregulatory response was significantly different between menstrual cycle phases. Therefore, we thought that causes other than Tc and cardiorespiratory strain could increase leukocyte concentrations in the luteal phase.

Some studies have found that menstrual cycle phase does indeed affect hormonal and metabolic responses to exercise [36,37], particularly in a CHO-depleted nutrition state [26,38]. It is possible that high concentrations of sex hormones in the luteal phase decrease gluconeogenesis and blood glucose concentrations, which, in turn, may lead to an increase in circulating cortisol concentrations and leukocytosis. In this study, the blood glucose concentration at 90 min in the LA trial was lower compared with that in the other trials. Moreover, the high correlation between serum free fatty acid concentration and leukocyte concentration may suggest this mechanism. It is possible that the CHO beverage maintained blood glucose concentrations and prevented the mobilization of stress hormones that cause leukocytosis. Thus, the increase in leukocyte concentration in the LA might be due to the combined effect of exercise and differential substrate metabolism by sex hormones.

Table 3 Serum cytokine concentrations

	PRE	30 min	60 min	90 min	POST
IL-1β (pg/mL)					
FA	0.9 ± 3.0	0.9 ± 2.5	1.0 ± 3.2	0.9 ± 2.8	0.7 ± 2.9
FC	0.9 ± 3.9	1.0 ± 4.9	1.0 ± 3.3	1.2 ± 3.7	1.4 ± 3.3
LA	0.9 ± 3.1	1.0 ± 2.8	0.8 ± 2.8	1.1 ± 3.0	1.1 ± 2.8
LC	1.2 ± 2.5	1.1 ± 2.7	0.9 ± 2.4	1.1 ± 2.7	1.3 ± 2.2
IL-1ra (pg/mL)					
FA	186 ± 109	196 ± 131	203 ± 154	256 ± 77	267 ± 130
FC	159 ± 59	173 ± 51	234 ± 95	214 ± 121	212 ± 89
LA	203 ± 103	200 ± 100	202 ± 83	196 ± 61	269 ± 152
LC	234 ± 117	219 ± 138	209 ± 81	224 ± 125	177 ± 115
IL-6 (pg/mL)					
FA	0.2 ± 1.5	0.1 ± 1.3	0.6 ± 2.3	2.6 ± 3.9[a]	6.3 ± 12.9[b,d]
FC	0.1 ± 0.5	0.2 ± 0.3	0.8 ± 1.5	1.9 ± 3.6	2.9 ± 8.8[a,c]
LA	0.2 ± 0.2	0.2 ± 0.1	0.5 ± 0.8	1.5 ± 4.0[a]	2.2 ± 9.2[b,d]
LC	0.2 ± 0.4	0.2 ± 0.2	0.9 ± 1.2	2.3 ± 2.0[a,c]	4.0 ± 6.6[b,d]
IL-8 (pg/mL)					
FA	1.2 ± 0.5	1.5 ± 0.5	1.3 ± 0.7	1.7 ± 0.7	2.0 ± 0.9
FC	1.5 ± 0.5	1.3 ± 0.5	1.0 ± 0.4	1.5 ± 0.5	1.4 ± 0.6
LA	0.8 ± 0.4	1.1 ± 0.4	1.2 ± 0.7	1.2 ± 0.4	1.1 ± 0.5
LC	1.1 ± 0.4	1.5 ± 0.6	1.1 ± 0.5	1.6 ± 0.9	1.8 ± 0.7
IL-10 (pg/mL)					
FA	5.3 ± 4.1	3.8 ± 3.8	5.1 ± 3.8	4.2 ± 1.6	2.8 ± 2.0
FC	2.6 ± 2.3	3.0 ± 5.0	3.2 ± 1.3	2.5 ± 2.7	2.9 ± 3.2
LA	4.5 ± 8.5	3.3 ± 2.4	3.5 ± 3.2	3.5 ± 3.0	4.9 ± 3.4
LC	3.4 ± 3.5	3.7 ± 3.5	3.9 ± 5.6	3.7 ± 2.4	3.4 ± 2.5
IL-12p40 (pg/mL)					
FA	37 ± 8	44 ± 11	36 ± 6	38 ± 9	43 ± 5
FC	29 ± 5	36 ± 4	43 ± 8	27 ± 6	36 ± 6
LA	43 ± 7	37 ± 6	32 ± 4	30 ± 10	35 ± 5
LC	32 ± 8	32 ± 3	33 ± 3	30 ± 3	34 ± 4
Calprotectin (ng/mL)					
FA	21 ± 14	26 ± 19	27 ± 24	47 ± 28	95 ± 147[b]
FC	18 ± 46	21 ± 121	25 ± 137	39 ± 196[b]	43 ± 267[b,c]
LA	23 ± 32	42 ± 29	62 ± 67	170 ± 181[b]	240 ± 117[b,d]
LC	26 ± 17	40 ± 45	60 ± 53	64 ± 42[a]	103 ± 276[b,c]
MPO (ng/mL)					
FA	17 ± 2	20 ± 3	20 ± 1	27 ± 4	46 ± 11[#]
FC	20 ± 5	26 ± 8	25 ± 5	38 ± 13	39 ± 9[#]
LA	10 ± 2	26 ± 4	24 ± 2	34 ± 3	46 ± 5[#]
LC	17 ± 2	21 ± 3	19 ± 3	30 ± 7	34 ± 8[#]
TNF-α (pg/mL)					
FA	0.3 ± 0.2	0.3 ± 0.1	0.3 ± 0.1	0.3 ± 0.1	0.4 ± 0.2

Table 3 Serum cytokine concentrations *(Continued)*

FC	0.3 ± 0.2	0.3 ± 0.2	0.3 ± 0.2	0.3 ± 0.1	0.3 ± 0.1
LA	0.3 ± 0.1	0.3 ± 0.1	0.3 ± 0.1	0.3 ± 0.1	0.3 ± 0.1
LC	0.3 ± 0.1	0.3 ± 0.1	0.2 ± 0.1	0.3 ± 0.1	0.3 ± 0.1

Data for IL-8, IL-12p40 and MPO are shown as mean ± SEM; data for IL-1β, IL-1ra, IL-6, IL-10, Calprotectin and TNF-α are shown as median ± quartile deviation [a]Significantly different from PRE ($P < 0.05$). [b]Significantly different from PRE ($P < 0.01$). [c]Significantly different from 30 min ($P < 0.05$). [d]Significantly different from 30 min ($P < 0.01$). [#]Main effect in time ($P < 0.01$).

Abbreviations: *FA* follicular phase placebo trial, *FC* follicular phase carbohydrate trial, *IL* interleukin, *LA* luteal phase placebo trial, *LC* luteal phase carbohydrate trial, *MPO* myeloperoxidase, *POST* high intensity time trial performance test, *PRE* before exercise, *TNF* tumor necrosis factor.

Previous studies on male subjects have consistently reported that ingesting CHO during exercise suppresses the rise in circulating neutrophils, most likely by reducing the secretion of stress hormones that regulate neutrophil mobilization by maintaining high blood glucose [13-15]. The results of this study may support these previous studies.

Muscle-derived IL-6 appears to be at least partly responsible for the elevated secretion of cortisol during endurance exercise. Infusion of recombinant human IL-6 into resting humans to mimic the exercise-induced plasma concentrations of IL-6 has been shown to increase plasma cortisol in a similar manner [35,39]. In this study, an increase in IL-6 concentration was observed in all trials, but there were no significant differences between menstrual cycle phases or CHO ingestion at any time point. These results suggest that factors other than IL-6 may be more related to changes in leukocyte concentrations, consistent with a previous study [9].

Most [13,15,17,21,40], but not all, studies [18,41,42] report that carbohydrate ingestion attenuates plasma IL-6 concentration following exercise. The increase in plasma IL-6 concentration observed following all trials in our study could be due to release of IL-6 from the skeletal muscle [43,44]. However, consistent plasma IL-6 concentration between trials was most likely due to consistent release of IL-6 from the skeletal muscle during exercise and suggests that there was no difference in muscle glycogen concentration [45].

Elevated serum MPO concentration after exercise likely reflects neutrophil degranulation because MPO is contained in azurophilic granules within neutrophils. MPO is an important contributor to neutrophil microbicidal activity. Serum MPO concentration depends on exercise intensity [46] and temperature [6]. In the present study, serum MPO concentration was significantly increased at POST compared with PRE, but there were no significant differences between trials. In this study, consistent with other findings [47], CHO intake did not influence change in serum MPO concentration.

Calprotectin is secreted from monocytes and neutrophils in response to a variety of inflammatory conditions [48]. In the present study, serum calprotectin concentration was significantly increased at POST compared with PRE, but there were no significant differences between trials. These results are in agreement with a previous study, in which the effect of heat stress during exercise on change in serum calprotectin concentration was reported [6]. The mechanisms regulating calprotectin release and the biological role of calprotectin during exercise are currently uncertain. We incorporated the POST in the experimental protocol assuming that participants would attempt a sprint similar to that in actual competitions. The study results show that menstrual cycle phase and beverage type had no significant effect on the timed performance test. In this study, cardiorespiratory responses were not significantly different between trials; therefore, no differences in performance between trials could be observed. This result supports a previous study [12], in which menstrual cycle phase did not affect the endurance performance at moderate temperatures.

One of the limitations of this study is the absence of cortisol, growth hormone, catecholamine, and muscle glycogen measurements during exercise, which would have allowed a better understanding of the relationships among hormone concentrations, glucose availability, and differential leukocyte concentrations. Even though we found that menstrual cycle phase significantly affected leukocyte concentration, we cannot rule out the possibility that the small cohort of subjects used in this study might have had a negative impact on some of the other measurements, rendering them non-significant. The small number of subjects may not have provided adequate statistical power to detect real, but relatively small, differences in some of the measured variables.

Conclusions

Menstrual cycle phase affected circulating leukocyte concentrations during endurance exercise while ingesting a placebo. The degree of leukocyte mobilization was greater in the luteal phase compared with the follicular phase. Ingestion of the CHO beverage eliminated the effect of menstrual cycle phase on leukocyte concentration, which may be explained by the effect of sex hormones on substrate utilization. However, there was no effect of menstrual cycle phase on cytokines during exercise.

The results of this study demonstrate that menstrual cycle changes do alter leukocyte concentration during exercise when subjects consume CHO beverage. Indeed, as the placebo trials progressed, differences became more pronounced, indicating that as endogenous CHO reserves were depleted the effect of menstrual cycle changes become more evident. This was further supported by the absences of difference in immune response between the FC and LC trials.

In women undergoing endurance training for recreational purposes, prolonged exercise in the luteal phase may lead to larger immune disturbances compared to the follicular phase if they ingest water alone during the duration of the exercise. Therefore, we recommend ingesting carbohydrate beverages to attenuate immune disturbances especially in the luteal phase, even though they are unlikely to enhance test performance. However, the total subject number is small and does not constitute a representative sample, and the results need further validation using larger cohorts.

Abbreviations

CHO: Carbohydrate; POST: high intensity time trial performance test; Tc: core temperature; RER: Respiratory exchange rate; HR: Heart rate; RPE: Rating of perceived exertion; FA: Follicular phase placebo trial; FC: Follicular phase carbohydrate trial; LA: Luteal phase placebo trial; LC: Luteal phase carbohydrate trial; PRE: Before exercise.

Competing interests

At the time of writing this article, one of the authors was employed at Asahi Soft Drinks Company, which manufactured and supplied the beverage for this study.

Authors' contributions

HH, TI, KS, and MH conceived and designed the study. HH, TI, and HH performed the experiments. KS performed blood sampling. HH, TI, and HH carried out immunoassay. HH analyzed the data and wrote the manuscript. All authors read and approved the final manuscript.

Author details

[1]Faculty of Sport Sciences, Waseda University, Saitama, Japan. [2]Products Research & Development Laboratory, Asashi Soft Drinks Co., Ltd, Ibaraki, Japan. [3]School of Human Culture, The University of Shiga Prefecture, Shiga, Japan. [4]Faculty of Health Promotional Sciences, Tokoha University, Shizuoka, Japan.

Refences

1. Tarnopolsky MA: **Gender differences in substrate metabolism during endurance exercise.** *Can J Appl Physiol* 2000, **25**:312–327.
2. Hicks AL, Kent-Braun J, Ditor DS: **Sex differences in human skeletal muscle fatigue.** *Exerc Sport Sci Rev* 2001, **29**:109–112.
3. Kaciuba-Uscilko H, Grucza R: **Gender differences in thermoregulation.** *Curr Opin Clin Nutr Metab Care* 2001, **4**:533–536.
4. Davis SN, Galassetti P, Wasserman DH, Tate D: **Effects of gender on neuroendocrine and metabolic counterregulatory responses to exercise in normal man.** *J Clin Endocrinol Metab* 2000, **85**:224–230.
5. Gabriel H, Schwarz L, Steffens G, Kindermann W: **Immunoregulatory hormones, circulating leucocyte and lymphocyte subpopulations before and after endurance exercise of different intensities.** *Int J Sports Med* 1992, **13**:359–366.
6. Peake J, Peiffer JJ, Abbiss CR, Nosaka K, Okutsu M, Laursen PB, Suzuki K: **Body temperature and its effect on leukocyte mobilization, cytokines and markers of neutrophil activation during and after exercise.** *Eur J Appl Physiol* 2008, **102**:391–401.
7. Mestre-Alfaro A, Ferrer MD, Banquells M, Riera J, Drobnic F, Sureda A, Tur JA, Pons A: **Body temperature modulates the antioxidant and acute immune responses to exercise.** *Free Radic Res* 2012, **46**:799–808.
8. Marshall J: **Thermal changes in the normal menstrual cycle.** *Br Med J* 1963, **1**:102–104.
9. Timmons BW, Hamadeh MJ, Devries MC, Tarnopolsky MA: **Influence of gender, menstrual phase, and oral contraceptive use on immunological changes in response to prolonged cycling.** *J Appl Physiol* 2005, **99**:979–985.
10. Sunderland C, Nevill M: **Effect of the menstrual cycle on performance of intermittent, high-intensity shuttle running in a hot environment.** *Eur J Appl Physiol* 2003, **88**:345–352.
11. Tenaglia SA, McLellan TM, Klentrou PP: **Influence of menstrual cycle and oral contraceptives on tolerance to uncompensable heat stress.** *Eur J Appl Physiol Occup Physiol* 1999, **80**:76–83.
12. Janse DEJXA, Thompson MW, Chuter VH, Silk LN, Thom JM: **Exercise performance over the menstrual cycle in temperate and hot, humid conditions.** *Med Sci Sports Exerc* 2012, **44**:2190–2198.
13. Nieman DC, Davis JM, Henson DA, Gross SJ, Dumke CL, Utter AC, Vinci DM, Carson JA, Brown A, McAnulty SR, McAnulty LS, Triplett NT: **Muscle cytokine mrna changes after 2.5 h of cycling: Influence of carbohydrate.** *Med Sci Sports Exerc* 2005, **37**:1283–1290.
14. Nieman DC, Nehlsen-Cannarella SL, Fagoaga OR, Henson DA, Utter A, Davis JM, Williams F, Butterworth DE: **Effects of mode and carbohydrate on the granulocyte and monocyte response to intensive, prolonged exercise.** *J Appl Physiol* 1998, **84**:1252–1259.
15. Bishop NC, Gleeson M, Nicholas CW, Ali A: **Influence of carbohydrate supplementation on plasma cytokine and neutrophil degranulation responses to high intensity intermittent exercise.** *Int J Sport Nutr Exerc Metab* 2002, **12**:145–156.
16. Nehlsen-Cannarella SL, Fagoaga OR, Nieman DC, Henson DA, Butterworth DE, Schmitt RL, Bailey EM, Warren BJ, Utter A, Davis JM: **Carbohydrate and the cytokine response to 2.5 h of running.** *J Appl Physiol* 1997, **82**:1662–1667.
17. Nieman DC, Davis JM, Henson DA, Walberg-Rankin J, Shute M, Dumke CL, Utter AC, Vinci DM, Carson JA, Brown A, Lee WJ, McAnulty SR, McAnulty LS: **Carbohydrate ingestion influences skeletal muscle cytokine mrna and plasma cytokine levels after a 3-h run.** *J Appl Physiol* 2003, **94**:1917–1925.
18. Nieman DC, Henson DA, Smith LL, Utter AC, Vinci DM, Davis JM, Kaminsky DE, Shute M: **Cytokine changes after a marathon race.** *J Appl Physiol* 2001, **91**:109–114.
19. Bishop NC, Blannin AK, Walsh NP, Robson PJ, Gleeson M: **Nutritional aspects of immunosuppression in athletes.** *Sports Med* 1999, **28**:151–176.
20. Mitchell JB, Costill DL, Houmard JA, Flynn MG, Fink WJ, Beltz JD: **Influence of carbohydrate ingestion on counterregulatory hormones during prolonged exercise.** *Int J Sports Med* 1990, **11**:33–36.
21. Nieman DC, Fagoaga OR, Butterworth DE, Warren BJ, Utter A, Davis JM, Henson DA, Nehlsen-Cannarella SL: **Carbohydrate supplementation affects blood granulocyte and monocyte trafficking but not function after 2.5 h or running.** *Am J Clin Nutr* 1997, **66**:153–159.
22. Matute ML, Kalkhoff RK: **Sex steroid influence on hepatic gluconeogenesis and glucogen formation.** *Endocrinology* 1973, **92**:762–768.
23. Sladek CD: **Gluconeogenesis and hepatic glycogen formation in relation to the rat estrous cycle.** *Horm Metab Res* 1974, **6**:217–221.
24. Hatta H, Atomi Y, Shinohara S, Yamamoto Y, Yamada S: **The effects of ovarian hormones on glucose and fatty acid oxidation during exercise in female ovariectomized rats.** *Horm Metab Res* 1988, **20**:609–611.
25. Ellis GS, Lanza-Jacoby S, Gow A, Kendrick ZV: **Effects of estradiol on lipoprotein lipase activity and lipid availability in exercised male rats.** *J Appl Physiol* 1994, **77**:209–215.
26. Lavoie JM, Dionne N, Helie R, Brisson GR: **Menstrual cycle phase dissociation of blood glucose homeostasis during exercise.** *J Appl Physiol* 1987, **62**:1084–1089.
27. Suzuki K, Hashimoto H, Oh T, Ishijima T, Mitsuda H, Peake J, Sakamoto S, Muraoka I, Higuchi M: **The effects of sports drink osmolality on fluid intake and immunoendocrine responses to cycling in hot conditions.** *J Nutr Sci Vitaminol* 2013, **59**:206–212.
28. American College of Sports, Sawka MN, Burke LM, Eichner ER, Maughan RJ, Montain SJ, Stachenfeld NS: **American college of sports medicine position stand. Exercise and fluid replacement.** *Med Sci Sports Exerc* 2007, **39**:377–390.
29. Borg G: **Perceived exertion as an indicator of somatic stress.** *Scand J Rehabil Med* 1970, **2**:92–98.

30. Jeukendrup A, Saris WH, Brouns F, Kester AD: **A new validated endurance performance test.** *Med Sci Sports Exerc* 1996, **28:**266–270.
31. Dill DB, Costill DL: **Calculation of percentage changes in volumes of blood, plasma, and red cells in dehydration.** *J Appl Physiol* 1974, **37:**247–248.
32. Oosthuyse T, Bosch AN: **The effect of the menstrual cycle on exercise metabolism: Implications for exercise performance in eumenorrhoeic women.** *Sports Med* 2010, **40:**207–227.
33. Landgren BM, Unden AL, Diczfalusy E: **Hormonal profile of the cycle in 68 normally menstruating women.** *Acta Endocrinologica* 1980, **94:**89–98.
34. Gunzer W, Konrad M, Pail E: **Exercise-induced immunodepression in endurance athletes and nutritional intervention with carbohydrate, protein and fat-what is possible, what is not?** *Nutrients* 2012, **4:**1187–1212.
35. Gleeson M: **Immune function in sport and exercise.** *J Appl Physiol* 2007, **103:**693–699.
36. Hackney AC: **Influence of oestrogen on muscle glycogen utilization during exercise.** *Acta Physiol Scand* 1999, **167:**273–274.
37. Campbell SE, Angus DJ, Febbraio MA: **Glucose kinetics and exercise performance during phases of the menstrual cycle: Effect of glucose ingestion.** *Am J Physiol. Endocrinol Metab* 2001, **281:**E817–E825.
38. Bonen A, Haynes FJ, Watson-Wright W, Sopper MM, Pierce GN, Low MP, Graham TE: **Effects of menstrual cycle on metabolic responses to exercise.** *J Appl Physiol* 1983, **55:**1506–1513.
39. Starkie RL, Arkinstall MJ, Koukoulas I, Hawley JA, Febbraio MA: **Carbohydrate ingestion attenuates the increase in plasma interleukin-6, but not skeletal muscle interleukin-6 mrna, during exercise in humans.** *J Physiol* 2001, **533:**585–591.
40. Steensberg A, Fischer CP, Keller C, Moller K, Pedersen BK: **IL-6 enhances plasma IL-1ra, IL-10, and cortisol in humans.** *Am J Physiol. Endocrinol Metab* 2003, **285:**E433–E437.
41. Suzuki K, Naganuma S, Totsuka M, Suzuki KJ, Mochizuki M, Shiraishi M, Nakaji S, Sugawara K: **Effects of exhaustive endurance exercise and its one-week daily repetition on neutrophil count and functional status in untrained men.** *Int J Sports Med* 1996, **17:**205–212.
42. Starkie RL, Angus DJ, Rolland J, Hargreaves M, Febbraio MA: **Effect of prolonged, submaximal exercise and carbohydrate ingestion on monocyte intracellular cytokine production in humans.** *J Physiol* 2000, **528:**647–655.
43. Keller C, Steensberg A, Pilegaard H, Osada T, Saltin B, Pedersen BK, Neufer PD: **Transcriptional activation of the il-6 gene in human contracting skeletal muscle: Influence of muscle glycogen content.** *FASEB J* 2001, **15:**2748–2750.
44. Febbraio MA, Steensberg A, Keller C, Starkie RL, Nielsen HB, Krustrup P, Ott P, Secher NH, Pedersen BK: **Glucose ingestion attenuates interleukin-6 release from contracting skeletal muscle in humans.** *J Physiol* 2003, **549:**607–612.
45. Pedersen BK: **Muscular interleukin-6 and its role as an energy sensor.** *Med Sci Sports Exerc* 2012, **44:**392–396.
46. Peake J, Wilson G, Hordern M, Suzuki K, Yamaya K, Nosaka K, Mackinnon L, Coombes JS: **Changes in neutrophil surface receptor expression, degranulation, and respiratory burst activity after moderate- and high-intensity exercise.** *J Appl Physiol* 2004, **97:**612–618.
47. Peake J, Peiffer JJ, Abbiss CR, Nosaka K, Laursen PB, Suzuki K: **Carbohydrate gel ingestion and immunoendocrine responses to cycling in temperate and hot conditions.** *Int J Sport Nutr Exerc Metab* 2008, **18:**229–246.
48. Foell D, Wittkowski H, Vogl T, Roth J: **S100 proteins expressed in phagocytes: A novel group of damage-associated molecular pattern molecules.** *J Leukoc Biol* 2007, **81:**28–37.

Effect of supplementation with chokeberry juice on the inflammatory status and markers of iron metabolism in rowers

Anna Skarpańska-Stejnborn[1*], Piotr Basta[2], Justyna Sadowska[3] and Łucja Pilaczyńska-Szcześniak[4]

Abstract

Background: The aim of this study was to analyze the effect of supplementation with chokeberry (*Aronia melanocarpa*) juice on the levels of pro-inflammatory cytokines, hepcidin, and selected markers of iron metabolism in rowers subjected to exhaustive exercise.

Methods: This double-blind study included 19 members of the Polish Rowing Team. The subjects were randomly assigned to the supplemented group (n = 10), receiving 150 mL of chokeberry juice for 8 weeks, or to the placebo group (n = 9). The participants performed a 2000-m test on a rowing ergometer at the beginning and at the end of the preparatory camp. Blood samples were obtained from the antecubital vein prior to each exercise test, one minute after completing the test, and after a 24-hour recovery period. The levels of hepcidin, interleukin 6 (IL-6), tumor necrosis factor alpha (TNF-alpha), ferritin, iron, uric acid, and myoglobin were determined, as well as the total iron-binding capacity, unbound iron-binding capacity, and total antioxidant capacity (TAC).

Results: Post-exercise, there was a significant increase in IL-6 and a significant decrease in the TAC in both groups, prior to and after supplementation with chokeberry juice. At the end of the experiment, the supplemented athletes showed significantly lower post-exercise levels of TNF-alpha and significantly higher TACs and iron levels than the controls.

Conclusion: Supplementation with chokeberry juice results in an increase in the antioxidant activity of plasma and contributes significantly to reducing the TNF-alpha level.

Keywords: Exercise, Rowers, Supplementation, Chokeberry, Iron, Interleukin

Physical exercise, especially an exhaustive activity, results in a number of unfavorable changes, such as a prooxidant shift in the prooxidant-oxidant balance, hyperthermia, metabolic acidosis, hypoglycemia, and hemoconcentration [1,2]. These processes contribute to a decrease in the osmotic resistance of erythrocytes and their greater susceptibility to hemolysis. This results in an increase in the free iron level, which not only induces free radical-mediated processes, but also enhances inflammation [3,4]. Recent studies showed that inflammatory conditions lead to a decrease in the level of iron, which seems to be analogous to the post-exercise drop off in iron observed in athletes and manifesting as the so-called "sports anemia". It is likely that this phenomenon is triggered by an acute phase response, which is associated with an increase in the level of cytokines and the resultant enhancement of hepcidin synthesis. The overproduction of hepcidin leads to an accumulation of plasma iron in macrophages and hepatocytes, reduced intestinal absorption of iron by enterocytes, and a decreased plasma level; inevitably, all these processes lead to anemia [5].

The protective role of flavonoids during inflammation may be associated with their ability to sequestrate iron [6] and the regulatory effect they exert on immune components involved in inflammatory processes [7]. An animal model study conducted by Ohgami et al. [8] showed that chokeberry extract exerts strong anti-inflammatory effects during endotoxin-induced uveitis in rats. The authors of

* Correspondence: ankass@poczta.onet.pl
[1]Department of Morphological and Health Sciences; Faculty of Physical Culture in Gorzów Wlkp, University School of Physical Education in Poznań, 13 Estkowskiego Str., 66 – 400 Gorzów Wlkp, Poland
Full list of author information is available at the end of the article

this study documented a significant, dose-dependent decrease in the number of inflammatory cells, concentration of protein, and levels of nitric oxide, pyrogenic prostaglandin E_2 and tumor necrosis factor alpha (TNFα) in the aqueous humor of the chokeberry extract-treated animals. The beneficial effects of chokeberry extract supplementation were also documented in humans [9].

The number of published research documenting anti-inflammatory effects of flavonoids in the context of exercise-induced changes is sparse. Therefore, there is a need to verify if and to what extent, supplementation with polyphenol-rich chokeberry juice may alter the inflammatory indices of elite athletes subjected to intensive exercise load. Moreover, we verified if active compounds of the chokeberry juice may influence the markers of iron metabolism in athletes during the competitive phase of their training cycle. We hypothesized that implementation of the chokeberry juice to athletes' diet may modulate their post-exercise plasma levels of IL-6 and TNFα, and stimulate favorable changes in iron metabolism parameters.

Materials and methods

The study included 19 male members of the Polish Rowing Team (16 heavyweight and 3 lightweight rowers). The basic characteristics and sport classes of the athletes are presented in Table 1. The study was conducted between May and July, during an 8-week training camp taking place between the preparatory and competitive phase of a yearly training cycle. The characteristics of a training profile, such as intensity, volume (in minutes), and type (specific, i.e. rowing: endurance, technical, speed, etc., and nonspecific: jogging, strength) were recorded on a daily basis. The intensity of the training was classified in relation to the lactic acid (LA) threshold (4 mmol/L): as an extensive (below the LA threshold) or intensive (above the LA threshold) workload (Table 2).

Food intake

Throughout the entire study period, the athletes resided and took their meals exclusively at one of the Olympic Games Training Centers. Their regular menu consisted of a mixed diet, providing the recommended dietary allowance (RDA) of carbohydrates, proteins, fats, and micronutrients (vitamins and minerals), as stated in the Polish Nutrition Society guidelines [10]. The athletes' daily food, caloric, and fruit and vegetable intakes were constant throughout the study period. All the athletes declared that they refrained from drugs, medications, and nutritional supplements for at least two weeks prior to the study and throughout the entire study period.

Table 1 Basic characteristics of the studied groups (mean ± standard deviation)

Parameters	Supplemented group (n = 10)	Control group (n = 9)
Age (years)	20.5 ± 0.97	20.8 ± 1.09
Body mass (kg)	86.7 ± 1.72	90.2 ± 12.11
Body height (cm)	188.5 ± 1.71	195.8 ± 8.07
Duration of training (years)	5.4 ± 1.1	5.7 ± 1.7

P = NS for all between-group comparisons.

Experimental procedure

The athletes who were randomized to the supplemented group (n = 10) received 50 mL of chokeberry juice three times a day for 8 weeks. The anthocyanin content of the chokeberry juice (24 mg/mL) was determined spectrophotometrically. The contents of the other compounds (Table 3) were determined by means of Rapid Resolution Liquid Chromatography (RRLC), using the parameters summarized in Table 4. The controls (n = 9) were given 50 mL of placebo three times a day for 8 weeks. The placebo, which contained a 6.6% solution of betaine [(CH3+)3 N+ · CH2COO−] and 1% solution of citric acid, was identical to the chokeberry juice in terms of appearance and taste. Both the chokeberry juice and the placebo were manufactured by Europlant PhytoPharm Klęka S.A. (Poland). To minimize any possible bias caused by subjective factors, both the solutions were placed in identical dark bottles labelled with encoded information on the type of preparation and its recommended dosage. An appropriate measure was affixed to each bottle. The label codes were decoded after completion of the study. All subjects received information about the nature of the investigation and provided their written informed consent to participate in the study. The protocol of the study was approved by the Local Ethics Committee at the Poznań University of Medical Sciences.

Training program

Training volumes (expressed in minutes per day) during the weeks preceding the first and the second assessments (referred to as Trial I and Trial II, respectively), which included extensive rowing, intensive rowing, kilometers, and extensive nonspecific training, are shown in Table 2. In the load training phase (before the first assessment), the training volume amounted to 1020 $min \cdot wk^{-1}$, of which approximately 41% was extensive rowing, 21% was nonspecific training such as power training, and the rest was intensive rowing. The total training volume before the second assessment was 880 $min \cdot wk^{-1}$ and comprised approximately 53% extensive rowing, 18% intensive rowing, and 11% land training.

Rowing performance test

The athletes performed a controlled 2000-m time test on the first day (prior to supplementation) and at the end of the training camp (after supplementation). Each

Table 2 Training schedules during the weeks preceding blood sample collections before (Trial 1) and after (Trial 2) the supplementation period

	Days before trial I						
	1	**2**	**3**	**4**	**5**	**6**	**7**
Total training time, min/day	200	110	210	120	190	110	80
Time rowed, min/day	80	90	110	100	75	90	
Distance rowed, km/day	18	20	24	22	18	20	
Training for force development, min/day	80		80		85		
Extensive endurance rowing training time, min/day	80	60	90	100	30	60	
High intensity endurance rowing training time, min/day		30	20		45	30	
Unspecific training (running, etc.), min/day	40	10	20	20	30	20	80
	Days before trial II						
	1	**2**	**3**	**4**	**5**	**6**	**7**
Total training time, min/day		90	220	110	170	190	100
Time rowed, min/day		80	130	100	150	110	80
Distance rowed, km/day		16	26	22	30	24	18
Training for force development, min/day			70			60	
Extensive endurance rowing training time, min/day		60	75	100	95	80	60
High intensity endurance rowing training time, min/day			55		65	20	20
Unspecific training (running, etc.), min/day		10	20	10	20	20	20

subject had to cover the distance on a rowing ergometer (Concept II, USA) in the shortest time possible. The results of both tests were taken into consideration during the selection to the championship team; therefore, the athletes were well motivated to perform both tests at maximal effort. Before each test, subjects performed a 5-minute individual warm-up.

Sample treatment

Blood samples were obtained from the antecubital vein, with dipotassium ethylene diamine tetra-acetic acid (K_2EDTA) used as an anticoagulant. The samples were collected before each 2000-m test (in the morning after an overnight fast), one minute after completing the test, and after a 24-hour recovery period. The samples were centrifuged immediately after obtaining to separate red blood cells from plasma. Serum was frozen immediately and stored at −80°C until use. Additionally, capillary blood samples were obtained from a finger prick before and after each exercise test to assess athletes' LA levels.

Table 3 Content levels of phenolic compounds in extracts from black chokeberry

Phenolic compounds	mg x L^{-1}
Chlorogenic acid	2181.05 ± 48.32
Rutin	498.80 ± 8.84
Caffeic acid	53.85 ± 0.50
Ferulic acid	15.09 ± 0.14
Quercetin	117.60 ± 1.45

Measurements

Serum IL-6 was measured using a commercially available enzyme-linked immunosorbent assay (ELISA; Quantikine HS, R&D Systems, Minneapolis, USA) with an assay range of 0.38-10 pg/mL. Serum concentrations of TNF-α (in pg/mL) were quantified using a commercially available enzyme immunoassay (Quantikine, cat. no. DTA00C Human TNF-alpha). Serum hepcidin was measured using a commercially available ELISA kit (Wuhan EIAab Science Co., China) with an assay range of 0.187-12 ng/mL^{-1}.

The iron concentration and total iron-binding capacity (TIBC) were determined using the colorimetric method with chromogens (Randox, cat. no. SI257 and TI1010) and the results were expressed in μg/dL. The unsaturated iron-binding capacity (UIBC) was calculated from the formula: UIBC = TIBC − Fe. The myoglobin concentration

Table 4 Basic chromatographic parameters

Method	
Mobile phase A: H_2O: acetic acid (98:2)	
Mobile phase B: H_2O: methanol: acetic acid (48:50:2)	
Time (min)	**% B**
0	0
22	80
26	80
28	0
31	0
Flow rate 1.1 mL x min^{-1}	

was determined immunochemically, with an aid of the Myoglobin ELISA kit (Biocom, cat. no. 11170) and the results were expressed in ng/mL. Serum ferritin levels were determined immunochemically, with the aid of a commercially available diagnostic kit (Demeditec, Germany, cat. no. DE7750) and the results were expressed in ng/mL. All the results were adjusted for changes in hematocrit level. The total antioxidant capacity (TAC), considered a marker of the plasma antioxidant capacity, was assessed with a commercially available kit (Cayman, cat no. Antioxidant Assay 709001–96, USA) and the results were expressed as mmol/L. The average intra-assay CV was < 9.0% for all the parameters. The concentration of LA in capillary blood was determined immediately after obtaining the sample, using a commercially available kit (Dr Lange, Germany, cat. no. LKM 140); LA concentrations were expressed in mmol/L.

Chemicals and reagents

The following reagents were obtained from Sigma: phenolic acids: caffeic, o-coumaric, p-coumaric, ferulic, gallic, and p-hydroxybenzoic; flavonoids: catechin, quercetin, and rutin.

Chromatography

The RRLC was performed with an Agilent Technologies 1200 series system comprising an autosampler (model G1329B), a pump (model G1312B0), and a diode array detector (model G1315C). The RRLC system was controlled by a ChemStation for LC 3D system. Spectral data from all peaks were recorded from 190–400 nm. Chromatograms were recorded at 280 nm for gallic acid, p-hydroxybenzoic acid, and catechin; at 320 nm for caffeic, p-coumaric, o-coumaric, sinapic, and ferulic acids; and at 360 nm for rutin and quercetin. Compounds were separated on a 50 mm x 4.6 mm, 1.8 µm particle, SB-C18 column (Agilent). This column was thermostatted at 25°C (Table 4).

Statistical analysis

Statistical analyses were performed using the STATISTICA v. 10.0 software package (StatSoft, Cracow, Poland). All parameters were compared using 2 (supplemented and placebo groups) × 3 (times of measurement) repeated measures analysis of variance (ANOVA). The data distribution was analyzed using the Shapiro-Wilk test. If significant changes were observed in ANOVA tests, Fisher's *post-hoc* test was applied to locate the source of significant differences. Student's unpaired t-test was used to compare the anthropometric characteristics of the study groups. Except for the rowing time, the results of the 2000-m tests performed prior to and after the supplementation were subjected to intragroup comparisons with Student's paired t-test, and for intergroup comparisons with Student's unpaired t-test. The results achieved during the 2000-m simulated rowing test were subjected to a one-way analysis of variance (ANOVA). Correlations were determined by using the parametric Pearson-R test. Values are reported as the means ± SD. The threshold of statistical significance was set at $P < 0.05$ for all the tests.

Results

The subjects form the supplemented group and the controls did not differ significantly in terms of mean age, body height, body weight, and years of training (Table 1). The mean power output and total run time during the 2000-m test performed at the beginning of the training camp did not differ between the study groups. Furthermore, no significant differences in the pre- and post-test blood lactate levels were documented when the results for Trial I were compared to those of Trial II (Table 5).

The pre- and post-test values of IL-6 are presented in Figure 1A. The analysis of variance documented significant exercise-induced changes of this parameter, with no significant effect on the study group. The post-exercise serum level of IL-6 was significantly higher the pre-exercise level, both prior to and after the supplementation period (P < 0.05). In contrast, a significant supplementation effect (main effect $P < 0.02$) and lack of the exercise effect were documented for TNF-alpha levels (Figure 1B). The pre-exercise level of TNF-alpha after supplementation was significantly lower than prior to supplementation. Furthermore, the post-supplementation level of TNF-alpha at recovery was significantly lower than the respective parameter of the placebo group.

The comparative analysis results of the TAC are presented in Figure 2A. A significant interaction effect of exercise was documented by ANOVA in both groups ($P < 0.001$). Irrespective of the group, the post-exercise TACs were significantly lower than the respective pre-exercise values, both prior to and after supplementation. At the end of the study, the athletes from the supplemented group showed significantly higher TACs at recovery than the individuals from the placebo group. Both prior to and after supplementation, a significant increase in the concentration of uric acid (UA) was observed in both groups when the post-exercise values were compared with the respective levels determined at recovery (Figure 2B).

Exercise had a significant effect on the hepcidin level by ANOVA ($P < 0.001$). Both groups demonstrated a post-exercise increase in hepcidin level at Trial II (Figure 3A). In addition, the results of ANOVA confirmed that supplementation with chokeberry juice exerted a significant effect on the plasma level of iron ($P < 0.05$). The level of iron determined during the recovery period of Trial II turned out to be significantly higher in the supplemented

Table 5 Changes in 2,000 m rowing ergometer performance before and after supplementation

Parameters	Supplemented group (n=10)		Control group (n= 9)	
	Before	After	Before	After
Power (watt)	441 ± 30.8	443 ± 34.9	437 ± 35.9	444 ± 38.5
(W x kg^{-1})	5.11 ± 0.23	5.13 ± 0.24	4.88 ± 0.31	4.94 ± 0.29
LA_{min} (mmol x L^{-1})^a	1.9 ± 0.16	1.8 ± 0.43	1.9 ± 0.12	1.9 ± 0.35
LA_{max} (mmol x L^{-1})^a	15.2 ± 2.62	15.8 ± 2.09	14.6 ± 2.30	14.8 ± 3.67
Time (s)	370.4 ± 9.58	369.5 ± 10.44	373.8 ± 15.84	371.2 ± 10.33

Values represent the mean ± standard deviation. [a]LA, lactic acid. There were no significant differences after supplementation relative to before supplementation ($P < 0.05$).

group than in the controls (Figure 3B). Moreover, physical exercise induced significant changes in the myoglobin levels of the study subjects (main effect $P < 0.02$). A post-exercise increase in myoglobin concentration was observed at Trial I, but not at Trial II (Table 6). No significant interaction effects were documented by ANOVA when comparing the supplementation and exercise groups, with regards to the ferritin, TIBC, and UIBC levels (Table 6).

Discussion

In this study, we verified the hypothesis that supplementation with chokeberry juice (50 mg three times a day for 6 weeks) may prevent or at least attenuate the consequences of inflammation associated with intensive physical exercise, and exerts beneficial effects on the parameters of iron metabolism. The hereby documented favorable changes after supplementation with the chokeberry juice likely reflected chemical composition of the latter and

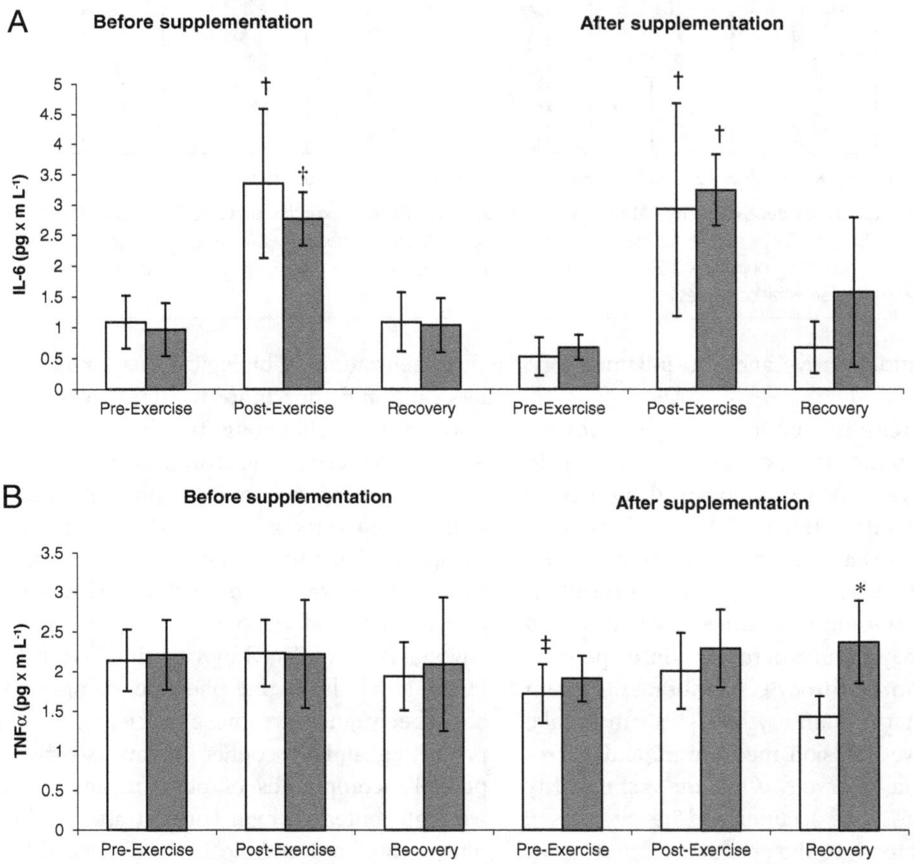

Figure 1 Changes in interleukin 6 (A) and tumor necrosis factor alpha (B) levels during exercise tests performed before and after the supplementation (mean ± *SD*). *Note*: IL-6 = interleukin 6; TNF α = tumor necrosis factor alpha; (gray square) - PLA = placebo group; □ - SUPL = supplemented group; **P* < .05 compared to the placebo group; † *P* < .05 compared to the pre-exercise values. ‡ P < .05 compared to the pre-supplementation values.

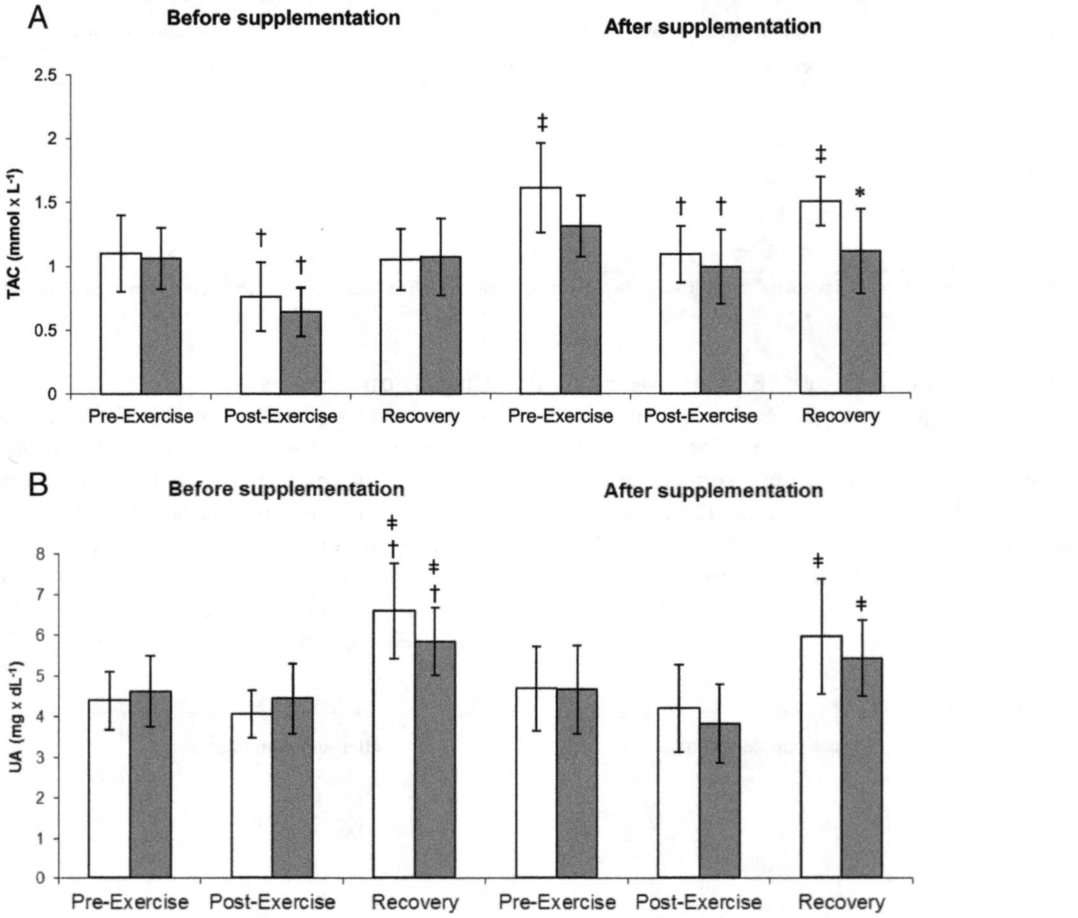

Figure 2 Changes in the total antioxidant capacity (A) and uric acid (B) levels during exercise tests performed before and after the supplementation (mean ± *SD*). *Note*: TAC = total antioxidant capacity; UA = uric acid; (gray square) - PLA = placebo group; □ - SUPL = supplemented group; $*P < .05$ compared to the placebo group; † $P < .05$ compared to the pre-exercise values; ǂ $P < .05$ compared to the post-exercise values; ǂ $P < .05$ compared to the pre-supplementation values.

resultant pleotropic, antioxidative and anti-inflammatory, effects.

The ergometric exercise test performed by our rowers was reflected by a significant post-exercise decrease in the TAC of the plasma, which was observed both prior to and after supplementation (Figure 2A). Previous studies also showed that exhaustive physical exercise can lead to reduction of the plasma TAC [11] and a resultant increase in the concentration of insufficiently neutralized free radicals, which may induce peroxidation of polyunsaturated fatty acids in erythrocyte membranes. Fiorani et al. [12], revealed that human erythrocytes can uptake flavonoids via a passive diffusion mechanism, and, therefore, constitute a specific reservoir. While the vast majority of flavonoids (up to 85%) are accumulated in the cytosol, they are also incorporated into the erythrocyte membrane. According to Arora et al. [13] and Erlejman et al. [14], the flavonoids accumulate at a lipid bilayer-aqueous phase interface, similar to cholesterol and alpha-tocopherol. Due to this intracellular location, flavonoids play vital roles in the stabilization of biological membranes, which become less fluid and thus more resistant to oxidation [15]. It is also worth highlighting the interactions of flavonoids, alpha-tocopherol, and ascorbic acid.

Flavonoids were shown to prevent intracellular oxidation of alpha-tocopherol and convert oxidized alpha-tocopherol back to its radical form (similar to vitamin C). Moreover, flavonoids protect ascorbic acid against oxidative injury and vice versa; thus, the protective effect of flavonoids is enhanced by vitamin C [16,17]. According to Heidi et al. [18], the phenolic compounds present in chokeberry juice are more efficient in regenerating and protecting alpha-tocopherol than ascorbic acid and the phenolic compounds of blackcurrant. These differences were attributed to high concentrations of two anthocyanins, cyanidin-3-arabinoside and cyanidin-3-galactoside, in chokeberry juice and the lack of these compounds in blackcurrants. In turn, Hwang et al. [19], suggested that the strong antioxidant and radical-scavenging activities of black chokeberry extract can be associated with its high

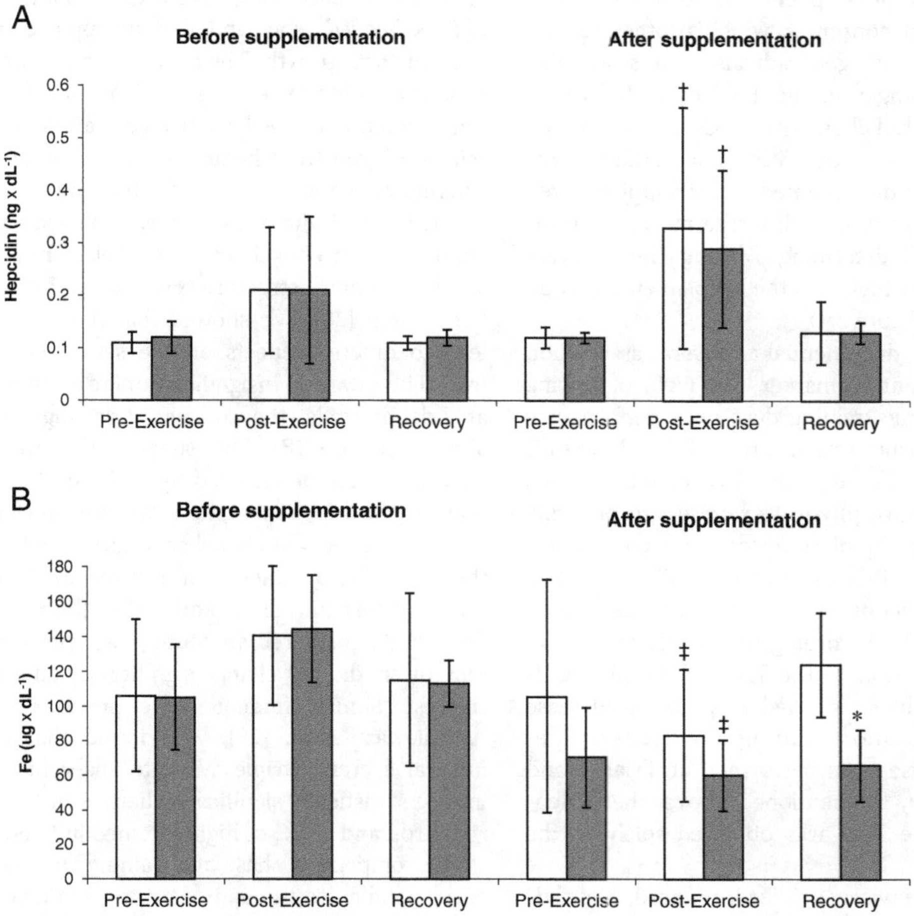

Figure 3 Changes in hepcidin (A) and serum iron (B) levels during exercise tests performed before and after the supplementation (mean ± *SD*). *Note*: Fe = iron; (gray square) - PLA = placebo group; □ - SUPL = supplemented group; * $P < .05$ compared to the placebo group; † $P < .05$ compared to the pre-exercise values; ‡ $P < .05$ compared to the pre-supplementation values.

Table 6 Changes in iron metabolism during exhaustive exercise before and after supplementation

Variables	*Before supplementation*			*After supplementation*			*P (ANOVA)*		
	Pre-exercise x ± SD	*Post-exercise x ± SD*	*Recovery x ± SD*	*Pre-exercise x ± SD*	*Post-exercise x ± SD*	*Recovery x ± SD*	*Exercise*	*supplement*	*Exercise × supplement*
Myoglobin (ng x mL^{-1})							0.0129	0.835	0.982
SUPL	203 ± 63.8	346 ± 169.5*	230 ± 68.6	228 ± 168.7	405 ± 283.5	300 ± 110.5			
PLA	216 ± 21.0	318 ± 109.4*	201 ± 39.6	267 ± 192.5	409 ± 340.2	348 ± 233.4			
Ferritin (ng x dL^{-1})							0.062	0.083	0.069
SUPL	74.25 ± 51.18	71.22 ± 29.23	80.00 ± 52.15	80.87 ± 31.02	89.67 ± 33.14	82.44 ± 28.54			
PLA	87.80 ± 27.25	91.00 ± 32.34	87.20 ± 18.58	76.80 ± 24.27	84.00 ± 33.35	77.80 ± 19.25			
TIBC (ug x dL^{-1})							0.087	0.865	0.076
SUPL	320.8 ±32.83	334.2 ± 34.57	325.2 ± 26.82	326.8 ±52.63	339.2 ± 24.37	320.5 ± 31.72			
PLA	316.7 ± 26.36	331.4 ± 25.97	328.3 ± 24.3	330.4 ± 48.3	349.5 ± 48.3	329.8 ± 40.6			
UIBC (ug x dL^{-1})							0.498	0.693	0.735
SUPL	175.0 ± 17.92	189.3 ± 18.87	177.6 ± 14.66	183.5 ± 39.72	194.6 ± 54.87	179.7 ± 38.95			
PLA	179.3 ± 11.62	192.3 ± 28.41	173.4 ± 15.54	190.1 ± 43.34	198.3 ± 49.73	188.43 ± 43.65			

The values represent the mean ±SD. *Abbreviations: TIBC* total iron-binding capacity, *UIBC* unsaturated iron-binding capacity, *PLA* placebo group, *SUPL* supplemented group; *$P < 0.05$ relative to pre-exercise - post-exercise.

levels of antioxidants (total phenolics, total flavonoids, and proanthocyanidin contents), which protect against damage from reactive oxygen radicals. Our study also showed favorable changes in the TAC of athletes who supplemented with chokeberry juice. Compared to the respective pre-supplementation values, a significant increase in the TAC was documented in the supplemented group during the recovery period; furthermore, the post-supplementation TAC determined during the recovery period was significantly higher in the supplemented group than in the controls (Figure 2A).

Braakhuis et al. [20], documented an inverse association between the antioxidant biomarker, the TAC, of rowing athletes and the chronic training dose on a performance test. A similar relationship was also reported by Margonis et al. [21]. The changes in the plasma level of antioxidants, observed after exhaustive physical exercise, are probably associated with a transfer of some of these compounds from tissues to plasma. Previous *in vivo* studies identified uric acid, an end-product of purine metabolism, as a major plasma antioxidant [22]. According to Wayner et al. [23], the uric acid contribution to the TAC of the plasma is about 35-65%. Our athletes showed a significant increase in uric acid concentrations during the recovery periods after the exercise tests performed at Trials I and II (Table 6). However, as mentioned above, the concomitant increase in the TAC was observed solely in the supplemented group.

A relative balance between oxidized, reduced, and radical forms of antioxidants is maintained by flavonoids and constitutes an important element of protection against increased concentrations of reactive oxygen species. However, the role of flavonoids in the chelation of iron ions seems even more important, as this prevents formation of a highly reactive hydroxyl radical, a potent inductor of peroxidation of polyunsaturated fatty acids and polymerization of proteins, which are both present in erythrocyte membranes at high concentrations.

Previous studies [24,25] revealed that structural alterations of erythrocyte membranes, resulting from enhanced generation of free radicals in response to exhaustive or long-term physical exercise, may lead to severe post-exercise hemolysis, which results in an increase in the plasma level of free iron. Under physiological conditions, the iron of heme proteins (hemoglobin, myoglobin, cytochromes) is protected inside a cell. However, it can be released as a result of cellular injury. Therefore, control of free Fe ions represents an important aspect of iron metabolism. Two important biological mechanisms are postulated to be involved in this process. The first is associated with preventing formation of highly toxic reactive oxygen species via the control of free or weakly-bound iron ions, and the second is aimed at protection of iron resources against bacterial degradation [26,27]. A number of bacterial species (e.g. *Mycobacterium tuberculosis, Salmonella* spp., and *Yersinia* spp.) require Fe^{3+}/Fe^{2+} ions for their growth. The decrease in pH, associated with exhaustive physical exercise and post-exercise inflammation (secretion of LA by activated granulocytes) promotes release of iron from hemoglobin, ferritin, and transferrin. Therefore, binding Fe^{+2} and other intermediate metals seems to be of vital importance. Anthocyanins, the major component of chokeberry, can chelate iron due to their specific chemical structure (presence of hydroxyl group in the C-ring) [28]. We showed that the same exercise test lead to different effects on the serum concentration of iron. There was an insignificant increase in this parameter at Trial I; while, the concentration slightly decrease at Trial II (Figure 3B). This suggests that the dynamics of serum iron are determined by a phase of training, rather than by the supplementation. We also did not document significant effects of chokeberry juice supplementation on the remaining parameters of iron metabolism, namely the levels of ferritin, TIBC and UIBC (Table 6). Although ferritin is considered an acute phase protein, its level in our rowers did not change significantly after the ergometric test. Similar findings were previously reported by Antosiewicz et al. [29], who found that high-intensity interval exercise (triple Wingate anaerobic test) did not induce statistically significant changes in the levels of ferritin, iron and TIBC of highly trained judo athletes.

The competitive phase of a training cycle (i.e. the period corresponding to the end of our experiment) was characterized by a markedly greater proportion of high-intensity training (Table 4) and a higher severity of post-exercise inflammation. This was also reflected by a post-exercise increase in the TNF-alpha level (Figure 1B). Other authors [30,31] also observed elevated TNF-alpha levels in rowing athletes exposed to intensive training loads.

At the end of our experiment, the levels of iron determined during the recovery period were significantly higher in the supplemented rowers than in the controls (Figure 3B). In addition, we documented a significantly lower pre-exercise level of TNF-alpha in the supplemented group when compared to the pre-supplementation level. Furthermore, the TNF-alpha level at recovery turned out to be significantly lower in the supplemented group than in the controls (Figure 1B). We also observed an inverse correlation between the post-supplementation levels of iron and TNF-alpha (−0.476; $p < 0.05$). According to a prior report, anthocyanins can attenuate the activity of major inflammatory enzymes, and prevent adhesion of leukocytes and their interaction with vascular endothelial cells via inactivation with TNF-alpha [32]. The administration of blackcurrant extract (equivalent to 48 g of blackcurrants) to individuals performing 30-minutes of exercise on a rowing ergometer with an intensity corresponding to 80% VO_{2max} was reflected by a markedly less pronounced post-exercise increase in TNF-alpha and IL-6 levels [33]. We did not document a significant influence of chokeberry juice on the level of IL-6 (Figure 1A). However, the concentration of this cytokine proved to be significantly modulated by physical exercise, which caused an increase in this parameter, irrespective of the analyzed group and trial. The level of IL-6 was positively correlated with the hepcidin level, both prior to (0.737; $p < 0.05$) and after the supplementation (0.506; $p < 0.05$). Hepcidin is considered an acute phase protein, as its synthesis in hepatocytes is induced by IL-6 [34]. This hormone is postulated to be an important mediator of post-exercise iron deficiency, which is observed in response to a number of physiological processes, such as inflammation, hypoxia, and an elevated concentration of Fe resulting from enhanced hemolysis, e.g. due to oxidative injury of erythrocyte membranes [3,35]. We observed a post-exercise increase in the activity of hepcidin solely at Trial II, i.e. after supplementation (Figure 3A). Perhaps, this was the reason behind the post-exercise decreases in the serum level of iron observed after supplementation.

We are well aware of potential limitations of the study. While we measured the parameters of iron metabolism, also determination of the markers of post-exercise hemolysis and its severity, such as bilirubin, haptoglobin, methemalbumin and free hemoglobin, would add considerably to our knowledge of beneficial effects of chokeberry juice in elite athletes.

Conclusions

We showed that the administration of a natural plant preparation with strong antioxidant potential, chokeberry juice, lead to an increase in the TAC of the plasma, as well as a decrease in the TNF-alpha level during the recovery period. Moreover, we observed a concomitant significant increase in the serum level of iron in the supplemented athletes. These results confirm the beneficial effects of chokeberry juice compounds in reducing the consequences of an intensive training load. Our findings justify the use of chokeberry juice in the supplementation of athletes undergoing maximal exercise.

Abbreviations

ELISA: Enzyme-linked immunosorbent assay; IL-6: Interleukin 6; LA: Lactic acid; RDA: Recommended dietary allowance; RRLC: Rapid resolution liquid chromatography; TAC: Total antioxidant capacity; TIBC: Total iron-binding capacity; TNF-alpha: Tumor necrosis factor alpha; UIBC: Unsaturated iron-binding capacity.

Competing interests

The authors declare that they have no competing interests.

Authors' contributions

ASS designed and supervised the study, secured funding, analyzed the data and drafted the manuscript. PB covered all practical aspects of the study and performed the statistical analysis. ŁPS conceived the study, participated in its design, coordinated and assisted in drafting the manuscript. JS determined the chromatographic parameters. All authors read and approved the final manuscript.

Acknowledgments

This work was supported by the State Committee for Scientific Research under Grant 4 P05D 02915.

Author details

[1]Department of Morphological and Health Sciences; Faculty of Physical Culture in Gorzów Wlkp, University School of Physical Education in Poznań, 13 Estkowskiego Str., 66 – 400 Gorzów Wlkp, Poland. [2]Department of Water Sports; Branch in Gorzów Wlkp, Faculty of Physical Culture, Gorzów, Poland. [3]School of Humanities, King Stanislaw Leszczynski in Leszno, Leszno, Poland. [4]Department of Hygiene, University School of Physical Education in Poznań, Poznań, Poland.

References

1. Chatard JC, Mujika II, Guy CC, Lacour JR: **Anaemia and iron deficiency in athletes: practical recommendations for treatment.** *Sports Med* 1999, **27**(4):229–240.
2. Reeder B, Wilson M: **The effects of pH on the mechanism of hydrogen peroxide and lipid hydroperoxide consumption by myoglobin: a role for the protonated ferryl species.** *Free Radic Biol Med* 2001, **30**(11):1311–1318.
3. Peeling P, Dawson B, Goodman C, Landers G, Trinder D: **Athletic induced iron deficiency: new insights into the role of inflammation, cytokines and hormones.** *Eur J Appl Physiol* 2008, **103**(4):381–391.
4. Peeling P, Dawson B, Goodman C, Landers G, Wiegerinck E, Swinkels D, Trinder D: **Training surface and intensity: inflammation, hemolysis, and hepcidin expression.** *Med Sci Sports Exerc* 2009, **41**(5):1138–1145.
5. Kong W, Gao G, Chang Y: **Hepcidin and sports anemia.** *Cell Biosci* 2014, **4**:19.
6. Seeram NP, Nair MG: **Inhibition of lipid peroxidation and structure-activity-related studies of the dietary constituents anthocyanins, anthocyanidins, and catechins.** *J Agric Food Chem* 2002, **50**(19):5308–5312.
7. Qin B, Anderson R: **An extract of chokeberry attenuates weight gain and modulates insulin, adipogenic and inflammatory signalling pathways in epididymal adipose tissue of rats fed a fructose-rich diet.** *Br J Nutr* 2012, **108**(4):581–587.
8. Ohgami K, Ilieva I, Shiratori K, Koyama Y, Jin X, Yoshida K, Kase S, Kitaichi N, Suzuki Y, Tanaka T, Ohno S: **Anti-inflammatory effects of aronia extract on rat endotoxin-induced uveitis.** *Invest Ophthalmol Vis Sci* 2005, **46**(1):275–281.
9. Naruszewicz M, Laniewska I, Millo B, Dłuzniewski M: **Combination therapy of statin with flavonoids rich extract from chokeberry fruits enhanced reduction in cardiovascular risk markers in patients after myocardial infraction (MI).** *Atherosclerosis* 2007, **194**(2):e179–e184.
10. Ziemlański S: **Norm of the man's nutrition.** Warszawa: PZWL; 2001.
11. Groussard CC, Rannou BF, Machefer GG, Chevanne MM, Vincent SS, Sergent OO, Cillard J, Gratas DA: **Changes in blood lipid peroxidation markers and antioxidants after a single sprint anaerobic exercise.** *Eur J Appl Physiol* 2003, **89**(1):14–20.
12. Fiorani M, Accorsi A, Cantoni O: **Human red blood cells as a natural flavonoid reservoir.** *Free Radic Res* 2003, **37**(12):1331–1338.
13. Arora AA, Strasburg GM, Nair MG, Byrem TM: **Modulation of liposomal membrane fluidity by flavonoids and isoflavonoids.** *Arch Biochem Biophys* 2000, **373**(1):102–109.
14. Erlejman A, Verstraeten S, Fraga C, Oteiza P: **The interaction of flavonoids with membranes: potential determinant of flavonoid antioxidant effects.** *Free Radic Res* 2004, **38**(12):1311–1320.
15. Bonarska-Kujawa D, Pruchnik H, Oszmiański J, Sarapuk J, Kleszczyńska H: **Changes caused by fruit extracts in the lipid phase of biological and model membranes.** *Food Biophys* 2011, **6**(1):58–67.
16. Clemetson CB: **Vitamin C/author, C. Alan B. Clemetson.** Boca Raton, Fla: CRC Press; 1989.
17. Block G, Henson D, Levine M: **Vitamin C: a new look.** *Ann Intern Med* 1991, **114**(10):909–910.
18. Heidi G, Eleonora B, Leif S, Mogens A: **Antioxidant synergism between fruit juice and α -tocopherol. A comparison between high phenolic black chokeberry (Aronia melanocarpa) and high ascorbic blackcurrant (Ribes nigrum).** *Eur Food Res Technol* 2008, **226**(4):737–743.

19. Hwang S, Yoon W, Lee O, Cha S, Kim J: **Radical-scavenging-linked antioxidant activities of extracts from black chokeberry and blueberry cultivated in Korea.** *Food Chem* 2014, **146:**71–77.
20. Braakhuis A, Hopkins W, Lowe T: **Effects of dietary antioxidants on training and performance in female runners.** *Eur J Sport Sci* 2014, **14**(2):160–168.
21. Margonis K, Fatouros I, Jamurtas A, Nikolaidis M, Douroudos I, Chatzinikolaou A, Mitrakou A, Mastorakos G, Papassotiriou I, Taxildaris K, Kouretas D: **Oxidative stress biomarkers responses to physical overtraining: implications for diagnosis.** *Free Radic Biol Med* 2007, **43**(6):901–910.
22. Kaur H, Halliwell B: **Action of biologically-relevant oxidizing species upon uric acid. Identification of uric acid oxidation products.** *Chem Biol Interact* 1990, **73**(2–3):235–247.
23. Wayner D, Burton G, Ingold K, Barclay L, Locke S: **The relative contributions of vitamin E, urate, ascorbate and proteins to the total peroxyl radical-trapping antioxidant activity of human blood plasma.** *Biochim Biophys Acta* 1987, **924**(3):408–419.
24. Aaseth J, Birketvedt G: **Hemolysis and rhabdomyolysis after marathon and long distance running.** *Immunol End Metabol Agents – Med Chem* 2012, **12**(1):8–13.
25. Kobayashi Y, Nakatsuji A, Aoi W, Wada S, Kuwahata M, Kido Y: **Intense exercise increases protein oxidation in spleen and liver of mice.** *Nutr Metab Insights* 2010, **7:**1–6.
26. Cisowska A, Wojnicz D, Hendrich A: **Anthocyanins as antimicrobial agents of natural plant origin.** *Nat Prod Commun* 2011, **6**(1):149–156.
27. Ward R, Crichton R, Taylor D, Della Corte L, Srai S, Dexter D: **Iron and the immune system.** *J Neural Transm* 2011, **118**(3):315–328.
28. Hider R, Liu Z, Khodr H: **Metal chelation of polyphenols.** *Methods Enzymol* 2001, **335:**190–203.
29. Antosiewicz J, Kaczor J, Kasprowicz K, Laskowski R, Kujach S, Luszczyk M, Radziminski L, Ziemann E: **Repeated "all out" interval exercise causes an increase in serum hepcidin concentration in both trained and untrained men.** *Cell Immunol* 2013, **283**(1–2):12–17.
30. Rämson R, Jürimäe J, Jürimäe T, Mäestu J: **The influence of increased training volume on cytokines and ghrelin concentration in college level male rowers.** *Eur J Appl Physiol* 2008, **104**(5):839–846.
31. Main L, Dawson B, Grove J, Landers G, Goodman C: **Impact of training on changes in perceived stress and cytokine production.** *Res Sports Med* 2009, **17**(2):121–132.
32. Speciale A, Virgili F, Cimino F, Saija A, Canali R, Chirafisi J: **Cyanidin-3-O-glucoside Protection against TNF-Îł-Induced Endothelial Dysfunction: Involvement of Nuclear Factor-ÎōB Signaling.** *J Agric Food Chem* 2010, **58**(22):12048–12054.
33. Lyall KA, Hurst SM, Cooney JJ, Jensen DD, Lo KK, Hurst RD, Stevenson LM: **Short-term blackcurrant extract consumption modulates exercise-induced oxidative stress and lipopolysaccharide-stimulated inflammatory responses.** *Am J Physiol Regul Integr Comp Physiol* 2009, **66**(1):R70–R81.
34. Nemeth E, Valore E, Territo M, Schiller G, Lichtenstein A, Ganz T: **Hepcidin, a putative mediator of anemia of inflammation, is a type II acute-phase protein.** *Blood* 2003, **101**(7):2461–2463.
35. Nemeth E, Rivera S, Gabayan V, Keller C, Taudorf S, Pedersen BK, Ganz T: **IL-6 mediates hypoferremia of inflammation by inducing the synthesis of the iron regulatory hormone hepcidin.** *J Clin Invest* 2004, **113**(9):1271–1276.

20

Effect of an herbal/botanical supplement on recovery from delayed onset muscle soreness: a randomized placebo-controlled trial

Corey A Rynders[2], Judy Y Weltman[1], Sara D Rynders[3], James Patrie[1], John McKnight[1], Frank I Katch[1], Jay Hertel[1] and Arthur Weltman[1*]

Abstract

Background: We examined the effects of a proprietary herbal/botanical supplement (StemSport, Stemtech, San Clemente, CA.) suggested to increase circulating stem cells, decrease inflammation, and attenuate exercise induced muscle damage on recovery from delayed onset muscle soreness (DOMS).

Methods: Sixteen subjects (male = 7, female = 9; age 23.8 ± 10 years; height 171.9 ± 10 cm, mass 72.2 ± 15 kg) were randomized in a crossover, double-blind, placebo controlled trial to receive a placebo or StemSport supplement (6150 mg/day) for 14 days. DOMS was induced on day 7 for both placebo and active conditions in the non-dominant elbow flexor group with repeated eccentric repetitions. Muscle swelling (biceps girth), elbow flexor isometric strength (hand held dynamometer), muscle pain/tenderness (visual analog scale), range of motion (active elbow flexion and extension), and inflammation (hsCRP, IL6, and TNF-α) were measured at baseline and at 24 h, 48 h, 72 h, and 168 h (1 week) post eccentric exercise. The crossover washout period was ≥14 days.

Results: No significant condition-by-time interactions between placebo and StemSport supplementation were observed with regard to measures of pain ($p = 0.59$), tenderness ($p = 0.71$), isometric strength ($p = 0.32$), elbow flexion ($p = 0.45$), muscle swelling ($p = 0.90$), or inflammation ($p > 0.90$). Decrements in elbow extension range of motion 48 h post-exercise were less after StemSport supplementation (Δ elbow extension 48 h post; StemSport, −2.0 deg; placebo, −10 deg; $p = 0.003$).

Conclusions: These data suggest that compared to placebo, StemSport supplementation does not improve outcome measures related to muscle recovery after acute upper-arm induced DOMS.

Keywords: DOMS, Blue-green algae, Eccentric exercise

Background

Delayed onset muscle soreness (DOMS) occurs following a bout of unaccustomed exercise in both novice and experienced athletes. DOMS is associated with muscle pain, decreased range of motion, muscle fiber disruption, altered joint kinematics, decreased strength, and acute tissue damage; each of which contribute to an impairment in future athletic performance and/or predispose individuals to injury [1,2]. Activities that involve high force eccentric muscle loading (e.g. plyometric exercises, the lowering phase of resistance training, and downhill running) induce the most severe cases of muscle damage. Symptoms of diffuse pain and tenderness associated with DOMS typically subside within 5 to 7 days after the inciting event. As such, studies evaluating the time course of DOMS typically include post-exercise data collection intervals as long as 168-h (1-wk) into the recovery period.

Delayed onset muscle soreness is a multi-factorial process and potential mechanistic theories include both anatomical/physiological and biochemical components. For example, anatomical/physiological mechanisms include connective tissue damage and muscular micro-trauma, and biochemical mechanisms include inflammation, and

* Correspondence: alw2v@virginia.edu
[1]Department of Kinesiology Exercise Physiology Core Laboratory, University of Virginia, Charlottesville, Virginia, USA
Full list of author information is available at the end of the article

oxidative stress. Acute elevations in perceived pain and tenderness are the result of nociceptor stimulation in damaged muscle fibers and surrounding connective tissue [3]. Chronic symptoms of pain and tenderness are likely due to increased intramuscular pressure from the local pro-inflammatory response (e.g. IL-1β, hsIL-6, TNF-α, hsCRP, and others) which peaks in the early phase of recovery and typically persists for 5–7 days after eccentric exercise [3-5].

Therapeutic modalities for the management of DOMS related symptoms are numerous and include cryotherapy, stretching, massage, compression, ultrasound, oral non-steroidal anti-inflammatory drugs (NSAIDS), and exercise [2]. In addition, several dietary supplements have been tested (e.g. protein powders, vitamin C, fish oil, and chondroitin sulfate) with varying success (see review by Connolly et al. [6]). The present placebo-controlled study examined the effects of a proprietary supplement, StemSport (StemSport, Stemtech, San Clemente, CA.), on the severity and time course of DOMS following acute eccentric upper arm exercise. StemSport contains an extract from the botanical Aphanizomenon flos-aquae (AFA; blue-green algae), which has recently been shown to elevate human bone marrow derived stem cells [7]. Jensen et al. reported that a novel compound from AFA binds to the ligand-binding area of human L-selectin. L-selectin appears to play a role in cell adhesion and the release of bone marrow stem cells into the circulation [7]. Drapeau et al. recently hypothesized that bone marrow-derived stem cells may accelerate the tissue regeneration process in some animal models of injury and may play a role in recovery from muscle damaging exercise [8].

StemSport also contains a proprietary blend of herbal antioxidants, and anti-inflammatory substances (Table 1). Preliminary data suggest that supplementation with StemSport may accelerate tissue repair and restore muscle function earlier than would occur otherwise [7]. The manufacturer of StemSport claims that "by assisting in increasing the number of adult stem cells in the bloodstream the StemSport concept may help your body naturally repair, rebuild and recover faster, so you can return to activity and athletic participation more quickly" [9].

Many commercially available supplements are often promoted without conclusive research demonstrating their efficacy. This present randomized, placebo-controlled, crossover study examined the effects of StemSport supplementation on the inflammatory response, muscle function, and perceptions of pain and tenderness associated with upper arm delayed onset muscle soreness (DOMS). We hypothesized that compared to placebo, StemSport would accelerate the rate of DOMS recovery.

Methods

Subjects

Subjects were healthy males (n = 7) and females (n = 9) between the ages 20 and 38 years. Subjects were of normal weight (mean ± SD, Mass = 72.2 ± 14 kg; Body Fat = 24.4 ± 5%) and not currently participating in a structured resistance or aerobic endurance training program (resistance exercise was performed ≤ 30 min/day, 1 day/week and low to moderate aerobic exercise was performed ≤ 30 min/day, 3 days/week; subjects were asked to refrain from performing high intensity exercise resistance/aerobic training for the duration of the study). Exclusion criteria included a history of vascular disease, pregnancy, recent injury or surgery to their non-dominant elbow or upper arm musculature, soft tissue compression complications such as open wounds/broken skin of the non-dominant shoulder, arm, wrist or hand, neurological impairments, such as paresthesia or peripheral neuropathies, circulatory insufficiencies, such as diabetes, hemopheila, thrombophlebitis or phlebothrombosis, and regular use of over-the-counter and prescription pain and inflammation medications, or any agent known to treat the pain and tenderness associated with DOMS. The Institutional Review Board at the University of Virginia approved the study and subjects provided written informed consent prior to participation.

Table 1 StemSport ingredient list and purported benefits

Ingredient	Amount per serving	Purported benefit
1. Aphanizomenon flos-aquae extract	1000 mg	Increase the number of circulating stem cells; muscle repair [7,8]
2. Proprietary Herbal/Botanical Blend*	1575 mg	
Cats Claw	–	Antioxidant [16]
Mangosteen	–	Antioxidant [17]
Rehmannia	–	Anti-inflammatory [18]
Berry extracts	–	Antioxidant
Nattokinase	–	Anti-inflammatory/fibrinolytic [19,20]
Serrapeptase	–	Anti-inflammatory/fibrinolytic [20]
Curcumin	–	Antioxidant/anti-inflammatory [21,22]

*Specific doses not provided by the manufacturer.

Design

A study timeline is provided in Figure 1. Subjects were initially examined by the study physician in the General Clinical Research Center (GCRC) at UVA to ensure pre-screening eligibility. Eligible subjects were given a 14 day supply of StemSport or a placebo. Subjects and members of the study team were blinded to the treatment condition. After 7-days of lead-in supplementation, subjects returned to the GCRC to complete baseline tests of upper arm swelling, range of motion, and visual analog scales to evaluate perceptions of elbow flexor pain and tenderness. Blood samples were obtained for analysis of highly sensitive C-reactive protein (hsCRP), tissue necrosis factor-alpha (TNF-α), and interleukin-6 (IL-6). After baseline testing, subjects performed an upper-arm DOMS exercise protocol. Tests of upper arm swelling, range of motion, pain and tenderness visual analog scales, and blood draws were repeated 24 h, 48 h, 72 h, and 168 h (1 week) after the DOMS exercise protocol in each condition (StemSport/Placebo).

StemSport and placebo supplementation

The StemSport ingredient list is presented in Table 1. Subjects were instructed to adhere to the following daily dosing schedule according to manufacturer recommendations: 1000 mg of Aphanizomenon flos-aquae extract 3 times per day in conjunction with food (breakfast, lunch, and dinner) and 1575 mg of a proprietary herbal/botanical blend twice per day in conjunction with food (breakfast and dinner). Prior to the DOMS protocol subjects ingested an extra 1000 mg dose of Aphanizomenon flos-aquae and an extra 1575 mg dose of the herbal/botanical blend. The extra dose was ingested with water at least 1-hour prior as per manufacturer instructions. No food was ingested because the pre-DOMS blood samples were collected in the fasted state. The placebo was visually similar to StemSport but consisted of a biologically inactive substance (1000 mg of encapsulated corn starch). The time of day that the supplements were taken was standardized to meal time (e.g. breakfast, lunch, and dinner). Subjects were required to maintain a pill diary throughout the study and were instructed to forfeit any capsules not ingested during the study period. Over-the-counter analgesic and anti-inflammatory medications (i.e. Tylenol, Advil, Ibuprofen, Motrin, Bextra, Celebrex, etc.) were prohibited during the supplementation period.

An independent manufacturer (StemSport, Stemtech, San Clemente, CA.) packaged and the supplements/placebo. Supplements (placebo/active) were stored and distributed to subjects by the University Investigational Pharmacy. None of the members of the study team (except the pharmacist) knew the identity of the supplements during the study. The order of supplement consumption (placebo or active) was randomly assigned based on a code known only to the pharmacist and the study biostatistician.

Pain and tenderness

A pressure algometer (Wagner Instruments, Greenwich, CT) was used to assess the pressure sensitivity and pain tolerance of the soft-tissue 5 cm proximal to the elbow joint line of the biceps brachii muscle. Each subject received 0.91 kg of compression and recorded their perceived level of pain on a visual analog scale (VAS) from 0–10, 0 indicating no pain and 10 representing the worst pain ever experienced. Perceived tenderness of the biceps brachii was also assessed using the same visual analog scale. A standard plastic measurement tape with 1 mm gradations was used to measure the girth of the non-dominant arm 5 cm proximal to the elbow joint line.

Biceps peak force

Isomeric elbow flex strength of the dominant arm was measured at an angle of 90 degrees using a hand-held dynamometer (Hoggan Health Industries, West Jordan, Utah).

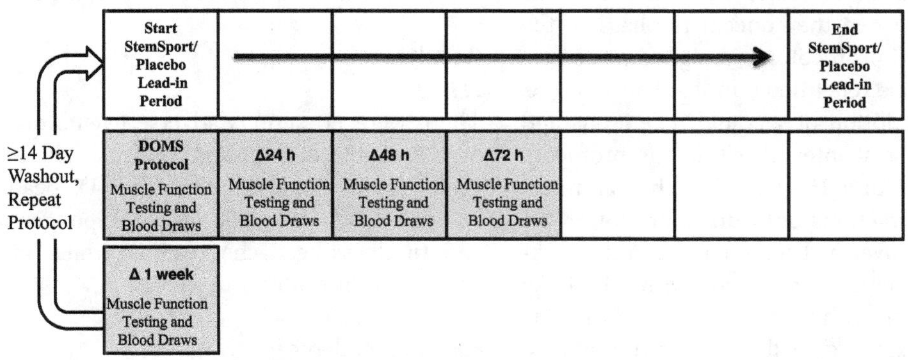

Figure 1 Study timeline. Subjects were administered either active or placebo for a 7 day lead in period. After the lead-in period, baseline measures of muscle function were assessed. Subjects then performed a standardized DOMS protocol for the upper arm. Stemsport/placebo supplementation continued for 7 days post-DOMS. Muscle function outcome measures were repeated for 3 consecutive days after the DOMS protocol and once again 7 days after the DOMS protocol. Subjects repeated the protocol (opposite condition) after a minimum 14-day washout period.

The test was performed in the standing position with the subject's upper arm resting against a wall to ensure exclusive contraction of the elbow flexors.

Range of motion

A standard goniometer (Model G300, Whitehall Manufacturing, City of Industry, CA) was used to measure the degrees of active elbow range of motion (extension and flexion).

Inflammatory assays

Subjects were fasted at least 6 hours prior to the blood draws at each time point. They were not allowed to consume any food and/or drink prior to the other baseline measurements or DOMS protocol. Water consumption was allowed, but the intake volume was not measured. TNF-alpha and IL-6 concentrations were measured in serum using high-sensitivity ELISA assays. The assay sensitivities were 0.5 pg · ml − 1 for TNF-α and 0.3 ng · ml − 1 for IL-6; the mean intra- and interassay coefficients of variation were 6.7% and 13.4% for TNF-α, and 7.4% and 7.8% for hsIL-6. CRP concentrations were measured by a chemiluminescent assay (Diagnostic Products Corporation, Immulite 2000, Los Angeles, CA), the assay sensitivity was 0.1 mg · l − 1 and the mean intra- and interassay coefficients of variation were 6.7%.

DOMS

After completion of the baseline tests above, subjects performed an upper arm DOMS protocol as described by Denegar et al. [10]. Proper positioning, timing, and form for the DOMs protocol were thoroughly explained by the study team and subjects were allowed to practice the protocol with light weights prior to the first supplementation period/actual day of testing. DOMS protocol prior to actually performing it. A preacher curl bench with adjustable height was used to isolate the biceps brachii muscle group of the non-dominant arm. Subjects repetitively performed all eccentric contractions, while study personnel performed the concentric phase of the bicep curl. The DOMS protocol was designed to be performed with continuous repetitions until exhaustion (i.e. there was not a prescription of sets and repetitions and there was no allotted rest interval within the protocol). Each subject started with a 15.91 kg dumbbell and performed eccentric contractions until unable to lower the weight under control over a three second count (if unable to perform one successful repetition with a 15.91 kg weight, subjects began with a 13.63 kg weight). The weight decreased in 2.27 kg (5 lbs) increments after a participant could no longer complete repetitions at a given weight all the way down to a final weight of 2.27 kg (5 lbs). The DOMS protocol was complete once the subject was unable to lower a 2.27 kg weight under control. Verbal cues were provided throughout the fatigue protocol, including encouragement to exert full strength and reminders about the minimum three second count. Upon completion of the DOMS protocol, each subject was provided with an arm sling to secure the non-dominant arm against the body with the elbow flexed at 90°. Subjects were asked to wear the sling up to the start of day 3 (72-hours post-DOMS exercise) and remove it only to perform activities of daily living (i.e. bathing, getting dressed, sleeping, driving).

Follow-up measures

Measures of pain and tenderness, muscle function, and blood draws for inflammatory markers were repeated 24-hours, 48-hours, 72-hours, and 168-hours (1-week) following DOMS protocol. After the 1-week post-exercise visit, subjects completed a 14-day washout period and then repeated the protocol exactly as outlined above with opposite treatment condition (StemSport or Placebo). Subjects were asked to maintain similar dietary patterns throughout the duration of the study.

Statistical analyses

Separate RM-ANOVA models were used to evaluate the effects of StemSport versus placebo on the primary outcomes. The primary outcome measures were change in perceived pain and tenderness (VAS scales), change in edema (girth), change in muscle function (range of motion and biceps peak force), and change in inflammation (hsCRP, TNF-alpha, and IL-6) 24-hours, 48-hours, 72-hours, and 168-hours post-DOMS. Treatment status (StemSport or placebo) was the between group factor and time was the within group factor. Baseline (pre-DOMS) values were used as covariates. Comparisons between conditions were tested by way of a Bonferoni adjusted linear contrast of means. A $p \leq 0.05$ decision rule was utilized as the null hypothesis rejection criterion for the individual adjusted statistical tests. SAS version 9.2 (SAS Institute Inc, Cary, NC, USA) was used to conduct the data analyses.

Results

Safety

There were no serious adverse events during the study period. Subjects reported unusual urine oder ($n = 1$), tiredness ($n = 1$), dry mouth ($n = 1$), headaches ($n = 2$), and nausea ($n = 1$) while on StemSport supplementation and tiredness/headaches ($n = 1$) while on the placebo. There were no subject dropouts.

Pain and tenderness

Perceived ratings of muscle pain and tenderness were significantly increased in both conditions for 72 hours post-exercise ($p < 0.001$; Figure 2A and B). There were no differences in pain or tenderness ratings between

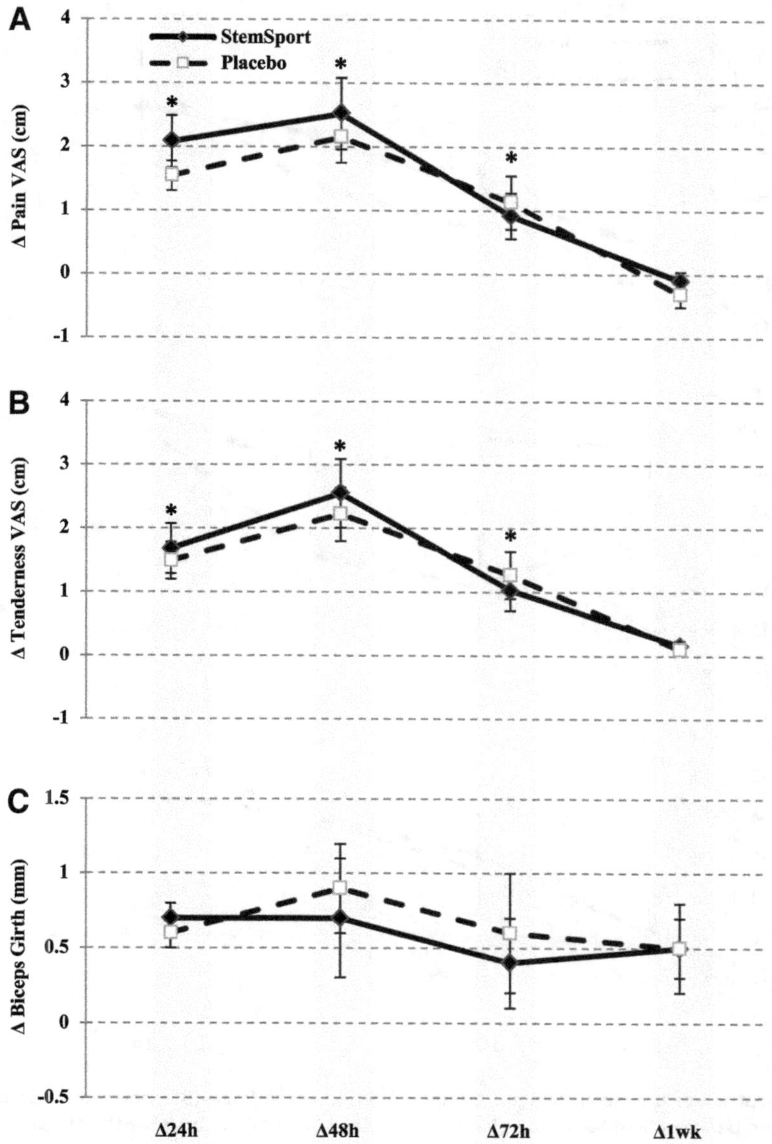

Figure 2 Baseline adjusted comparison of the mean change (±SEM) in (A) elbow flexor pain and (B) tenderness, and (C) biceps girth between StemSport and placebo at 24, 48, 72 and 168 hours post-DOMS exercise. *Perceived ratings of muscle pain and tenderness were significantly increased in both conditions for 72 hours post-exercise ($p < 0.001$; **A** and **B**).

conditions at any time point (baseline adjusted comparison of the mean change in pain and tenderness at 24, 48, 72, and 168 hours post-exercise, $p = 0.99$). Biceps girth, a measure of local tissue swelling, was increased for 48-hours post-exercise in both conditions ($p < 0.03$; Figure 2C).

Measures of muscle function

Biceps peak force was decreased for 72 hours in both the placebo ($p < 0.02$; Figure 3A) and StemSport condition ($p < 0.05$; Figure 3A). Significant decrements in elbow extension range of motion were observed for 72 hours during the placebo ($p < 0.001$; Figure 3B), and range of motion tended to be reduced during StemSport supplementation ($p < 0.14$; Figure 3B). Elbow flexion range of motion was significantly reduced in both groups for 72 hours ($p < 0.03$; Figure 3C). The only significant difference in muscle function between conditions was elbow extension range of motion (placebo, 10 degree decrement in elbow extension range of motion at 48 hours post-exercise versus StemSport, 2 degree decrement in elbow extension range of motion; $p = 0.003$; Figure 3B). Overall, less extension range of motion decrement post-exercise was found with supplementation of StemSport versus the placebo up to 72-hrs post exercise. All measures of muscle function returned to baseline values 1 week post-exercise ($p > 0.07$; Figure 3A-C).

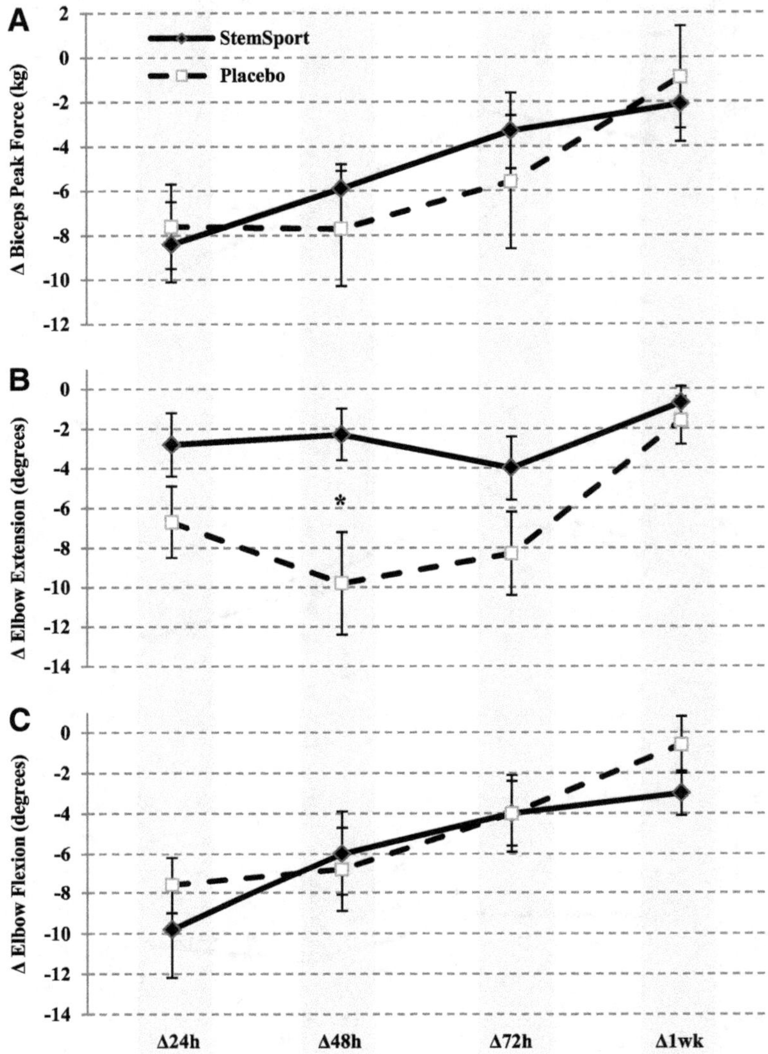

Figure 3 Baseline adjusted comparison of the mean change (±SEM) in (A) biceps peak force, (B) elbow extension range of motion, and (C) elbow flexion range of motion between StemSport and placebo at 24, 48, 72 and 168 hours post-DOMS exercise. *p = 0.003, significantly different from placebo. For biceps peak force, 0.91 kg equates to 2 pounds or 8.9 Newtons.

Inflammatory markers

Complete blood work was completed on 14 of 16 subjects and the data are presented in Figure 4A-C (missing data due to difficulties with blood draws and laboratory analysis). Systemic markers of inflammation did not significantly change from baseline values in either condition (hsCRP, p-value for time = 0.24; IL-6, p-value for time = 0.05; TNF-α, p-value for time = 0.24). There were no differences between groups for plasma markers of inflammation (p = 0.90).

Discussion

The main finding of the present study is that StemSport did not accelerate recovery from an acute bout of single upper-arm eccentric exercise in non-resistance trained adults.

StemSport contains the fresh water blue-green algae, AFA, which has been studied primarily for its antioxidant/anti-inflammatory properties [11]. The effects of AFA on inflammation are limited to animal studies [11]. To our knowledge, the present study is the first to examine the effects of AFA on systemic inflammation and other markers of DOMS in humans.

Most recently, AFA has been suggested to be a potential bone marrow stem cell mobilizer [7]. Studies from Jensen et al. (2007) and Drapeau et al. (2010) indicate that a novel compound from AFA appears to play a role in the release of bone marrow stem cells into the circulation, and it has been suggested that bone marrow-derived stem cells may accelerate the tissue regeneration process in some animal models of injury [7,8]. It has been further hypothesized that AFA plays a role in

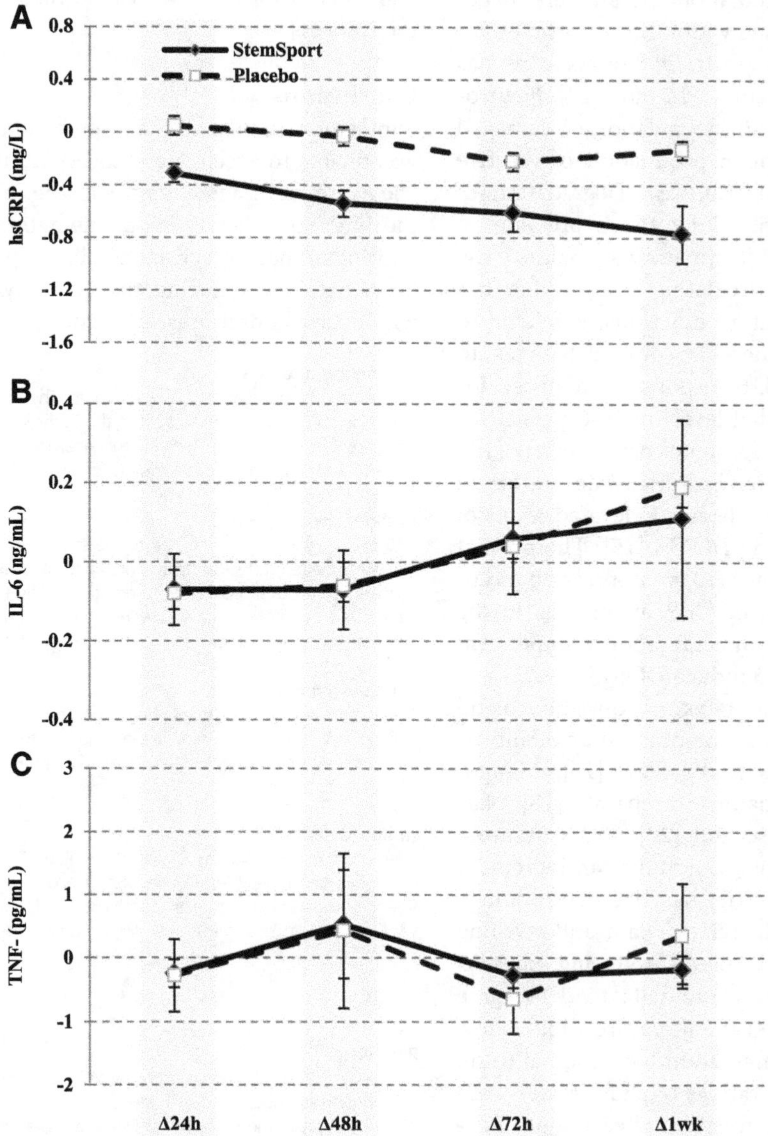

Figure 4 Baseline adjusted comparison of the mean change (±SEM) in (A) hsCRP, (B) IL-6, and (C) TNF-α between StemSport and placebo at 24, 48, 72 and 168 hours post-DOMS exercise.

recovery from muscle damaging exercise via increasing bone marrow-derived stem cells, although this has not been tested directly in humans [8].

In a placebo-controlled double-blind crossover study, a 5:1 concentrate of AFA concentrate fed to healthy volunteers (n = 12) produced a 25 ± 1% increase in number of circulating CD34+ stem cells at 60 minutes ($p < 0.0001$) [7]. In contrast, the placebo only produced minor fluctuations in levels of stem cells in the blood circulation over 2 hours. It has been hypothesized that acute increases in post-exercise circulating levels of stem cells may be beneficial for tissue regeneration and recovery [8]. Stem cell counts (e.g. CD34+) were not specifically measured in the present study, however, given that recovery of muscle function was similar between conditions, it is unlikely that any AFA induced change in circulating stem cells plays a major role in recovery from upper arm DOMS.

In agreement with previous studies in the literature, we did not observe an association between circulating inflammatory markers and others markers of DOMS (e.g. pain and tenderness) [12,13]. However, this may be related to the relatively small muscle mass utilized in our DOMS protocol which may not have been a potent stimulus for increasing circulating cytokines. Future studies should attempt to study AFA supplementation in response to an eccentric exercise protocol designed to produce a much larger inflammatory response (i.e. downhill running).

Leukocytes, neutrophils, and monocytes/macrophages are attracted to damaged tissue within hours of tissue injury and remain present for up to 24 hours, or as has been shown in macrophages, up to 14 days [14]. Neutrophils and macrophages assist in degradation of damaged muscle tissue primarily through production of reactive oxygen and nitrogen species (RONS). Degradation of damaged tissue is also initiated by the expression of many local pro- and anti-inflammatory cytokines (e.g. IL-6, TNF-α, IL-1β, etc.). Circulating IL-6, which has both pro- and anti-inflammatory functions, is related to the level of DOMS, and there is some debate as to whether the post-exercise IL-6 response is required for muscle adaptation [5]. Elevated levels of IL-6 persist for at least 48 hours after eccentric upper arm exercise [15]. Less is known about the post-exercise time course of TNF-α, although studies have detected elevated levels of TNF-α for up to 5 days during DOMS [15]. The present data do not support a role of AFA in suppressing circulating levels of IL-6, TNF-α, or CRP in humans in the basal state or in response to an acute bout of upper arm eccentric exercise designed to induce DOMS.

Besides AFA, StemSport contains a proprietary blend of several herbal substances potential antioxidant or anti-inflammatory properties (Cat's Claw [16], Mangosteen juice [17], Radix Rehmanniae Preparata [18], Nattokinase [19,20], Serrapeptase and [20], and Curcumin [21]; see Table 1). For example, Curcumin, an ingredient derived from the spice Tumeric, has been shown in a few studies to reduce DOMS related pain and swelling [17,22] and has a potential role is reducing obesity-related inflammation. However, our data tend to agree with the majority of studies in the literature which show that oral antioxidant supplementation has minimal to no effect on reducing subjective ratings of pain, tissue swelling, or decrements in muscle function after a bout of eccentric exercise [2,23-25]. It should be noted that data in the literature now support an inhibitory effect of oral antioxidant supplementation on the skeletal muscle adaptations exercise [26]. In addition, supplementation with the popular antioxidant ascorbic acid has been shown to delay the recovery process [24].

A possible limitation of this study was the use of DOMS to examine the utility of StemSport. It is possible that the amount of tissue damage associated with the DOMS protocol may have been too great for StemSport to have an effect. It is possible that if a less disruptive regimen was applied (e.g. strength training) StemSport supplementation may enhance chronic adaptations to whole body resistance training. Also, future studies may consider investigating the effects of AFA, independent or in combination with the other herbal substances. Strengths include study design (placebo-controlled, double-blinded, randomized trial) and measurement of both subjective markers of DOMS as well as bio-markers of the inflammatory process.

Conclusions

Supplementation with StemSport compared to a placebo was unable to accelerate recovery from upper arm eccentric exercise. In agreement with the majority of studies in the literature, dietary supplementation with antioxidant/anti-inflammatory substances likely provides minimal to no benefit for reducing the acute symptoms associated with delayed onset muscle soreness.

Competing interests

The authors declare that they have no competing interests. The study was funded in part by an urestricted gift to the Curry School of Education Exercise Physiology Fund from StemTech International, Inc. San Clemente, CA. FIK, JH, and AW served as scientific consultants for StemTech International.

Authors' contributions

CAR, JH, FIK, and AW contributed to the study conception and design, SDR and JM screened the subjects and provided medical oversight, CAR, JYW acquired the data, JP performed the data analysis, CAR, JH, FIK, and AW interpreted the data; All authors were involved in drafting the manuscript and have given final approval of the published version.

Acknowledgments

The authors would like to thank the subjects for their participation and the nursing staff of the UVA Clinical Research Center for assistance with the blood draws. We would also like to thank Noelle Selkow, PhD for her assistance with data collection.

Author details

[1]Department of Kinesiology Exercise Physiology Core Laboratory, University of Virginia, Charlottesville, Virginia, USA. [2]Department of Human Movement Sciences, Human Performance Laboratory, Old Dominion University, Norfolk, VA, USA. [3]Jordan Young Institute, Virginia Beach, VA, USA.

References

1. Lewis PB, Ruby D, Bush-Joseph CA: **Muscle soreness and delayed-onset muscle soreness.** *Clin Sports Med* 2012, **31**:255–262.
2. Cheung K, Hume P, Maxwell L: **Delayed onset muscle soreness: treatment strategies and performance factors.** *Sports Med* 2003, **33**:145–164.
3. Smith LL: **Acute inflammation: the underlying mechanism in delayed onset muscle soreness?** *Med Sci Sports Exerc* 1991, **23**:542–551.
4. Smith LL, Anwar A, Fragen M, Rananto C, Johnson R, Holbert D: **Cytokines and cell adhesion molecules associated with high-intensity eccentric exercise.** *Eur J Appl Physiol* 2000, **82**:61–67.
5. Pedersen BK, Toft AD: **Effects of exercise on lymphocytes and cytokines.** *Br J Sports Med* 2000, **34**:246–251.
6. Connolly DA, Sayers SP, McHugh MP: **Treatment and prevention of delayed onset muscle soreness.** *J Strength Cond Res* 2003, **17**:197–208.
7. Jensen GS, Hart AN, Zaske LA, Drapeau C, Gupta N, Schaeffer DJ, Cruickshank JA: **Mobilization of human CD34+ CD133+ and CD34+ CD133(–) stem cells in vivo by consumption of an extract from Aphanizomenon flos-aquae–related to modulation of CXCR4 expression by an L-selectin ligand?** *Cardiovasc Revasc Med* 2007, **8**:189–202.
8. Drapeau C, Antarr D, Ma H, Yang Z, Tang L, Hoffman RM, Schaeffer DJ: **Mobilization of bone marrow stem cells with StemEnhance improves muscle regeneration in cardiotoxin-induced muscle injury.** *Cell Cycle* 2010, **9**:1819–1823.
9. **StemSport® advanced formula.** http://www.stemtechbiz.com/StemSport.aspx.
10. Denegar CR, Perrin DH: **Effect of transcutaneous electrical nerve stimulation, cold, and a combination treatment on pain, decreased range of motion, and strength loss associated with delayed onset muscle soreness.** *J Athl Train* 1992, **27**:200–206.

11. Benedetti S, Benvenuti F, Pagliarani S, Francogli S, Scoglio S, Canestrari F: **Antioxidant properties of a novel phycocyanin extract from the blue-green alga Aphanizomenon flos-aquae.** *Life Sci* 2004, **75:**2353–2362.
12. Phillips T, Childs AC, Dreon DM, Phinney S, Leeuwenburgh C: **A dietary supplement attenuates IL-6 and CRP after eccentric exercise in untrained males.** *Med Sci Sports Exerc* 2003, **35:**2032–2037.
13. Houghton D, Onambele GL: **Can a standard dose of eicosapentaenoic acid (EPA) supplementation reduce the symptoms of delayed onset of muscle soreness?** *J Int Soc Sports Nutr* 2012, **9:**2.
14. Malm C, Nyberg P, Engstrom M, Sjodin B, Lenkei R, Ekblom B, Lundberg I: **Immunological changes in human skeletal muscle and blood after eccentric exercise and multiple biopsies.** *J Physiol* 2000, **529**(Pt 1):243–262.
15. Peake J, Nosaka K, Suzuki K: **Characterization of inflammatory responses to eccentric exercise in humans.** *Exerc Immunol Rev* 2005, **11:**64–85.
16. Sandoval M, Okuhama N, Zhang X-J, Condezo L, Lao J, Angeles F, Musah R, Bobrowski P, Miller M: **Anti-inflammatory and antioxidant activities of cat's claw are independent of their alkaloid content.** *Phytomedicine* 2002, **9:**325–337.
17. Udani JK, Singh BB, Singh VJ, Sandoval E: **BounceBack capsules for reduction of DOMS after eccentric exercise: a randomized, double-blind, placebo-controlled, crossover pilot study.** *J Int Soc Sports Nutr* 2009, **6:**14.
18. Tan W, Yu K-q, Liu Y-y, Ouyang M-z, Yan M-h, Luo R, Zhao X-s: **Anti-fatigue activity of polysaccharides extract fromRadix Rehmanniae Preparata.** *Int J Biol Macromolec* 2012, **50:**59–62.
19. Kim JY, Gum SN, Paik JK, Lim HH, Kim K-c, Ogasawara K, Inoue K, Park S, Jang Y, Lee JH: **Effects of nattokinase on blood pressure: a randomized, controlled trial.** *Hypertens Res* 2008, **31:**1583–1588.
20. Fadl N, Ahmed H, Booles H, Sayed A: **Serrapeptase and nattokinase intervention for relieving Alzheimer's disease pathophysiology in rat model.** *Hum Exp Toxicol* 2013, **32:**721–735.
21. Kim T, Davis J, Zhang AJ, He X, Mathews ST: **Curcumin activates AMPK and suppresses gluconeogenic gene expression in hepatoma cells.** *BBRC* 2009, **388:**377–382.
22. Menon VP, Sudheer AR: **Antioxidant and anti-inflammatory properties of curcumin.** *Adv Exp Med Biol* 2007, **595:**105–125.
23. Bloomer RJ, Goldfarb AH, McKenzie MJ, You T, Nguyen L: **Effects of antioxidant therapy in women exposed to eccentric exercise.** *Int J Sport Nutr Exerc Metab* 2004, **14:**377–388.
24. Close GL, Ashton T, Cable T, Doran D, Holloway C, McArdle F, MacLaren DP: **Ascorbic acid supplementation does not attenuate post-exercise muscle soreness following muscle-damaging exercise but may delay the recovery process.** *Br J Nutr* 2006, **95:**976–981.
25. Gomez-Cabrera MC, Ristow M, Vina J: **Antioxidant supplements in exercise: worse than useless?** *Am J Physiol Endocrinol Metab* 2012, **302:**E476–E477. author reply E478-479.
26. Gomez-Cabrera MC, Domenech E, Romagnoli M, Arduini A, Borras C, Pallardo FV, Sastre J, Vina J: **Oral administration of vitamin C decreases muscle mitochondrial biogenesis and hampers training-induced adaptations in endurance performance.** *Am J Clin Nutr* 2008, **87:**142–149.

The influence of commercial energy shots on response time and power output in recreational cyclists

John G Seifert* and David A Connor

Abstract

Background: Caffeine based energy shot products accounted for $1.3 billion in sales in 2011. Caffeine has been shown to confer numerous benefits during exercise and is oftentimes combined with ingredients such as carbohydrates and taurine in the hope of further performance improvement. The purpose of this project was to compare auditory response time, power output, and physiological responses between the ingestion of a CHO, PRO, caffeine supplement (CPC), a caffeine-taurine-niacin based supplement (CTN), and a placebo (PL) in commercially formulated products that make claims as to improving performance.

Methods: Fourteen subjects cycled an interval exercise of 70% VO_2max for 13 minutes and 90% of VO_2max for two minutes for a total of 120 minutes which was then followed by a six-minute power output (PO) task. Subjects ingested a total of 45 g CHO, 7.5 g PRO, and 375 mg caffeine for CPC while 512 mg caffeine and 1200 mg taurine were ingested for CTN throughout the exercise. The treatments were administered in a double blind, randomly assigned protocol. Response time was assessed by auditory response. Significance was set at $p < 0.05$.

Results: Average PO was significantly greater for CPC: 309 ± 60 W than CTN: 290 ± 57 W and PL: 282 ± 63 W. Response time was significantly faster for the CPC: 0.219 ± .049 s than CTN: 0.232 ± .060 s and PL: 0.228 ± .047 s. HR was significantly greater for CTN: 143 ± 16 bpm than CPC: 139 ± 16 bpm. RPE was significantly lower for CPC: 13.0 ± 1.7 than CTN: 13.5 ± 1.2 and PL: 13.8 ± 1.9. Blood glucose was greater for CPC: 5.5 ± 0.8 mM/L than CTN: 4.9 ± 0.7 mM/L and PL: 4.6 ± 1.1 mM/L. No significant differences were observed for RER.

Conclusions: The co-ingestion of CPC improved both cycling power output and auditory response time following 2 hours of moderate and high intensity interval cycling compared to CTN and PL. It is possible that the CPC treatment conferred not only a positive peripheral effect, but also a central effect. Even with a large caffeine dose, the combination of caffeine, taurine, niacin led to an inhibitory pattern which did not improve power output or response time performances over a PL.

Keywords: Performance, Energy shots, Caffeine, Taurine, Carbohydrates

Background

Caffeine is a widely used supplement. Caffeine based energy shot products accounted for $1.3 billion in sales in 2011 [1]. In the athletic realm, Del Coso et al. reported that 74% of elite level athletes reported ingesting caffeine prior to competition [2]. Caffeine may confer numerous benefits such as improved endurance performance, strength performance, reaction time, fat oxidation, and a reduction in subjective perceived exertion [3-8]. As with caffeine research, the ingestion of carbohydrate during exercise has also been extensively studied. Endurance and high intensity performance and carbohydrate oxidation are generally improved while markers of central fatigue are mitigated with the ingestion of carbohydrates [9-13].

There has been interest in whether the combining of carbohydrates and caffeine would have a synergistic effect. The supplied carbohydrate serves as a potential substrate while caffeine serves as a neurological stimulant. Hulston and Jeukendrup reported that the co-ingestion of caffeine

* Correspondence: john.seifert@montana.edu
Movement Science Laboratory, Montana State University, Bozeman, MT 59717, USA

and carbohydrate led to a 4.6% improvement over carbohydrate-only solution in endurance performance [14]. Those authors reported that caffeine increases the oxidation of exogenous carbohydrate during exercise. Acker-Hewitt et al. reported a synergistic effect when carbohydrates and caffeine were combined compared to either of the components separately and a placebo during a short term, high intensity cycling exercise [15].

Most of the previous caffeine research has focused on supplying caffeine in a powder or capsule form. Additionally, caffeine has been typically dosed on a per kg body weight either before or during the exercise. It is unlikely, however, that athletes and recreational athletes dose their supplement ingestion based upon their body weight. Such dosing may not be truly representative of athletes' habits during training or competition. Rather, products are typically ingested by a given serving size or volume of a given commercially available product.

It is quite rare, however, that one would find a caffeine-only product in the energy shot and drink market. Oftentimes, caffeine is combined with ingredients such as carbohydrates, taurine, and niacin in the hope of improving performance. Taurine is a non-essential amino acid which is found throughout the brain and skeletal muscle and serves as a neurotransmitter and neuromodulator [16,17]. In theory, combining caffeine and taurine, in the proper dose, should improve brain and muscle functions. Niacin is another common additive. It serves as a precursor to NAD and could have an influence in energy production.

Therefore, the purpose of this project was to compare auditory response time, power output, heart rate, and rating of perceived exertion between the ingestion of a carbohydrate + protein + caffeine supplement (CPC), a caffeine-taurine-niacin based supplement (CTN), and a non-caloric placebo in commercially formulated products that make claims as to improving performance.

Methods

Following approval from the Montana State University IRB, 14 subjects provided informed consent to participate in this project. Subjects' average age was 30.1 ± 3.9 y while average weight 74.9 ± 9.5 kg. Four females (mean weight and VO_2max were 66.7 ± 6.2 kg and 42.8 + 2.3 mL/kg/min) and 10 males (mean weight and VO_2max were 80.8 ± 6.4 kg and 51.6 ± 7.0 mL/kg/min) participated. Oxygen uptake was assessed using a three-minute ramped protocol to volitional exhaustion with the highest attained VO_2 used to calculate experimental workloads. All subjects were recreational cyclist who exercised regularly, but did not compete in races.

The two experimental treatments were a commercially available sports CPC shot containing carbohydrate, protein, and caffeine (Body Glove Surge®, 18 grams CHO, 3 grams PRO, and 150 mg caffeine per serving; PacificHealth Laboratories, Inc., Matawan, NJ), a commercially available caffeine-based shot (5 Hour Energy®; ~205 mg caffeine, ~480 mg taurine, 30 mg niacin per 57 mL serving; Living Essentials, LLC, Farm Hills, MI), and a non-caloric liquid placebo (PL) served as the control. Total caffeine ingested during the exercise was 375 mg for CPC and 512 mg for CTN. Subjects ingested a half of a serving (28 mL) at 30 minutes of exercise and then one serving (57 mL) of the given treatment after 60 minutes of exercise and then another serving (57 mL) after 90 minutes of exercise. The goal of this administration was an attempt to have maximal caffeine levels for the performance tests at the end of the two hour exercise.

Along with the given treatment, subjects also ingested 75 mL plain water. Treatments were administered in a double blind, randomly assigned fashion in a crossover, counterbalanced protocol. Seven to 10 days elapsed between experimental days. The PL was flavored similar to that of CPC and CTN. To further blind the subjects to the treatments, multiple flavors of each treatment were used.

Subjects cycled for 120 minutes which was then followed by a six-minute time trial performance task (see Figure 1 for a schematic of the protocol). The 120 min segment was divided into eight - 15 minute intervals. Each interval required the cyclists to pedal at a workload corresponding to 70% of their maximal oxygen uptake for 13 minutes followed by cycling for two minutes at a workload corresponding to 90% of their maximal oxygen uptake. Heart

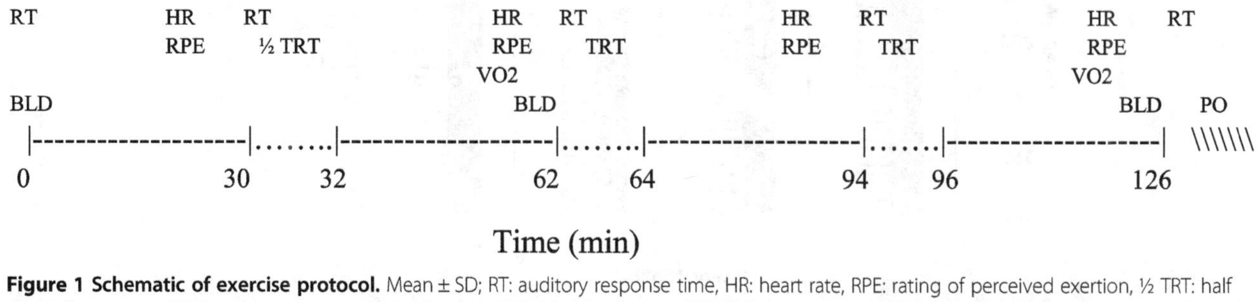

Figure 1 Schematic of exercise protocol. Mean ± SD; RT: auditory response time, HR: heart rate, RPE: rating of perceived exertion, ½ TRT: half dose of treatment, VO2: oxygen consumption collection, BLD: blood collection, TRT: full dose treatment, PO: six minute power output test.

rate (HR) and rating of perceived exertion (RPE) were collected at the 28 minute mark of each 30 minute phase. Rating of perceived exertion (RPE) was collected on the 6–20 Borg scale. Each 30 min phase was separated by a two minute break. Following the 120 minute reaction test, subjects completed a time trial test where they attempted to produce and maintain as great of power output as possible during the six minute test. A Monark 868 ergometer and SMI Power program were used to assess power output. Cycling resistance was set at 5% of BW.

During each 30 min break, an auditory response time test was completed by the subjects. Subjects dismounted the ergometer and sat in a nearby chair to complete the test. Subjects wore headphones that were connected to a computer. A computer based program was used to assess auditory response time (BioPac Systems, Coleta, CA). The response time test is a simple auditory response time test where subjects pushed a switch upon hearing 10 randomly spaced beeps. Times were analyzed by computing the average of the 10 beeps that were collected through the program. All subjects practiced and were experienced with the timing apparatus for this test.

Blood glucose was monitored by a fingerstick sample taken pre-exercise, 60, and 120 minutes (Bayer Contour, Whippany, NJ). Blood samples were measured in duplicate with the mean used for analysis. Expired air was collected for five minutes at 55 minutes and 110 minutes with data from the final three minutes of each interval averaged and analyzed for respiratory exchange ratio (RER; ParvoMedics, Salt Lake City, UT).

Subjects entered the lab four hours post prandial. Laboratory temperature was 21°C with 28% RH. All subjects ingested caffeine in their diets at some point during their normal day. The lowest intake was about 90 mg/day while the highest was about 270 mg/day. Subjects were instructed to consume similar diets and minimize exercise for 24 hour prior to each of their trials. Caffeine ingestion was not allowed on the day of testing. All subjects exercised either in the late morning or early afternoon to minimize diurnal variation.

Data were analyzed using a repeated measures ANOVA. Upon a significant interaction, Tukey's post hoc test was used to differentiate means at a given time point. Significance level was set at $p < 0.05$. All data are listed as mean (±SD).

Results

Data from one subject were not included in the analyses as he entered his final trial extremely dehydrated. He did not complete the final trial. Therefore, data was analyzed using 13 subjects.

Power output

Subjects ingesting CPC completed the 6 min time trial with a statistically greater average power output than when ingesting CTN and PL (Figure 2). Average power outputs during the time trial were 309.1 ± 60 W for the CPC trial, 290.2 ± 57 W for CTN trial, and 282.4 ± 63.1 W for PL trial. These differences amounted to 6.5% between CPC and CTN while the difference between CPC and PL was 8.8%. No statistical difference was observed between CTN and PL ($p = .08$). No significant differences were observed for the main effect of time or for the interaction of treatment by time.

Response time

Average auditory response time for the CPC trial was significantly faster than that of CTN and PL trials (Figure 3). Average response times were 0.219 ± 0.049 s for the CPC trial, 0.232 ± 0.060 s for CTN, and 0.228 ± 0.047 s for the PL trial. As with power output, no statistical difference was observed between CTN and PL ($p = 0.06$). The differences amount to 5.7% between CPC and CTN, 2.2% between CPC and PL, and 2.6% between CTN and PL. No

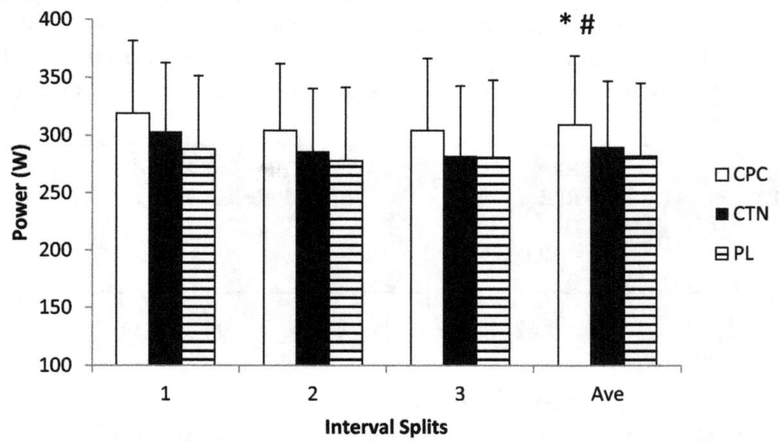

Figure 2 Power output. Mean ± SD; *: main effect of treatment, CPC is significantly faster than CTN and PL.

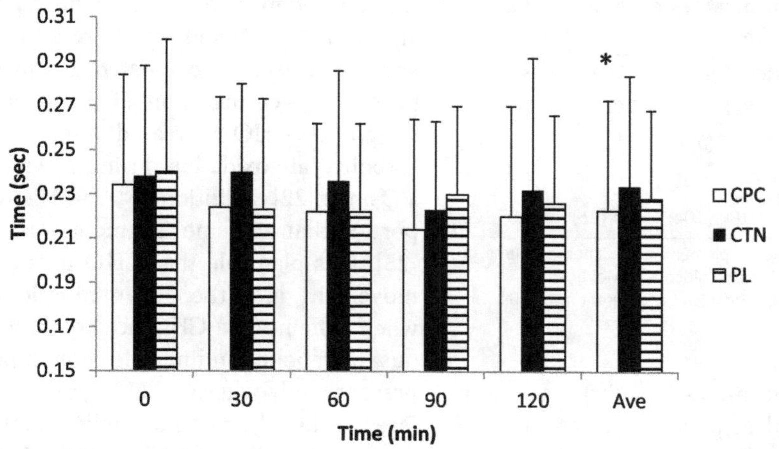

Figure 3 Auditory response time. Mean ± SD; *: main effect of treatment, CPC is significantly faster than CTN and PL.

significant differences were observed for the main effect of time or for the interaction of treatment by time.

Heart rate

Over the course of the 120 min exercise, the ingestion of the CPC led to a significantly lower average HR than CTN (Figure 4). Average HR for the CPC trial was 138.5 ± 16.0 bpm, 143.1 ± 15.6 bpm for CTN, and 141.0 ± 14.5 bpm for PL. No difference was observed between CPC and PL ($p = 0.08$) or for CTN vs. PL ($p = 0.09$). No interaction of treatment by time was observed. There was however, a main effect of time was observed where the average HR value at 120 min was significantly greater that at 30 min.

RPE

Average RPE for CPC, CTN, and PL were 13.0 ± 1.7, 13.5 ± 1.2, and 13.8 ± 1.9, respectively. Rating of perceived exertion for the CPC was significantly lower than CTN and PL. There was no difference between CTN and PL ($p = 0.1$).

Blood glucose and RER

Blood glucose (Table 1) at 120 min was significantly greater for CPC (5.5 ± 0.8 mMol/L) than CTN (4.9 ± 0.7 mMol/L) and PL (4.6 ± 1.1 mMol/L). No difference was observed between CTN vs. PL at either time point for blood glucose. No differences were observed between treatments, or time, for RER during the exercise (Table 1). Average RER for CPC was 0.87 ± 0.04), 0.87 ± 0.04 for CTN, and 0.86 ± 0.04 for PL.

Discussion

The primary purpose of this study was to investigate the effects of commercially available products, containing caffeine, on response time and cycling performance. The major finding of the present study is that a low dose carbohydrate, protein, and caffeine supplement (22.5 g/hr

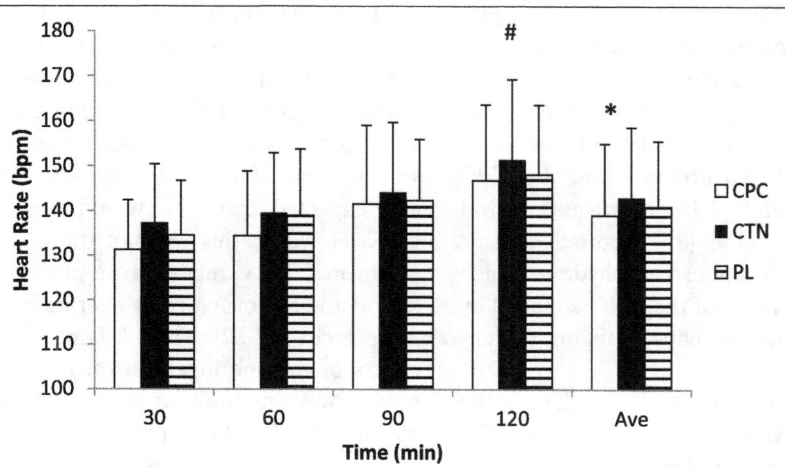

Figure 4 Heart rate during experimental ride. Mean ± SD; #: main effect of time, group average is significantly greater than 30 min group average. *: main effect of treatment, average HR for CPC is significantly lower than CTN.

Table 1 Blood glucose and respiratory exchange ratio values during 120 min of cycling

	0 minutes		60 minutes		120 minutes	
	BG	RER	BG	RER	BG	RER
CPC	4.6 (0.5)	-	5.0 (0.7)	0.87 (0.04)	5.5 (0.8)*	0.87 (.04)
CTN	5.0 (0.6)	-	4.8 (0.4)	0.88 (0.03)	4.9 (0.7)	0.86 (.04)
PL	4.6 (0.6)	-	4.7 (0.7)	0.88 (0.04)	4.6 (0.5)	0.85 (.04)

CPC: carbohydrate, protein, and caffeine supplement, CTN: Caffeine, taurine, and niacin supplement; PL: Placebo; BG: blood glucose (mMol/L), RER: respiratory exchange ratio; Mean (±SD); *: significantly different from CTN and PL.

CHO, 3.5 g/hr PRO and 188 mg caffeine/hr) resulted in improved power output and response time over that of CTN treatment (256 mg caffeine/hr) even though the CPC contains 27% less caffeine than the CTN treatment. In the present study, 10 of 13 subjects had a greater power output during the time trial when ingesting CPC compared to CTN, while 12 out of the 13 subjects had a significantly faster average response time at 120 min during the CPC trial compared to CTN. In contrast to previously published reports, even with the high dose of caffeine, the CTN treatment did not confer statistically significant power output or response time performance advantages over PL [5,18,19], although there were strong trends for CTN to result in improved performances ($p = 0.08$ and $p = 0.06$, respectively). However, the current results do support other reports that have shown no significant difference between caffeine and placebo [5,20,21].

Results of the present study support previous findings that there is a synergistic effect of the co-ingestion of CHO and caffeine on performance [14,15,22]. Power output was improved in the present study with CPC ingestion by 6.5% over CTN and 8.8% over the PL. Hulston and Jeukendrup reported that the co-ingestion of caffeine (5.3 mg/kg BW) with CHO during exercise enhanced the 45 min time trial performance by 4.6% compared with CHO only and 9.0% compared with a water placebo [14]. Those authors noted that caffeine increased exogenous CHO oxidation and glucose kinetics during steady state exercise. The results of the present study are rather surprising given the fact that the CTN treatment provided 256 mg/hr of caffeine while the CPC provided 188 mg/hr of caffeine. However, as Hulston and Jeukendrup [14] and Yeo et al. [22] reported, caffeine increases the oxidation of exogenous carbohydrate which would point to the fact that more of the CHO supplied by the CPC was oxidized for fuel, perhaps changing the endogenous substrate input.

The improvement in performance with the CPC in the present study cannot be explained by changes in RER, although blood glucose concentration was greater with the CPC than the CTN and PL trials. The RER data supports those findings reported by Graham and Spriet. [23] and Graham et al. [24] who reported that 9 mg/kg and 6 mg/kg caffeine ingestion did not alter RER during endurance exercise compared to a placebo. Yeo et al. reported that co-ingestion of 5 mg/kg BW caffeine with 48 g/h of CHO increased the rate of the exogenous carbohydrate oxidation during 120 min of cycling at 64% VO_2max [22]. Additionally, Van Nieuwenhoven et al. reported that caffeine augments carbohydrate kinetics [25]. It is plausible that CHO uptake from the gut and movement into the active muscle may be enhanced when caffeine and CHO are combined. However, previous metabolic findings do not support those of the present study where CTN ingestion did not lead to differences in substrate metabolism between treatments as assessed by RER and blood glucose levels. Thus, there must be an confounding interaction of ingredients in CTN.

While it was expected that the CPC treatment would most likely improve performance, due to the CHO content, it was surprising that the CTN treatment did not improve power output or response time performance over the PL, in contrast to numerous other studies [3-8,26,27]. Although the present study did not attempt to establish the mechanism of performance changes, there are a number of possibilities as to why performance was not improved with CTN. The 6.2 mg/kg and 7.5 mg/kg caffeine doses in the present study are on the high end of dosing that has been reported to induce positive results [4,26,27]. There is the possibility that the combination of taurine and niacin found in CTN minimized the influence of caffeine. Jia et al. [28] demonstrated that taurine reduced the excitability of thalamocortical relay neurons and activated the extrasynaptic $GABA_A$ receptors. GABA receptors are well known as inhibitory receptors. These authors reported that taurine actually exhibits a sedative effect on the brain. Barthel et al. noted that taurine neutralized the positive effects of caffeine in the premovement brain potentials in both the frontal and parietal regions [29]. Additionally, Lin et al. reported that a high ratio of taurine to caffeine induced lethargy and sleepiness [30]. The CTN product used in the present study contains 476 mg of taurine and 207 mg caffeine per serving which would be considered a high ratio. It was also expected that RER would favor fat oxidation with CTN. However, this was not the case. It is possible that niacin in CTN exhibited a negative influence on physiological and performance by altering the FFA response during exercise [31,32]. Thus, it is plausible that any positive effects of caffeine ingestion on response time and power output were neutralized by the addition of taurine and niacin to the CTN product.

The present study opted to use an auditory system to assess central fatigue. This would minimize the influence of gross motor movement patterns on this type of performance. Souissi et al. [33] fed subjects 5 mg of caffeine/kg BW and found that visual reaction time increased as well as peak and mean power with caffeine ingestion compared to the placebo trial. That study was performed with subjects completing a 30 sec Wingate test in the early morning hours without consuming breakfast. Subjects in the Souissi et al. [33] study also improved reaction time with caffeine ingestion by about 11% over the placebo trial. In contrast, subjects in the present study were four hours post prandial while response time was improved for the CPC treatment by nearly 6% over the CTN treatment. Ingredients of the supplements, exercise intensities (Wingate vs. 2 hr interval work), pre-exercise feeding minimizes the effect of caffeine on muscle energetics, and the type of response test used (visual vs. auditory) all may explain the differences in these two studies' results.

Conclusions

In conclusion, the present study attempted to mimic real life conditions by providing commercially available energy shots in doses that are used in 'real world' settings, by allowing subjects to be fed four hours before their experimental rides, and by assessing performance based on measuring peripheral, or muscular, and central fatigue. Although other rigorous assessments of central fatigue were not used, the use of auditory response time added practicality to the study. Study results demonstrate that, following two hours of moderate and high intensity interval cycling, ingestion of carbohydrate, protein and caffeine containing shot produced positive peripheral and central effects by significantly improving cycling power output and auditory response time compared to a caffeine-taurine-niacin shot and a non-caloric placebo. While response time is a novel measure of central fatigue, it may be considered a limitation of this study when compared to other tests. The expected responses on power output and response time were not observed when caffeine was combined with taurine and niacin. Although not statistically significant different from PL, there was a strong trend for CTN to result in improved performance. This poses the practical significance implications of this supplement. Additional research of commercial supplements is needed to not only further elucidate performance characteristics, but also on the mechanisms of possible antagonistic interactions. However, the results of these studies indicate that the combination of carbohydrate, protein, and caffeine improves exercise performance and would be of benefit for individuals participating in moderate to intense exercise. The caffeine-taurine-niacin combination may be problematic since the results of the present study indicate no performance improvement, either peripherally or centrally, when compared to a non-caloric placebo.

Competing interests

The authors declare that they have no competing interests. JS designed protocol, completed data analysis, and took primary writing responsibilities. DC assisted in protocol design, led data collection, and assisted in assays and data analysis.

Authors' contribution

JS designed study protocol, assisted in data collection, completed the data analyses, and led the writing of the manuscript. DC assisted in protocol design, led the data collection, directed data entry, and assisted in writing the manuscript. Both authors read and approved the final manuscript.

Acknowledgements

The authors would like to thank the subjects for their efforts. This project was supported financially by PacificHealth Laboratories, Inc. PacificHealth Laboratories was not involved in study design or data analyses of this study.

References

1. **5-hour-energy-places-400 mm-in-notes-to-fund-major-expansion** [http://www.forbes.com/sites/clareoconnor/2012/02/08/manoj-bhargava-the-mystery-monk-making-billions-with-5-hourenergy/]
2. Del Coso J, Muñoz G, Muñoz-Guerra J: **Prevalence of caffeine use in elite athletes following its removal from the World Anti-Doping Agency list of banned substances.** *Appl Physiol Nutr Metab* 2011, **36:**555–561.
3. Costill DL, Dalsky GP, Fink WJ: **Effects of caffeine ingestion on metabolism and exercise performance.** *Med Sci Sports* 1978, **10:**155–158.
4. Cole KJ, Costill DL, Starling RD, Goodpaster BH, Trappe SW, Fink WJ: **Effect of caffeine ingestion on perception of effort and subsequent work production.** *Int J Sport Nutr* 1996, **6:**14–23.
5. Del Coso J, Salinero JJ, González-Millán C, Abián-Vicén J, Pérez-González B: **Dose response effects of a caffeine-containing energy drink on muscle performance: a repeated measures design.** *J Int Soc Sports Nutr* 2012, **9:**21.
6. Desbrow B, Biddulph C, Devlin B, Grant GD, Anoopkumar-Dukie S, Leveritt MD: **The effects of different doses of caffeine on endurance cycling time trial performance.** *J Sports Sci* 2012, **30:**115–120.
7. Ivy JL, Costill DL, Fink WJ, Lower RW: **Influence of caffeine and carbohydrate feedings on endurance performance.** *Med Sci Sports* 1979, **11:**6–11.
8. Kovacs EM, Stegen JHCH, Brouns F: **Effect of caffeinated drinks on substrate metabolism, caffeine excretion, and performance.** *J Appl Physiol* 1998, **85:**709–715.
9. Coyle EF: **Fluid and fuel intake during exercise.** *J Sports Sci* 2004, **22:**39–55.
10. Davis JM: **Carbohydrates, branched-chain amino acids, and endurance: the central fatigue hypothesis.** *Int J Sport Nutr* 1995, **5**(Suppl):S29–S38.
11. Ivy JL, Res PT, Sprague RC, Widzer MO: **Effect of a carbohydrate-protein supplement on endurance performance during exercise of varying intensity.** *Int J Sport Nutr Exerc Metab* 2003, **13:**382–395.
12. Saunders MJ, Luden ND, Herrick JE: **Consumption of an oral carbohydrate-protein gel improves cycling endurance and prevents postexercise muscle damage.** *J Strength Cond Res* 2007, **21:**678–684.
13. Seifert JG, Kipp RW, Amann M, Gazal O: **Muscle damage, fluid ingestion, and energy supplementation during recreational alpine skiing.** *Int J Sport Nutr Exerc Metab* 2005, **15:**528–536.
14. Hulston CJ, Jeukendrup A: **Substrate metabolism and exercise performance with caffeine and carbohydrate intake.** *Med Sci Sports Exerc* 2008, **40:**2096–2104.
15. Acker-Hewitt TL, Shafer BM, Saunders MJ, Goh Q, Luden ND: **Independent and combined effects of carbohydrate and caffeine ingestion on aerobic cycling performance in the fed state.** *Appl Physiol Nutr Metab* 2012, **37:**276–283.
16. Neuringer M, Sturman J: **Visual acuity loss in rhesus monkey infants fed a taurine-free human infant formula.** *J Neurosci Res* 1987, **18:**597–601.
17. Turner O, Phoenix J, Wray S: **Developmental and gestational changes of phosphoethanolamine and taurine in rat brain, striated and smooth muscle.** *Exp Physiol* 1994, **79:**681–689.
18. Duncan MJ, Oxford SW: **Acute caffeine ingestion enhances performance and dampens muscle pain following resistance exercise to failure.** *J Sports Med Phys Fitness* 2012, **52:**280–285.

19. Turley KR, Rivas JD, Townsend JR, Morton AB, Kosarek JW, Cullum MG: **Effects of caffeine on anaerobic exercise in boys.** *Pediatr Exerc Sci* 2012, **24:**210–219.
20. Dean S, Braakhuis A, Paton C: **The effects of EGCG on fat oxidation and endurance performance in male cyclists.** *Int J Sport Nutr Exerc Metab* 2009, **19:**624–644.
21. Ryan EJ, Kim CH, Muller MD, Bellar DM, Barkley JE, Bliss MV, Jankowski-Wilkinson A, Russell M, Otterstetter R, Macander D, Glickman EL, Kamimori GH: **Low-dose caffeine administered in chewing gum does not enhance cycling to exhaustion.** *J Strength Cond Res* 2012, **26:**844–850.
22. Yeo SE, Jentjens RL, Wallis GA, Jeukendrup AE: **Caffeine increases exogenous carbohydrate oxidation during exercise.** *J Appl Physiol* 2005, **99:**844–850.
23. Graham TE, Spriet LL: **Performance and metabolic responses to a high caffeine dose during prolonged exercise.** *J Appl Physiol* 1991, **71:**2292–2298.
24. Graham TE, Helge JW, MacLean DA, Kiens B, Richter EA: **Caffeine ingestion does not alter carbohydrate or fat metabolism in human skeletal muscle during exercise.** *J Physiol* 2000, **529:**837–847.
25. Van Nieuwenhoven MA, Brummer RM, Brouns F: **Gastrointestinal function during exercise: comparison of water, sports drink, and sports drink with caffeine.** *J Appl Physiol* 2000, **89:**1079–1085.
26. Del Coso J, Estevez E, Mora-Rodriguez R: **Caffeine effects on short-term performance during prolonged exercise in the heat.** *Med Sci Sports Exerc* 2008, **40:**744–751.
27. Stuart GR, Hopkins WG, Cook C, Cairns SP: **Multiple effects of caffeine on simulated high-intensity team-sport performance.** *Med Sci Sports Exerc* 2005, **37:**1998–2005.
28. Jia F, Yue M, Chandra D, Keramidas A, Goldstein PA, Homanics GE, Harrison NL: **Taurine is a potent activator of extrasynaptic GABA(A) receptors in the thalamus.** *J Neurosci* 2008, **28:**106–115.
29. Barthel T, Mechau D, Wehr T, Schnittker R, Liesen R, Weiss M: **Readiness potential in different states of physical activation and after ingestion of taurine and/or caffeine containing drinks.** *Amino Acids* 2001, **20:**63–73.
30. Lin FJ, Pierce MM, Sehgal A, Wu T, Skipper DC, Chabba R: **Effect of taurine and caffeine on sleep-wake activity in *Drosophila melanogaster*.** *Nat Sci Sleep* 2010, **2:**221–231.
31. Howlett KF, Spriet LL, Hargreaves M: **Carbohydrate metabolism during exercise in females: effect of reduced fat availability.** *Metabolism* 2001, **50:**481–487.
32. Murray R, Bartoli WP, Eddy DE, Horn MK: **Physiological and performance responses to nicotinic-acid ingestion during exercise.** *Med Sci Sports Exerc* 1995, **27:**1057–1062.
33. Souissi M, Abedelmalek S, Chtourou H, Atheymen R, Hakim A, Sahnoun Z: **Effects of morning caffeine' ingestion on mood States, simple reaction time, and short-term maximal performance on elite judoists.** *Asian J Sports Med* 2012, **3:**161–168.

22

Nine–month nutritional intervention improves restoration of menses in young female athletes and ballet dancers

Karolina Łagowska[1*], Karina Kapczuk[2] and Jan Jeszka[1]

Abstract

Background: We hypothesized that an intervention designed to increase the energy and nutrient intake could serve as an efficacious method to restore normal menstrual functions in athletes and ballet dancers.

Methods: In this study, a 9-month nutritional intervention (NI) was conducted in 21 dancers and 31 athletes with menstrual disorders. Analyses of the body composition were performed, and the levels of LH, FSH, P, E2, TSH, T, PRL, SHBG, leptin, resting metabolic rate (RMR), energy and nutrient intake, total energy expenditure were estimated. The NI was based on an individual diet. The effects of the NI were controlled after 3, 6 and 9 months of use.

Results: The NI resulted in a significant change of the energy and nutrient intake. After 9 months, a significant increase in the LH level among dancers was observed, while in female athletes this effect was seen after 3 months of the NI use. The 9-month NI resulted in the restoration of regular menses in 3 dancers and 7 athletes, respectively. Women with regular cycles had a higher percentage of the fat mass (FM).

Conclusions: A non-pharmacological intervention in female athletes and ballet dancers with menstrual disorders can restore regular menstrual cycles, although restoration of menses may take more than 1 year. An increase in the body fat mass may be one of the most important predictors of restoration of menses.

Keywords: Body composition, Metabolism, Nutrition

Background

It has been shown that energy and nutrient values of daily diets (DD) and energy availability have an important place in the etiology of menstrual disorders in female athletes. Due to the start of physical training at a young age and high daily energy expenditure combined with strict weight limits ballet dancers are also in a high-risk group of such disturbances. Furthermore, the results of studies performed by other authors, regarding ballet dancers and female athletes from different sports disciplines, confirm that the knowledge on the potential effects of untreated menstruation disorders is limited [1,2].

There are several reports regarding the outcomes of a non-pharmacological nutritional intervention in female athletes with menstrual disorders. Arends et al. [3] indicated that a weight gain or BMI increase may be important predictors of menses restoration. These results were based on the outcomes taken from a 5-year retrospective study of 373 female athletes treated with non-pharmacological therapies, including an increased dietary intake and/or decreased exercise expenditure. In a case report, Mallinson et al. [4] compared and contrasted the responses of two exercising women with amenorrhea of varying duration to a 12-month nutritional intervention including an increased energy intake; however, without changes in the total energy expenditure (TEE) and training volume. The restoration of menses occurred on day 23 and 74 of the intervention for women with short- and long-term amenorrhea, respectively; however, the onset of ovulation and regular cycles was associated not only with an energy intake increase, but also with a weight gain increase. Those authors suggested that further research in larger samples is necessary to determine the primary contributors of menses resumption

* Correspondence: karolina@up.poznan.pl
[1]Department of Human Nutrition and Hygiene, Poznan University of Life Sciences, Poznan, Poland
Full list of author information is available at the end of the article

in exercising women with amenorrhea. Our study could be an answer to this suggestion. We previously identified 31 female athletes with hypothalamic menstrual disorders, in whom treatment with a nutritional intervention included an individual diet and nutritional recommendations without any change in the volume and intensity of training. Three months of a nutritional intervention resulted in a significant increase of energy and nutrient intakes, increase of energy availability and energy balance. Also the LH level and the FSH to LH ratio elevations, but without changes in the menses rhythm, were observed [5]. Then, we decided to include ballet dancers to this study and continue the controlled nutritional intervention to assess the extent to which long-term improvement in the nutritional status would allow for menstruation recovery. To our knowledge, this is the first study in which ballet dancers with menstrual disorders were treated with a non-pharmacological nutritional intervention.

Methods

Subjects

In this study, 45 well-trained female athletes with menstrual disorders (18 rowers, 12 synchronized swimmers, 15 triathlonists) from different sports clubs in Poznan and 27 ballet dancers from the Secondary Ballet School in Poznan were enrolled. The inclusion criteria were as follows: menstrual disorders within the last 12 months, at least 3-year training period, training session frequency > 4/wk., no serious medical conditions, no use of hormonal contraception or other medications that might interfere with the hypothalamic-pituitary-gonadal axis, no clinical diagnosis of eating disorders, no history of primary ovarian failure, hyperprolactinemia, thyroid dysfunction or polycystic ovary syndrome and non-smoking. Finally, 31 female athletes and 21 dancers completed a nine-month NI period (1 female athlete with hypothyroidism was excluded from the analysis, 2 athletes were excluded because of sports injuries, 11 withdrew their consent and 6 discontinued dropped out ballet school). A written informed consent was obtained from all participants and their parents. The study was approved by the Poznan Medical Ethics Committee (No.: 334/09).

Menstrual status

Each subject completed a questionnaire. In the first part of the questionnaire, questions were focused on menstruation: age at menarche, length of menses and history of amenorrhea. The second part of the questionnaire referred to sport activities: age at the beginning of training, training period, number of training sessions per week, hours of training per day and per week. Primary amenorrhea was diagnosed in females without the onset of menses by the age of 15, while secondary amenorrhea was diagnosed in subjects without menstruation for a 6-month period. Menstrual periods occurring with intervals of more than 35 days were defined as oligomenorrhea [6]. Similarly to Mallinson et al. [4], we described the recovery of menstrual function as the resumption of menses followed by at least 2 menses of less than 36 days in duration. Each subject underwent a gynaecological evaluation, including pelvic ultrasound and luteinizing hormone (LH), follicle-stimulating hormone (FSH), progesterone (P), estradiol (E2), prolactin (PRL), thyroid-stimulating hormone (TSH), testosterone (T), and sex-hormone-binding globulin (SHBG) levels assessment in order to exclude independent causes of amenorrhea or oligomenorrhea (such as pregnancy, primary ovarian failure, hyperprolactinaemia, thyroid dysfunction or polycystic ovary syndrome). The serum leptin level was also measured. In subjects with possible polycystic ovary syndrome, hyperandrogenism (elevated testosterone levels or LH to FSH ratio >3:1), thyroid dysfunction (normal range for TSH was established at 0.4–4.0 mIU/L), hyperprolactinaemia (PRL >25 ng/mL), other examinations to diagnose or exclude other causes of amenorrhea and oligomenorrhea were also performed [7,8].

Blood sampling and biochemical analyses

In subjects with irregular cycles, blood samples were collected between day 2 and 5 of the menstrual cycle (in the early follicular phase), and in amenorrheic subjects the samples were taken in a random manner. Blood samples were drawn between 6.00 a.m. and 9.00 a.m., following overnight fasting and rest. Subjects were instructed to abstain from caffeine and alcohol during a 24-hour period prior to blood sampling, and to refrain from strenuous exercise on the day of sampling. The levels of LH, FSH, E2, P, PRL, TSH, T and SHBG were measured by immunochemical methods using Chemiluminescent Microparticle Immunoassay (CMIA) and Microparticle Chemiflex Flexible assay protocols, and diagnostic sets and an ARCHITECT automatic analyser. The serum leptin levels were estimated using the Human Leptin Elisa by LINCO Research. All hormones levels were determined in a duplicate.

Body weight and body composition measurements

Height and body weight (BW) were measured using an anthropometer coupled with a WPT 200 OC verified medical scale (Rad Wag). During measurements, all participants were dressed minimalistically, and the obtained results were rounded to the nearest 0.5 kg and 0.5 cm, respectively. The analysis of the body fat mass (FM) and fat-free mass (FFM) was performed in the morning, following overnight fasting, in subjects lying in a supine position, using BODYSTAT 1500, as described by Heyward et al. [9].

Resting metabolic rate

Resting metabolic rate (RMR) was assessed by using a portable indirect calorimeter for 25 minutes (Cosmed K4b2, Cosmed, Italy). A face mask (Hans Rudolph, Kansas City, MO) covering the mouth and nose of the participant was attached to a bidirectional digital turbine flow-meter and fastened to the participant using a mesh hairnet with Velcro straps. To guarantee an airtight seal, a disposable gel seal (Hans Rudolph) was positioned between the inside of the face mask and the skin. The Cosmed K4b2 system was calibrated prior to each individual test according to the manufacturer's guidelines. Breath-by-breath O_2 and CO_2 gas exchange was measured and recorded in the portable unit's computer system. On completion of each test, the stored data were transferred to the Cosmed K4b2 version 6 computer software running on a Windows-based laptop computer. The data were then averaged over 15 second intervals and transferred to Microsoft *Excel* for further analysis. The morning before the RMR measurements, the Cosmed K4b2 was calibrated with a calibration gas mixture (16% O_2, 5% CO_2). The test was carried out with the participant in a comfortable supine position, at an environmental temperature of 21–22°C. All measurements were done in the morning (between 6 and 9 a.m.) following a 12 hours fast and a minimum of 8 hours of rest. The results of the RMR measurement were compared with the RMR predicted by the Harris-Benedict equation [10] and the RMR(kcal)/FFM(kg) ratio was also calculated. In anorexic women, a reduced ratio of measured REE value to REE value calculated with the use of Harris–Benedict prediction equation amounting to 0.60–0.80 during periods of low BW and prior to refeeding has been reported [11,12]. In this study, a ratio <0.90 correlated with energy deficiency.

Total energy expenditure and energy availability

Similarly to study by Reguła et al. [13] and ours previously study [5], each subject was wearing a heart rate monitor (HR) (Polar Sport Tester, RS 400, Finland), during a 3-day period, in order to estimate the total energy expenditure (TEE). The 24-hour energy balance (EB) was calculated as the difference between the mean of 24-hour energy intake, taken from seven consecutive days, and the mean of TEE calculated on the basis of three-day measurement. Energy availability (EA) was calculated by subtracting the exercise energy expenditure (EEE) from the total daily energy intake, and was adjusted for the FFM (kg) [6].

Nutritional intervention

Under the supervision of dieticians, dietary records from 7 consecutive days were obtained. Subjects had a regular contact with a registered dietician, who instructed them how to record a nutrient intake. All meals (including recipes and weights of products), snacks, beverages and fluids were recorded in a diary form using a Photographic Album of Products and Dishes [14]. DD were analysed with regard to their energy and nutrient levels (fat, protein, carbohydrate, calcium, vitamin D) using the *Dietician* computer software package, based on Polish food composition tables [15]. Next, all participants were informed about nutritional mistakes in their current diets and about consequences of nutritional deficiencies. Subsequently, as a part of the nutritional intervention (NI), we prepared an individual diet for each subject. During first months of nutritional intervention, the baseline energy value was increased by 20-30% per month, until zero energy balance and energy availability >40 kcal/kg FFM/d were obtained. Thus, the energy value of recommended diets ranged from 2500 to 3500 kcal per day. The wide range of values was dependant on individual features, such as: anthropometric measurements, age and sport discipline or actual training period and associated training intensity. Female triathlonists had the highest energy requirements, while in dancers the energy requirements were the lowest. The recommended level of nutrients intake was determined in accordance with the recommendations of the ACSM Female Athlete Triad Position Stand [6] and Jarosz et al. [16]. Also, the percentage of nutrients was mainly dependant on sport discipline, however female triathlonists received a diet providing minimum 60% of energy from carbohydrates. The percentage of energy taken from fats was 25-30% with saturated fats intake less than 10%; while proteins covered 16-18% of energy requirements, and at least one half of protein was of animal origin. During diet composition, the individual food preferences of each competitor and dancer, daily schedule, training hours, aversions and food intolerances were taken into account. However, highly-processed food, sweets, savoury snacks and fast foods were excluded. Diets were composed of 5 or 6 meals, including 3 main meals (breakfast, lunch, dinner) with additionally pre- and post training snacks. Also, an adequate fluid intake, including isotonic drinks, with a volume depending on quantity, length and intensity of trainings was considered. During dietary counselling sessions, issues concerning special foods for athletes, sports beverages, supplements, shopping tips, low-fat and low-calorie food, food preparation, dining out, iron, calcium and vitamins content in foods were also elaborated. After every month of NI use, the monitoring of following parameters was performed. Repeated assessments of TEE (1 day), EA, energy and nutrient values of DD (3 days) were conducted (data no shown). Next, after 3, 6 and 9 months NI effect follow-up was performed, and subsequently TEE (3 day), EA, energy and nutrient values of subject's daily diets (DD) (7 days), LH, FSH, E2 and P levels were reassessed. Those data were used for the purpose of statistical analysis.

Statistical analysis

Means and standard deviations of quantitative variables were calculated. The normality of the distribution was checked. Comparisons between data obtained pre and post 3-, 6- and 9-month time point of the nutritional intervention were carried out with the use of repeated measures analysis of variance. Comparisons between dancers and female athletes groups were carried out using a *t*-test for independent variables. Statistical analyses were performed using *Statistica 8.0* software (StatSoft, 2008). *P*-values below 0.05 level were considered statistically significant.

Results

The characteristics of subjects who completed the study are shown in Table 1. The duration of training period differed significantly between two study groups, being significantly longer for dancers. The daily training load was also significantly higher in ballet dancers; and they also obtained significantly lower, predicted and measured, RMR values. RMR/FFM ratios *100% also differed significantly between two above mentioned study groups. The age at menarche and T level, between dancers and female athletes, were also significantly different. The serum leptin level did not differ significantly between the groups, but both dancers and athletes had a lower value than the predicted laboratory range. In the group of ballet dancers, as early as after 3 months of NI, a significant increase of DD energy value associated with an increase of fat, protein and carbohydrates intakes was observed. The comparison of dancers' diet before and after the 9-month NI revealed significant differences with regard to energy value and an increased intake of all macronutrients. Therefore, significant changes in EB and EA were observed. In addition, EA was over the critical level of 30 kcal//kg FFM/d. After three months of NI use in the group of dancers, no statistically significant changes in body composition were seen. After another 3-month period, differences in BW, BMI and FFM (kg) turned out to be significant, which was also maintained at 9-month time point. After 3 months of NI in the group of female athletes, apart from significant energy intake increase, an important increase of total protein and carbohydrates intake, eliminating discrepancies between TEE and energy intake, and simultaneously the EA increase over the critical value of 30 kcal/kg FFM/d were observed. In contrast to dancers, no significant changes in BW, BMI and body composition, during the nine-month NI in female athletes were seen (Table 2). Amenorrhea was diagnosed in 5 out of all eligible dancers, and oligomenorrhea in 16 subjects. The nine-month NI use resulted in regular menses recovery in 3 ballerinas and in the lower number of dancers with amenorrhea. At the

Table 1 Baseline characteristics of study participants M ± SD

Parameters	Ballet dancers	Female athletes	P-value
Baseline characteristics			
Age (years)	17.1 ± 0.9	18.1 ± 2.6	NS
Age at menarche (years)	167.1 ± 4.5	13.0 ± 1.2	0.018
Age at the beginning of training (years)	6.7 ± 0.5	11.2 ± 3.5	< 0.001
Training period (years)	10.7 ± 1.2	6.8 ± 3.3	< 0.001
Number of training sessions per week (n/d)	5.2 ± 0.5	5.2 ± 1.0	NS
Hours of training per day (hours/d)	4.7 ± 1.1	4.0 ± 1.8	NS
Hours of training per week (hours/week)	24.9 ± 6.9	19.5 ± 7.2	0.009
RMR predicted (kcal/d)	1399 ± 60	1458 ± 56	< 0.001
RMR measured (kcal/d)	1198 ± 142	1354 ± 151	0.001
RMR measured/predicted × 100%	85.6 ± 9.1	92.8 ± 10.0	0.011
RMR measured – RMR predicted (kcal/d)	−201.0 ± 122.1	−105.0 ± 146.8	0.017
RMR/FFM (kcal/kg)	28.2 ± 3.6	29.0 ± 3.6	NS
Hormonal parameters			
TSH (μlU/mL)	1.96 ± 1.33	1.74 ± 0.80	NS
PRL (ng/mL)	16.38 ± 8.88	13.0 ± 9.33	NS
T (ng/dL)	72.95 ± 25.92	37.28 ± 21.85	< 0.001
SHBG (nmol/L)	71.62 ± 22.03	62.79 ± 41.91	NS
Leptin (ng/mL)	4.59 ± 2.78	6.25 ± 4.94	NS

Table 2 Effects of the 9-month nutritional intervention on the energy and nutrients intake, TEE, BW and composition M ± SD

Ballet dancers										
	0	**3**	**6**	**9**	**0 vs. 3**	**3 vs. 6**	**0 vs. 6**	**3 vs. 9**	**6 vs. 9**	**0 vs. 9**
Energy (kcal)	1640 ± 412	2130 ± 503	2300 ± 290	2368 ± 182	< 0.001	NS	< 0.001	0.03	NS	< 0.001
Fat (g)	57.0 ± 18.9	71.0 ± 19.7	72.6 ± 17.2	73.2 ± 15.9	<0.001	NS	<0.001	NS	NS	<0.001
Protein (g)	58.8 ± 13.3	77.3 ± 17.5	82.7 ± 9.7	85.3 ± 9.3	<0.001	NS	<0.001	NS	NS	<0.001
Carbohydrate (g)	222.8 ± 55.7	295.7 ± 72.0	328.9 ± 50.9	342.0 ± 33.2	<0.001	NS	<0.001	0.004	NS	<0.001
TEE (kcal/d)	2038 ± 279	2170 ± 372	2276 ± 236	2292 ± 245	NS	NS	0.005	NS	NS	0.002
EB (kcal/d)	−384 ± 267	−40 ± 267	24 ± 111	75 ± 147	NS	NS	<0.001	NS	NS	<0.001
EEE (kcal/d)	731 ± 207	758 ± 315	737 ± 129	750 ± 113	<0.001	NS	NS	NS	NS	NS
EA (kcal/kg FFM/d)	21.7 ± 7.2	32.8 ± 6.8	35.9 ± 5.5	37.2 ± 4.2	0.NS	NS	<0.001	0.017	NS	<0.001
BW (kg)	52.9 ± 5.8	53.2 ± 5.7	54.4 ± 5.0	54.2 ± 4.7	<0.001	0.001	<0.001	0.003	NS	0.001
BMI (kg/m^2)	18.9 ± 1.7	19.0 ± 1.7	19.5 ± 1.5	19.4 ± 1.4	NS	0.001	<0.001	0.003	NS	0.001
FM (%)	18.7 ± 3.2	19.2 ± 3.2	19.5 ± 3.7	19.3 ± 3.3	NS	NS	NS	NS	NS	NS
FM (kg)	9.9 ± 2.2	10.2 ± 2.3	10.6 ± 2.4	10.5 ± 2.1	NS	NS	NS	NS	NS	NS
FFM (%)	81.3 ± 3.2	80.8 ± 3.2	80.5 ± 3.7	80.7 ± 3.3	NS	NS	NS	NS	NS	NS
FFM (kg)	43.0 ± 4.8	42.8 ± 4.6	43.8 ± 4.4	43.7 ± 4.0	NS	0.042	NS	0.040	NS	NS
Female athletes										
	0	**3**	**6**	**9**	**0 vs. 3**	**3 vs. 6**	**0 vs. 6**	**3 vs. 9**	**6 vs. 9**	**0 vs. 9**
Energy (kcal)	2354 ± 539	2588 ± 557	2803 ± 387	2800 ± 321	0.041	NS	< 0.001	NS	NS	< 0.001
Fat (g)	92.2 ± 27.5	84.2 ± 20.4	95.0 ± 19.7	87.4 ± 11.1	NS	0.034	NS	NS	NS	NS
Protein (g)	75.6 ± 14.8	85.5 ± 15.6	90.8 ± 12.7	93.0 ± 10.7	0.004	NS	<0.001	0.038	NS	<0.001
Carbohydrate (g)	305.4 ± 78.0	372.2 ± 86.3	395.9 ± 59.8	410.2 ± 56.9	<0.001	NS	<0.001	0.038	NS	<0.001
TEE (kcal/d)	2642 ± 348	2638 ± 421	2744 ± 348	2741 ± 328	NS	NS	NS	NS	NS	NS
EB (kcal/d)	−288 ± 477	−51 ± 224	59 ± 72	59 ± 89	0.002	NS	<0.001	NS	NS	<0.001
EEE (kcal/d)	959 ± 174	905 ± 337	898 ± 283	868 ± 275	NS	NS	NS	NS	NS	NS
EA (kcal/kg FFM/d)	52.9 ± 5.8	35.8 ± 12.3	41.0 ± 8.6	40.9 ± 8.2	0.011	0.001	<0.001	0.001	NS	<0.001
BW (kg)	59.3 ± 5.3	59.6 ± 5.3	59.5 ± 5.7	59.4 ± 5.8	NS	NS	NS	NS	NS	NS
BMI (kg/m^2)	20.6 ± 1.4	20.7 ± 1.5	20.7 ± 1.6	20.6 ± 1.7	NS	NS	NS	NS	NS	NS
FM (%)	20.6 ± 3.7	21.0 ± 3.5	21.3 ± 3.4	21.2 ± 3.1	NS	NS	NS	NS	NS	NS
FM (kg)	12.2 ± 2.4	12.5 ± 2.4	12.7 ± 2.7	12.6 ± 2.5	NS	NS	NS	NS	NS	NS
FFM (%)	79.4 ± 3.7	79.0 ± 3.7	78.7 ± 3.4	78.8 ± 3.1	NS	NS	NS	NS	NS	NS
FFM (kg)	47.1 ± 4.9	47.1 ± 4.8	46.8 ± 4.2	46.8 ± 4.3	NS	NS	NS	NS	NS	NS

0 - before nutritional intervention, 3 – after 3 months of the nutritional intervention, 6 – after 6 month of the nutritional intervention, 9 – after 9 month of the nutritional intervention (post –study).

study end, changes in hormone levels (increased LH) were visible. On the other hand, amenorrhea was diagnosed in 5 subjects from the group of female athletes, while oligomenorrhea was observed in 26 females. The nine-month NI resulted in regular menstruation recovery in 7 female athletes. As early as after 3 months of the NI, LH levels and LH to FSH ratio changes were visible (Table 3). As the 9-month NI did not result in resumption of regular menstruation in all examined subjects, EB, EA, BW and body composition values, as well as the levels of selected hormones, were compared between two groups created on the basis of the above mentioned criterion, i.e. recovery of regular menstrual cycle. Even before the NI start, statistically significant intergroup differences concerning EB, EA, FM and FFM values were observed. Additionally, women with potential recovery of the regular menstrual cycle had almost normal EB, higher EA, higher FM, and lower FFM. Discrepancies in the above mentioned parameters were also visible at the NI end, when higher rate of FM and no changes in BW were observed. Moreover, the nine-month NI use resulted in significant increase of LH levels in both groups, whereas in the group with restored menstruation this value was higher (Table 4).

Table 3 Hormone levels in study participants after and during the nutritional intervention M ± SD

	0	3	6	9	*P-value*					
					0 vs 3	3 vs 6	0 vs 6	3 vs 9	6 vs 9	0 vs 9
Ballet dancers										
Eumenorrhea	0	0	1	3						
Amenorrhea	5	4	3	1						
Oligomenorrhea	16	17	17	17						
LH (mIU/mL)	3.00 ± 1.51	4.17 ± 2.29	4.63 ± 2.47	4.81 ± 1.64	NS	NS	NS	NS	NS	0.026
FSH (mIU/mL)	5.23 ± 2.32	4.95 ± 1.67	4.67 ± 2.16	4.90 ± 1.08	NS	NS	NS	NS	NS	NS
E_2 (pg/mL)	39.9 ± 21.7	43.7 ± 23.6	42.0 ± 20.0	42.3 ± 18.9	NS	NS	NS	NS	NS	NS
P (ng/mL)	0.53 ± 0.50	0.41 ± 0.63	0.24 ± 0.12	0.25 ± 0.09	NS	NS	NS	NS	NS	NS
LH to FSH ratio	0.72 ± 0.54	0.81 ± 0.49	1.03 ± 0.57	0.92 ± 0.22	NS	NS	NS	NS	NS	NS
Female athletes										
Eumenorrhea	0	0	4	7						
Amenorrhea	5	5	5	4						
Oligomenorrhea	26	26	22	20						
LH (mIU/mL)	3.04 ± 1.63	4.59 ± 2.53	4.67 ± 2.49	4.89 ± 1.99	0.009	NS	0.005	NS	NS	0.001
FSH (mIU/mL)	5.01 ± 2.37	5.00 ± 2.08	4.99 ± 2.01	5.04 ± 1.86	NS	NS	NS	NS	NS	NS
E_2 (pg/mL)	36.5 ± 19.4	36.2 ± 15.3	39.2 ± 18.4	34.4 ± 11.7	NS	NS	NS	NS	NS	NS
P (ng/mL)	0.54 ± 0.99	0.68 ± 0.77	0.46 ± 0.32	0.36 ± 0.38	NS	NS	NS	NS	NS	NS
LH to FSH ratio	0.84 ± 0.56	0.96 ± 0.52	0.98 ± 0.49	0.97 ± 0.29	0.001	NS	0.003	NS	NS	0.033

0 - before nutritional intervention, 3 – after three month of the nutritional intervention, 6 – after six month of the nutritional intervention 9 – after nine month of the nutritional intervention (post – study).

Discussion

Our results confirm the role of a non-pharmacological NI comprising increased energy and nutrition intakes and dietitian consultations, without any TEE changes, in treatment not only of female athletes, but also dancers with hypothalamic amenorrhea and oligomenorrhea.

The evaluation of subject's eating habits performed prior to the beginning of the NI, indicated deficiencies in energy and nutritional values of DD which may, among others, impair the endocrine functions of the FM associated with leptin secretion, and therefore lead to menstrual disturbances [17]. In 90.5% of ballet dancers and 64.5% of female athletes the serum leptin levels were below the laboratory norms what is consistent with results obtained by other authors [18,19]. However, in 9.5% of ballet dancers and 29% of female athletes higher leptin levels were observed. It has been reported that a diet composition has a significant effect on the leptin

Table 4 Baseline and post-study characteristic among study participants with and without return of menses M ± SD

	Return of menses (n = 10)			No return of menses (n = 42)			0 vs. 0	9 vs. 9
	0	9	0 vs. 9 p	0	9	0 vs. 9 p	p	p
EB (kcal/day)	−44 ± 508	121 ± 188.0	NS	−395 ± 352.7	52 ± 87.5	< 0.001	0.01	NS
EA (kcal/kg FFM/d)	31.0 ± 8.3	42.0 ± 7.8	<0.001	24.5 ± 8.8	38.9 ± 6.9	<0.001	0.05	NS
BW (kg)	57.4 ± 4.8	57.5 ± 4.1	NS	56.6 ± 6.6	57.2 ± 6.8	NS	NS	NS
BMI (kg/m^2)	20.7 ± 1.2	20.8 ± 0.9	NS	19.7 ± 1.9	19.9 ± 2.0	NS	NS	NS
FM (%)	22.0 ± 2.9	22.8 ± 0.9	NS	19.3 ± 3.6	19.9 ± 3.4	NS	0.04	0.01
FM (kg)	12.6 ± 2.0	13.1 ± 1.1	NS	10.9 ± 2.6	11.4 ± 2.7	NS	NS	NS
FFM (%)	78.0 ± 2.9	77.2 ± 0.9	NS	81.7 ± 3.6	80.1 ± 3.7	NS	0.04	0.01
FFM (kg)	44.8 ± 4.0	44.4 ± 3.2	NS	45.7 ± 5.5	45.8 ± 4.7	NS	NS	NS
LH (mIU/mL)	2.78 ± 1.60	5.33 ± 1.97	0.016	3.22 ± 1.71	4.53 ± 1.61	0.002	NS	NS
FSH (mIU/mL)	5.02 ± 2.38	6.08 ± 1.91	NS	5.16 ± 2.34	5.19 ± 1.53	NS	NS	NS

0 - before nutritional intervention, 9 – after 9 month of the nutritional intervention (post – study).

synthesis, whereas in subjects on a high-energy diet higher leptin levels may be observed. Therefore, it may explain higher leptin levels in some female athletes because this group is known to use the type of a diet mentioned above. Mantzoros et al. [20] report that late high-energy evening meal consumption may also induce an increase in the leptin levels by 40-60%, persisting up to 12 hours. Despite the fact that all subjects were instructed not to consume high-energy meals late in the evening on the day before blood collection, it was impossible to verify their compliance. Genetic factors may also have a significant impact on the leptin levels. Therefore, it is difficult to unanimously determine the cause of high leptin levels observed in some subjects. Moreover, not all factors responsible for the serum leptin levels are known.

Energy intake restrictions are also regarded as the main reason for RMR reduction [21,22]. This study also demonstrates significant intergroup differences in the RMR rate. In ballet dancers, compared to female athletes, EB and EA were lower what potentially confirms the diet impact on the RMR value. The above-mentioned results are similar to those obtained by Lebenstedt et al. [23] who in female athletes with menstrual disturbances demonstrated lower RMR values by 114 kcal/d. Also Myburgh et al. [24] reported that reduced RMR, observed in dancers, was associated with menstrual disorders. Kaufman et al. [25] demonstrated that the RMR depended not only on diet composition, but also on the leptin levels. Moreover, Welt et al. [26] claimed that the insufficient energy intake and low serum leptin levels resulted in synthesis and frequency of gonadotropic hormone pulses reduction, and thus lead to ovulation inhibition. Furthermore, Kelesidis et al. [27] stated that the leptin deficit was responsible for reduced LH secretion and delayed menarche in patients with menstruation disorders. A similar conclusion was emphasized by Ackerman et al. [18] who indicated that low leptin levels may contribute to changes in the LH pulse frequency resulting in amenorrhoea.

During a nutritional intervention, an individual meal schedule was based on the real energy expenditure, current nutritional status, and in case of female athletes, on a current training stage. After a NI had started, the intervention was followed up every month. This follow-up demonstrated significant changes in a subject's diet (a statistical analysis comprised data obtained before the start and 3, 6 and 9 months after the intervention start). Mean values indicated an energy and nutrient intake increase and high standard deviations; they also indicated that not all dancers and female athletes followed NI guidelines what indicates an important difficulty associated with implementation of an individual diet in this population. However, in subsequent NI follow-ups, the standard deviation value was gradually lower indicating progressive implementation of dietetic changes. However, the rate of such changes was different than expected. Thus, in both dancers and female athletes the EB value was compensated and the EA level exceeded the critical threshold of 30 kcal/kg FFM/d, below which, according to other authors [28,29], the menstruation disorders become more intense and the risk of bone mineral density reduction increases. Unfortunately, even after 9 months of the NI use the recommended level of vitamin D intake was not achieved neither in dancers nor in female athletes. This could be explained by a high demand standard accepted based on the ACSM recommendations [6,30,31]. However, the principal aim of this paper was to follow the guidelines of an individual diet without the need for additional vitamin and mineral supplementation. Nevertheless, in dancers and female athletes at the risk of a triad syndrome, additional vitamin D supplementation may be necessary in the nearest future.

In our study, the return of menses was observed in 3 ballet dancers and 7 female athletes. Moreover, after a 9-month NI there were less subjects with secondary amenorrhea. Among hormones responsible for the maintenance of a regular menstrual cycle a significant increase in the LH levels was observed in dancers on the third follow-up visit monitoring the effects of a nutritional intervention (after 9 months of the NI). On the other hand, in female athletes beneficial changes in the levels of this hormone were observed as early as after the third month of a diet. Results obtained may indicate that increased energy and nutrient consumption has a positive effect on the hormone status in young women with menstruation disorders. It is extremely important to note that a 9-month diet used in the group of female athletes did not result in any changes of the BW value and body composition. However, in a group of ballet dancers an increase in the BW and BMI values was visible as early as after a 3-month diet and resulted in an FFM increase. Changes of the body weight in a group of ballet dancers during a 9-month nutritional intervention were 1.3 kg. It has to be emphasised that a more negative energy balance and lower energy availability were observed in this group before the start of the nutritional intervention. Additionally, ballet dancers had a lower resting metabolism rate. Results obtained may indicate that this group is malnourished to a greater extent and it may account for more significant changes in their body weight. The comparison of a nutritional status, EB and EA values between a group with recovered menses and a group with menstrual disturbances suggests that resumption of menstruation can be obtained when the FM level reaches a specific value, i.e. 22%. This observation seems to confirm the hypothesis of Frish et al. [32] who showed that a BW increase alone was not so important. These findings are inconsistent with prior studies conducted by Zanker et al. [33] who demonstrated an association between BW and resumption of menses in female athletes with hypothalamic amenorrhea. In their study, Arends et al. [3] demonstrated that regular menstruation recovery in female athletes depends on the BW and BMI increase. Unfortunately, the publication by Arends et al. [3] does not provide the parameters of female athletes' body composition, therefore a full comparison of those results with results obtained herein is impossible. It is difficult to overestimate practical implications of our observations confirming that a relatively low difference in the FM amount, potentially obtained without a significant BW increase, may result in regular menstruation recovery. Our studies included girls practicing disciplines in which a silhouette is of vital importance. Thus, the NI implementation in dancers was a significant problem due to a belief that a BW increase may potentially translate into subjective ratings received from judges and lower scores for visual performance and artistic image; while in triathlonists or rowers it may reduce their speed or physical capability. In our study, a 9-month nutritional intervention, similarly to other studies, was used. Dueck et al. [34] and Knopp-Woodroffe et al. [35] demonstrated menses resumption in female athletes after approximately 6 months and 9–12 weeks, respectively. However, based on our results, we can suggest that the mean time to menses recovery could be longer than 1 year. Also Arends et al. [3] suggested that a non-pharmacological intervention in female athletes with menstrual disturbances might restore regular cycles, although the restoration of menses may take more than 1 year.

It may be suggested that limitations associated with regular menses restoration in the study population, both in our paper and in other authors' studies, may be due to the fact that there are many overlapping factors contributing to above-mentioned disturbances. Bruni et al. [36] state that an inappropriate diet, increased physical effort and stress are basic factors differentiating women suffering from menstruation disturbances. Therefore, it is not recommended to combine the general population suffering from such conditions into one group. In our studies, young eligible women form a specific population in which all factors predisposing to above-mentioned dysfunctions seem to be combined. Papers by Nattiv et al. [6] and Manore et al. [37] emphasized that an appropriately balanced diet with simultaneous limitation of the training volume and intensity is one of many potential possibilities that may be used to reduce menstrual disorders in dancers and female athletes. The above-mentioned papers were significant because they emphasized an appropriately planned and individualized diet including daily load with physical training. Moreover, the effects were obtained without any changes in the volume and intensity of training, taking into account the fact that it might have been an argument against participation in these studies.

Conclusion

Menstruation disorders reduction, in dancers and female athletes, is possible without any pharmacological intervention only by following the guidelines of an appropriately planned NI comprising balanced energy balance and higher energy availability. However, time period duration with possibility of complete menstruation recovery, due to non-pharmacological NI use, depends to a large extent on women's "baseline characteristics" including their body composition, nutritional status, earlier nutritional habits and metabolic state. When the baseline amount of FM is low, i.e. below 20%, the need of longer NI use, even >1 year, should be considered. The regulation of gonadotropic hormone levels alone may not translate into immediate restoration of regular menses, although it would definitely make menstrual disorders less severe. Further research is needed in larger samples to determine the primary contributors to resumption of menses in amenorrheic and oligomenorreic, exercising women.

Competing interests

The authors declare that they have no competing interests.

Authors' contributions

KŁ, KK, JJ. All authors read and approved the final manuscript.

Acknowledgement

The project was financed by Ministry of Science and Higher Education under a number N N312 239738.

Author details

[1]Department of Human Nutrition and Hygiene, Poznan University of Life Sciences, Poznan, Poland. [2]Department of Perinatology and Gynecology, Poznan University of Medical Sciences, Poznan, Poland.

References

1. Hoogenboom BJ, Morris J, Morris C, Schaefer K: **Nutritional knowledge and eating behaviors of female, collegiate swimmers.** *N Am J Sports Phys Ther* 2009, **4**(3):139–148.
2. Miller SM, Kukuljan S, Turner AI, van der Pligt P, Ducher G: **Energy deficiency, menstrual disturbances, and low bone mass: what do exercising Australian women know about the female athlete triad?** *Int J Sport Nutr Exerc Metab* 2012, **22**(2):131–138.
3. Arends JC, Cheung MY, Barrack MT, Nattiv A: **Restoration of menses with Nonpharmacologic therapy in collegiate athletes with menstrual disturbances: a 5 year retrospective study.** *Int J Sport Nutr Exerc Metab* 2012, **22**(2):98–108.
4. Mallinson RJ, Williams NI, Olmsted MP, Scheid JL, Riddle ES, De Souza MJ: **A case report of recovery of menstrual function following a nutritional intervention in two exercising women with amenorrhea of varying duration.** *J Int Soc Sports Nutr* 2013, **10**:34.
5. Lagowska K, Kapczuk K, Friebe Z, Bajerska J: **Effects of dietary intervention in young female athletes with menstrual disorders.** *J Int Soc Sports Nutr* 2014, **26**(11):21.
6. Nattiv A, Loucks AB, Manore MM, Sanborn CF, Sundgot-Borgen J, Warren MP: **American College of Sports Medicine. The female athlete triad. Position stand.** *Med Sci Sports Exerc* 2007, **39**(10):1867–1882.
7. Yang Y, Li Q, Guo L, Cui M, Bao T, Zhang Z, Wang C, Ni Y, Zhang J: **A retrospective analysis of thyroid cancer in China.** *Asian Pac J Cancer Prev* 2011, **12**(9):2245–2249.
8. Majumdar A, Mangal NS: **Hyperprolactinemia.** *J of Hum Reprod Sci* 2013, **6**(3):168–175.

9. Heyward VH, Wagner DL: *Applied Body Composition Assessment.* Champaign, IL: Human Kinetics; 2003.
10. Harris JA, Benedict FA: *A biometric study of basal metabolic rate in man.* Washington, DC: Carnegie Institute of Washington, DC (Pub No 279); 1919:370–373.
11. Konrad KK, Carels RA, Garner DM: **Metabolic and psychological changes during refeeding in anorexia nervosa.** *Eat Weight Disord* 2007, **12**(1):20–26.
12. Polito A, Fabbri A, Ferro-Luzzi A, Cuzzolaro M, Censi L, Ciarapica D, Fabbrini E, Giannini D: **Basal metabolic rate in anorexia nervosa: relation to body composition and leptin concentrations.** *Am J Clin Nutr* 2000, **71**(6):1495–1502.
13. Reguła J, Jeszka J, Gramza A: **Effectiveness of weight reduction program in adolescents under sanatorium conditions in Poland including the role of diet and energy balance.** *Asia Pac J Clin Nutr* 2007, **16**(1):353–358.
14. Szponar L, Wolnicka K, Rychlik E: *Album Fotografii Produktów i Potraw.* Warsaw: Wydawnictwo IŻŻ; 2000.
15. Kunachowicz H, Nadolna I, Przygoda B, Ivanow K: *Tables of Nutritional Value of Foodstuffs and Dishes 3rd Extended and Update Edition.* Warsaw: Wydawnictwo IŻŻ; 2005.
16. Jarosz M, Bułhak-Jachymczyk B: *Normy Żywienia Człowieka. Podstawy Prewencji Otyłości i Chorób Niezakaźnych.* Wydawnictwo Lekarskie PZWL: Warsaw IŻŻ; 2011.
17. Ahima RS, Osei SY: **Leptin signaling.** *Physiology Behaviour* 2004, **81**:223–241.
18. Ackerman KE, Slusarz K, Guereca G, Pierce L, Slattery M, Mendes N, Herzog DB, Misra M: **Higher ghrelin and lower leptin secretion are associated with lower LH secretion in young amenorrheic athletes compared with eumenorrheic athletes and controls.** *Am J Physiol Endocrinol Metab* 2012, **302**(7):800–806.
19. Christo K, Prabhakaran R, Lamparello B, Cord J, Miller KK, Goldstein MA, Gupta N, Herzog DB, Klibanski A, Misra M: **Bone metabolism in adolescent athletes with amenorrhea, athletes with eumenorrhea, and control subjects.** *Pediatrics* 2008, **121**(6):1127–1136.
20. Mantzoros CS, Magkos F, Brinkoetter M, Sienkiewicz E, Dardeno TA, Kim SY, Hamnvik OP, Koniaris A: **Leptin in human physiology and pathophysiology.** *Am J Physiol Endocrinol Metab* 2011, **301**(4):567–584.
21. Doyle-Lucas AF, Akers JD, Davy BM: **Energetic efficiency, menstrual irregularity, and bone mineral density in elite professional female ballet dancers.** *J Dance Med Sci* 2010, **14**(4):146–154.
22. Sterling WM, Golden NH, Jacobson MS, Ornstein RM, Hertz SM: **Metabolic assessment of menstruating and nonmenstruating normal weight adolescents.** *Int J Eat Disord* 2009, **42**(7):658–663.
23. Lebenstedt M, Platte P, Pirke KM: **Reduced resting metabolic rate in athletes with menstrual disorders.** *Med Sci Sports Exerc* 1999, **31**(9):1250–1256.
24. Myburgh KH, Berman C, Novick I, Noakes T, Lambert E: **Decreased resting metabolic rate in ballet dancers with menstrual irregularity.** *Int J Sport Nutr* 1999, **9**(3):285–294.
25. Kaufman BA, Warren MP, Dominguez JE, Wang J, Heymsfield SB, Pierson RN: **Bone density and amenorrhea in ballet dancers are related to a decreased resting metabolic rate and lower leptin levels.** *J Clin Endocrinol Metab* 2002, **87**(6):2777–2783.
26. Welt CK, Chan JL, Bullen J, Murphy R, Smith P, DePaoli AM, Mantzoros CS: **Recombinant human leptin in women with hypothalamic amenorrhoea.** *N Engl J Med* 2004, **351**(10):987–997.
27. Kelesidis T, Kelesidis I, Chou S, Mantzoros CS: **Narrative review: the role of leptin in human physiology: emerging clinical applications.** *Ann Intern Med* 2010, **152**(2):93–100.
28. Loucks AB, Thuma JR: **Luteinizing hormone pulsatilityis disrupted at a threshold of energy availability in regularly menstruating women.** *J Clin Endocrinol Metab* 2003, **88**(1):297–311.
29. Ihle R, Loucks AB: **Dose – response relationships between energy availability and bone turnover in young exercising women.** *J Bone Miner Res* 2004, **19**(8):1231–1240.
30. Rodriguez NR, Di Marco NM, Langley S: **American college of sports medicine position stand. Nutrition and athletic performance. American Dietetic Association; Dietitians of Canada; american College of Sports Medicine.** *Med Sci Sports Exerc* 2009, **41**(3):709–731.
31. Roupas ND, Georgopoulos NA: **Menstrual function in sports.** *Hormones* 2011, **10**(2):104–116.
32. Frish RE, Mc Arthur JW: **Menstrual cycles: fatness as a determinacy of minimum weight and height necessary for their maintenance or oncet.** *Science* 1974, **185**(4155):849–860.
33. Zanker CL, Cooke CB, Truscott JG, Oldroyd B, Jacobs HS: **Annual changes of bone density over 12 years in an amenorrheic athlete.** *Med Sci Sports Exerc* 2004, **36**(1):137–142.
34. Dueck CA, Matt KS, Manore MM, Skinner JS: **Treatment of athletic amenorrhea with a diet and training intervention program.** *Int J Sport Nutr* 1996, **6**(1):24–40.
35. Kopp-Woodroffe SA, Manore MM, Dueck CA, Skinner JS, Matt KS: **Energy and nutrient status of amenorrheic athletes participating in a diet and exercise training intervention program.** *Int J Sport Nutr* 1999, **9**(1):70–88.
36. Bruni V, Dei M, Morelli C, Schettino MT, Balzi D, Nuvolone D: **Body composition variables and leptin levels in functional hypothalamic amenorrhea and amenorrhea related to eating disorders.** *J Pediatr Adolesc Gynecol* 2011, **24**(6):347–352.
37. Manore MM, Kam LC, Loucks AB: **The female athlete triad: components, nutrition issues, and health consequences.** *J Sports Sci* 2007, **25**:61–71.

Effects of a carbohydrate-electrolyte solution on cognitive performance following exercise-induced hyperthermia in humans

Jason KW Lee[1,2,3*†], Wee Hon Ang[1†], Jonathan WX Ng[2†], Priscilla WP Fan[1†], Ya Shi Teo[1†], Heinrich W Nolte[4†] and Yvonne YW Yeo[2†]

Abstract

Background: There is limited information on the effects of sports drinks on cognitive function after exercise in the heat. We aimed to investigate the effects of ingesting a commercially available carbohydrate-electrolyte (CHO) solution on cognitive performance following exercise-induced hyperthermia.

Methods: Twelve participants completed three practices of cognitive tests, one full familiarisation and two experimental trials in an environmental chamber (dry bulb temperature: 30.2 ± 0.3°C, relative humidity: 70 ± 3%). The experimental trials consisted of five cognitive tests (symbol digit matching, search and memory, digit span, choice reaction time and psychomotor vigilance test) performed before and after a 75-min run on a treadmill at 70% VO_2 max. One ml/kg body mass of a 6.8% CHO solution or placebo was consumed at the start, every 15 min during exercise and between cognitive tests after exercise. Core temperature, heart rate, blood glucose concentrations, subjective ratings and cognitive performance were assessed (symbol digit matching, search and memory, digit span, choice reaction time and psychomotor vigilance).

Results: Participants were hyperthermic at the end of the run (placebo: 39.5 ± 0.4°C, CHO: 39.6 ± 0.5°C; Mean ± SD; $p = 0.37$). The change in blood glucose was higher with CHO ingestion (1.6, 0.7 to 4.5 mmol/L) (median, range) than with placebo ingestion (0.9, -0.1 to 4.7 mmol/L; $p < 0.05$). CHO ingestion reduced the maximum span of digits memorized, in contrast to an increase in maximum span with placebo ingestion ($p < 0.05$). CHO solution had no effect on other cognitive tests ($p > 0.05$).

Conclusions: These results suggest that CHO solution ingestion may impair short-term memory following exertional heat stress.

Background

Diminished cognitive ability is of concern to a wide variety of people who are routinely engaged in physical activity under heat stress. Examples of such occupations include professional athletes, soldiers, and civil defense personnel. Cognitive performance has been shown to degrade following exercise-induced hyperthermia [1].

Bursill [2] studied the effects of exertional hyperthermia on attention in 18 heat-acclimatised individuals. He observed that a funneling of peripheral awareness towards the central field of vision occurred in a high proportion of participants and inhibited their ability to respond appropriately to the presented stimuli. In a more recent study, Morley et al. [3] investigated the effect of treadmill exercise while wearing thermal protective clothing on cognitive function. While cognitive performance did not change immediately after exercise, short term memory was reduced 60 and 120 min after exercise. Furthermore, the mean of the 10 slowest reaction times increased 120 min after exercise. It was noteworthy that while 50 min of treadmill exercise in thermal protective clothing resulted in near maximal physiological strain, alterations

* Correspondence: lkaiwei@dso.org.sg
†Equal contributors
[1]Combat Protection and Performance Programme, Defence Medical and Environmental Research Institute, DSO National Laboratories, Singapore, Republic of Singapore
[2]Department of Physiology, National University of Singapore, Singapore, Republic of Singapore
Full list of author information is available at the end of the article

in neurocognitive performance were not observable until an hour or more following exercise.

There are several possible reasons explaining impaired cognitive function following exercise-induced heat stress. These include dehydration [4], competition for attentional resources [5], and the availability of blood glucose to power cognitive processes [6]. All cellular activities in the body require energy in the form of ATP to sustain, including the brain cells. Most of the ATPs used by the brain are derived from the oxygen-dependent metabolism of glucose. Since the brain is the most metabolically active organ in the body, it is particularly vulnerable to the disruption of energy resources. In addition, it is also noteworthy that the brain possesses paradoxically limited stores of glycogen, which without replenishment are exhausted in up to 10 min [7]. Depletion of ATP at the cellular level can cause failure of membrane ion-transport systems due to neuron depolarization. Therefore, neural dysfunction due to inadequate blood glucose may be one important underlying mechanism of cognitive impairment following exercise-induced hyperthermia.

The role of glucose in the modulation of cognitive processes is well established. Beneficial effects of glucose supplementation have been observed across different populations under various experimental conditions. For example, it has been demonstrated that glucose supplementation can enhance learning and memory in healthy young and aged humans [8,9]. Enhanced cognitive performance caused by elevated plasma glucose levels has also been reported in schizophrenia patients [10]. Improved glycemic control was shown to enhance performance on selective areas of cognition [7]. Although glucose has beneficial effects on a range of cognitive tasks, evidence from the literature suggests that glucose has the most prominent effects on memory performance [7].

To our knowledge, there is limited information available on the effects of sports drinks on cognitive function after exercise in the heat [11]. The objective of this study was to investigate the effects of ingesting sports drinks on cognition following exertional heat stress. We hypothesized that the ingestion of sports drinks, as compared with a placebo, will alleviate the degree of cognitive impairment following exercise-induced hyperthermia.

Methods

Twelve male endurance athletes (age: 23.8 ± 1.7 years; VO_2 max: 59.4 ± 5.3 mL/kg/min) participated in this study that was approved by the DSO Institutional Review Board. Following an informed consent session explaining the nature, benefits and risks of the study, participants gave their consent verbally and in writing. Participants were certified fit for participation in this study by a physician. Before the commencement of each trial, participants completed a health status questionnaire to ensure that they were well.

Each participant visited the laboratory on five separate sessions. The first two sessions were conducted to familiarise participants with the cognitive test battery. Anthropometric measurements and peak aerobic capacity (VO_2 max) were also determined during the first and second sessions respectively. Participants completed a full familiarisation trial (exercise and cognitive test battery) in the third session prior to the experimental trials with either the carbohydrate-electrolyte (CHO) solution or placebo in a counterbalanced manner.

Height was measured to the nearest 0.1 cm using a stadiometer (Seca, Brooklyn, N.Y., USA) and body mass was obtained to the nearest 0.05 kg using a digital scale (ID1 Plus/KCC150, Mettler-Toledo, Germany) during the first session. Skin-fold measurements were taken at four sites (biceps, triceps, subscapular and suprailiac) using skin-fold calipers (Model HSK-BI-3; Baty International, West Sussex, UK). Body density [12] and percent body fat [13] were calculated.

Peak aerobic capacity was measured during the second session. Each participant ran at four different speeds on a treadmill (h/p/cosmos Mercury, Germany), starting at a speed 1 km/h slower than his expected pace for a 10 km race, with increments of 1 km/h every 3 min, for a total of 12 min. Heart rate (HR) and ratings of perceived exertion (RPE) were recorded during the last 10 s of each 3 min stage. Oxygen uptake (VO_2) was assessed over the final min of each 3 min stage through a mouthpiece connected to a metabolic cart (Cortex Metalyser 3B, Germany). Following the 12 min-run, participants were given 5 – 10 min rest before they started on a continuous treadmill run with an initial gradient of 1%, which increased by 1% every one min until volitional exhaustion [14]. Heart rate was measured continuously by short-range telemetry using a HR monitor (Model S810i; Polar Electro, Oy, Kempelem, Finland). Maximum oxygen uptake (VO_2 max) was recorded as the mean oxygen uptake over the last min before volitional exhaustion. The relationship between VO_2 and speed was determined and the speed corresponding to 70% VO_2 max for each participant was used in subsequent experimental trials.

Trials were separated by at least seven days to allow recovery. Participants were required to standardize their dietary intake, as well as to refrain from alcohol consumption and strenuous activity 24 hours prior to each trial. A dietary record sheet was provided to aid them in standardising their dietary intake. Each participant ingested a Jonah temperature capsule (Mini Mitter Co., Inc., Bend, OR, USA) at least 8 hours prior to the commencement of trial as a measurement of core temperature (T_c). They were also requested to consume 500 mL of water 90 min before the commencement of each trial and refrain from drinking thereafter. A schematic of the experimental protocol is shown in Figure 1.

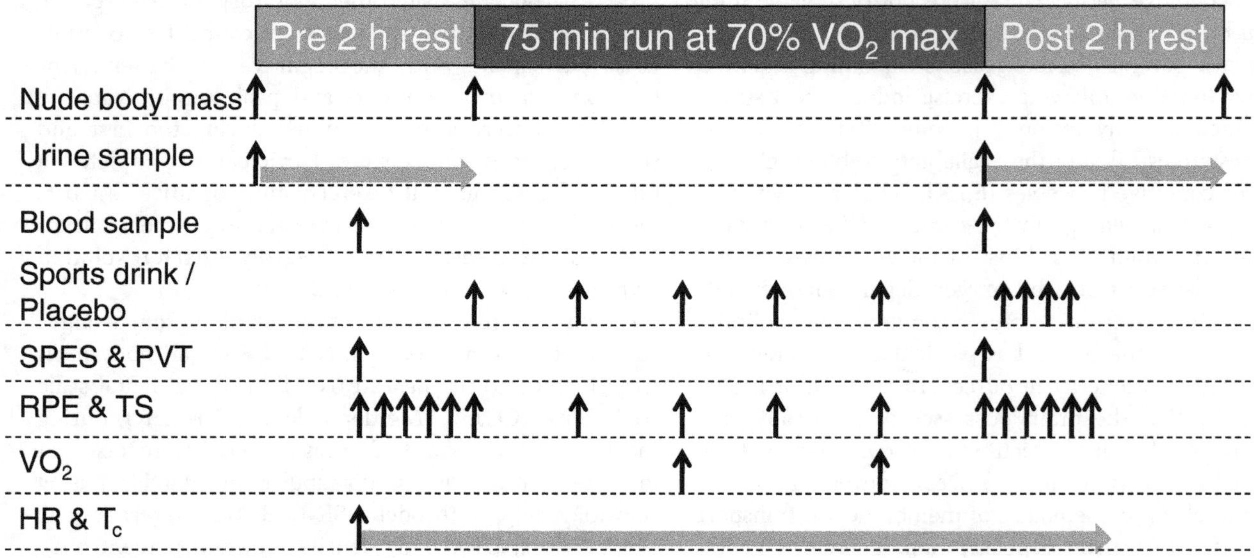

Figure 1 Experimental protocol.

Upon arrival at the laboratory for each experimental trial, urine sample was collected before measurement of nude body mass. Urine osmolality was measured using freezing point depression (Osmomat 030-D, Gonotec, Germany). The VitalSense® temperature logger (Mini Mitter Co. Inc., Bend, OR, USA) was sealed in a waterproof bag fitted into a padded pouch, and worn on a customised lightweight harness around the waist positioned in the lumbar region of the participant. Each participant also wore a chest band and wrist watch HR monitor. A climatic monitoring device (Squirrel 2020 data logger, Grant Instruments, United Kingdom) was used to measure dry bulb temperature and relative humidity during the experimental trials.

Participants entered an environmental chamber (Heraeus Votsch, Germany) programmed to maintain a dry bulb temperature of 30°C and 70% relative humidity. A baseline blood sample was obtained after participants stood for 10 min. Participants commenced with the Swedish Performance Evaluation System (SPES) [15] that assessed a variety of cognitive functions such as symbol digit matching, search and memory, digit span, choice reaction time, followed by the Psychomotor Vigilance Test (PVT) [16]. The total duration of the cognitive test battery took approximately 40 min. The test battery was performed before and immediately after exercise in the environmental chamber.

Participants performed a run at 70% VO_2 max for 75 min on a motorized treadmill following completion of the baseline cognitive test battery. Participants were required to consume 1 ml/kg body mass of sports drinks (100Plus, F&N, Singapore; CHO trial) or placebo (control) before the start, every 15 min during, immediately after exercise and in between the cognitive tests after exercise. The nutritional compositions of the sports drink and placebo are shown in Table 1. Ratings of perceived exertion and thermal sensation (RTS) were assessed before the start, every 15 min during exercise, at the beginning and the end of each cognitive test. Trials were terminated prematurely when a participant's core temperature reached 40°C, in adherence with pre-determined ethical guidelines. Following completion of the 75 min run, blood sampling, body mass measurements and urine sampling were performed before participants completed the post-exercise cognitive test battery. Sweat loss was estimated from the difference in body masses, corrected for fluid intake and urine production: (pre-exercise body mass – post-exercise body mass) + ingested fluid – urine output.

Table 1 Energy content and composition of placebo and sports drink

Drink contents	Placebo	Sports drink
Energy value (kcal/L)*	6	270
Fat (g/L)	0	0
Protein (g/L)	0	0
Carbohydrate (g/L)	0	68
Sucrose (g/L)	0	48
Glucose (g/L)	0	20
Osmolality (mOsmol/kg)*	29 ± 1	349 ± 11
Sodium (mmol/L)	0	18 ± 3
Potassium (mmol/L)	0	3 ± 0

*There may be trace amounts of sugars present in the placebo drink which could not be detected by our analysis, thus explaining the energy and osmolality values despite the absence of carbohydrates.

Venous blood samples (4.5 mL each) were collected from the participants' forearm after they stood for 10 min and immediately after the run. The blood was dispensed into an anticoagulant-free tube and blood glucose concentrations were assessed using a commercial glucose analyser (Acc-Chek® Advantage, Roche, Germany).

The Statistical Package for Social Sciences version 15.0 was used to perform all statistical computations. Normality of experimental trial data was assessed using the Shapiro-Wilk test. Paired t-test was performed on data that were normally distributed. Data that did not follow the normal distribution were analyzed using Wilcoxon matched-pair signed rank test. A 5% level of significance was used for all statistical analyses. Results with normal distribution were reported in mean and standard deviation while those that did not follow a normal distribution were reported in median and range.

Results

Environmental conditions and pre-trial hydration status

There were no differences in dry bulb temperature (placebo: 30.2 ± 0.3°C vs. CHO: 30.2 ± 0.3°C; $p = 0.86$) and relative humidity (placebo: 72 ± 2% vs. CHO: 69 ± 3%; $p = 0.10$) between the placebo and CHO trials. Participants were considered euhydrated prior to each trial as indicated by their urine osmolality (placebo: 163, 74 to 669 mOsmol/kg [median, range]; CHO: 205, 102 to 621 mOsmol/kg; $p = 0.41$).

Exercise intensity and duration during run

Participants ran at similar exercise intensity with placebo (70 ± 5% VO_2 max) and CHO ingestion (71 ± 5% VO_2 max, $p = 0.12$). Eight subjects terminated exercise early during one or both experimental trials. Out of these eight subjects, two terminated exercise early as their core temperature has reached the approved ethical limit of 40°C. Six subjects stopped running before 75 min due to exhaustion. Statistical analysis revealed similar exercise duration between the placebo (67 ± 8 min) and the CHO trials (66 ± 13 min, $p = 0.73$). Removal of these participants from the analysis of cognitive, physiological and blood data had no effect on the interpretation of results, hence their data were included.

Core temperature

No difference was found in core temperature between the placebo and CHO trials at the start of the run (placebo: 36.7 ± 0.2°C vs. CHO: 36.7 ± 0.2°C; $p = 0.79$), at end of the run (placebo: 39.5 ± 0.4°C vs. CHO: 39.6 ± 0.5°C; $p = 0.37$), at the beginning of the post-exercise cognitive test battery (placebo: 38.9 ± 0.4°C vs. CHO: 38.8 ± 0.5°C; $p = 0.93$), and at the end of the post-exercise cognitive test battery (placebo: 37.3 ± 0.3°C vs. CHO: 37.4 ± 0.5°C; $p = 0.37$).

Heart rate

Heart rate was similar between the placebo and CHO trials at the start of the run (placebo: 58 ± 7 bpm vs. CHO: 59 ± 7 bpm; $p = 0.19$), at end of the run (placebo: 171 ± 10 vs. CHO: 171 ± 10 bpm; $p = 0.97$), at the beginning of the post-exercise cognitive test battery (placebo: 99 ± 16 bpm vs. CHO: 98 ± 14 bpm; $p = 0.73$), and the end of the post-exercise cognitive test battery (placebo: 82 ± 10 bpm vs. CHO: 85 ± 10 bpm; $p = 0.14$).

Ratings of thermal sensation (RTS) and perceived exertion (RPE)

No difference was found in mean RTS between the placebo (4.1 ± 0.9) and CHO trials (4.1 ± 0.8; $p = 0.49$). Mean RPE was also similar between the placebo (13 ± 4) and CHO trials (13 ± 4; $p = 0.08$).

Blood glucose

Comparing the placebo and the CHO trials, the intra-subject increase in blood glucose (pre-exercise to post-exercise) was higher with CHO ingestion (1.6, 0.7 to 4.5 mmol/L [median, range]) than with placebo ingestion (0.9, -0.1 to 4.7 mmol/L; $p < 0.05$).

Sweat rate and fluid balance

Sweat rate was similar between the placebo (1.77 ± 0.47 L/h) and CHO trials (1.72 ± 0.35 L/h, $p = 0.83$). Body mass loss during the run was similar between the placebo (1.4 ± 0.6 kg) and CHO trials (1.4 ± 0.5 kg; $p = 0.94$).

Cognitive tests

Results of the cognitive tests are shown in Table 2. Test scores from the symbol digit matching, search and memory, choice reaction time, and PVT showed no differences between the placebo and CHO trials ($p > 0.05$). CHO ingestion reduced the maximum span of digits memorized in the digit span test ($p < 0.05$), in contrast to an increase in maximum span with placebo ingestion ($p < 0.05$; Figure 2). Out of our 12 participants, only one performed better for the digit span test during the CHO trial while performance was similar between trials in three other participants.

Discussion

This study assessed the efficacy of ingesting a commercially available carbohydrate-electrolyte solution (CHO) on cognitive performance following exercise-induced hyperthermia. Prior to the main experimental trials, all participants underwent three practices of the cognitive test battery to minimize learning effect. The study indicated that ingestion of CHO solution resulted in a decrease in the longest string of digits memorized in the digit span test, but had no effect on the performance of

Table 2 Cognitive test summary (n = 12)

Cognitive test	Measures	Pre-placebo	Post-placebo	Change	Pre-CHO	Post-CHO	Change
Symbol Digit Matching	Mean Reaction Time (ms)	1624 ± 279	1490 ± 232	-134 ± 154	1693 ± 265	1525 ± 276	-169 ± 139
	No. of Errors	2 ± 3	2 ± 2	0 ± 4	2 ± 2	2 ± 3	0 ± 3
Search & Memory	Mean Reaction Time (ms)	4437 ± 1661	4311 ± 1309	-126 ± 807	4464 ± 1666	4411 ± 1707	-53 ± 603
Level 1	No. of Errors	0 ± 1	1 ± 1	0 ± 1	1 ± 1	1 ± 1	0 ± 1
Search & Memory	Mean Reaction Time (ms)	6984 ± 2406	6693 ± 3331	-291 ± 1955	7256 ± 2552	6862 ± 2782	-393 ± 1007
Level 2	No. of Errors	1 ± 1	2 ± 2	1 ± 2	2 ± 1	2 ± 2	1 ± 2
Search & Memory	Mean Reaction Time (ms)	9711 ± 3799	9384 ± 4314	-328 ± 2077	9936 ± 3658	9317 ± 4381	-619 ± 2337
Level 3	No. of Errors	1 ± 2	1 ± 2	0 ± 1	3 ± 2	3 ± 2	0 ± 3
Digit Span	Maximum Span	10 ± 2	11 ± 2	1 ± 2	11 ± 2	10 ± 2	-1 ± 1
	No. of Directional Changes	8 ± 2	9 ± 2	1 ± 3	8 ± 1	9 ± 2	1 ± 2
Choice Reaction Time	Number of Correct Responses	121 ± 6	120 ± 15	-1 ± 13	122 ± 5	122 ± 9	0 ± 6
	Mean Reaction Time (ms)	574 ± 88	522 ± 71	-51 ± 84	562 ± 74	546 ± 96	-16 ± 57
Psychomotor Vigilance	Median Reaction Time (ms)	262 ± 55	244 ± 46	-18 ± 30	254 ± 42	236 ± 47	-18 ± 19
	No. of Errors	3 ± 3	1 ± 2	-2 ± 3	2 ± 2	2 ± 4	0 ± 4

the other cognitive tests (symbol digit matching, search and memory, choice reaction time and PVT). This suggests that CHO ingestion led to a degradation in short-term memory after a 75 min run in the heat but had no effect on perceptual capacity and speed, executive control functioning, speed of decision making, vigilance, and response latency. There are several possible reasons why ingestion of a CHO drink would impair short-term memory, including glycemic index and rapid swings in blood glucose levels.

The rate of glucose delivery depends on physicochemical properties of the food, which can be summarized by the glycemic index (GI), a parameter that reflects the rate and extent of the postprandial rise and fall in blood glucose [17]. Glucose, which was ingested by our participants during the CHO trials, is a carbohydrate with high GI. This is significant as high GI foods can induce rapid changes in blood glucose levels, which have been associated with fatigue and reduced cognitive function [18,19]. Furthermore, there is evidence to support the notion that foods with lower glycemic loads are associated with better performances on aspects of cognitive functioning [6,20,21]. A study conducted by Nilsson et al. [21] examined the

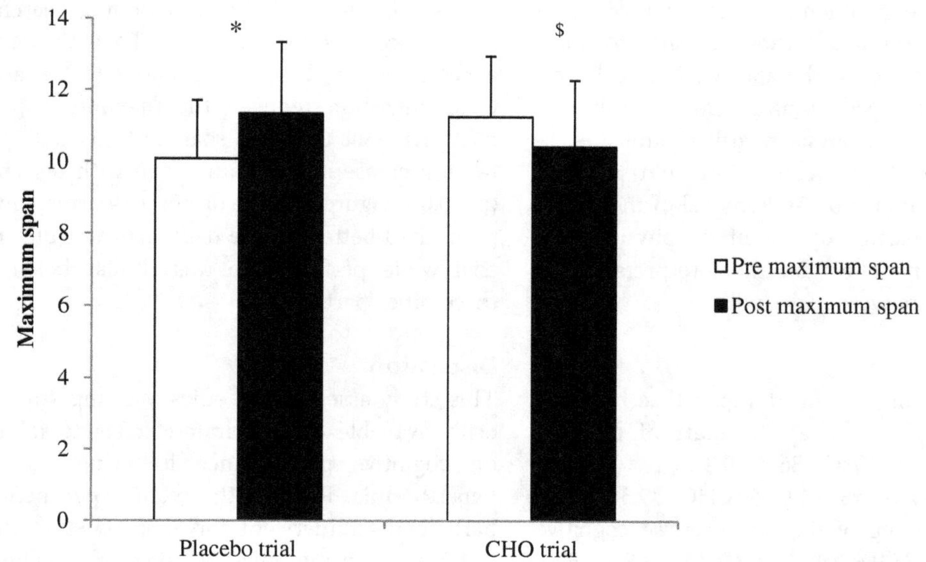

Figure 2 Effect of placebo and CHO ingestion on short-term memory (n = 12). * indicates increased in maximum span of digits memorized from pre- to post-exercise for the placebo trial ($p < 0.05$). $ indicates decreased in maximum span of digits memorized from pre- to post-exercise for the CHO trial ($p < 0.05$).

effects of GI on cognitive performance. In that study, a white wheat bread enriched with guar gum was able to produce a low but sustained blood glucose net increment. Working memory and selective attention were subsequently evaluated with this white wheat bread enriched with guar gum in the postprandial period against a high GI white wheat bread only. It was found that cognitive performance was improved in participants who ingested the white wheat bread enriched with guar gum. Similarly, Benton et al. [17] also showed that consuming a high GI meal resulted in poorer memory performance when compared to a low GI meal in both humans and rats. The influence of the GI of breakfast on verbal memory of adults was measured throughout the morning and it was found that a low GI diet (vs. a high GI diet) improved memory, especially in the late morning (150 and 210 min after breakfast). After 3 h following breakfast, it was found that rats displayed better learning performance after they were fed with a low GI diet.

The interaction between blood glucose and memory function has been shown to follow an inverted U-shaped dose-response curve; best memory performance was observed when increase in blood glucose was between 0.6 – 2.8 mmol/L [22]. Although the rise in blood glucose levels following CHO ingestion (1.6, 0.7 to 4.5 mmol/L) was within the optimum range for memory performance, it was unknown if this increase persisted throughout the entire cognitive test battery. Further increase in blood glucose levels caused by ingesting more CHO solution following exercise could have stimulated a higher insulin response in our study. A sharper profile of postprandial insulin release induced by high GI diets is likely to result in more glucose being directed towards insulin-sensitive tissues such as muscles, liver and white adipose tissue. As a consequence to the insulin surge, blood glucose levels may decrease which can lead to disruption of glucose delivery to the brain, thus slowing down local energy recruitment in the brain when cognitive demand occurs [17,21]. Since blood glucose was only analyzed immediately after exercise in this study, we do not know the glucose level during the actual cognitive tests.

The lack of significant effect of CHO ingestion on the other cognitive tests in this study could be due to the cognitive test battery being not demanding enough for the participants. Studies have suggested that ingestion of carbohydrate is more likely to improve cognitive function of higher complexity [23-25]. Glucose ingestion was found to enhance verbal episodic memory performance in studies that employed a divided attention protocol [26,27], but not in studies lacking in this protocol [28-30]. The divided attention protocol involved participants performing a secondary task during encoding of a supraspan memory list. The difficulty of cognitive test is also relative to the age of the participant as glucose was found to have greater enhancing effects in older adults than younger adults, and also in tasks with high levels of difficulty or that require divided attention [6,7,23]. This may be related to the notion that healthy young adults are operating at their 'cognitive peak'; therefore, a cognitive enhancer would only be effective when individuals experienced an increase in cognitive demands [31,32]. Since participants in our study were mainly young adults (age: 23.8 ± 1.7 years), one possible reason for the lack of cognitive benefits after CHO could be due to low task difficulty.

Participants in our placebo group experienced an increase in blood glucose levels after exercise (0.9, -0.1 to 4.7 mmol/L). During exercise, plasma glucagon is known to increase in response to the decreasing blood glucose and insulin levels [33]. Glucagon acts on the liver to break down glycogen stores and release glucose into the bloodstream, maintaining blood glucose levels during exercise. The increased blood glucose levels after exercise observed in this study could be due to a spillover effect of the increased plasma glucagon induced by exercise. This increased blood glucose level may be sufficient to allow the placebo group to handle the difficulty of the cognitive tests, thus achieving similar results as the CHO group. Additional intake of glucose (as seen in the CHO group) may be unnecessary for the brain during the cognitive tests, and may even have detrimental effects on cognitive performances due to high insulin response as discussed above.

Conclusions

In conclusion, these results suggest that CHO solution ingestion may impair short-term memory following exertional heat stress but does not have any effect on working memory, executive control function, speed of decision making and vigilance. Commercially available sports drink may thus offer negligible cognitive benefits.

Competing interests

The authors declare that they have no competing interests.

Authors' contributions

JKWL, PWPF, YST and HWN designed the study. YYY, PWPF, YST and WHA performed the experiments. JKWL, YYY, WHA, JWXN and PWPF performed the statistical analyses. JKWL, WHA, JWXN and YYY drafted the manuscript. JKWL, WHA and HWN reviewed the manuscript. All the authors read and approved the final manuscript.

Authors' information

JKWL, PWPF, WHA, YST are from Combat Protection and Performance Programme, Defence Medical and Environmental Research Institute, DSO National Laboratories, Republic of Singapore. JKWL, JWXN and YYY are from the Department of Physiology, National University of Singapore, Republic of Singapore. JKWL is also from Lee Kong Chian School of Medicine, Nanyang Technological University, Republic of Singapore. HWN is from ERGOnomics TECHnologies, Research and Development, Armscor, Pretoria, South Africa.

Acknowledgements

The authors expressed their gratitude to Ms. Lydia Law, Dr. Frederick Tey and Ms. Tan Ying Ying from DSO National Laboratories for their inputs on the selection of cognitive tests. We would also like to thank Mr. Glen Liu (from National University of Singapore), Ms. Jacinta Yeo and Mr. David Fun (from DSO National Laboratories) for their assistance during data collection. The authors would also like to thank all participants for their commitment to the study. The study was funded by DSO National Laboratories, Singapore and the National University of Singapore. All authors declared they had no conflict of interest.

Author details

[1]Combat Protection and Performance Programme, Defence Medical and Environmental Research Institute, DSO National Laboratories, Singapore, Republic of Singapore. [2]Department of Physiology, National University of Singapore, Singapore, Republic of Singapore. [3]Lee Kong Chian School of Medicine, Nanyang Technological University, Singapore, Republic of Singapore. [4]ERGOnomics TECHnologies, Research and Development, Armscor, Pretoria, South Africa.

References

1. Maughan RJ, Shirreffs SM, Watson P: **Exercise, heat, hydration and the brain.** *J Am Coll Nutr* 2007, **26**(5 Suppl):604S–6012S.
2. Bursill AE: **The restriction of peripheral-vision during exercise to hot and humid conditions.** *Q J Exp Psychol* 1958, **10**(3):113–129.
3. Morley J, Beauchamp G, Suyama J, Guyette FX, Reis SE, Callaway CW, Hostler D: **Cognitive function following treadmill exercise in thermal protective clothing.** *Eur J Appl Physiol* 2012, **112**(5):1733–1740.
4. Grandjean AC, Grandjean NR: **Dehydration and cognitive performance.** *J Am Coll Nutr* 2007, **26**(5 Suppl):549s–554s.
5. Hancock PA, Vasmatzidis I: **Human occupational and performance limits under stress: the thermal environment as a prototypical example.** *Ergonomics* 1998, **41**(8):1169–1191.
6. Gibson EL: **Carbohydrates and mental function: feeding or impeding the brain?** *Nutr Bull* 2007, **32**:71–83.
7. Owen L, Sunram-Lea SI: **Metabolic agents that enhance ATP can improve cognitive functioning: a review of the evidence for glucose, oxygen, pyruvate, creatine, and L-carnitine.** *Nutrients* 2011, **3**(8):735–755.
8. Hall JL, Gonder-Frederick L, Chewning W, Silveira J, Gold P: **Glucose enhancement of performance of memory tests in young and aged humans.** *Neuropsychologia* 1989, **27**:1129–1138.
9. Craft S, Murphy C, Wemstrom J: **Glucose effects on complex memory and nonmemory tasks: The influence of age, sex, and glucoregulatory response.** *Psychobiology* 1994, **22**:95–105.
10. Newcomer JW, Craft S, Fucetola R, Moldin SO, Selke G, Paras L, Miller R: **Glucose-induced increase in memory performance in patients with schizophrenia.** *Schizophr Bull* 1999, **25**(2):321–335.
11. Welsh RS, Davis JM, Burke JR, Williams HG: **Carbohydrates and physical/mental performance during intermittent exercise to fatigue.** *Med Sci Sports Exerc* 2002, **34**(4):723–731.
12. Durnin JV, Womersley J: **Body fat assessed from total body density and its estimation from skinfold thickness: measurements on 481 men and women aged from 16 to 72 years.** *Br J Nutr* 1974, **32**:77–97.
13. Siri WE: **The gross composition of the body.** *Adv Biol Med Phys* 1956, **4**:239–280.
14. Yeo ZW, Fan PW, Nio AQ, Byrne C, Lee JK: **Ice slurry on outdoor running performance in heat.** *Int J Sports Med* 2012, **33**(11):859–866.
15. Iregren A, Gamberale F, Kjellberg A: **SPES: a psychological test system to diagnose environmental hazards. Swedish Performance Evaluation System.** *Neurotoxicol Teratol* 1996, **18**(4):485–491.
16. Loh S, Lamond N, Dorrian J, Roach G, Dawson D: **The validity of psychomotor vigilance tasks of less than 10-minute duration.** *Behav Res Methods Instrum Comput* 2004, **36**(2):339–346.
17. Benton D, Ruffin MP, Lassel T, Nabb S, Messaoudi M, Vinoy S, Desor D, Lang V: **The delivery rate of dietary carbohydrates affects cognitive performance in both rats and humans.** *Psychopharmacology (Berl)* 2003, **166**(1):86–90.
18. Hopkins RO, Suchyta MR, Snow GL, Jephson A, Weaver LK, Orme JF: **Blood glucose dysregulation and cognitive outcome in ARDS survivors.** *Brain Inj* 2010, **24**(12):1478–1484.
19. Kakos LS: **Improving Cognitive Function Following Exercise-Induced Dehydration: Role of Sports Drink Supplementation.** In *Unpublished PhD thesis.* Kent, Ohio, United States: Kent State University; 2013:123.
20. Nabb S, Benton D: **The influence on cognition of the interaction between the macro-nutrient content of breakfast and glucose tolerance.** *Physiol Behav* 2006, **87**(1):16–23.
21. Nilsson A, Radeborg K, Björck I: **Effects on cognitive performance of modulating the postprandial blood glucose profile at breakfast.** *Eur J Clin Nutr* 2012, **66**(9):1039–1043.
22. Gold PE, Vogt JA, Hall JL: **Glucose effects on memory: Behavioral and pharmacological characteristics.** *Behav Neural Biol* 1986, **46**:145–155.
23. Giles GE, Mahoney CR, Brunyé TT, Gardony AL, Taylor HA, Kanarek RB: **Differential cognitive effects of energy drink ingredients: caffeine, taurine, and glucose.** *Pharmacol Biochem Behav* 2012, **102**(4):569–577.
24. Kennedy DO, Scholey AB: **Glucose administration, heart rate and cognitive performance: effects of increasing mental effort.** *Psychopharmacology (Berl)* 2000, **149**(1):63–71.
25. Scholey AB, Harper S, Kennedy DO: **Cognitive demand and blood glucose.** *Physiol Behav* 2001, **73**(4):585–592.
26. Riby LM, McMurtrie H, Smallwood J, Ballantyne C, Meikle A, Smith E: **The facilitative effects of glucose ingestion on memory retrieval in younger and older adults: is task difficulty or task domain critical?** *Br J Nutr* 2006, **95**(2):414–420.
27. Sünram-Lea SI, Foster JK, Durlach P, Perez C: **The influence of fat co-administration on the glucose memory facilitation effect.** *Nutr Neurosci* 2004, **7**(1):21–32.
28. Riby LM, McLaughlin J, Riby DM, Graham C: **Lifestyle, glucose regulation and the cognitive effects of glucose load in middle-aged adults.** *Br J Nutr* 2008, **100**(5):1128–1134.
29. Riby LM, Sünram-Lea SI, Graham C, Foster JK, Cooper T, Moodie C, Gunn VP: **P3b versus P3a: an event-related potential investigation of the glucose facilitation effect.** *J Psychopharmacol* 2008, **22**(5):486–492.
30. Scholey AB, Kennedy DO: **Cognitive and physiological effects of an "energy drink": an evaluation of the whole drink and of glucose, caffeine and herbal flavouring fractions.** *Psychopharmacology (Berl)* 2004, **176**(3–4):320–330.
31. Foster JK, Lidder PG, Sünram SI: **Glucose and memory: fractionation of enhancement effects?** *Psychopharmacology (Berl)* 1998, **137**(3):259–270.
32. Smith MA, Riby LM, Eekelen JA, Foster JK: **Glucose enhancement of human memory: a comprehensive research review of the glucose memory facilitation effect.** *Neurosci Biobehav Rev* 2011, **35**(3):770–783.
33. Gyntelberg F, Rennie MJ, Hickson RC, Holloszy JO: **Effect of training on the response of plasma glucagon to exercise.** *J Appl Physiol Respir Environ Exerc Physiol* 1977, **43**(2):302–305.

Lactose-free milk prolonged endurance capacity in lactose intolerant Asian males

Kriyot Sudsa-ard[1†], Kallaya Kijboonchoo[1*†], Visith Chavasit[1], Rungchai Chaunchaiyakul[2], Amanda Qing Xia Nio[3] and Jason Kai Wei Lee[4,5,6]

Abstract

Background: Several studies on Caucasian volunteers have proven that milk is an effective recovery drink for athletes. Such benefit, however, cannot be directly applied to the lactose-intolerant Asian population. This study investigated the effects of ingesting water (WT), sports drink (SPD) and lactose-free milk (LFM) on cycling capacity.

Methods: Ten healthy young men completed 3 randomized experimental trials. Each trial consisted of an intermittent glycogen depleting session, a 2 h recovery period during which they ingested the test drink, followed by cycling at 70% of their maximum oxygen consumption (VO_2max) to volitional exhaustion. Each trial was separated by at least one week.

Results: There were no complaints or symptoms of lactose intolerance during any of the trials. The cycling periods were different ($p < 0.05$) amongst the 3 trials, namely, lactose-free milk (LFM; 69.6 ± 14.0 min), sports drink (SPD; 52.1 ± 11.6 min), and water (WT; 36.0 ± 11.1 min), respectively. The VO_2 and VCO_2 of LFM (30 ± 4 and 29 ± 4 ml/kg/min) were lower ($p < 0.05$) than that of SPD (34 ± 4 and 34 ± 4 ml/kg/min) and WT (35 ± 4 and 33 ± 5 ml/kg/min). There were no differences ($p = 0.45$) in VO_2 and VCO_2 between SPD and WT. Mean rating of perceived exertion was lowest in LFM (14 ± 5; $p < 0.05$), while no difference was found between the other two trials (SPD: 16 ± 4 and WT: 16 ± 4; $p = 0.18$).

Conclusion: Lactose-free milk is likely to be an effective recovery drink for enhancing subsequent cycling capacity in lactose intolerant Asian males.

Keywords: Lactose intolerance, Hydration, Recovery drink, Cycling, Endurance capacity, Asian population

Introduction

Nutrition is one aspect of an athlete's lifestyle that can be modified to enhance sporting performance. This encompasses individualized interventions adopted before, during, and after exercise. Appropriate nutrition after exercise can enhance recovery and augment performance in the subsequent exercise bout, which may in turn, encourage greater physiological adaptation to exercise training and result in improved performance during competition.

Milk has been proven to be an effective post-exercise drink for endurance activities [1-7]. Milk contains several ergogenic nutrients including carbohydrate, protein, fat, vitamins, and minerals. Following an exhaustive bout of exercise, athletes who drank milk could recover faster and exhibit better exercise performance compared with those who had commercial sports drinks or carbohydrate replacement drink [5,6]. Moreover, an electrolyte drink that was fortified with carbohydrate and protein could increase muscle glycogen by 128% more than a 6% carbohydrate drink [8]. Beradi et al. [9] explained that muscle glycogen resynthesis was greater following 6 h of recovery due to the addition of protein to the recovery drink.

Unfortunately, the benefits of protein and carbohydrate, especially from milk, in enhancing the recovery period of athletes are not applicable to lactose intolerance individuals, such as Asians. Symptoms of lactose intolerance can include nausea, vomiting, and diarrhea, with the severity of symptoms dependent on the level of

* Correspondence: kallaya.kij@mahidol.ac.th
†Equal contributors
[1]Institute of Nutrition, Mahidol University, Salaya, Phutthamonthon, Nakhon Pathom 73170, Thailand
Full list of author information is available at the end of the article

lactose intolerance. Such an effect will likely impair exercise performance. A study performed in indigenous Asians in Singapore showed that all of the sampled 22 subjects aged 15–42 y were lactose-intolerant [10]. Asmawi et al. [11] reported hypolactasia in 88% of Malaysian Malays, 91% of Malaysian Chinese, and 83% of Malaysian Indians. A study using the breath-hydrogen test after oral intake of 25 g lactose in Thai adults demonstrated that almost half of the cohort was lactose intolerant [12].

Lactose-free milk (LFM) may be potentially ergogenic as a recovery beverage for lactose intolerant individuals. We hypothesized that a LFM drink could extend cycling time to exhaustion. To our knowledge, there is no study of LFM on prolonged exercise. We investigated the effects of LFM on endurance cycling capacity in healthy Thai males.

Methods

Study participants

Ten healthy males volunteered for this study (Table 1). Experimental procedures were approved by Mahidol University Institutional Review Board, Thailand. Participants received a verbal explanation about the study before providing written informed consent.

Laboratory protocol

Participants arrived at the laboratory in the morning following an overnight fast. Each participant completed four visits to the laboratory (ambient temperature: 25 ± 1°C; relative humidity: 56% ± 2): a maximal incremental exercise test and three randomized experimental trials ingesting water (WT), a commercial sports drink (SPD), or lactose-free milk (LFM; manufactured by the Institute of Nutrition, Mahidol University, Thailand; Table 2).

Lactose-free milk was produced by adding 500 ppm β-galactosidase (lactase) enzyme (Ha-Lactase 5200 NLU/g, Chr-Hansen, Horsholm, Denmark) to an in-house low-fat pasteurized milk. The inoculated milk was incubated at 8°C for 24 h before pasteurization at 72°C for 15 s. The pasteurized milk was cooled to room temperature and fortified with sodium and potassium to increase its

Table 1 Physical and physiological characteristics of the participants (n = 10)

	Mean ± SD	Range
Age (yr)	21.2 ± 0.8	20–22
Height (cm)	174 ± 3	168–178
Body weight (kg)	66.8 ± 4.6	60.8–73.8
BMI (kg/m^2)	22.1 ± 1.5	20.3–24.8
Body fat (%)	12.6 ± 4.3	9.7–19.7
VO_2max (ml/kg/min)	44 ± 2	40–47
Peak power output (W)	288 ± 41	280–320

Table 2 Nutritional content in 250 mL of each test drink

Contents	Water	Sports drink	Lactose-free milk
Energy (kcal)	-	100	100
Carbohydrate (g)	-	25.0	12.5
Protein (g)	-	-	8
Fat (g)	-	-	2
Sodium (g)	-	0.092	0.439
Potassium (g)	-	0.015	0.518
Osmolality (mosmol/kg)	-	415	352

osmolality which was initially much lower than the sports drink.

The experimental trial consisted of an exercise-induced glycogen depletion session, a 2-h recovery period during which the test drink was ingested, and an endurance capacity test. Each trial was separated by 1–2 weeks. Dietary intake in the three days prior to the first experimental trial was recorded and repeated for subsequent trials. The macronutrients ingested were calculated using an in-house dietary software programme (INMUCAL, Institute of Nutrition, Mahidol University, Thailand). Urine specific gravity (Refractometer model 300CL, Atago Inc, Japan) was recorded as a measure of hydration status before each experimental trial.

Maximal incremental exercise test

Participants completed a standardized 2-min warm-up (cadence 60 revolutions [rev]/min, workload 0.5kp) on a cycle ergometer (Ergomedic 828 E, Sweden) followed by an incremental cycling test to volitional exhaustion at a cadence of 80 rev/min. Workload was increased by 1 kp every 2 min. Oxygen uptake was determined using a metabolic cart (Vmax Sensor Medics Metabolic, SensorMedics® Corporation, USA). Heart rate (Polar RS800CX POLAR®, Finland) was measured. The test was accepted if at least two of following criteria were met: i) respiratory exchange ratio (RER) greater than 1.1; ii) heart rate above 90% of age-predicted maximum heart rate; and iii) a VO_2 increase of less than 0.15 l/min from the previous workload [13]. Maximum power output (Pmax) was defined as the power output attained during the final completed stage.

Glycogen depletion session

The glycogen depletion exercise consisted of 2-min intervals at 60%–90%Pmax interspersed with 50%Pmax recovery at 80 rev/min [5]. Participants commenced the exercise with 2-min intervals at 90%Pmax and the workload was subsequently reduced to 80%Pmax when their cadence fell below 70 rev/min for more than 30 s. This criterion was repeated for further reductions to 70%

Pmax and 60%Pmax, respectively. Participants continued cycling with the alternating 2 min periods at each work interval at 50%Pmax with 80 rev/min until they could no longer maintain the required cadence over a minute. Heart rate was monitored every minute. Height, weight, body fat, and body mass index (BMI) were measured using a body composition analyzer (Inbody 720, Biospace, Korea) before and immediately after the glycogen depletion session. Blood lactate was measured before and after the endurance capacity test using a lactate scout analyzer (SensLab, LSSY-170407-E, Germany). VO_2, VCO_2 and RER (Vmax Sensor Medics Metabolic, SensorMedics®, USA) were measured continuously during the endurance capacity test.

Recovery period

After completing the glycogen depletion session, participants rested for 2 h in the laboratory. The volume of LFM provided was calculated such that participants received 1 g of CHO/kg BM [5,6] during the recovery period. For example, if the participant had a body mass of 66 kg, he would receive 1320 ml of LFM (12.5 g CHO/250 ml LFM). By selecting a commercially available sports drink with a caloric content similar to LFM, both volume and caloric content of test drinks ingested during the SPD and LFM trials were matched. An equal volume of water was provided during the WT trial. Each test drink was administered in three aliquots during the recovery period: 50% at 0 min, 25% at 30 min and the remaining 25% at 60 min. [14,15].

Endurance capacity test

Following the recovery period, participants completed a standardized warm-up (2 min at 60 rev/min, workload of 0.5 kp) before embarking on the endurance capacity test at 80 rev/min at $70\%VO_2max$. The test was terminated when the participant's cadence fell below 70 rev/min for more than 30 s twice [5]. VO_2, VCO_2, and RER were measured during the endurance capacity test. Heart rate was recorded continuously. Time to exhaustion was measured. Rating of perceived exertion (RPE) were measured every 5 min [16]. Body weight and blood lactate were measured at the start and immediately at the end of the trial.

Data analysis

Statistical analyses were performed using SPSS (IBM® Corp, SPSS®Statistics Version 21, USA). One-way repeated measures analysis of variance (ANOVA) was used to compare all variables (e.g. heart rate, oxygen uptake and cycle time to exhaustion) between trials (i.e. WT, SPD and LFM). Data were presented as mean ± standard deviation (SD). Alpha was set *a priori* at 0.05.

Results

Physical and physiological characteristics of participants are shown in Table 1. Participants were similarly euhydrated (urine specific gravity; WT: 1.014 ± 0.004, SPD: 1.014 ± 0.004, LFM: 1.020 ± 0.003; $p = 0.57$) and had similar absolute (WT: 2019 ± 573, SPD: 1722 ± 487, LFM: 2113 ± 389 kcal/day; $p = 0.95$) and relative caloric intakes (WT: 30 ± 3, SPD: 26 ± 8, LFM: 31 ± 6 kcal/kg/day; $p = 0.39$) prior to undertaking the experimental trials.

Heart rate was similar across all three experimental trials (Table 3). Whilst oxygen consumption and RER were similar during all three glycogen depletion sessions, oxygen uptake was lower in LFM ($p < 0.05$) during the endurance capacity test than in SPD and WT. In addition, RER was lower in WT than SPD during the endurance capacity test ($p < 0.05$).

Time to exhaustion was greatest in LFM ($p < 0.05$), followed by SPD and WT (Figure 1). The longer exercise duration in LFM also elicited the greatest body mass loss compared to the other two trials (LFM 1.0 ± 0.3 kg; SPD 0.8 ± 0.3 kg; WT 0.6 ± 0.3 kg; $p < 0.05$). Blood lactate was higher after the endurance capacity test with WT (2.4 ± 1.9 mmol/dl) than SPD (1.0 ± 0.7 mmol/dl; $p < 0.05$), but neither was significantly different in comparison to LFM (1.7 ± 1.4 mmol/dl; $p > 0.05$).

Discussion

Our study is the first to demonstrate the ergogenic effects of ingesting lactose-free milk on endurance cycling capacity in young adults. The ingestion of lactose-free milk during recovery after glycogen depleting exercise almost doubled (93% increase) the subsequent cycle time to exhaustion in comparison with water, and further extended exercise duration by 34% compared to sports drink. Despite identical workloads during the endurance capacity test with all three drinks, the oxygen uptake

Table 3 Physiological responses during each trial

	Water	Sports drink	Lactose-free milk
Glycogen depletion session			
Heart rate (beats/min)	136 ± 7	139 ± 6	135 ± 7
VO_2 (ml/min/kg)	38 ± 1	38 ± 1	36 ± 1
VCO_2 (ml/min/kg)	42 ± 2	43 ± 2	41 ± 2
RER	1.11 ± 0.02	1.11 ± 0.01	1.12 ± 0.02
Endurance performance test			
Heart rate (beats/min)	153 ± 13	153 ± 13	152 ± 13
VO_2 (ml/min/kg)	35 ± 4	34 ± 4	30 ± 4*#
VCO_2 (ml/min/kg)	33 ± 5	34 ± 4	29 ± 4*#
RER	0.95 ± 0.05	0.99 ± 0.05*	0.97 ± 0.03
RPE	16 ± 4	16 ± 4	14 ± 5

*$p < 0.05$ compared with water; # $p < 0.05$ compared with sports drink.

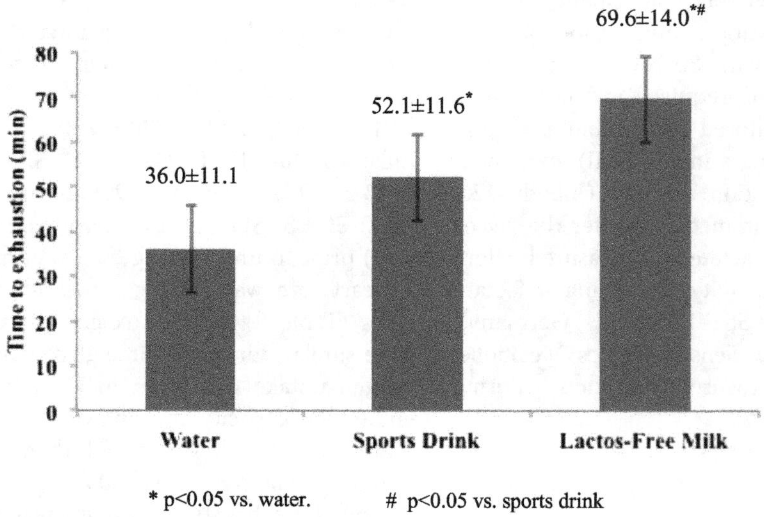

Figure 1 Endurance capacity between trials. *$p < 0.05$ vs. water. #$p < 0.05$ vs. sports drink.

and concomitant expired carbon dioxide during exercise was lower after the ingestion of lactose-free milk compared to water and sports drink. This may indicate that the ingestion of lactose-free milk during recovery enhances metabolic efficiency during the subsequent exercise bout.

Although muscle glycogen resynthesis was not measured in the present study, this may have been enhanced with the ingestion of lactose-free milk compared to the isocaloric sports drink [9,17]. Previous work has generally shown a greater muscle glycogen resynthesis with carbohydrate-protein drinks compared to carbohydrate-only drinks [8,18], although mixed results exist [19]. The interpretation of these results, however, is limited by a higher caloric content in the carbohydrate-protein drinks than the carbohydrate-only drinks. Whilst it has been suggested that a greater carbohydrate intake may enhance glycogen resynthesis to match that after carbohydrate-protein intake [20], other comparisons of isocaloric carbohydrate-only and carbohydrate-protein drinks nevertheless demonstrate a more efficient replenishment of muscle glycogen after carbohydrate-protein intake [9,17]. Moreover, drinks containing too much carbohydrate (8–10%), similar to the sports drink in the present study, may also delay gastric emptying and fluid absorption [15]. This could result in reduced muscle and liver glycogen stores. Taken together, it is thus possible that muscle glycogen resynthesis was enhanced with ingestion of lactose-free milk compared to sports drink (and water) in the present study. An improved glycogen repletion would enable a better metabolic efficiency during the cycle ride to exhaustion after ingestion of lactose-free milk and explain, in part, the lower oxygen uptake required to sustain exercise and the resultant extension in exercise duration [8].

Differences in the type of carbohydrate in lactose-free milk compared to sports drink could also have contributed to the lower oxygen consumption observed during the cycle ride to exhaustion in the present study. Whilst SPD contained 6% glucose and 4% sucrose, LFM consisted of 2.5% glucose and 2.5% galactose. Exogenous glucose oxidation during exercise has a maximum of 1.0–1.1 g/min, whereas galactose utilization is limited to ~0.4 g/min [14]. This lower oxidation rate of galactose compared to glucose and sucrose [21] is due to the conversion of glucose in the liver, before subsequent utilization by the skeletal muscles. The ingested galactose may also have been synthesized to form glycogen during the recovery period. It is thus possible that the galactose in lactose-free milk slowed the oxidation process, resulting in the lowered oxygen consumption and carbon dioxide production observed [4].

A reduction in muscle damage (i.e. creatine phosphokinase levels [18]) with lactose-free milk ingestion is another likely candidate to explain the physiological differences observed during the cycle ride to exhaustion in the present study. This may be achieved via a reduced rate of protein breakdown (i.e. improved whole body net protein balance [22]) and greater myofibrillar muscle protein synthesis through p70S6K, downstream of mTOR [23], following the ingestion of protein after exercise. Whether the performance benefits associated with lactose-free milk ingestion in the present study are also relevant to a more aerobically fit population (e.g. VO2peak 65 ± 7 mL/min/kg [24]) is unclear, and requires further investigation.

Whilst the underlying mechanism(s) for the lower oxygen consumption and carbon dioxide production with LFM cannot be elucidated from the present study, our results nonetheless clearly demonstrate the efficacy of LFM as a recovery drink to enhance subsequent exercise performance. The extended time to exhaustion after LFM ingestion observed in the present study is in agreement with previous work that have investigated chocolate milk as a recovery drink [5,6]. Those studies have reported that the ingestion of chocolate milk as a recovery drink results in at least comparable, if not better, subsequent exercise performance compared to other commercially available fluid- and carbohydrate-replacement drinks [5,6].

Further work is necessary to determine the mechanism(s) underlying the extended endurance capacity duration after lactose-free milk ingestion, compared to an isocaloric and isovolumic sports drink. In the present study, participants could not be blinded to the test drink and this may have psychologically affected them during the cycle ride to exhaustion. Whilst the efficacy of lactose-free milk as a recovery drink is clear, the product used the present study was manufactured in-house and fortified with sodium and potassium. This is a key limitation for the immediate applicability of our results to the lactose intolerant population, as the lactose-free milk investigated in the present study is not currently commercially available.

Conclusion

This study demonstrates an increased cycle time to exhaustion after ingesting lactose-free milk as a recovery drink, as compared to water and sports drink. The extended exercise duration may be explained by a greater metabolic efficiency, as the amount of oxygen consumed and carbon dioxide produced were both reduced with lactose-free milk. Consequently, lactose-free milk may be appropriate as a recovery drink for the general population and can be used as a substitute for normal milk in lactose intolerant individuals.

Competing interests

The authors declare that they have no competing interests.

Authors' contributions

KS was the investigator, supervised subject recruitment, data acquisition, data specimen collection, and data analysis (30% of total contribution). KK wrote the proposal, obtained grant funds, designed the study, interpreted data, and prepared the manuscript (30%). VC supervised and prepared lactose free-milk and interpreted data (10%). RC designed the study and interpreted data (10%). AN (10%) and JKWL (10%) contributed to the study design and prepared the manuscript. All authors read and approved the final manuscript.

Acknowledgements

We would like to thank the Sports Authority of Thailand for their financial support.

Author details

[1]Institute of Nutrition, Mahidol University, Salaya, Phutthamonthon, Nakhon Pathom 73170, Thailand. [2]College of Sports Science and Technology, Mahidol University, Salaya, Phutthamonthon, Nakhon Pathom 73170, Thailand. [3]School of Sport, Cardiff Metropolitan University, Cardiff, UK. [4]Defence Medical and Environmental Research Institute, DSO National Laboratories, Singapore, Singapore. [5]Yong Loo Lin School of Medicine, National University of Singapore, Singapore, Singapore. [6]Lee Kong Chian School of Medicine, Nanyang Technological University, Singapore, Singapore.

References

1. Cockburn E, Stevenson E, Hayes PR, Robson-Ansley P, Howatson G: **Effect of milk-based carbohydrate-protein supplement timing on the attenuation of exercise induced muscle damage.** *Appl Physiol Nutr Metab* 2010, **35**:270–277.
2. Shirreffs SM, Watson P, Maughan RJ: **Milk as an effective post-exercise rehydration drink.** *Bri J Nutr* 2007, **98**:173–180.
3. Watson P, Love TD, Maughan RJ, Shirreffs SM: **A comparison of the effects of milk and a carbohydrate-electrolyte drink on the restoration of fluid balance and exercise capacity in a hot, humid environment.** *Eur J Appl Physiol* 2008, **104**:633–642.
4. Lee JK, Maughan RJ, Shirreffs SM: **Effects of milk ingestion on prolonged exercise capacity in young healthy men.** *Nutrition* 2008, **24**:340–347.
5. Karp JR, Johnston JD, Tecklenburg S, Mickleborough TD, Fly AD, Stager JM: **Chocolate milk as a post-exercise recovery aid.** *Int J Sport Nutr Exer Metab* 2006, **16**:78–91.
6. Thomas K, Morris P, Stevenson E: **Improved endurance capacity following chocolate milk consumption compared with 2 commercially available sport drinks.** *Appl Physiol Nutr Metab* 2009, **34**:78–82.
7. Pritchett K, Bishop P, Pritchett R, Green M, Katica C: **Acute effects of chocolate milk and commercial recovery beverage on postexercise recovery indices and endurance cycling performance.** *Appl Physiol Nutr Metab* 2009, **34**:1017–1022.
8. Williams MB, Raven PB, Fogt DL, Ivy JL: **Effects of recovery beverages on glycogen restoration and endurance exercise performance.** *J Strength Cond Res* 2003, **17**(1):12–19.
9. Beradi JM, Price TB, Noreen EE, Lemon PW: **Postexercise muscle glycogen recovery enhanced with a carbohydrate-protein supplement.** *Med Sci Sport Exer* 2006, **38**(6):1106–1113.
10. Bolin TD, Davis AE, Seah CS, Chua KL, Yong V, Kho KM, Siak CL, Jacob E: **Lactose intolerance in Singapore.** *Gastroenterology* 1970, **59**:76–84.
11. Asmawi MZ, Seppo L, Vapaatalo H, Korpela R: **Hypolactasia and lactose intolerance among three ethnic groups in Malaysia. Indian.** *J Med Res* 2006, **124**:697–704.
12. Densupsoontorn N, Jirapinyo P, Thamonsiri N, Wongarn R: **Lactose intolerance in Thai adults.** *J Med Assoc Thai* 2004, **87**(12):1501–1505.
13. Taylor HL, Buskirk E, Henschel A: **Maximal oxygen make objective measure of cardio-respiratory performance.** *J Appl Physiol* 1955, **8**(1):73–80.
14. Jeukendrup AE, Jentjens R: **Oxidation of carbohydrate feedings during prolonged exercise current thoughts, Guidelines and directions for future research.** *Sports Med* 2000, **29**(6):407–422.
15. Murray R, Seifert JG, Eddy DE, Paul GL, Halaby GA: **Carbohydrate feeding and exercise: effect of beverage carbohydrate content.** *Eur J Appl Physiol* 1989, **59**:152–158.
16. Borg G: *Borg's Perceived Exertion and Pain Scales.* Champaign, IL: Human Kinetic; 1998.
17. Ivy JL, Goforth HW Jr, Damon BM, McCauley TR, Parsons EC, Price TB: **Early postexercise muscle glycogen recovery is enhanced with a carbohydrate-protein supplement.** *J App Physiol* 2002, **93**(4):1337–1344.
18. Saunders JM, Kane DM, Todd KM: **Effects of a carbohydrate-protein beverage on cycling endurance and muscle damage.** *Med Sci Sports Exer* 2004, **36**(7):1233–1238.
19. Wojcik JR, Walberg-Rankin J, Smith LL, Gwazdauskas FC: **Comparison of carbohydrate and milk-based beverage on muscle damage and glycogen following exercise.** *Int J Sport Nutr Exer Metab* 2001, **11**:406–419.
20. van Loon LJ, Saris WH, Kruijshoop M, Wagenmakers AJ: **Maximizing postexercise muscle glycogen synthesis: carbohydrate supplementation and the application of amino acid or protein hydrolysate mixtures.** *Am J Clin Nutr* 2000, **72**:106–111.
21. Leijssen DPC, Saris WH, Jeukendrup AE, Wagenmaker AJM: **Oxidation of orally ingested [13C]-glucose and [13C]-galactose during exercise.** *J Appl Physiol* 1995, **79**:720–725.

22. Howarth KR, Moreau NA, Phillips SM, Gibala MJ: **Coingestion of protein with carbohydrate during recovery from endurance exercise stimulates skeletal muscle protein synthesis in humans.** *J App Physiol* 2009, **106**(4):1394–1402. doi:10.1152/japplphysiol.90333.2008.
23. Breen L, Philp A, Witard OC, Jackman SR, Selby A, Smith K, Baar K, Tipton KD: **The influence of carbohydrate-protein co-ingestion following endurance exercise on myofibrillar and mitochondrial protein synthesis.** *J Physiol* 2011, **589**(Pt 16):4011–4025. doi:10.1113/jphysiol.2011.211888.
24. Goh Q, Boop CA, Luden ND, Smith AG, Womack CJ, Saunders MJ: **Recovery from cycling exercise: effects of carbohydrate and protein beverages.** *Nutrients* 2012, **4**(7):568–584. doi:10.3390/nu4070568.

Ergogenic effects of caffeine and sodium bicarbonate supplementation on intermittent exercise performance preceded by intense arm cranking exercise

Matthaus Marriott[1], Peter Krustrup[1,2] and Magni Mohr[3,4*]

Abstract

Background: Caffeine and sodium bicarbonate ingestion have been suggested to improve high-intensity intermittent exercise, but it is unclear if these ergogenic substances affect performance under provoked metabolic acidification. To study the effects of caffeine and sodium bicarbonate on intense intermittent exercise performance and metabolic markers under exercise-induced acidification, intense arm-cranking exercise was performed prior to intense intermittent running after intake of placebo, caffeine and sodium bicarbonate.

Methods: Male team-sports athletes (n = 12) ingested sodium bicarbonate ($NaHCO_3$; 0.4 g.kg^{-1} b.w.), caffeine (CAF; 6 mg.kg^{-1} b.w.) or placebo (PLA) on three different occasions. Thereafter, participants engaged in intense arm exercise prior to the Yo-Yo intermittent recovery test level-2 (Yo-Yo IR2). Heart rate, blood lactate and glucose as well as rating of perceived exertion (RPE) were determined during the protocol.

Results: CAF and $NaHCO_3$ elicited a 14 and 23% improvement ($P < 0.05$), respectively, in Yo-Yo IR2 performance, post arm exercise compared to PLA. The $NaHCO_3$ trial displayed higher [blood lactate] ($P < 0.05$) compared to CAF and PLA (10.5 ± 1.9 vs. 8.8 ± 1.7 and 7.7 ± 2.0 mmol.L^{-1}, respectively) after the Yo-Yo IR2. At exhaustion CAF demonstrated higher ($P < 0.05$) [blood glucose] compared to PLA and $NaHCO_3$ (5.5 ± 0.7 vs. 4.2 ± 0.9 vs. 4.1 ± 0.9 mmol.L^{-1}, respectively). RPE was lower ($P < 0.05$) during the Yo-Yo IR2 test in the $NaHCO_3$ trial in comparison to CAF and PLA, while no difference in heart rate was observed between trials.

Conclusions: Caffeine and sodium bicarbonate administration improved Yo-Yo IR2 performance and lowered perceived exertion after intense arm cranking exercise, with greater overall effects of sodium bicarbonate intake.

Keywords: Yo-Yo IR2 test performance, Fatigue, Blood lactate, Rating of perceived exertion, Team sport athletes

Introduction

Fatigue during high-intensity intermittent exercise is complex and multifaceted. Early speculation regarding the aetiology of fatigue commends that high rate of lactic acid production and a concomitant fall in blood and muscle pH [1], which may have multiple indirect and direct impairing effects on centrally and peripherally mediated fatigue-resistance. Caffeine and sodium bicarbonate ($NaHCO_3$) are two supplements frequently consumed to elicit ergogenic effects on high-intensity exercise performance [2].

Effects of caffeine on intense intermittent exercise performance have for example been studied by Stuart et al. [3] demonstrating improved repeated sprint performance during a simulated rugby game trial. Moreover, team-sport athletes improved both total work and mean power output during an intermittent cycle sprint protocol [4] and Yo-Yo IR2 performance by 16% after caffeine intake [5]. However, Glaister et al. [6] showed that although the fastest sprint time in a repeated sprint test was observed with caffeine intake, the magnitude of

* Correspondence: magnim@setur.fo
[3]Faculty of Natural and Health Sciences, University of the Faroe Islands, Jónas Broncks gøta 25. 3rd floor, Tórshavn, Faroe Islands
[4]Center of Health and Human Performance, Department of Food and Nutrition, and Sport Science, University of Gothenburg, Gothenburg, Sweden
Full list of author information is available at the end of the article

fatigue in the caffeine condition appeared to be greater compared to a placebo trial. Furthermore, no ergogenic effect has been found on sprint performance during the Loughborough intermittent shuttle test [7]. Thus, the effects of caffeine intake on intense intermittent exercise protocols are equivocal.

$NaHCO_3$ ingested 90–150 min prior exercise has been used as an ergogenic aid for athletic events highly dependent on anaerobic glycolysis, since the ergogenic potential that $NaHCO_3$ might elicit is suggested to depend upon the demands of the activity being sufficient to induce performance inhibiting levels of metabolic acidosis [8]. $NaHCO_3$ ingestion has been reported to improve competitive and laboratory-based protocols lasting 1–7 min including swimming, middle distance running, rowing and repeated sprinting [9]. In addition, improvement in performance during a repeated sprint protocol is reported [10]. However, other studies are less affirmative and demonstrating no performance enhancing effects on high-intensity intermittent cycling [11]. Further discrepancies have been illustrated by Cameron et al. [12] whereby no benefits were observed during a high-intensity rugby-specific training session followed by a repeated-sprint test. The absence of effects within the aforementioned studies is potentially due to insufficient metabolic taxation.

The Yo-Yo Intermittent Recovery test level 2 (Yo-Yo IR2) consists of 20-m shuttle runs at progressive running speed and has a high anaerobic energy turnover [13]. Thus, in order to examine the effect of caffeine and $NaHCO_3$ intake on high-intensity intermittent exercise the Yo-Yo IR2 test can be utilized. Moreover, engaging in intense arm exercise prior to repeated high-intensity running elevates the levels of leg muscle and blood [lactate] and [H^+] [14], as well as increasing the accumulation rate in muscle interstitial [K^+] resulting in decreased knee extensor exercise performance [15]. Therefore, intense upper-body exercise prior to running exercise can be applied to induce pre-exercise muscle acidosis and high metabolic disturbance without exercising the legs.

Thus, the aim of the present study was therefore to compare the effects of caffeine and $NaHCO_3$ supplementation 70–90 min prior to exercise, respectively, on Yo-Yo IR2 performance and physiological response to intense intermittent exercise with prior metabolic acidosis induced by intense arm cranking exercise.

Methods

Participants

Twelve healthy male participants involved in sub-elite team-sports (age: 20.8 ± 1.4 (±SD) yrs.; height: 183 ± 7 cm; body mass: 78.9 ± 5.4 kg) volunteered to participate in this study. Participants gave their written informed consent to participate prior to the experimental procedures and the study conforms the ethical guidelines of the Declaration of Helsinki. The study was approved by the University of Exeter Ethics Committee.

Design

The participants reported to the laboratory on five separate occasions with at least four days between visits. On the initial visit to the laboratory the participants were familiarised to the arm exercise protocol conducted on an upper body arm cranking ergometer (Lode BV, Angio, Netherlands) to determine individual specific power outputs as previously described [15]. On the second occasion participants performed a baseline, control (CON) Yo-Yo IR2 that they were familiarized to prior to the study [13]. The CON-trial was performed without any supplementation or prior arm-exercise. Participants were then assigned in a single-blind, randomized, crossover design to receive placebo (PLA; plain flour), caffeine (CAF) or sodium bicarbonate ($NaHCO_3$) supplementation.

Experimental procedure

On each experimental visit, participants were asked to report to the laboratory 100 min prior to the initiation of the Yo-Yo IR2 in a fully hydrated state and ≥2 h postprandial. The tests were carried out at the same time of the day (±1 h). The participants were not permitted to consumed alcohol 24 h prior to testing or to take any other form of dietary supplements for the duration of the study and to avoid strenuous exercise 24 h preceding each experimental trial. In addition the participants were asked to avoid food items containing caffeine prior to the experimental days. Moreover, the food intake was noted the day prior to the first test trial and replicated prior to the remaining trials. Upon arrival to the laboratory participants were fitted with a heart rate (HR) monitor (Polar Electro, Kempele, Finland) and a baseline fingertip capillary blood sample was obtained. Participants were then given either CAF or PLA (blinded) or $NaHCO_3$ to orally ingest under the supervision of the researchers. 70 min before the start of the Yo-Yo IR2 either CAF or PLA was taken orally in gelatine capsule (6 $mg.kg^{-1}$ body mass; 474 ± 31 mg; see Mohr et al. [5]). $NaHCO_3$ was ingested orally in 21–25 gelatine capsules (0.4 $g.kg^{-1}$ body mass; 31.6 ± 1.6 g) and supplementation began 90 min prior to the start of the Yo-Yo IR2 with 7 $ml.kg^{-1}$ of water drank ad libitum over a 30 min period as described by Carr et al. [9]. The respective $NaHCO_3$ intake protocol has in a pilot study been demonstrated to markedly raise the blood HCO_3^- concentration (data not shown).

The arm exercise protocol lasted for 17 min, during which the participants maintained a constant cadence (80 ± 5 RPM) at individualised power outputs (157.6 ±

7.4 W). The protocol, adapted from others [14,15] consisting of 4×1-min and 1×1.5-min exercise periods separated by 0.5-min recovery, followed by 4.5 min of recovery and a final 1-min exercise period. Immediately after completion of the arm exercise, a blood sample was taken. The Yo-Yo IR2 began 4 min after the completion of the arm exercise protocol corresponding to 70 min post CAF and PLA intake and 90 min after the $NaHCO_3$ ingestion. The Yo-Yo IR2 test was completed on a wooden surface and consists of repeated two 20-m runs at a progressively increased speed controlled by audio bleeps from a CD player [13]. The test-leader controlling the Yo-Yo IR2 test was blinded in relation to drug-treatment.

Fingertip capillary 300 μL blood samples were collected in heparin-fluoride coated Microvette CB 300 tubes (Sarstedt Ltd, UK) which were immediately stored on ice and subsequently analysed to determine blood [lactate] and [glucose] after the protocol [5] using a YSI 2500 Lactate Analyser (YSI, Yellow Springs, US) having a test-retest coefficient of variance of <2%. Blood samples were obtained: prior to supplementation on arrival to the laboratory, immediately after arm exercise, immediately after Yo-Yo IR2 exhaustion, 1, 3 and 5 min post exhaustion. Heart rate was determined during the entire protocol while rating of perceived exertion (RPE) values using the Borg scale [16] were recorded during the Yo-Yo IR2 at 160, 280, 440, 600 m and at exhaustion.

Statistical analyses

Differences between baseline Yo-Yo IR2 performance and PLA Yo-Yo IR2 after arm exercise were analysed using a paired-samples *t*-test. A one-way repeated measures ANOVA was used to determine the influence of supplementation on the performance in the Yo-Yo IR2 after intense arm exercise. Where analyses revealed a significant main effect, the origin of this effect was determined by Bonferroni adjusted post hoc paired *t*-tests. Differences in plasma [glucose], [lactate], HR and RPE between the three conditions (PLA, CAF and $NaHCO_3$) were analysed using multiple separate two-way repeated measures ANOVAs (supplement x time). Significant main effects were further analysed by Bonferroni adjusted post hoc paired *t*-tests. All repeated measures data was checked for the assumption of sphericity using Mauchly's test. All data were analysed using the statistical software package SPSS (version 20). Statistical significance was accepted at $P < 0.05$. Results are presented as means ± SD.

Results

Performance

Yo-Yo IR2 performance was reduced (P < 0.05) by 41% when the test was preceded by an intense intermittent arm cranking (CON: 696 ± 185 m vs. PLA: 413 ± 121 m; $P < 0.01$, Figure 1A). However, after CAF and $NaHCO_3$ supplementation Yo-Yo IR2 performance was 14 and 23% higher (P < 0.05) compared to PLA (480 ± 113 and 540 ± 138 m, respectively), with a greater (P < 0.05) improvement in $NaHCO_3$ than CAF (Figure 1B).

Blood metabolites

Baseline blood [Lactate] was similar (0.9 ± 0.3, 1.0 ± 0.5 and 0.9 ± 0.6 $mmol.L^{-1}$; P > 0.05) for PLA, CAF and $NaHCO_3$, respectively, but increased ($P < 0.01$) post arm crank (7.3 ± 1.8, 7.4 ± 1.5 and 8.3 ± 1.8 $mmol.L^{-1}$, respectively, Figure 2A) with no significant differences between the three trials, although there was a trend ($P = 0.09$) for higher blood [lactate] for the $NaHCO_3$ trial. Blood [lactate] did not change ($P > 0.05$) during Yo-Yo IR2 for PLA at exhaustion (7.7 ± 2.0 $mmol.L^{-1}$), but rose ($P < 0.05$) for both CAF and $NaHCO_3$ (8.8 ± 1.7 vs. 10.5 ± 1.9 $mmol.L^{-1}$, respectively, Figure 2A). Between group comparisons revealed that blood [lactate] values were similar between PLA and CAF, but higher ($P < 0.01$) for the $NaHCO_3$ trial compared to PLA and CAF trials at exhaustion (Figure 2A). At 1 min post exhaustion PLA blood [lactate] rose (9.4 ± 1.8 $mmol.L^{-1}$; $P < 0.05$) compared to exhaustion whereas CAF and NaHCO3 remained unchanged ($P > 0.05$) and blood [lactate] in the $NaCHO_3$ trial still remained higher (11.6 ± 1.7 $mmol.L^{-1}$; $P < 0.01$) when compared to PLA and CAF. At 3 min post Yo-Yo IR2 [lactate] was not different between groups (8.1 ± 1.9, 8.5 ± 2.2 and 8.8 ± 1.7 $mmol.L^{-1}$; $P > 0.05$) PLA, CAF and $NaHCO_3$, respectively. At 5 min into recovery Yo-Yo IR2 blood [lactate] was reduced in the PLA trial when compared to CAF and $NaHCO_3$ (7.2 ± 2.2 vs. 8.5 ± 2.3 and 9.1 ± 1.9 $mmol.L^{-1}$; $P < 0.05$, respectively) whereas CAF and $NaCHO_3$ were similar at this time point ($P > 0.05$).

Baseline blood [glucose] was not significantly different between trials (4.5 ± 0.5 vs. 4.2 ± 0.4 vs. 4.4 ± 0.9 $mmol.L^{-1}$; $P > 0.05$, Figure 2B) for PLA, CAF and $NaHCO_3$, respectively. For all trials at Yo-Yo IR2 exhaustion there was no difference ($P > 0.05$) in blood [glucose] within and between the supplements (3.9 ± 0.9 vs. 4.5 ± 1.1 vs. 4.2 ± 0.8 $mmol.L^{-1}$, respectively, Figure 2B). In the PLA and $NaHCO_3$ trials blood [glucose] rose (P < 0.05) between exhaustion and 1 min post Yo-Yo IR2 (4.9 ± 0.9 and 4.9 ± 0.7 $mmol.L^{-1}$). In the CAF trial blood [glucose] rose by 30% at the end of the protocol (Figure 2B), compared to the PLA ($P < 0.05$). However, no differences ($P > 0.05$) were in [glucose] between PLA and $NaHCO_3$ at any protocol time points (Figure 2B). Between group comparisons revealed that at 5 min post Yo-Yo IR2 blood [glucose] in the CAF trial was greater ($P < 0.05$) compared to the PLA and $NaHCO_3$ (5.5 ± 0.7 vs. 4.2 ± 0.9 and 4.1 ± 0.9 $mmol.L^{-1}$, respectively).

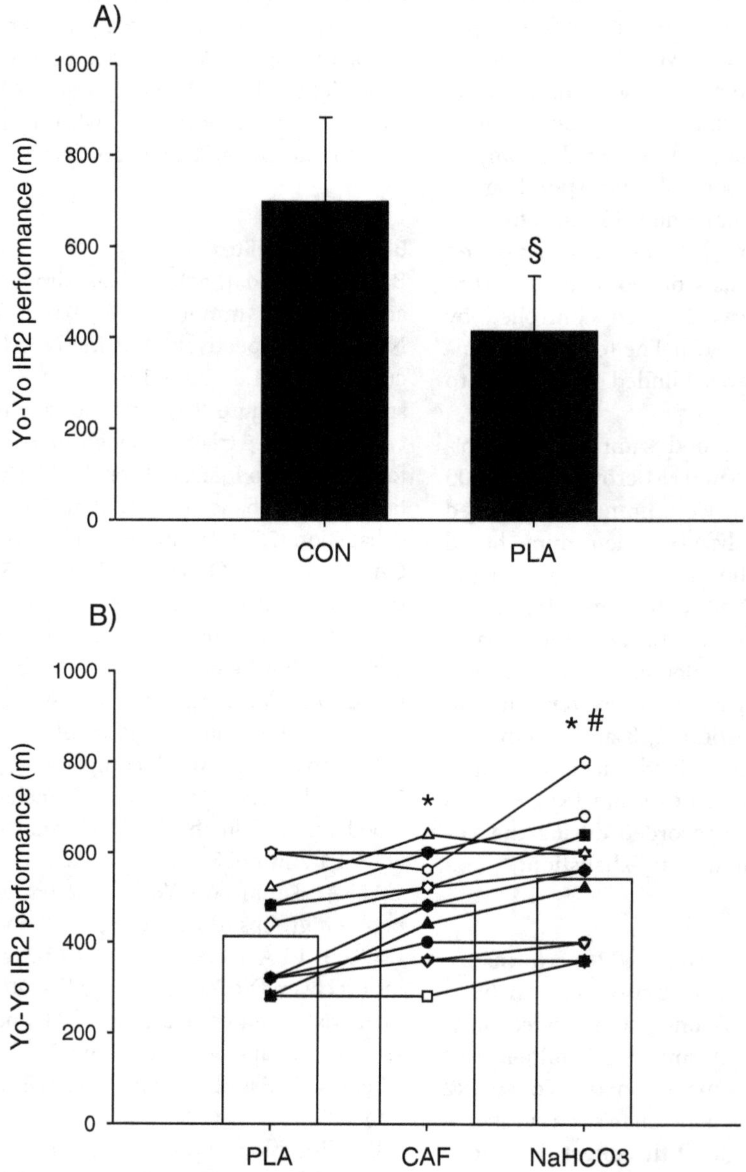

Figure 1 Yo-Yo Intermittent Recovery level 2 test (Yo-Yo IR2) performance in control (CON) and placebo (PLA) trials (A) and individual Yo-Yo IR2 performance during PLA and after caffeine (CAF) and sodium bicarbonate ($NaHCO_3$) supplementation (B) (n = 12). §: Denotes a significant difference from CON. *Denotes a significant difference from PLA. # Denotes a significant difference from CAF. Significance level $P < 0.05$.

Rating of perceived exertion and heart rate loading

Between group comparisons revealed that RPE was reduced ($P < 0.05$) in the $NaHCO_3$ trials at both 160 m and 280 m (160 m: 15.3 ± 2.3 and 15.0 ± 1.6 vs. 13.1 ± 2.0), (280 m: 17.8 ± 1.2 and 17.3 ± 1.8 vs. 15.8 ± 1.5) for PLA, CAF and $NaHCO_3$, respectively (Figure 3). No differences ($P > 0.05$) were observed at Yo-Yo IR2 exhaustion (19.3 ± 1.0, 19.3 ± 0.9 and 19.3 ± 0.7 in PLA, CAF and $NaHCO_3$, respectively, Figure 3). Arm exercise caused a rise ($P < 0.01$) in heart rate during all trials (179 ± 7, 178 ± 8 and 177 ± 9 bts.min^{-1}) for PLA, CAF and $NaHCO_3$, respectively. At Yo-Yo IR2 exhaustion a further rise ($P < 0.05$) in heart rate for CAF and $NaHCO_3$ was observed (187 ± 7 and 186 ± 7 bts.min^{-1}, respectively). Comparisons between trials revealed that there was no difference between PLA, CAF and $NaHCO_3$ at any time points during the testing protocol.

Discussion

The principle findings of the present study were that Yo-Yo IR2 performance after intense arm cranking exercise was markedly reduced compared to a control trial, while both caffeine and $NaHCO_3$ intake improved fatigue resistance during the Yo-Yo IR2 test. $NaHCO_3$

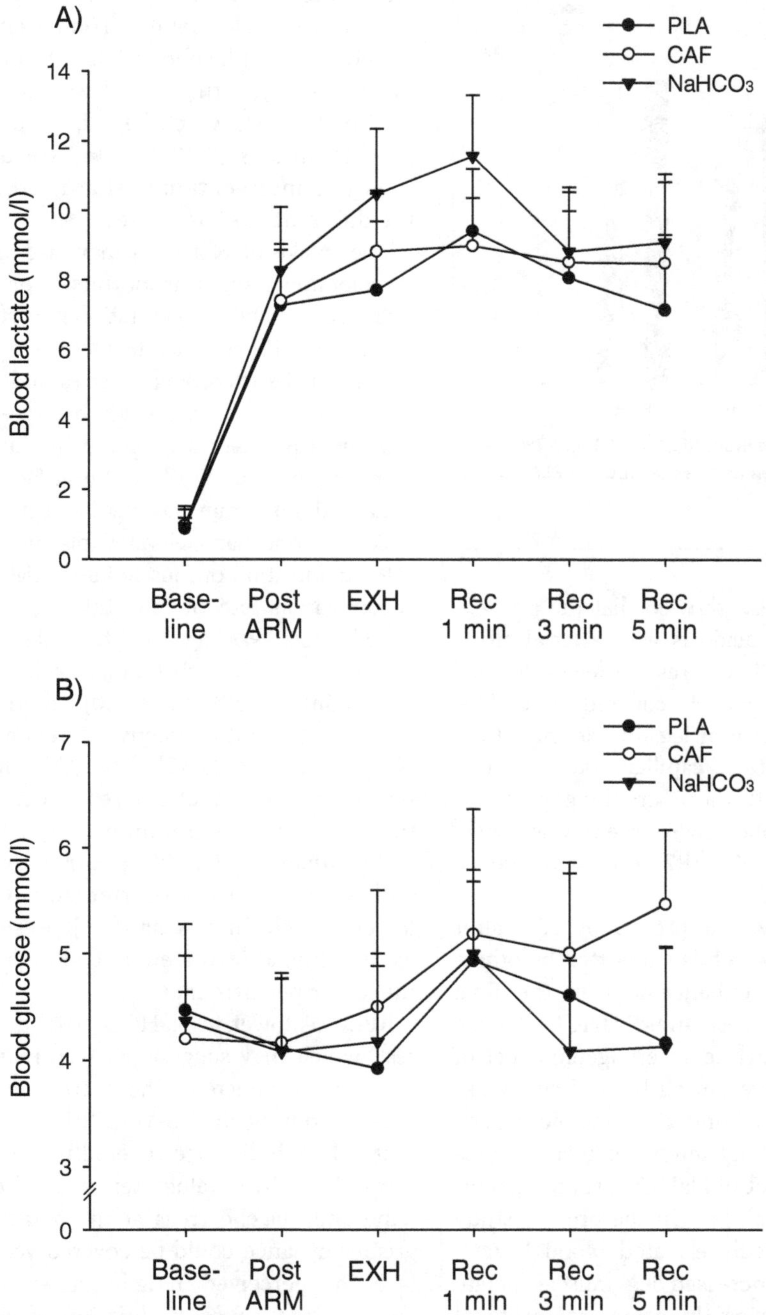

Figure 2 Capillary blood lactate (A) and glucose (B) concentrations before, during and after the Yo-Yo IR2 test protocol (n = 12) in the placebo (PLA), caffeine (CAF) and sodium bicarbonate ($NaHCO_3$) trials.

intake elicited a further ergogenic effect on Yo-Yo IR2 performance when performed after intense arm cranking exercise compared to that of caffeine. The present study is the first to report performance effects of caffeine and $NaHCO_3$ intake using high-intensity intermittent running exercise preceded by intense arm cranking exercise and to demonstrate additional performance and perceptual benefits of $NaHCO_3$ beyond that of caffeine.

The reduction in high-intensity running performance when performed after intense arm cranking exercise is consistent with previous research studying isolated muscle performance [14,15]. In the present study, Yo-Yo IR2 performance was reduced by 41% when preceded by arm exercise, which is of a similar magnitude as the performance decrements of 35% and ~48%, respectively, observed during intense exhaustive one-legged knee extensor exercise performed after intense arm cranking

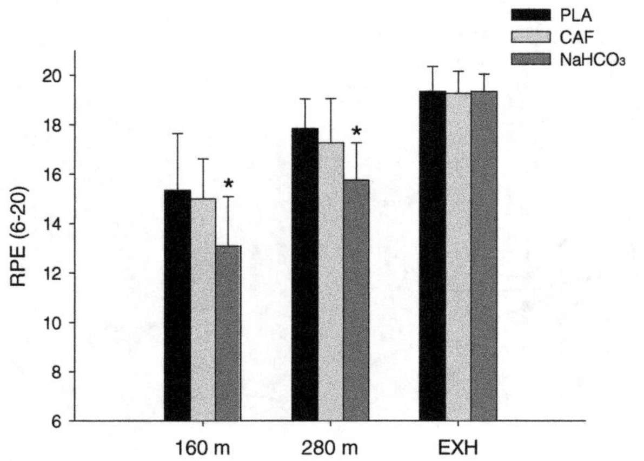

Figure 3 Rating of Perceived Exertion (RPE) at 160 and 280 m during the Yo-Yo IR2 test, as well as at exhaustion in PLA, CAF and $NaHCO_3$. *Denotes a significant difference from PLA. Significance level $P < 0.05$.

[14,15]. These two studies also showed that the arm exercise resulted in metabolic acidosis with arterial blood lactate being elevated by ~11-fold resting levels, as well as higher leg muscle lactate and H^+ concentrations [14] and elevated accumulation rate of leg muscle interstitial $[K^+]$ [15]. In the present study capillary blood lactate was elevated ~8-fold after the arm cranking protocol, confirming that the metabolic environment was markedly altered prior to the Yo-Yo IR2 test compared to baseline conditions.

Yo-Yo IR2 performance was improved by 23% after $NaHCO_3$ supplementation, which is supported by others [9,10]. Indeed performance enhancement in the final sprints of a repeated sprint test after $NaHCO_3$ intake has been reported [10], indicating an ergogenic effect of $NaHCO_3$ on fatigue resistance during high intensity exercise conditions performed under metabolic stress. However, some studies applying intense exercise protocols report no beneficial effect of $NaHCO_3$ supplementation (for review see Carr et al. [9]). In the present study intense arm cranking markedly elevated blood lactate, confirming findings of an increased leg muscle lactate and H^+ concentration following the same arm protocol [14]. Part of the longer exercise time level in the $NaHCO_3$-trial may be explained by an elevated $NaHCO_3$ induced buffer capacity in the blood, which will increase the muscle-to-blood H^+ and lactate gradient. Since the monocarboxylate transporters (MCT) are gradient dependent [17], this will increase the removal of H^+ and lactate ions from the leg muscles before and during the Yo-Yo IR2 test. This may reduce the degree of intramuscular acidification and corresponding fatigue development [1]. The higher blood lactate levels were observed in the $NaHCO_3$-trial, may also partly be a direct consequence of the greater fatigue resistance, and thereby higher glycolytic contribution and concomitant muscle lactate production compared to the caffeine and placebo trials. A limitation with the present study is that blood was not drawn during the Yo-Yo IR2 test, which have been done on other comparable studies [5,13], so we are unable to compare the three intervention trial at fixed time points due to the different exercise times.

The intake of $NaHCO_3$ may also affect the activity of sarcolemmal ion transporters. For example elevated extracellular Na^+ concentration may stimulate the Na^+/H^+ exchangers [18] and thereby increase the efflux of hydrogen ions from the exercising muscles and attenuate intramuscular acidification. In a study by Street et al. [19] muscle interstitial pH decreased gradually during graded exercise comparable to the Yo-Yo IR2 test. However, in a follow-up study sodium citrate was ingested prior to intense exercise, which on one hand elevated plasma HCO_3^- and lowered the accumulation of muscle interstitial H^+ [18]. Finally, the accumulation rate of interstitial K^+ was significantly reduced, which was suggested to relate to less opening probability of the K_{ATP} channels, which tend to open during intracellular acidification [20]. In addition, the elevated systemic Na^+ may directly stimulate the activity in the Na^+-K^+ ATPase [1,18]. Thus, the intake of $NaHCO_3$ may have elevated fatigue resistance by inducing maintenance of a more optimum intracellular pH [21] and/or by enhancing Na^+/K^+ pump activity and potentially $Na^+/K^+/2Cl^-$ co-transporter activity, contributing to lower muscle interstitial $[K^+]$ preserving sarcolemma excitability, allowing enhanced high intensity repeated muscular performance [1].

RPE was lower in $NaHCO_3$-trial during the Yo-Yo IR2 test, which may suggest that centrally mediated mechanisms were affected. The participants experienced less exertion during the Yo-Yo IR2 in the $NaHCO_3$-trial, and that although distance covered before exhaustion was increased the RPE values remained the same as the caffeine and placebo trials at the point of fatigue. Thus, a greater distance could be covered yet reporting an equal level of perceived fatigue at exhaustion. Peripheral changes may cause modulation of neural strategies via group III and IV muscle afferents which are widely distributed through the muscle and are responsive to chemical stimuli such as altered H^+ and K^+ [22]. Different mechanisms have been proposed by which such peripheral inputs might lead to modulation of motor neuron firing rates and muscle function including facilitation or inhibition of spinal reflexes, pre-synaptic inhibition of the group Ia afferents thus reducing inhibitory input into the motoneurons, and altered supraspinal drive [22]. Thus, part of the improved performance after $NaHCO_3$ treatment may relate to less negative feedback from the muscle and thereby less effect on the descending drive to the motoneurons [22,23].

In the present study caffeine increased Yo-Yo IR2 performance by 14% compared to the placebo-trial, which is in line with other findings [3,4]. Caffeine has multiple physiological effects that may promote fatigue resistance during intense exercise, such as elevating the catecholamine levels [24] and reducing muscle interstitial K^+ accumulation [5]. Peak blood glucose concentrations were higher in the caffeine-trial than placebo, which is in accordance with findings by others [5], indicating an elevated catecholamine response, which may facilitate the Na^+-K^+ ATPase activity [25]. The arm protocol has been shown to increase the accumulation of interstitial potassium during leg exercise [15], and caffeine may reduce this effect by increasing the pump activity in the Na^+-K^+ APTase directly or via an elevated catecholamine response [5,25]. Finally caffeine may have an effect on central mechanisms associated with fatigue [23,26], however, the RPE rating were not different between the caffeine and placebo trials in the present study. Caffeine is well-known to affect the central nervous system response mediated via antagonism of adenosine receptors, which dampens pain perception and attenuates fatigue [27]. However, during high-intensity intermittent exercise caffeine-induced effects on RPE appear to be negated [6], which is supported by this study.

Intriguingly, there were no differences in HR between the trials, suggesting that the aerobic demands were similar, yet participant's perception of fatigue was attenuated during the $NaHCO_3$-trial, indicating that $NaHCO_3$ in contrast to caffeine might impact upon central fatigue as well as peripheral fatigue.

The possibility of a 'high-responders' and 'low-responders' phenomena for both caffeine and $NaHCO_3$ has been previously reported [27-29]. This effect was apparent in the present study, whereby three subjects and one subject, respectively, after caffeine and $NaHCO_3$ intake, showed no improvement compared to PLA. Moreover five of the subjects reported experiencing some form of gastrointestinal discomfort after sodium bicarbonate intake; however this was apparently not detrimental to exercise performance.

Conclusions

The present study demonstrates that high-intensity intermittent exercise performance is impaired when preceded by intense arm exercise. However, fatigue resistance can be markedly improved by caffeine and $NaHCO_3$ administration 70–90 min prior to exercise. Moreover, for the first time $NaHCO_3$ has been shown to elicit an improvement above that of caffeine in a sport-specific high-intensity intermittent test with concomitant reductions in RPE and higher blood lactate levels. This study suggests that caffeine and $NaHCO_3$ might be effective ergogenic aids for intermittent high-intensity exercise performance in sub-elite team sport athletes.

Competing interests

The authors declare that they have no competing interests.

Authors' contributions

MM and MM participated in the design of the study, and carried out the data collection in cooperation with PK. MM, PK and MM performed the data treatment including statistical analyses. MM and MM drafted the manuscript with help from PK. All authors read and approved the manuscript.

Acknowledgement

The authors would like to thank the athletes for committed participation. Moreover, we thank Dr. Nikolai Nordsborg, Dr. Sarah R. Jackman and Giorgios Ermidis for excellent technical assistance. The authors have no conflict of interest in relation to the study.

Author details

[1]Sport and Health Sciences, College of Life and Environmental Sciences, St. Luke's Campus, University of Exeter, Exeter, UK. [2]Department of Nutrition, Exercise and Sports, Section of Human Physiology, Copenhagen Centre for Team Sport and Health, University of Copenhagen, Copenhagen, Denmark. [3]Faculty of Natural and Health Sciences, University of the Faroe Islands, Jónas Broncks gøta 25. 3rd floor, Tórshavn, Faroe Islands. [4]Center of Health and Human Performance, Department of Food and Nutrition, and Sport Science, University of Gothenburg, Gothenburg, Sweden.

References

1. Fitts R. Cellular mechanism of muscle fatigue. Physiol Rev. 1994;74:49–94.
2. Kilding AE, Overton C, Gleave J. Effects of caffeine, sodium bicarbonate, and their combined ingestion on high-intensity cycling performance. Int J Sport Nutr Exerc Metab. 2012;22:175–83.
3. Stuart GR, Hopkins WG, Cook C, Cairns SP. Multiple effects of caffeine on simulated high-intensity team-sport performance. Med Sci Sports Exerc. 2005;37:1998–2005.
4. Schneiker KT, Bishop D, Dawson B, Hackett LP. Effects of caffeine on prolonged intermittent-sprint ability in team-sport athletes. Med Sci Sports Exerc. 2006;38:578–85.
5. Mohr M, Nielsen JJ, Bangsbo J. Caffeine intake improves intense intermittent exercise performance and reduces muscle interstitial potassium accumulation. J Appl Physiol. 2011;111:1372–9.
6. Glaister M, Howatson G, Abraham CS, Lockey RA, Goodwin JE, Foley P, et al. Caffeine supplementation and multiple sprint running performance. Med Sci Sports Exerc. 2008;40:1835–40.
7. Foskett A, Ali A, Gant N. Caffeine enhances cognitive function and skill performance during simulated soccer activity. Int J Sport Nutr Exerc Metab. 2009;19:410–23.
8. McNaughton LR, Siegler J, Midgley A. Ergogenic effects of sodium bicarbonate. Curr Sports Med Rep. 2008;7:230–6.
9. Carr AJ, Slater GJ, Gore CJ, Dawson B, Burke LM. Effect of sodium bicarbonate on [HCO_3-], pH, and gastrointestinal symptoms. Int J Sport Nutr Exerc Metab. 2011;21:189–94.
10. Bishop D, Edge J, Davis C, Goodman C. Induced metabolic alkalosis affects muscle metabolism and repeated-sprint ability. Med Sci Sports Exerc. 2004;36:807–13.
11. Bishop D, Claudis B. Effects of induced metabolic alkalosis on prolonged intermittent-sprint performance. Med Sci Sports Exerc. 2005;37:759–67.
12. Cameron SL, McLay-Cooke RT, Brown RC, Gray AR, Fairbairn KA. Increased blood pH but not performance with sodium bicarbonate supplementation in elite rugby union players. Int J Sport Nutr Exerc Metab. 2010;20:307–21.
13. Krustrup P, Mohr M, Nybo L, Nielsen JJ, Jensen JM, Bangsbo J. The Yo-Yo IR2 test: physiological response, reliability, and application to elite soccer. Med Sci Sports Exerc. 2006;38:1666–73.
14. Bangsbo J, Madsen K, Kiens B, Richter EA. Effect of muscle acidity on muscle metabolism and fatigue during intense exercise in man. J Physiol. 1996;495:587–96.

15. Nordsborg N, Mohr M, Pedersen LD, Nielsen JJ, Langberg H, Bangsbo J. Muscle interstitial potassium kinetics during intense exhaustive exercise: effect of previous arm exercise. Am J Physiol Regul Integr Comp Physiol. 2003;285:143–8.
16. Borg G. Borg's perceived exertion and pain scales. IL, USA: Champaign; 1998.
17. Juel C, Klarskov C, Nielsen JJ, Krustrup P, Mohr M, Bangsbo J. Effect of high-intensity intermittent training on lactate and H+ release from human skeletal muscle. Am J Physiol Endocrinol Metab. 2004;286:e245–51.
18. Street D, Nielsen JJ, Bangsbo J, Juel C. Metabolic alkalosis reduces exercise-induced acidosis and potassium accumulation in human skeletal muscle interstitium. J Physiol. 2005;566:481–9.
19. Street D, Bangsbo J, Juel C. Interstitial pH in human skeletal muscle during and after dynamic graded exercise. J Physiol. 2001;537:993–8.
20. Davis NW, Standen NB, Stanfield PR. ATP-dependent potassium channels of muscle cells: their properties, regulation, and possible functions. J Bioenerg Biomembr. 1991;23:509–35.
21. Raymer GH, Marsh GD, Kowalchuk JM, Thompson RT. Metabolic effects of induced alkalosis during progressive forearm exercise to fatigue. J Appl Physiol. 2004;96:2050–6.
22. Gandevia SC. Spinal and supraspinal factors in human muscle fatigue. Physiol Rev. 2001;81:1725–89.
23. Nybo L, Secher NH. Cerebral perturbations provoked by prolonged exercise. Prog Neurobiol. 2004;72:223–61.
24. Greer F, McLean C, Graham TE. Caffeine, performance, and metabolism during repeated Wingate exercise tests. J Appl Physiol. 1998;85:1502–8.
25. Clausen T. Na^+-K^+ pump regulation and skeletal muscle contractility. Physiol Rev. 2003;83:1269–324.
26. Del Coso J, Muñoz-Fernández VE, Muñoz G, Fernández-Elías VE, Ortega JF, Hamouti N, et al. Effects of a caffeine containing energy drink on simulated soccer performance. PLoS One. 2012;7:e31380.
27. Davis JK, Green JM. Caffeine and anaerobic performance: ergogenic value and mechanisms of action. Sports Med. 2009;39:813–32.
28. Wu CL, Shih MC, Yang CC, Huang MH, Chang CK. Sodium bicarbonate supplementation prevents skilled tennis performance decline after a simulated match. J Int Soc Sports Nutr. 2010;7:33–41.
29. Siegler JC, Marshall PW, Bray J, Towlson C, et al. Sodium bicarbonate supplementation and ingestion timing: does it matter? J Strength Cond Res. 2012;26:1953–8.

Body composition changes associated with fasted versus non-fasted aerobic exercise

Brad Jon Schoenfeld[1*], Alan Albert Aragon[2], Colin D Wilborn[3], James W Krieger[4] and Gul T Sonmez[1]

Abstract

It has been hypothesized that performing aerobic exercise after an overnight fast accelerates the loss of body fat. The purpose of this study was to investigate changes in fat mass and fat-free mass following four weeks of volume-equated fasted versus fed aerobic exercise in young women adhering to a hypocaloric diet. Twenty healthy young female volunteers were randomly assigned to 1 of 2 experimental groups: a fasted training (FASTED) group that performed exercise after an overnight fast (n = 10) or a post-prandial training (FED) group that consumed a meal prior to exercise (n = 10). Training consisted of 1 hour of steady-state aerobic exercise performed 3 days per week. Subjects were provided with customized dietary plans designed to induce a caloric deficit. Nutritional counseling was provided throughout the study period to help ensure dietary adherence and self-reported food intake was monitored on a regular basis. A meal replacement shake was provided either immediately prior to exercise for the FED group or immediately following exercise for the FASTED group, with this nutritional provision carried out under the supervision of a research assistant. Both groups showed a significant loss of weight ($P = 0.0005$) and fat mass ($P = 0.02$) from baseline, but no significant between-group differences were noted in any outcome measure. These findings indicate that body composition changes associated with aerobic exercise in conjunction with a hypocaloric diet are similar regardless whether or not an individual is fasted prior to training.

Background

Regimented exercise is considered an important component of a structured weight loss program [1]. Meta-analytic data show that a combined diet-plus-exercise program is more effective in promoting long-term weight loss than a diet-only program [2]. This is consistent with a compelling body of research showing that weight management is predicated on the balance between energy expenditure and intake [3]. Since human movement alters the expenditure side of the energy balance equation, it therefore follows that an increase in physical activity will be accompanied by a reduction in body mass provided energy intake remains constant. Interestingly and importantly, there is evidence in both animal [4] and human [5] models that regular exercise can preferentially reduce abdominal fat, which has been implicated as a primary factor in cardiometabolic risk [6].

The provision of nutrients prior to aerobic exercise has been shown to have a profound impact on the physiological response to the training bout [7,8]. Accordingly, a number of strategies have been devised to take advantage of this phenomenon. One such strategy involves training after an overnight fast to accelerate the loss of body fat [9]. In theory, low glycogen and insulin levels cause the body to shift energy utilization away from carbohydrates, thereby allowing greater mobilization of stored fat for fuel. Findings from several acute studies appear to support this contention, with exercise in the fed state resulting in a reduced entry of long-chain fatty acids in the mitochondria and a corresponding decrease in fat oxidation [10-12]. These results in the fed state have been attributed to an insulin-mediated attenuation of adipose tissue lipolysis, an increased glycolytic flux, and/or a decreased expression of genes involved in fatty acid transport and oxidation [12-14]. There also is evidence that consistent exercise while fasted results in chronic molecular adaptations favorable to fat oxidation. For example, 6 weeks of fasted aerobic training increased the content of intramuscular fatty acid binding protein and uncoupling-protein-3 content to a greater extent than training post-prandially [15]. In addition, regimented fasted training has been shown to promote superior improvements in whole-body glucose tolerance and insulin sensitivity as well as upregulating

* Correspondence: brad@workout911.com
[1]Department of Health Science, Lehman College, Bronx, NY, USA
Full list of author information is available at the end of the article

various lipolytic enzymes compared to exercising while fed [8,16].

Despite an apparent theoretical basis, evidence is scant as to whether fasted aerobic exercise results in greater fat loss over time compared to exercising in the post-prandial state. Although several studies have examined measures of body composition between exercise carried out fasted versus fed [7,8,16], to the authors' knowledge none have directly investigated this topic during periods of energy restriction. The purpose of this study therefore was to investigate changes in fat mass and fat-free mass following four weeks of volume-equated fasted versus fed aerobic exercise in young women adhering to a hypocaloric diet.

Methods

Subjects

Subjects were 20 healthy young female volunteers (age: 22.4 ± 2.8 yrs; height: 163.4 ± 4.7 cms; weight: 62.2 ± 6.5 kgs) recruited from a university population. This sample size was justified by *a priori* power analysis using a target effect size of 0.6, alpha of 0.05 and power of 0.80 with percent body fat as an outcome measure based on previously established results [17]. All participants reported performing aerobic exercise several days a week on a regular basis and several were off-season collegiate track and field athletes. Initial screening required that subjects were between the ages of 18–35, not classified as obese based on a body mass index (BMI; calculated as kg/m^2) of ≥30, and not involved in a resistance training program at the time of the study. Individuals meeting these criteria were invited to attend a familiarization session where a complete explanation of the study was provided, and a medical history and informed consent were obtained. Participants were excluded from the study if they are found to have any of the following: existing lower body injury; current participation in a resistance training program; metabolic or cardiovascular disorders (including coronary artery disease, cardiac arrhythmias, diabetes, thyroid disease, or hypertension); history of pregnancy within the past 6 months; any condition that would result in stratification as high risk based on criteria set forth by the American College of Sports Medicine [18], and/or taking a prescription or non-prescription weight-loss aid. Those meeting eligibility criteria and willing to participate in the study were scheduled for baseline testing. Approval for the study was obtained from the Institutional Review Board at Lehman College.

Testing sessions

Testing was carried out in the 24–48 hours prior to beginning the intervention and after the fourth week at completion of the study. For each testing session, subjects reported to the lab in the morning following an overnight fast having refrained from vigorous physical activity, alcohol intake, or consumption of over-the-counter medications for at least 12 hours. Baseline assessments included body mass, height, body composition, and waist circumference, After completion of testing, subjects were pair-matched based on initial body mass measurements and randomly assigned to 1 of 2 experimental groups: a fasted training (FASTED) group that performed exercise after an overnight fast (n = 10) or a post-prandial training (FED) group that consumed a meal prior to exercise (n = 10). The number of athletes and non-athletes were evenly distributed between groups.

Exercise training intervention

Training consisted of 1 hour of steady-state aerobic exercise performed 3 days per week on a LifeFitness, treadmill (model CLST-0100R-01, Brunswick Corporation, Rosemont, IL) at a 0% grade. Subjects performed a warm-up for the first 5 minutes at an intensity equating to 50% of maximal heart rate (MHR), determined by the formula 220 – age, then increased intensity to 70% MHR for the next 50 minutes, and finished with a 5 minute cool down at 50% MHR. Heart rate monitors (model F7U, Polar Electro Inc, Lake Success, NY) were used to ensure that exercise remained at the appropriate intensity. A low-to-moderate training intensity was used because it has been shown to maximize lipid oxidation during fasted aerobic exercise as compared to higher-training intensities [19]. All training sessions were supervised by research assistants who were upper level undergraduate students in exercise science. Subjects were instructed to refrain from performing any additional structured exercise for the duration of the study.

Dietary intervention

Subjects were provided with customized dietary plans prepared by one of the researchers (A.A.A.) for the length of the study. In order to facilitate weight loss, energy consumption was set so that subjects remained in a caloric deficit. The determination of energy intake was based on the Mifflin-St. Jeor Equation, which is considered an accurate formula for estimating resting metabolic rate [20]. The formula is as follows:

$$10 \times \text{weight (kg)} + 6.25 \times \text{height (cm)} - 5 \times \text{age (y)} - 161$$

The formula was multiplied by a moderate activity factor (1.5) to estimate energy balance, and the total was then reduced by 500 calories to impose a caloric deficit. Dietary protein intake was set at 1.8 g/kg of body mass, as higher protein consumption has been shown to help offset losses in lean tissue mass and promote greater adherence to the nutritional regimen [21,22]. After accounting for protein intake, dietary fat was 25-30% of total calories and the remaining calories were obtained from carbohydrate. Sample meal plans were provided to guide the participants in acceptable food choices.

Dietary plans included provision of a meal replacement shake (Pursuit Recovery, Dymatize Nutrition, Dallas, TX). The shake contained 250 calories consisting of 40 g carbohydrate, 20 g protein, and 0.5 g fat. On exercise days, FED consumed the shake immediately prior to the exercise bout and FASTED consumed the shake immediately after finishing the bout. Shakes were consumed under the supervision of a research assistant to ensure adherence within the context of the subject's respective participation in the fed or fasted protocol.

Dietary adherence was assessed by self-reported food records using MyFitnessPal.com (http://www.myfitnesspal.com), which were collected and analyzed during on a daily basis to ensure that intake was not based on recall. Subjects were instructed on how to properly record all food items and their respective portion sizes that were consumed for the designated period of interest. Each item of food was individually entered into the program, and the program provided relevant information as to total energy consumption, as well as amount of energy derived from proteins, fats, and carbohydrates over the length of the study. Continued nutritional guidance was provided to the subjects at the time of each training session by the research team to encourage dietary adherence.

Anthropometrics and body composition measurements

Height and body mass measurements were made using a double beam scale. Circumference measurements of the waist was made using an Intelametrix tape measure (Intelametrix Inc., Livermore, CA) according to established criteria [18]. Body mass index (BMI) was calculated as body mass in kg divided by height in meters squared. Percent fat mass and lean body mass was obtained via air displacement plethysmography (ADP) using the BodPod body composition analyzer (model 2000a, Life Measurement, Concord, CA) as per the user manual and described previously in the literature [23]. ADP has been shown to have good validity in measuring body fat percentage when compared to dual x-ray absorptiometry in the sampled population [24,25]. Subjects were tested in tight clothing (either compression shorts and a sports bra or a swimsuit) and Lycra swim cap. Based on body mass and volume as well as through body density, total fat mass, total fat free mass and body fat percentage were calculated by the BodPod system software.

Statistical analyses

Normality assumptions were checked using a one-sample Kolmogorov-Smirnov test; all data was found to meet normality assumptions. Independent t-tests were used to assess differences in baseline measurements between groups as well as energy and macronutrient intake over the length of the study period. Cohen's D effect sizes were calculated for all pre- to post-study outcome measures using the following formula:

$$M_1 - M_2/SD$$

where M_1 represents the pre-study mean, M_2 represents the post study mean, and; SD represents the pooled standard deviation.

All other data was modeled using a linear mixed model estimated by a restricted maximum likelihood algorithm. Treatment was included as the between-subject factor, time was included as the repeated within-subjects factor, and time x treatment was included as the interaction. Repeated covariance structures were specified as unstructured. All analyses were performed using S-Plus 8.2 (Tibco Spotfire, Boston, MA). Effects were considered significant at $P \leq 0.05$, and trends were declared at $0.05 < P \leq 0.10$. Data are reported as $\bar{x} \pm SD$.

Results

The FED group was significantly younger than the FASTED group (21 ± 1.7 yrs versus, 23.8 ± 3.0 yrs, respectively; p = 0.02). No other significant group differences were noted in any baseline measure. Total energy and macronutrient consumption was not different between groups over the length of the study period (see Table 1). FASTED reported consuming 1236 calories/day; FED reported consuming 1277 calories/day. The reported nutritional consumption for both groups was below that prescribed in the individual meal plans. Figures 1 and 2 display macronutrient percentage intake in FASTED and FED, respectively.

Pre- to post-study results for each outcome measure are presented below. Table 2 summarizes these findings.

Body mass

There was no significant interaction between time and group, and there was no significant effect of group. There was a significant effect of time (P = 0.0005), with a decrease in body mass from pre- to post.

BMI

There was no significant interaction between time and group and there was no significant effect of group. There was a significant effect of time (P = 0.0005), with a decrease in BMI from pre- to post.

Table 1 Nutritional intake between groups

Group	Calories	Carbohydrate (g)	Fat (g)	Protein (g)
FASTED	1236 ± 177	152 ± 38	37 ± 7	74 ± 15
FED	1277 ± 137	148 ± 19	41 ± 13	78 ± 21

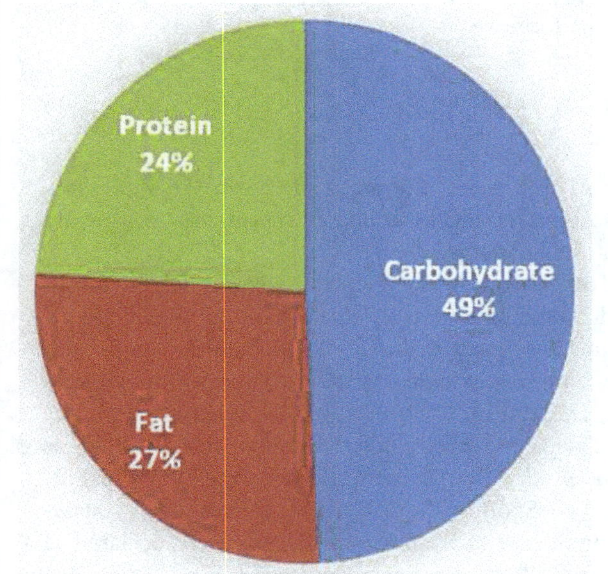

Figure 1 Percent macronutrient intake for FASTED.

Percent body fat

There was no significant interaction between time and group, and there was no significant effect of group. There was a trend for an effect of time ($P = 0.06$), with a trend for a decrease in percent body fat from pre- to post.

Waist circumference

There was no significant interaction between time and group, and no significant effect of group. There was a trend for an effect of time ($P = 0.07$), with a trend for a decrease in waist circumference from pre- to post.

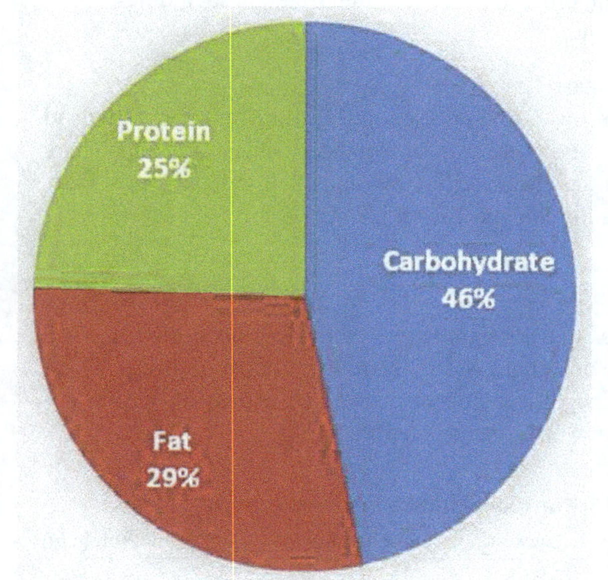

Figure 2 Percent macronutrient intake for FED.

Fat mass

There was no significant interaction between time and group, and no significant effect of group ($P = 0.88$). There was a significant effect of time ($P = 0.02$), with a decrease in fat mass from pre- to post.

Fat-free mass

There was no significant interaction between time and group, and no significant effects of group or time.

Discussion

To the authors' knowledge, this is the first study to investigate body composition changes associated with aerobic exercise performed in the fasted versus fed state while subjects maintained a caloric deficit. It has been hypothesized that exercising when fasted forces the body to rely on using fat as a substrate rather than carbohydrate, thereby reducing body fat to a greater extent than performance of post-prandial exercise. Our results refute the veracity of this hypothesis. Although both groups lost a significant amount of weight and fat mass, no differences were seen between conditions in any outcome measure regardless of pre-exercise feeding status.

Van Proeyen et al. [16] investigated the effects of fasted versus fed aerobic exercise on metabolic parameters and body composition in a convenience sample of physically active young men while maintaining an energy-matched hyper-caloric diet (~ + 30% kcal day^{-1}). Subjects performed a combination of moderately intense cycling and running exercise for 60–90 minutes, 4 days per week. After 6 weeks, the fed group significantly increased body mass by 1.4 kg while no significant increases were found in the fasted group, suggesting an attenuation of weight gain from fasted training. Follow-up work from the same lab employing the same basic training protocol but with subjects consuming an isocaloric diet (based on 4-day dietary analysis) showed no differences in body weight change between fasted versus fed conditions [8]. Recently, Gillen et al. [7] compared body composition changes associated with exercising in the fasted versus fed state in 16 overweight/obese women. Exercise consisted of high-intensity interval training (ten 60-second cycling intervals at 90% maximal heart rate with a 1:1 work/recovery ratio) performed 3 days per week for 6 weeks. Subjects were instructed to maintain their pre-intervention eating patterns throughout the study period. At study's end, body mass remained unchanged from baseline but lower body fat was noted both in the abdominal and leg regions as well as the whole body level in both groups. No significant differences were found between conditions.

Our results are novel in that subjects consumed a supervised hypocaloric diet throughout the intervention period. Loss of body mass is predicated on shifting energy balance to favor expenditure over intake [3]. This is

Table 2 Pre- vs. Post-study body composition measures

MEASURE	FASTED-PRE	FASTED-POST	ES	FED-PRE	FED-POST	ES
Weight (kg)	62.4 ± 7.8	60.8 ± 7.8*	0.21	62.0 ± 5.5	61.0 ± 5.7*	0.18
BMI	23.4 ± 2.9	22.8 ± 3.0*	0.20	23.3 ± 2.5	22.9 ± 2.5*	0.16
Body Fat%	26.3 ± 7.9	25.0 ± 7.7	0.17	24.8 ± 8.4	24.1 ± 8.5	0.08
Waist (cm)	77.5 ± 6.4	75.9 ± 6.9	0.24	77.7 ± 9.4	75.7 ± 8.6	0.22
Fat Mass (kg)	16.5 ± 5.5	15.4 ± 5.5*	0.20	15.7 ± 6.3	15.0 ± 6.1*	0.11
Fat Free Mass (kg)	45.9 ± 6.7	45.4 ± 6.1	0.08	46.3 ± 3.8	46.1 ± 4.3	0.05

An asterisk* indicates a significant effect from baseline values.

consistent with the First Law of Thermodynamics, which essentially states that energy is neither created nor destroyed, but rather changed from one form to another. Thus, our approach allowed for a controlled investigation of the effects of fasted exercise on body composition under conditions favorable for fat loss. Moreover, to optimize the proposed benefits of training while fasted, exercise was performed at low-to-moderate intensities. This is consistent with acute research showing that lipolysis is blunted during performance of higher- [14,26] but not lower-intensity exercise when carried out in the fed state [10,11,27]. Despite these accommodations, fasted exercise showed no beneficial effects compared to training post-prandially.

The theoretical basis behind a fat-burning advantage to fasted exercise is predicated on increasing lipid oxidation during training bout. However, this ignores the dynamic nature of the human body, which continually adjusts its use of substrate for fuel. There is evidence that a greater utilization of fat for fuel during a given time period is compensated by a greater carbohydrate utilization later in the day [28]. Hence, fat burning must be considered over the course of days — not on an hour to hour basis — to meaningfully assess its impact on body composition [29]. In support of this contention, Paoli et al. [30] compared differences in 24-hour fat metabolism associated with performance of moderate-intensity cardiovascular treadmill exercise in the fasted versus fed state. Food quantity and quality was identical between conditions over the ensuing 24-hour recovery period. Consumption of breakfast for the fed condition resulted in a significant increase in respiratory exchange ratio (RER) compared to fasting (0.96 vs. 0.84, respectively). However, at 12 hours post-exercise RER was significantly lower in the fed versus fasting condition and the difference remained significant after 24 hours.

Any potential increases in fat oxidation from fasted exercise might be neutralized by an increase in the thermic effect of exercise from eating pre-exercise. Lee et al. [31] compared the acute thermogenic effects of an exercise bout performed in either a fasted state or following ingestion of a glucose/milk (GM) beverage. Employing a within-subject design, 10 male college students performed four experimental conditions in randomized order: low intensity, long duration exercise with GM; low intensity, long duration exercise without GM; high intensity, short duration exercise with GM, and; high intensity, short duration exercise without GM. Results showed that consumption of the GM beverage increased excess post-exercise oxygen consumption to a significantly greater extent than exercise performed while fasted in both high and low intensity conditions. Similar findings have been reported in other controlled trials [32,33].

The study had several notable limitations that must be taken into account when attempting to draw evidence-based conclusions. First, the duration of the testing period was fairly short, lasting just four weeks. While this period is certainly sufficient to attain significant fat loss, it remains possible that subtle changes between protocols would take more time to manifest. Second, although every attempt was made to control the subject's nutritional intake, it remains possible that differences in energy and/or macronutrient intake may have confounded results. There is evidence that self-reported consumption of food can vary by as much as 18% even after being trained by dieticians [34]. The fact that food diaries were collected daily provides confidence that a lapse in memory did not influence what was reported, but the inability to accurately measure portions and/or intent to deliberately misreport intake cannot be ruled out. Given that mean weight loss across groups was somewhat less than anticipated, it seems reasonable to assume that subjects did in fact underreport the amount of calories consumed, which would explain the attenuated results. Similarly, although subjects were instructed not to partake in any other structured exercise other than activities of daily living, there is no way to assure that they adhered to this request. Third, the use of young women as participants raises the possibility of confounding by menstrual cycles. The fact that testing was carried out exactly one month apart provides some degree of confidence that this did not influence results. However, it is not uncommon for women to have irregular menses, which may have affected hydration status and thus altered body composition measures. Fourth, the FASTED subjects consumed nutrients immediately following training; it is not clear what, if any, impact would be seen on results by delaying consumption for longer periods post-exercise. Finally, results are specific to young, non-obese women and cannot necessarily be generalized to other populations. For example, employing fasted-state, low- to moderate-intensity aerobic exercise is a popular tactic in physique sports where pushing extremes of leanness is one of the primary aims of contest preparation [35]. The applicability of the present study's results to such endeavors remains open to question.

Conclusion

In conclusion, our findings indicate that body composition changes associated with aerobic exercise in conjunction with a hypocaloric diet are similar regardless whether or not an individual is fasted prior to training. Hence, those seeking to lose body fat conceivably can choose to train either before or after eating based on preference. It should be noted that given the small sample size and short study duration, we cannot rule out the possibility that either condition might confer a small benefit over the other with respect to fat loss. Further study is warranted in a longer term trial with a greater number of participants.

Competing interests

The authors declare that they have no competing interests.

Authors' contributions

BJS devised the study design, carried out the data collection, participated in the interpretation of data, and drafted the manuscript; AAA developed and implemented the nutritional protocol, participated in the interpretation of data and assisted in the writing the manuscript; CDW devised the dietary analysis, participated in the in the interpretation of data and assisted in the writing of the manuscript; JWK performed all statistical analysis, participated in the interpretation of data and assisted in the writing of the manuscript. All authors read and approved the final manuscript.

Acknowledgements

The authors gratefully acknowledge the contributions of Robert Harris, Fanny Chen, Saem You, Jasmine Springer, and Romaine Fearon for their indispensable role as research assistants in this study. We also would like to express our gratitude to Dymatize Nutrition for providing the meal replacement shakes used in this study.

Author details

[1]Department of Health Science, Lehman College, Bronx, NY, USA. [2]California State University, Northridge, CA, USA. [3]Exercise and Sport Science Department, University of Mary Hardin-Baylor, Belton, TX, USA. [4]Weightology, LLC, Redmond, WA, USA.

References

1. Donnelly JE, Blair SN, Jakicic JM, Manore MM, Rankin JW, Smith BK, American College of Sports Medicine: **American college of sports medicine position stand. Appropriate physical activity intervention strategies for weight loss and prevention of weight regain for adults.** *Med Sci Sports Exerc* 2009, **41**(2):459–471.
2. Wu T, Gao X, Chen M, van Dam RM: **Long-term effectiveness of diet-plus-exercise interventions vs. diet-only interventions for weight loss: a meta-analysis.** *Obes Rev* 2009, **10**(3):313–323.
3. Hall KD, Heymsfield SB, Kemnitz JW, Klein S, Schoeller DA, Speakman JR: **Energy balance and its components: implications for body weight regulation.** *Am J Clin Nutr* 2012, **95**(4):989–994.
4. Laye MJ, Thyfault JP, Stump CS, Booth FW: **Inactivity induces increases in abdominal fat.** *J Appl Physiol* 2007, **102**(4):1341–1347.
5. Hunter GR, Brock DW, Byrne NM, Chandler-Laney PC, Del Corral P, Gower BA: **Exercise training prevents regain of visceral fat for 1 year following weight loss.** *Obesity (Silver Spring)* 2010, **18**(4):690–695.
6. Calabro P, Yeh ET: **Intra-abdominal adiposity, inflammation, and cardiovascular risk: new insight into global cardiometabolic risk.** *Curr Hypertens Rep* 2008, **10**(1):32–38.
7. Gillen JB, Percival ME, Ludzki A, Tarnopolsky MA, Gibala MJ: **Interval training in the fed or fasted state improves body composition and muscle oxidative capacity in overweight women.** *Obesity (Silver Spring)* 2013, **21**(11):2249–2255.
8. Van Proeyen K, Szlufcik K, Nielens H, Ramaekers M, Hespel P: **Beneficial metabolic adaptations due to endurance exercise training in the fasted state.** *J Appl Physiol* 2011, **110**(1):236–245.
9. Kang J, Raines E, Rosenberg J, Ratamess N, Naclerio F, Faigenbaum A: **Metabolic responses during postprandial exercise.** *Res Sports Med* 2013, **21**(3):240–252.
10. Horowitz JF, Mora-Rodriguez R, Byerley LO, Coyle EF: **Lipolytic suppression following carbohydrate ingestion limits fat oxidation during exercise.** *Am J Physiol* 1997, **273**(4 Pt 1):E768–E775.
11. Ahlborg G, Felig P: **Influence of glucose ingestion on fuel-hormone response during prolonged exercise.** *J Appl Physiol* 1976, **41**(5 Pt. 1):683–688.
12. Civitarese AE, Hesselink MK, Russell AP, Ravussin E, Schrauwen P: **Glucose ingestion during exercise blunts exercise-induced gene expression of skeletal muscle fat oxidative genes.** *Am J Physiol Endocrinol Metab* 2005, **289**(6):E1023–E1029.
13. Coyle EF, Jeukendrup AE, Wagenmakers AJ, Saris WH: **Fatty acid oxidation is directly regulated by carbohydrate metabolism during exercise.** *Am J Physiol* 1997, **273**(2 Pt 1):E268–E275.
14. Horowitz JF, Mora-Rodriguez R, Byerley LO, Coyle EF: **Substrate metabolism when subjects are fed carbohydrate during exercise.** *Am J Physiol* 1999, **276**(5 Pt 1):E828–E835.
15. De Bock K, Derave W, Eijnde BO, Hesselink MK, Koninckx E, Rose AJ, Schrauwen P, Bonen A, Richter EA, Hespel P: **Effect of training in the fasted state on metabolic responses during exercise with carbohydrate intake.** *J Appl Physiol* 2008, **104**(4):1045–1055.
16. Van Proeyen K, Szlufcik K, Nielens H, Pelgrim K, Deldicque L, Hesselink M, Van Veldhoven PP, Hespel P: **Training in the fasted state improves glucose tolerance during fat-rich diet.** *J Physiol* 2010, **588**(Pt 21):4289–4302.
17. Arciero PJ, Ormsbee MJ, Gentile CL, Nindl BC, Brestoff JR, Ruby M: **Increased protein intake and meal frequency reduces abdominal fat during energy balance and energy deficit.** *Obesity (Silver Spring)* 2013, **21**(7):1357–1366.
18. American College of Sports Medicine: *ACSM's Guidelines for Exercise Testing and Prescription.* Baltimore, MD: Lippincott Williams & Wilkins; 2009.
19. Schoenfeld B: **Does cardio after an overnight fast maximize fat loss?** *Strength Cond J* 2011, **33**(1):23–25.
20. Frankenfield D, Roth-Yousey L, Compher C: **Comparison of predictive equations for resting metabolic rate in healthy nonobese and obese adults: a systematic review.** *J Am Diet Assoc* 2005, **105**(5):775–789.
21. Larsen TM, Dalskov SM, van Baak M, Jebb SA, Papadaki A, Pfeiffer AF, Martinez JA, Handjieva-Darlenska T, Kunesova M, Pihlsgard M, Stender S, Holst C, Saris WH, Astrup A, Diet, Obesity, and Genes (Diogenes) Project: **Diets with high or low protein content and glycemic index for weight-loss maintenance.** *N Engl J Med* 2010, **363**(22):2102–2113.
22. Pasiakos SM, Cao JJ, Margolis LM, Sauter ER, Whigham LD, McClung JP, Rood JC, Carbone JW, Combs GF Jr, Young AJ: **Effects of high-protein diets on fat-free mass and muscle protein synthesis following weight loss: a randomized controlled trial.** *FASEB J* 2013, **27**(9):3837–3847.
23. McCrory MA, Gomez TD, Bernauer EM, Mole PA: **Evaluation of a new air displacement plethysmograph for measuring human body composition.** *Med Sci Sports Exerc* 1995, **27**(12):1686–1691.
24. Maddalozzo GF, Cardinal BJ, Snow CA: **Concurrent validity of the BOD POD and dual energy x-ray absorptiometry techniques for assessing body composition in young women.** *J Am Diet Assoc* 2002, **102**(11):1677–1679.
25. Ballard TP, Fafara L, Vukovich MD: **Comparison of Bod Pod and DXA in female collegiate athletes.** *Med Sci Sports Exerc* 2004, **36**(4):731–735.
26. Febbraio MA, Chiu A, Angus DJ, Arkinstall MJ, Hawley JA: **Effects of carbohydrate ingestion before and during exercise on glucose kinetics and performance.** *J Appl Physiol* 2000, **89**(6):2220–2226.

27. Gonzalez JT, Veasey RC, Rumbold PL, Stevenson EJ: **Breakfast and exercise contingently affect postprandial metabolism and energy balance in physically active males.** *Br J Nutr* 2013, **110**(4):721–732.
28. de Venne WP V, Westerterp KR: **Influence of the feeding frequency on nutrient utilization in man: consequences for energy metabolism.** *Eur J Clin Nutr* 1991, **45**(3):161–169.
29. Hansen K, Shriver T, Schoeller D: **The effects of exercise on the storage and oxidation of dietary fat.** *Sports Med* 2005, **35**(5):363–373.
30. Paoli A, Marcolin G, Zonin F, Neri M, Sivieri A, Pacelli QF: **Exercising fasting or fed to enhance fat loss? influence of food intake on respiratory ratio and excess postexercise oxygen consumption after a bout of endurance training.** *Int J Sport Nutr Exerc Metab* 2011, **21**(1):48–54.
31. Lee YS, Ha MS, Lee YJ: **The effects of various intensities and durations of exercise with and without glucose in milk ingestion on postexercise oxygen consumption.** *J Sports Med Phys Fitness* 1999, **39**(4):341–347.
32. Davis JM, Sadri S, Sargent RG, Ward D: **Weight control and calorie expenditure: thermogenic effects of pre-prandial and post-prandial exercise.** *Addict Behav* 1989, **14**(3):347–351.
33. Goben KW, Sforzo GA, Frye PA: **Exercise intensity and the thermic effect of food.** *Int J Sport Nutr* 1992, **2**(1):87–95.
34. Mertz W, Tsui JC, Judd JT, Reiser S, Hallfrisch J, Morris ER, Steele PD, Lashley E: **What are people really eating? the relation between energy intake derived from estimated diet records and intake determined to maintain body weight.** *Am J Clin Nutr* 1991, **54**(2):291–295.
35. Helms ER, Aragon AA, Fitschen PJ: **Evidence-based recommendations for natural bodybuilding contest preparation: nutrition and supplementation.** *J Int Soc Sports Nutr* 2014, **11**:20-2783-11-20. eCollection 2014.

Effects of sports drinks on the maintenance of physical performance during 3 tennis matches: a randomized controlled study

Thibault Brink-Elfegoun[1], Sébastien Ratel[2,10], Pierre-Marie Leprêtre[3], Lore Metz[2,10], Gael Ennequin[2,10], Eric Doré[2,10], Vincent Martin[2,10], David Bishop[4,5], Nicolas Aubineau[6], Jean-François Lescuyer[6], Martine Duclos[7,8,9,10], Pascal Sirvent[2,10*] and Sébastien L Peltier[6]

Abstract

Background: Tennis tournaments often involve playing several consecutive matches interspersed with short periods of recovery.

Objective: The objective of this study was firstly to assess the impact of several successive tennis matches on the physical performance of competitive players and secondly to evaluate the potential of sports drinks to minimize the fatigue induced by repeated matches.

Methods: This was a crossover, randomized controlled study. Eight male regionally-ranked tennis players participated in this study. Players underwent a series of physical tests to assess their strength, speed, power and endurance following the completion of three tennis matches each of two hours duration played over three consecutive half-days (1.5 day period for each condition). In the first condition the players consumed a sports drink before, during and after each match; in the second, they drank an identical volume of placebo water. The results obtained were compared with the third 'rest' condition in which the subjects did not play any tennis. Main outcomes measured were maximal isometric strength and fatigability of knee and elbow extensors, 20-m sprint speed, jumping height, specific repeated sprint ability test and hand grip strength.

Results: The physical test results for the lower limbs showed no significant differences between the three conditions. Conversely, on the upper limbs the EMG data showed greater fatigue of the *triceps brachii* in the placebo condition compared to the rest condition, while the ingestion of sports drinks attenuated this fatigue.

Conclusions: This study has demonstrated for the first time that, when tennis players are adequately hydrated and ingest balanced meals between matches, then no large drop in physical performance is observed even during consecutive competitive matches.

Trial registration: ClinicalTrials.gov: NCT01353872.

Keywords: Tennis, Nutrition, Fatigue, Performance, Sports drinks

* Correspondence: pascal.sirvent@univ-bpclermont.fr
[2]Clermont Université, Université Blaise Pascal, EA 3533, Laboratoire des Adaptations Métaboliques à l'Exercice en conditions Physiologiques et Pathologiques (AME2P), Bâtiment Biologie B, 24 avenue des Landais, BP 80026F-63171 Aubière Cedex, France
[10]CRNH-Auvergne, Clermont-Ferrand F-63001, France
Full list of author information is available at the end of the article

Introduction

Tennis tournaments are quite complex due to their variability in terms of exercise duration and the type of effort required. One feature of competitive tennis is that the season is relatively long and that the ranking system pushes players to compete all year long. During a competition, players must sometimes play one or two matches a day on consecutive days. For many reasons the duration and intensity of these matches are highly variable, but it is not uncommon to see matches continue beyond three hours [1,2] and various studies have shown a drop in high-level tennis performance during extended matches [3-6]. Under these conditions, optimum recovery methods are needed to maintain a high level of performance over the duration of a match, tournament or season. Among the strategies used, nutrition appears to be an important element to consider [7].

The majority of studies on the impact of nutritional strategies on tennis performance have been conducted by taking measurements during or at the end of long matches. Some studies have suggested a beneficial effect of carbohydrates during prolonged tennis matches [4,5,8-10]. Caffeine has also been suggested as positively affecting performance, although the number of relevant studies is very limited [4,5,9]. Among less common nutritional strategies, one study has also demonstrated a beneficial effect of sodium bicarbonate [6]. On the other hand, creatine supplementation did not appear to lead to positive effects on tennis performance [11,12].

To our knowledge, no study has evaluated the effects of nutritional strategies on physical performance in the days following a series of matches, despite this being the reality of competitive tennis. Furthermore, studies conducted in the field of tennis nutrition have only been interested in the isolated effects of nutritional strategies before or during the match. However, it is increasingly common for competitive athletes to use sports drinks before, during and after matches to help maintain their performance over the duration of a tournament [13]. Different types of commercial beverages, specifically formulated to meet the needs of athletes before, during or after exercise, have been developed and introduced into the market in recent years, even though the claimed benefits of these advertised products have usually not been scientifically proven [14].

Recently, we have conducted a controlled, randomized, double-blind study to evaluate the impact of ingesting specially formulated pre-exercise, endurance, and recovery sports drinks on glycaemia and tennis performance indices during a simulated tennis tournament [15]. We observed that this nutritional strategy allowed higher stroke frequency during play, with decreased rates of perceived exertion. In this follow-up study we investigated the effects of this nutritional strategy on physical performance. Physical performance was assessed by a series of physical tests which determined strength, speed, power and endurance of the subjects following the end of the tennis tournament simulation in each condition (placebos and sports drinks). Our hypotheses were that physical performance would naturally decrease over the matches and that the sports drinks would limit this fatigue.

Methods

Trial design

This was a single-center, double-blind, placebo-controlled, cross-over trial conducted in France. It was performed according to Good Clinical Practice. This clinical trial was approved by the Southeast VI Ethics Committee for Human Research and by the French Health Products Safety Agency (2010-A00724-35). All procedures were in accordance with the ethical standards of the 1975 Helsinki Declaration, as revised in 1983. The study protocol was also registered at clinicaltrials.gov as NCT01353872.

Subjects

Eight well-trained male tennis players volunteered to participate in this study (age 26.0 ± 5.7 years; height 1.84 ± 0.70 m; body mass 82 ± 11 kg). The major inclusion criteria were as follows: men aged 18 – 35 years with a body mass index ≥ 18.5 $kg.m^{-2}$ and < 26 $kg.m^{-2}$, nonsmoking or consuming less than 5 cigarettes per day, reporting a moderate caffeine intake (1–2 cups of coffee or equivalent per day), stable weight for at least one month before the beginning of the study, training at least twice a week, being involved in tennis-based training for at least three months prior to the beginning of the study, and figuring in the regional ranking tables drawn up by French Tennis Federation. Furthermore, participants also needed to have stable eating patterns during the month preceding the beginning of the protocol and had to agree to maintain these dietary habits throughout the study. Principal exclusion criteria included high-level sporting activities other than tennis and those necessary for their training, injury during the three months prior to the beginning of the study, diabetes, whether treated or detected at the inclusion visit, vegetarians and vegans, subjects with extreme eating habits and/or with a significant history of anorexia nervosa, bulimia or other eating disorders, a history of diseases that could disrupt our tests or subjects taking diuretics or other medications that we felt might interfere with our tests, and subjects consuming more than two alcoholic beverages per day (every day). Each candidate selected was fully informed of the purpose and risks associated with the procedures, and their written informed consent was obtained.

Trial protocol

The experiment included three conditions, each of which consisted of a battery of physical performance tests: the first was after the "rest condition" (CON) and the other two were carried out following a tennis-tournament-type situation with matches played on 2 consecutive days during which the participants ingested either sports drinks (SPD) or placebos (PLA) (Figure 1). For each of the three conditions, the physical performance tests were performed at 3:00 PM on Sunday and 3 hours after the end of the last tennis match (for SPD and PLA). Each of the three test sessions was performed 2 hours and 30 minutes after a standardized meal. The order for the three conditions was randomized and each was separated by 2 weeks. All trials were performed on the same indoor, hard-surface (Greenset®) courts. The participants became familiar with the experimental procedures and courts during a training session which took place two weeks before their first test condition. The players were instructed to continue their usual dietary habits, refrain from any changes in food selections or exercise during the trial and asked not to consume any food supplements or functional foods during the study. From 48 hours before each session, training was not allowed and subjects were asked to refrain from consuming caffeine (coffee, tea, chocolate, cola), tobacco and alcohol. In order to minimize the influence of previous evaluation tests, the sequence of tests was selected to propose the most fatiguing tests at the end. The orders of testing and recovery times were the same in each condition: isometric handgrip strength, power (jump height), maximal 20-m sprints, repeated-sprint ability, maximal isometric strength and fatigability of knee and elbow extensors.

Dietary protocol

To verify diet stability, the subjects were instructed to record their food intake during the 48 hours prior to each session. For this purpose, an instruction booklet containing daily menu examples was given to each subject who was trained by a dietician how to keep their intake diary during the inclusion meeting. Food diary records from each session were analyzed using Nutrilog® 2.10 software (Nutrilog®, Marans, Fance); their analysis revealed no significant difference in total caloric and macronutrient levels (data not shown). During each day of experiments, the diet was standardized as follows: fat 25%, protein 15% and carbohydrate 65%, plus 200 mL of mineral water at each meal. The total energy provided by breakfast, lunch and dinner was 3197, 4443 and 4841 kJ, respectively. This standardization of meals was done to minimize variations in pre-exercise glycogen stocks.

On match days three drinks were taken: before, during and after each match. The pre-match drink consisted of 500 mL of liquid (either a sports drink or a placebo) taken in the hour preceding the match. During the match subjects drank 750 mL/h of their test drink and 250 mL just after the match. The placebo drinks were specially developed to be similar in color and taste to the sports drinks. Moreover, subjects were informed that they were testing two sports drinks similar in appearance but different in composition and were therefore unaware that they may be taking a placebo. The drinks were kept at 8–10°C. Using a 10-point scale as a measure of

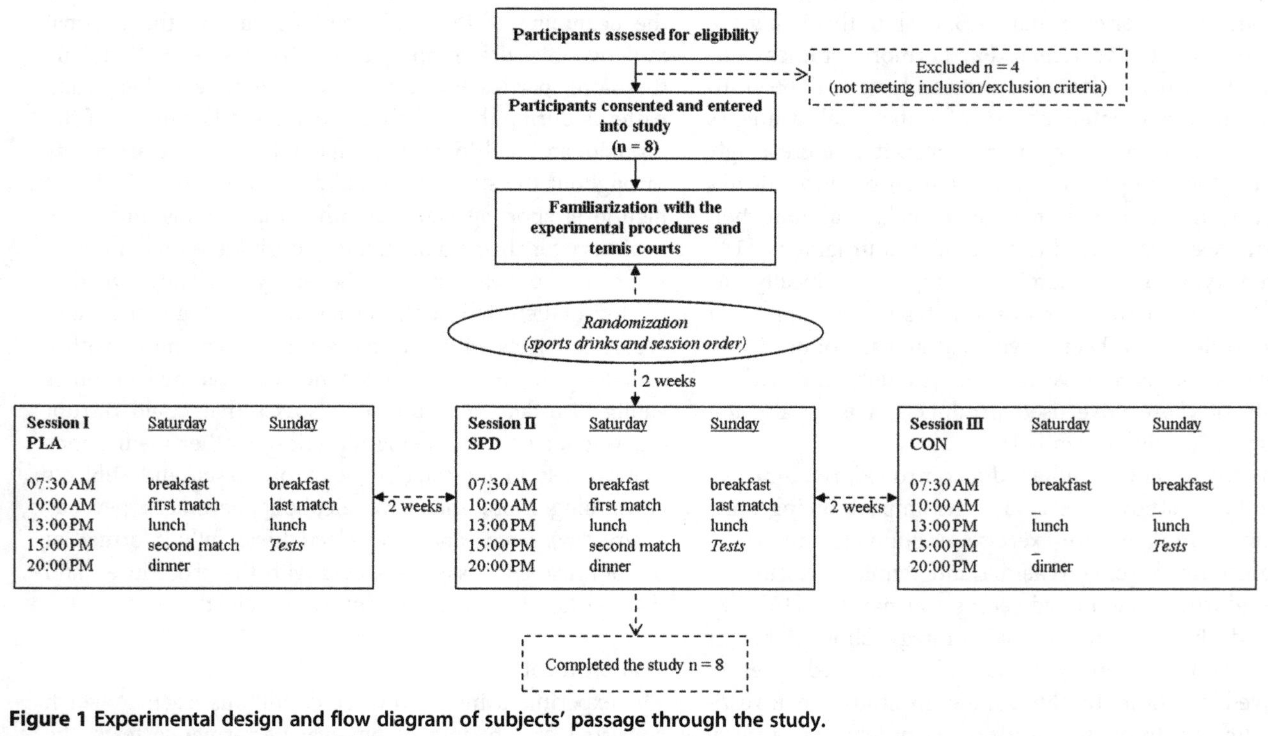

Figure 1 Experimental design and flow diagram of subjects' passage through the study.

gastrointestinal discomfort, the drinks were well tolerated (data not shown).

Composition of drinks

The nutritional composition of the pre-match drink was as follows: fructose 36 $g.L^{-1}$; maltodextrin 31 $g.L^{-1}$; hydroxycitrate 300 $mg.L^{-1}$; sodium citrate 7 $g.L^{-1}$; caffeine 140 $mg.L^{-1}$; vitamins B1 0.4 $mg.L^{-1}$, B2 0.4 $mg.L^{-1}$, B6 0.6 $mg.L^{-1}$ (70 $g.L^{-1}$, 1142 $kJ.L^{-1}$). Composition of the placebo pre-match drink: citric acid, natural grapefruit flavor, sucralose, acesulfame potassium, sillicium dioxide, maltodextrin, beetroot juice concentrate (amount of traces), tartrazine (3.0 $g.L^{-1}$, 35.8 $kJ.L^{-1}$). Match drink: maltodextrin 31.6 $g.L^{-1}$, dextrose 24.2 $g.L^{-1}$, fructose 12.8 $g.L^{-1}$, Branched-Chain Amino Acids 4 $g.L^{-1}$, curcumin 250 $mg.L^{-1}$, piperine 2.6 $mg.L^{-1}$, caffeine 75 $mg.L^{-1}$, sodium 884 $mg.L^{-1}$, magnesium 100 $mg.L^{-1}$, zinc 5 $mg.L^{-1}$, vitamins C 15 $mg.L^{-1}$, E 5 $mg.L^{-1}$, B1 0.7 $mg.L^{-1}$, B2 0.4 $mg.L^{-1}$, B3 9 $mg.L^{-1}$ (80 $g.L_{-1}$, 1254 $kJ.L^{-1}$). Placebo match drink: natural flavors, malic and citric acids, xanthan gum, acesulfame potassium, sucralose, silicium dioxide, yellow FCF, tartrazine (3.2 $g.L^{-1}$, 50 $kJ.L^{-1}$). Post-match drink: proteins 40 $g.L^{-1}$; glucose 28.8 $g.L^{-1}$; fructose 14.4 $g.L^{-1}$; lipids 7.2 $g.L^{-1}$; curcumin 680 mg.L-^{1}; piperine 7.6 $mg.L^{-1}$; sodium chloride 576 $mg.L^{-1}$; potassium 156 $mg.L^{-1}$; vitamins C 120 $mg.L^{-1}$; E 20 $mg.L^{-1}$; B1 5.6 $mg.L^{-1}$; B2 3.3 $mg.L^{-1}$; B3 72 $mg.L^{-1}$; B6 4 $mg.L^{-1}$ (64 $g.L^{-1}$, 2144 $kJ.L^{-1}$). Placebo post-match drink: natural flavors, titanium dioxide, tartrazine, maltodextrin, beetroot juice concentrate (amount of traces), citric acid, acesulfame potassium, sucralose, silicium dioxide (3.0 $g.L^{-1}$, 68 $kJ.L^{-1}$). All drinks were provided by Nutratletic (Aytré, France) and respected the current legislation for dietary products.

Tennis tournament simulation

Each tournament took place over a weekend. On the experiment days (SPD and PLA sessions), the players arrived at the tennis club at 07 h00 after an overnight fast. A standardized breakfast was given to the subjects. The eight players were randomly divided into two groups of four players. Every player in each group played randomly against each of the three other players. Therefore, each player played three matches. The first game began at 10 h00 on Saturday, the second game at 15 h00 and the third match was scheduled at 10 h00 on Sunday. A standardized breakfast, lunch and dinner was given to the subjects at 07 h30, 13 h00 and 20 h00 respectively. To maintain the competitive aspect, but play for similar periods, the format of each game was adapted to last 2 h. In practice, the players played 3 sets using the No Ad scoring system to limit variability in the duration of the games. The first 2 sets were played in 6 games with a tiebreak in case of a tie at 6 all. At the end of the first two sets, the format of the third set was adjusted to obtain an estimated final match time of 2 h. If the duration of the first two sets was less than 1 h 20 min, the third set took place in 6 games, like the first 2. If the first 2 sets lasted between 1 h 20 min and 1 h 40 min, the third set was played in 4 games, with a tiebreaker played in the event of a tie at four games all. Finally, if the duration of the first 2 sets was above 1 h 40 min, the third set was replaced by a super tiebreak of 10 points. This protocol resulted in matches very close to 2 h in duration and with very low variability, while avoiding games played "in time", which could have led to abnormal playing and have had a negative impact on the player motivation. No significant differences could be detected in the average duration of matches between the PLA and SPD sessions (data not shown).

Isometric handgrip strength

Three consecutive measurements for isometric handgrip strength of the dominant hand were made with a calibrated dynamometer (TK200, Takei®, Niigata, Japan). The best performance was recorded for each subject. The apparatus was reset to zero before each measurement. The measurements were conducted under standardized conditions: subject seated, the shoulder adducted and neutrally rotated, with the forearm and wrist in a neutral position and the elbow at 90° flexion. The subjects were verbally encouraged to perform three, 3-s maximum voluntary contractions (MVC) separated by at least 3 min of recovery in between.

Power (jump height)

All vertical jumps were performed using an optical measurement system (Optojump, Microgate®, Bolzano, Italy). A software program recorded jump height based on flight time. In order to ensure the validity of the test, participants were asked to have their knees as fully extended as possible and their ankles completely plantarflexed on both take-off and landing. Participants stood with their feet shoulder width apart and flat on the contact mat. The best jump from three attempts was recorded for both squat jumps (SJ) and countermovement jumps (CMJ). A 1-min recovery was provided between all jump trials. For both jump measurements, participants stood feet flat on the contact mat with hands on hips (no arm swing). For SJ measurements, participants held their knees flexed at 90° for two seconds, and were then told to jump as high as possible, avoiding the use of a stretch-shortening cycle as for CMJ. No specific instructions were given about the depth or speed of the countermovement for the CMJ test.

Maximal 20-m sprints

The running speed of participants was evaluated with a 5- and 20-m sprint effort using photocells (Racetime2,

Microgate®, Bolzano, Italy). The timing gates were positioned 5- and 20-m cross-wind from a pre-determined starting point. Participants were instructed to run as fast as possible along the 20-m distance from a standing start. Subjects started the test in their own time from a static position 30 cm behind the photocells, with timing starting once the beams of the first timing gate (0 m) were broken. The fastest time obtained from three trials was used in data analysis. There was a 2-min recovery period between trials. Time spent to cover 20-m was measured to the nearest 0.001 s.

Repeated sprint ability

The repeated sprint ability test, which attempts to quantify fatigue by comparing actual performance to an imagined "ideal performance", consisted of 6 times 24.69 m (3 times 8.23 m, corresponding to the width of the tennis court) of discontinuous sprints, interspersed with 30 s of walking recovery. The timing gates were positioned in the width of the court, at the opposite of the court's two single lines. Subjects were instructed to run as fast as possible from one side to another 3 times from an initial standing start. Subjects started the test from a static position 30 cm behind the photocells, with timing starting once the beams of the first timing gate (0 m) were broken. Speed was measured to the nearest 0.001 s. A photoelectric cell timing system (Racetime2, Microgate®, Bolzano, Italy) linked to a digital chronoscope was used to record each sprint and rest interval time with an accuracy of 0.001 s. Fatigability (percent decrease in time between the fastest and slowest sprints) and sprint decrement score (Sdec) were calculated from sprint times using the following formula : Fatigue (%) = –((slowest sprint-fastest sprint)/ fastest sprint)×100; Sdec (%) = –(((Sprint 1 time + Sprint 2 time + ... + Sprint 6 time)/Best sprint time × number of sprints)-1)×100 [16].

Knee and elbow extensors maximal isometric strength

The maximal isometric strength of the dominant knee extensors was measured from maximum voluntary contractions (MVC) performed on a custom-made ergometer. This ergometer was built in order to allow placement of the force transducer (Model F2712, 0- to 100-daN force range, Meiri Company, Bonneuil, France) at the level of the lateral malleolus and adjustment of the seat depth depending on the length of the thighs. The knee angle and the hip angle were set at 60° (0° is full extension). The knee was fixed at an angle of 60° of flexion since it has been demonstrated to be the angle of maximal isometric force generation for human muscles [17,18]. The dominant leg was defined as the preferred kicking leg. Subjects were secured to the chair by a strap slung over the shoulders to avoid any compensatory movement of the trunk. Subjects were also instructed to grip the seat during the voluntary contractions to further stabilize the pelvis. The subjects were verbally encouraged to perform three, 3-s MVCs separated by at least 3 min of recovery. Isometric MVC strength was determined as the best of three reproducible measurements. During each trial, subjects were instructed to contract the muscle as strongly as possible. Isometric MVC torque of the knee extensor muscles (KE MVC torque) was calculated as the product of maximal force and moment leg length; the latter being measured from the lateral malleolus to the lateral femoral condyle in resting conditions using a tape measure.

The isometric MVC strength of the dominant (arm holding the racket) elbow extensors was measured on a custom-made, home-built ergometer. This ergometer was built in order to place the subjects in a seated position and pull a grip connected to a force transducer with the elbow flexed at 90°. During each test, subjects were instructed to keep their chest in an upright position to avoid any compensatory movement of the trunk. The experimental protocol was the same as that previously described for the knee extensors. The subjects were encouraged to perform three, 3-s isometric MVCs separated by 3-min resting periods. Isometric MVC strength was determined as the best trial from three reproducible measurements. Isometric MVC torque of elbow extensors (EE MVC torque) was calculated as the product of maximal force and moment arm length, the latter being measured from the lateral epicondyle of the elbow to the ulna head in resting conditions using a tape measure. Force output was measured using a calibrated force transducer (Model F2712, 0- to 100-daN force range, Meiri Company, Bonneuil, France) and transmitted to a PC using an analog/digital card (National Instruments, NI USB-6211, France).

Knee and elbow extensors fatigability

The subjects performed a 90-s sustained isometric contraction at 25% MVC in order to evaluate the muscle fatigability of the main knee and elbow extensor muscles. Visual feedback about force was provided to the subject during the sustained contraction. Electromyographic signals (EMG) of the superficial heads of the knee extensors (*vastus lateralis*, *vastus medialis* and *rectus femoris*) and the *triceps brachii* muscle (medial and lateral heads) were recorded throughout the 90-s sustained contraction. EMG was quantified in the time domain using the Root Mean Square value (RMS). All the RMS values recorded during the 90-s contraction were normalized to a percentage of maximal Root Mean Square value (RMS_{max}) of the best MVC trial for each muscle.

Electromyography

The EMG signals were recorded using bipolar silver chloride surface electrodes (Kendall, Arbo, Tyco Healthcare,

Neustadt, Germany) during the MVCs and the fatigability test. The recording electrodes were taped lengthwise on the skin over the muscle belly following SENIAM recommendations [19], with an inter-electrode distance of 20 mm. The position of the electrodes was marked on the skin so that they could be fixed in the same place during the following test session. The reference electrode was attached to the patella or to the elbow. Low impedance ($Z < 5$ kΩ) at the skin-electrode surface was obtained by shaving, abrading the skin with thin sand paper and cleaning with alcohol. Electromyographic signals were amplified with a bandwidth frequency ranging from 10 Hz to 500 Hz and simultaneously digitized together with force signals using an acquisition card (National Instruments, NI USB-6211, Nanterre, France) and a custom made software (MatLab Version 7.5.0, R2007b). The sampling frequency was 1000 Hz.

Statistical analyses

Data are reported as mean values ± standard deviation (SD). The statistical analyses were done using GraphPad PRISM® 5.01 software (La Jolla, USA). A p-value < 0.05 was considered significant. Two-way ANOVA were used when the interaction between time and condition effects was tested (EMG data). Other endpoints were analyzed using non-parametric tests. To test for the condition effect (CON, PLA, SPD), the Kruskal-Wallis one-way test was used. In case of significant difference, the Wilcoxon signed-rank test was performed to compare all pairs of conditions.

Results

Eight subjects completed all three different test conditions without experiencing any complications. During the three test sessions, environmental conditions were not significantly different: ambient temperature was: 27.1 ± 0.4, 27.5 ± 0.5 and 28.0 ± 0.4°C in the CON, PLA and SPD sessions, respectively. The relative humidity was 38.0 ± 2.7, 40.0 ± 3.0 and 41.0 ± 3.3% in the CON, PLA and SPD trials, respectively.

Isometric handgrip strength

Average handgrip strength values for the CON, PLA and SPD were 51.18 ± 1.36, 47.23 ± 2.01 and 49.08 ± 0.88 kg respectively, with no significant difference between the 3 conditions (Figure 2).

Power (jump height)

Average CMJ height values for the CON, PLA and SPD were 34.98 ± 1.87, 34.55 ± 1.75 and 34.60 ± 1.78 cm, respectively, with no significant differences between these 3 conditions (Figure 3). Average SJ height values for the CON, PLA and SPD were 31.05 ± 1.91, 29.98 ± 1.93 and 31.20 ± 1.97 cm, respectively, with no significant difference between the three conditions (Figure 3).

Maximal 20-m Sprints

Average 5-m sprint time values for the CON, PLA and SPD were 1.16 ± 0.03, 1.34 ± 0.12 and 1.26 ± 0.03 s, respectively. Average 5 to 20-m sprint time values for the CON, PLA and SPD were 2.14 ± 0.04, 2.14 ± 0.05 and 2.13 ± 0.05 s, respectively. Average 20-m sprint time values for the CON, PLA and SPD were 3.29 ± 0.06, 3.48 ± 0.13 and 3.37 ± 0.06 s, respectively. No significant differences between the three conditions were observed for any of the sprint times (Figure 4).

Repeated sprint ability

Average best performance for the 3 × 8.23 m (24.69 m) repeated sprint test for the CON, PLA and SPD were 6.23 ± 0.21, 6.27 ± 0.24 and 6.19 ± 0.22 s, respectively, with no significant difference between the three conditions (Figure 5, Panel A). The fatigue index was also not significantly different between conditions (−4.69 ± 0.63, −4.58 ± 0.68 and −4.88 ± 0.68% for CON, PLA and SPD respectively) (Figure 5, Panel B). The sprint decrement score was also not different between the three conditions (−3.21 ± 0.50, −2.70 ± 0.58 and −2.98 ± 0.41% for CON, PLA and SPD respectively).

Knee and elbow extensors maximal isometric strength

Analysis of variance revealed no significant difference in knee extension and elbow extension MVC torque between the three experimental conditions (Figure 6).

Knee and elbow extensors fatigability

Electromyographic changes throughout the 90-s sustained isometric contraction were similar in the 3 conditions for all muscles, except for the lateral head of the *triceps brachii* whereby RMS values increased significantly less in the SPD group compared to the PLA group (Figure 7). No

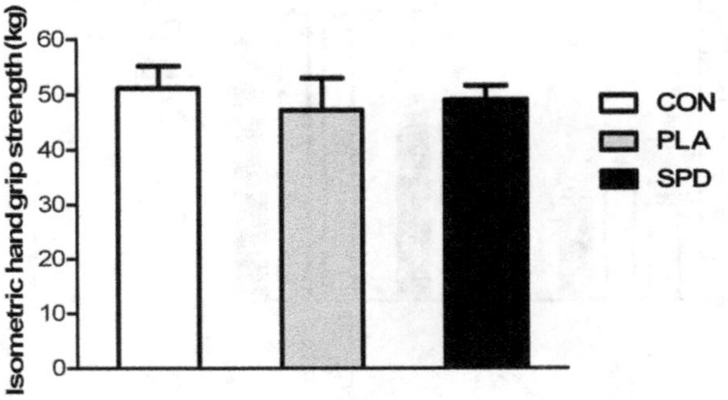

Figure 2 Mean (±SD) isometric hand grip strength with the dominant hand in the 3 conditions (CON, PLA and SPD). Inter-group analysis was carried out using the Kruskal-Wallis one-way analysis; no statistical difference was found.

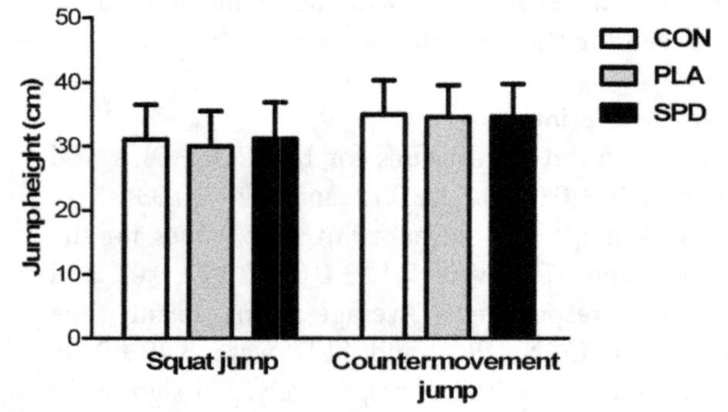

Figure 3 Mean (±SD) jump height for the squat (SJ) and countermovement (CMJ) jumps in the 3 conditions (CON, PLA and SPD). For SJ and CMJ, inter-group analysis was carried out using the Kruskal-Wallis one-way analysis; no statistical differences were found.

significant difference was observed for the *triceps brachii* between the SPD and CON conditions.

Discussion

The objective of this study was to evaluate the effects of a nutritional strategy on the physical performance of competitive tennis players. This strategy consisted of taking a pre-match drink, a match-drink and a post-match drink during every match of a simulated tennis tournament. Based on data in the literature, showing that a prolonged tennis match could induce muscle fatigue [20,21], our first hypothesis was that repeated tennis matches would induce a decrease in physical performance even after a few hours of recovery compared to the resting condition. Since some studies have also demonstrated that carbohydrate supplements during prolonged tennis matches delays the onset of fatigue [4,5,8-10], our second hypothesis was that drinking sports beverages before, during and after each tennis match would limit the decrease in physical performance

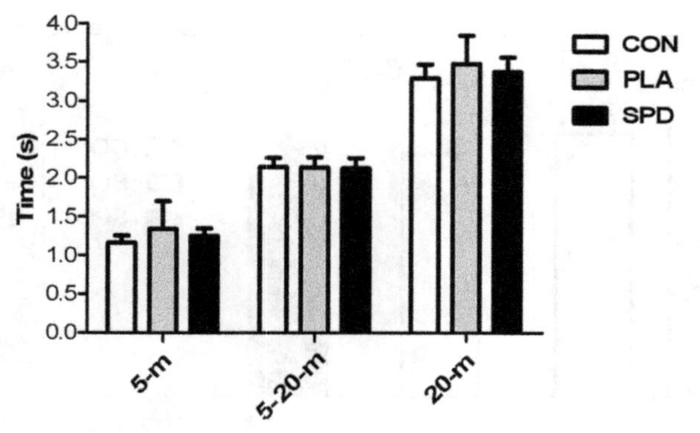

Figure 4 Average (±SD) time spent to cover 5-, 5 to 20- and 20-m sprint values for the 3 conditions (CON, PLA and SPD). Inter-group analysis was carried out using the Kruskal-Wallis one-way analysis; no statistical difference was found.

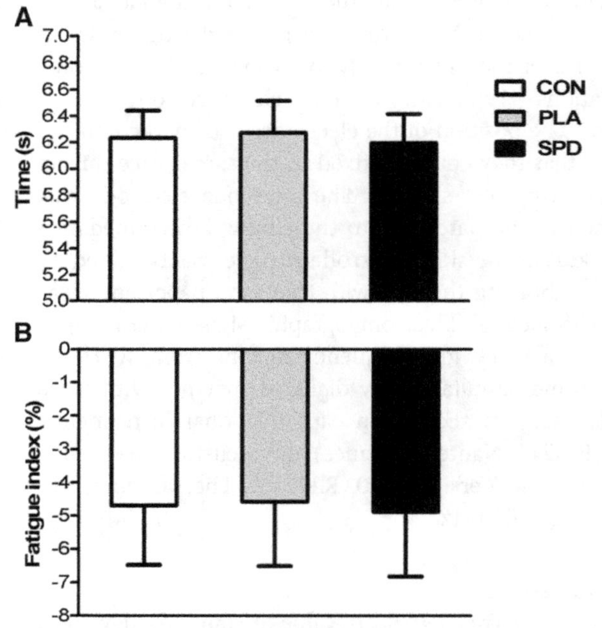

Figure 5 Repeated sprint best time and fatigue index. Average (±SD) best performance for the 3 x 8.23 m repeated sprints in the 3 conditions (CON, PLA and SPD) (Panel **A**). Mean (±SD) fatigue index in the 3 conditions (Panel **B**). Fatigue index was calculated by the percent decrease in time between the fastest and the slowest sprints. Inter-group analysis was carried out using the Kruskal-Wallis one-way analysis; no statistically difference was found.

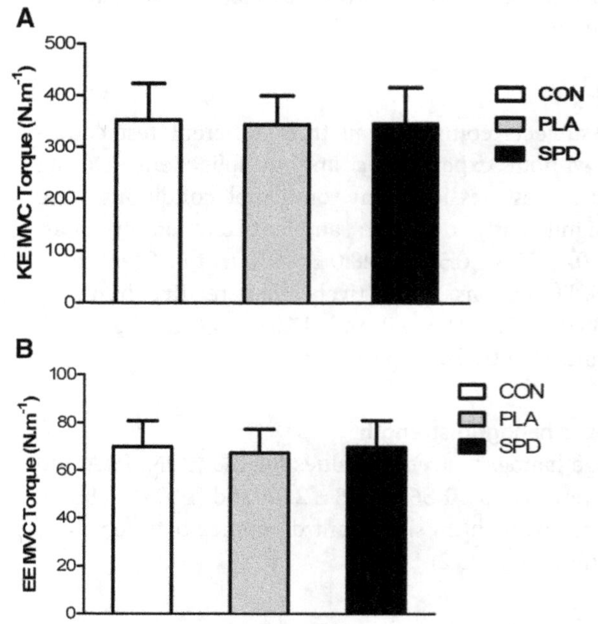

Figure 6 Mean (±SD) isometric maximal voluntary contraction torque of knee extensors (KE MVC Torque, Panel A) and of elbow extensors (EE MVC Torque, Panel B) in the 3 conditions (CON, PLA and SPD). For KE MVC Torque and EE MVC Torque, inter-group analysis was carried out using the Kruskal-Wallis one-way analysis; no statistical differences were found.

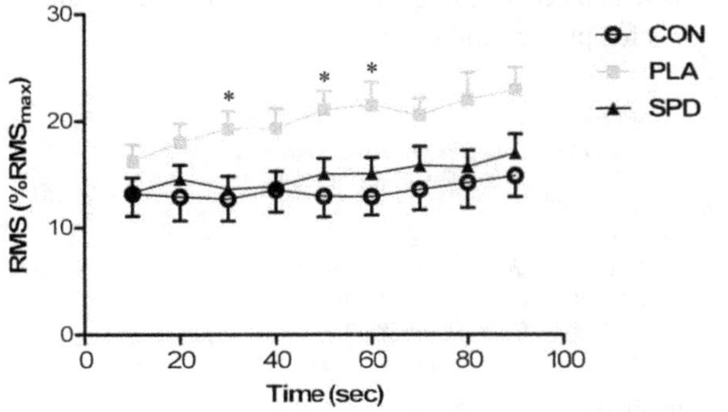

Figure 7 Time course of root mean square (RMS) values (expressed as a percentage of the maximal RMS of the best MVC trial) of the *triceps brachii* muscle (lateral head) throughout the 90-sec time trial. Results are expressed as mean values ± SD in the three conditions (CON, PLA and SPD). Two-way ANOVA was used (time and condition); time effect: $p < 0.001$, condition x time effect: $p = 0.0167$. Bonferroni post hoc analysis showed significant difference between PLA and SPD for time 30-, 50- and 60-sec ($p < 0.05$). Tendencies were observed for time 40-sec ($p = 0.07$), 80-sec ($p = 0.08$) and 90-sec ($p = 0.07$).

compared to conditions where the only fluid intake was water. The main results show that playing three simulated tennis matches in a thirty-six-hour period did not significantly decrease any of the physical performance measures 3 h after the last match.

Various studies have shown that prolonged tennis playing in competitions leads to the development of muscle fatigue that may impair skilled performance on the court [3-6]. However, all of these studies conducted performance tests during or immediately after the match. Given the characteristics of tennis tournaments, *i.e.* several matches in a limited time-frame interspersed with short recovery periods, it is important to consider whether these consecutive matches would finally result in decreased physical performance and whether ingesting sports drinks before, during and after each match would limit fatigue, facilitate recovery and so favor improved performance in subsequent matches. Considering that nutritional strategies can have an important influence on the capacity to recover [14,22], notably influencing muscle and hepatic glycogen stores [23], we have been careful in this study to precisely control the amount and type of nutrients ingested during the meals taken by the players in the different conditions studied. Thus the breakfasts, lunches and dinners eaten on study days were standardized and identical for each of the conditions.

The results of our study show that after playing three 2-hour matches within thirty-six hours, only 3 hours of passive recovery (including the ingestion of a standardized lunch) was sufficient to observe no significant decrease in physical performance parameters, compared to the rest condition. The only significant difference in physical performance was the increase in RMS values during the 90-s sustained isometric contraction at 25% MVC for the lateral head of the *triceps brachii* in the PLA condition compared to the CON condition. The increased RMS value under the placebo condition is an index of fatigue and indicative of the greater number of motor units required to maintain an equivalent level of force [24].

This study, the first to assess the influence of repeated tennis matches on physical performance, suggests that when the length of a match does not exceed 2 hours, when balanced meals are taken between matches, and when hydration during matches is sufficient, there is no major deleterious impact on physical performance of the lower-limb muscles. It has already been suggested that skilled tennis performance, which can be affected by prolonged match-induced fatigue [3,6], quickly returns to normal [21,25]. We can hypothesize that, if the measurements of physical performance had been carried out immediately after the end of the last match of a tournament, a significant decline in performance parameters would have been observed. For example, two recent studies [26,27] showed a decrease of 9 - 15% in the plantar flexor muscles' MVC immediately after 3-hour tennis matches. Nevertheless, two-hour tennis matches are not always associated with decreased performance. Indeed, McRae et al. were not able to show any significant decrease in a specific tennis skill-test following a 2-hour tennis match [10]. We can hypothesize that a succession of longer matches and/or more intense and/or performed under more constraining environmental conditions would have induced a decrease in physical performance even after several hours of recovery, but more studies are needed to address this hypothesis. Moreover, most of the studies exploring muscle fatigue following tennis matches have used an isometric device [26-32]. To date, only one study has evaluated the impact of tennis practice on muscle performance using isokinetic dynamometer in elite young tennis players [33]. They found that a 90 min practice session induced a 9 to 13% decrease in the knee extensors and flexors of the contractile joint moments evaluated at 60 and 180°.s^{-1}. Therefore, it would be particularly interesting to conduct more studies evaluating fatigue following tennis matches and practice sessions using isokinetic measurements, which represent more closely tennis activity muscle contraction pattern.

In this study, we evaluated physical performance through some simple tests of speed, strength, power and endurance. However, it is conceivable that complementary tests might have revealed fatigue, or that a specific assessment of tennis performance would have demonstrated a drop in performance. One explanation for the fact that the only fatigue observed in our study concerned the *triceps brachii* muscle could be the fiber composition of this muscle, as it has been recognized that this influences muscle fatigue [34]. It has also been shown that the *triceps brachii* muscle has a fast profile, with less than 20% of type I fibers [35], while the quadriceps muscle has a more mixed profile with more than 50% of type I fibers [36-38].

The second objective of this study was to assess whether supplementation with sports drinks before, during and after each match, compared with water alone, could limit the negative impact of the succession of matches on physical performance of the players. Since consecutive matches induced little or no drop in performance during the tests performed three hours after the last match, it is not surprising to observe almost no difference between the placebo and drinks conditions. Interestingly, in our study the only fatigue observed in the placebo condition compared with the rest condition (an increase in RMS of the *triceps brachii* muscle), was counteracted when the players were supplemented with sports drinks. The main active ingredients of the drinks consumed by the players were carbohydrates (pre-match drink, match-drink and post-match drink), caffeine (pre-match drink and match-drink), and proteins (match-drink and post-match drink). Some studies have already demonstrated the potential of carbohydrates and caffeine supplementation to positively affect performance of tennis players [4,5,8-10], while proteins have only been suggested [21]. In the context of repeated matches with short recovery periods, it is at least conceivable that a decrease in glycogen stocks may contribute to the development of muscle fatigue, and that supplementation with carbohydrate before, during and after each match could promote the use of exogenous substrates and the rate of resynthesis of glycogen stocks between matches and therefore finally enable better maintenance of performance over repeated matches. Given that a drop in tennis performance has been observed during extended matches (>3 h), further research is needed to investigate whether the current nutritional supplementation strategy would more effective under such conditions.

In conclusion, this study demonstrates that playing three 2-hour tennis matches in a day and a half does not induce any significant decrease in physical performance of the lower-limb muscles three hours after the end of the last match, when water-based hydration is sufficient and the meals are well-balanced. The only fatigue observed in the placebo condition compared with the rest condition involved the *triceps brachii* muscle, and this fatigue was counteracted when the players were supplemented with sports drinks, which allows one to hypothesize that this type of nutritional strategy could be effective in the more extreme conditions that occur during competitive tennis tournaments. Further studies are needed to address this hypothesis which could lead to interesting practical recommendations for players and coaches.

Competing interests

Nicolas Aubineau and Sébastien L Peltier are employees of Laboratoire Lescuyer-Nutratletic. Jean-François Lescuyer is the general director of the company.

This trial was carried out by Laboratoire des Adaptations Métaboliques à l'Exercice en conditions Physiologiques et Pathologiques (AME2P) and Laboratoire Lescuyer-Nutratletic as a joint venture.

The other authors have no competing interests.

Authors' contributions

TB: conception and design of the study, acquisition of data, analysis and interpretation of data, drafting manuscript. SR: conception and design of the study, acquisition of data (electromyographic measures), analysis and interpretation of data (electromyographic measures), drafting manuscript. PL: conception and design of the study, acquisition of data, analysis and interpretation of data, revising manuscript. LM: acquisition of data, dietary protocol management, revising manuscript. GE: acquisition of data, analysis and interpretation of data, revising manuscript. ED: conception and design of the study, acquisition of data, revising manuscript. VM: analysis and interpretation of data (electromyographic measures), revising manuscript. DB: design of the study, revising manuscript. NA: analysis and interpretation of data, revising manuscript. JL: conception and design of the study, revising manuscript. MD: conception and design of the study (main clinical investigator), acquisition of data, revising manuscript. PS: conception and design of the study (main project coordinator), acquisition of data, analysis and interpretation of data, drafting manuscript. SP: conception and design of the study (main project coordinator), analysis and interpretation of data, statistical analysis, drafting manuscript. All authors have read and approved the final manuscript.

Author details

[1]Division of Sport Medicine and Biology of Physical Activity, University of Athens Faculty of Physical Education and Sport Science, Antistasis 41Dafni 17237 Athens, Greece. [2]Clermont Université, Université Blaise Pascal, EA 3533, Laboratoire des Adaptations Métaboliques à l'Exercice en conditions Physiologiques et Pathologiques (AME2P), Bâtiment Biologie B, 24 avenue des Landais, BP 80026F-63171 Aubière Cedex, France. [3]Laboratoire de Recherche Adaptations Physiologiques à l'Exercice et Réadaptation à l'Effort, EA-3300, Faculté des Sciences du Sport, Université de Picardie Jules Verne, Amiens, France. [4]Institute of Sport, Exercise and Active Living (ISEAL), Victoria University, Melbourne, Australia. [5]College of Sport and Exercise Science, Victoria University, Melbourne, Australia. [6]Department of Research, Laboratoire Lescuyer, Nutratletic, Aytré, France. [7]Department of Sport Medicine and Functional Explorations, University-Hospital (CHU), G. Montpied Hospital, Clermont-Ferrand F-63003, France. [8]INRA, UMR 1019, Clermont-Ferrand F-63001, France. [9]University Clermont 1, UFR Médecine, Clermont-Ferrand F-63001, France. [10]CRNH-Auvergne, Clermont-Ferrand F-63001, France.

References

1. Fernandez J, Mendez-Villanueva A, Pluim BM: **Intensity of tennis match play.** *Br J Sports Med* 2006, **40**(5):387–391. discussion 391.
2. Hornery DJ, Farrow D, Mujika I, Young W: **An integrated physiological and performance profile of professional tennis.** *Br J Sports Med* 2007, **41**(8):531–536. discussion 536.
3. Davey PR, Thorpe RD, Williams C: **Fatigue decreases skilled tennis performance.** *J Sports Sci* 2002, **20**(4):311–318.
4. Hornery DJ, Farrow D, Mujika I, Young WB: **Caffeine, carbohydrate, and cooling use during prolonged simulated tennis.** *Int J Sports Physiol Perform* 2007, **2**(4):423–438.
5. Vergauwen L, Brouns F, Hespel P: **Carbohydrate supplementation improves stroke performance in tennis.** *Med Sci Sports Exerc* 1998, **30**(8):1289–1295.

6. Wu CL, Shih MC, Yang CC, Huang MH, Chang CK: **Sodium bicarbonate supplementation prevents skilled tennis performance decline after a simulated match.** *J Int Soc Sports Nutr* 2010, **7**:33.
7. Kovacs MS: **Carbohydrate intake and tennis: are there benefits?** *Br J Sports Med* 2006, **40**(5):e13.
8. Bergeron MF, Waller JL, Marinik EL: **Voluntary fluid intake and core temperature responses in adolescent tennis players: sports beverage versus water.** *Br J Sports Med* 2006, **40**(5):406–410.
9. Ferrauti A, Weber K, Struder HK: **Metabolic and ergogenic effects of carbohydrate and caffeine beverages in tennis.** *J Sports Med Phys Fitness* 1997, **37**(4):258–266.
10. McRae KA, Galloway SD: **Carbohydrate-electrolyte drink ingestion and skill performance during and after 2 hr of indoor tennis match play.** *Int J Sport Nutr Exerc Metab* 2012, **22**(1):38–46.
11. Eijnde BO, Vergauwen L, Hespel P: **Creatine loading does not impact on stroke performance in tennis.** *Int J Sports Med* 2001, **22**(1):76–80.
12. Pluim BM, Ferrauti A, Broekhof F, Deutekom M, Gotzmann A, Kuipers H, Weber K: **The effects of creatine supplementation on selected factors of tennis specific training.** *Br J Sports Med* 2006, **40**(6):507–511. discussion 511–502.
13. Maughan RJ, Depiesse F, Geyer H: **The use of dietary supplements by athletes.** *J Sports Sci* 2007, **25**(Suppl 1):S103–S113.
14. Rodriguez NR, Di Marco NM, Langley S: **American College of Sports Medicine position stand. Nutrition and athletic performance.** *Med Sci Sports Exerc* 2009, **41**(3):709–731.
15. Peltier SL, Lepretre PM, Metz L, Ennequin G, Aubineau N, Lescuyer JF, Duclos M, Brink T, Sirvent P: **Effects of pre-exercise, endurance and recovery designer sports drinks on performance during tennis tournament simulation.** *J Strength Cond Res* 2013, **27**(11):3076–3083.
16. Bishop D, Edge J: **Determinants of repeated-sprint ability in females matched for single-sprint performance.** *Eur J Appl Physiol* 2006, **97**(4):373–379.
17. Thorstensson A, Grimby G, Karlsson J: **Force-velocity relations and fiber composition in human knee extensor muscles.** *J Appl Physiol* 1976, **40**(1):12–16.
18. Tihanyi J, Apor P, Fekete G: **Force-velocity-power characteristics and fiber composition in human knee extensor muscles.** *Eur J Appl Physiol Occup Physiol* 1982, **48**(3):331–343.
19. Hermens HJ, Freriks B, Disselhorst-Klug C, Rau G: **Development of recommendations for SEMG sensors and sensor placement procedures.** *J Electromyogr Kinesiol* 2000, **10**(5):361–374.
20. Girard O, Millet GP: **Neuromuscular fatigue in racquet sports.** *Phys Med Rehabil Clin N Am* 2009, **20**(1):161–173. ix.
21. Hornery DJ, Farrow D, Mujika I, Young W: **Fatigue in tennis: mechanisms of fatigue and effect on performance.** *Sports Med* 2007, **37**(3):199–212.
22. Gilbert N: **Conference on "Multidisciplinary approaches to nutritional problems". Symposium on "Performance, exercise and health". Practical aspects of nutrition in performance.** *Proc Nutr Soc* 2009, **68**(1):23–28.
23. Lambert EV, Goedecke JH: **The role of dietary macronutrients in optimizing endurance performance.** *Curr Sports Med Rep* 2003, **2**(4):194–201.
24. Moritani T, Yoshitake Y: **1998 ISEK Congress Keynote Lecture: The use of electromyography in applied physiology. International Society of Electrophysiology and Kinesiology.** *J Electromyogr Kinesiol* 1998, **8**(6):363–381.
25. Mendez-Villanueva A, Fernandez-Fernandez J, Bishop D: **Exercise-induced homeostatic perturbations provoked by singles tennis match play with reference to development of fatigue.** *Br J Sports Med* 2007, **41**(11):717–722. discussion 722.
26. Fabre JB, Martin V, Gondin J, Cottin F, Grelot L: **Effect of playing surface properties on neuromuscular fatigue in tennis.** *Med Sci Sports Exerc* 2012, **44**(11):2182–2189.
27. Girard O, Racinais S, Micallef JP, Millet GP: **Spinal modulations accompany peripheral fatigue during prolonged tennis playing.** *Scand J Med Sci Sports* 2011, **21**(3):455–464.
28. Girard O, Lattier G, Maffiuletti NA, Micallef JP, Millet GP: **Neuromuscular fatigue during a prolonged intermittent exercise: Application to tennis.** *J Electromyogr Kinesiol* 2008, **18**(6):1038–1046.
29. Girard O, Lattier G, Micallef JP, Millet GP: **Changes in exercise characteristics, maximal voluntary contraction, and explosive strength during prolonged tennis playing.** *Br J Sports Med* 2006, **40**(6):521–526.
30. Girard O, Racinais S, Periard JD: **Tennis in hot and cool conditions decreases the rapid muscle torque production capacity of the knee extensors but not of the plantar flexors.** *Br J Sports Med* 2014, **48**(Suppl 1):i52–i58.
31. Ojala T, Hakkinen K: **Effects of the tennis tournament on players' physical performance, hormonal responses, muscle damage and recovery.** *J Sports Sci Med* 2013, **12**(2):240–248.
32. Rota S, Morel B, Saboul D, Rogowski I, Hautier C: **Influence of fatigue on upper limb muscle activity and performance in tennis.** *J Electromyogr Kinesiol* 2014, **24**(1):90–97.
33. Malliou VJ, Beneka AG, Gioftsidou AF, Malliou PK, Kallistratos E, Pafis GK, Katsikas CA, Douvis S: **Young tennis players and balance performance.** *J Strength Cond Res* 2010, **24**(2):389–393.
34. Westerblad H, Bruton JD, Katz A: **Skeletal muscle: energy metabolism, fiber types, fatigue and adaptability.** *Exp Cell Res* 2010, **316**(18):3093–3099.
35. Liu Y, Schlumberger A, Wirth K, Schmidtbleicher D, Steinacker JM: **Different effects on human skeletal myosin heavy chain isoform expression: strength vs. combination training.** *J Appl Physiol* 2003, **94**(6):2282–2288.
36. Guadalupe-Grau A, Perez-Gomez J, Olmedillas H, Chavarren J, Dorado C, Santana A, Serrano-Sanchez JA, Calbet JA: **Strength training combined with plyometric jumps in adults: sex differences in fat-bone axis adaptations.** *J Appl Physiol* 2009, **106**(4):1100–1111.
37. Holm L, Reitelseder S, Pedersen TG, Doessing S, Petersen SG, Flyvbjerg A, Andersen JL, Aagaard P, Kjaer M: **Changes in muscle size and MHC composition in response to resistance exercise with heavy and light loading intensity.** *J Appl Physiol* 2008, **105**(5):1454–1461.
38. Luden N, Minchev K, Hayes E, Louis E, Trappe T, Trappe S: **Human vastus lateralis and soleus muscles display divergent cellular contractile properties.** *Am J Physiol Regul Integr Comp Physiol* 2008, **295**(5):R1593–R1598.

28

Nutritional knowledge and eating habits of professional rugby league players: does knowledge translate into practice?

Ieva Alaunyte[1,2*], John L Perry[1] and Tony Aubrey[1]

Abstract

Background: Adequate nutrient intake is important to support training and to optimise performance of elite athletes. Nutritional knowledge has been shown to play an important role in adopting optimal nutrition practices. The aim of the present study was to investigate the relationship between the level of nutritional knowledge and dietary habits in elite English rugby league players using the eatwell plate food categories.

Method: General nutritional knowledge questionnaires were collected during the Super League competitive season in the first team squad of 21 professional Rugby league players (mean age 25 ± 5 yrs, BMI 27 ± 2.4 kg/m2, experience in game 6 ± 4 yrs). According to their nutritional knowledge scores, the players were assigned to either good or poor nutritional knowledge group (n = 11, n = 10, respectively). Their dietary habits were assessment using a food frequency questionnaire.

Results: The findings revealed that nutritional knowledge was adequate (mean 72.82%) in this group of athletes with the highest scores in dietary advice section (85.71%), followed by food groups (71.24%) and food choice (69.52%). The majority of athletes were not aware of current carbohydrate recommendations. This translated into their dietary habits as many starchy and fibrous foods were consumed only occasionally by poor nutritional knowledge group. In terms of their eating habits, the good nutritional knowledge group consumed significantly more fruit and vegetables, and starchy foods ($p < .05$). Nutritional knowledge was positively correlated to fruit and vegetables consumption ($r_s = .52$, $p < .05$) but not to any other eatwell plate categories.

Conclusions: The study identified adequate general nutritional knowledge in professional rugby league players with the exception of recommendation for starchy and fibrous foods. Players who scored higher in nutritional knowledge test were more likely to consume more fruits, vegetables and carbohydrate-rich foods.

Keywords: Diet, Elite, Rugby league, Athletes, Sport

Background

Rugby League is a physically demanding sport that is characterised by repeated changes in exercise intensity, from low-speed activity such as standing and walking to high-intensity bouts such as sprints and tackles [1]. These physiological demands place heavy requirements on body's fuel stores. An adequate nutritional intake is essential for promoting overall health as well as for optimal training and competition performance of professional rugby league players.

Despite the increased interest in nutrition amongst many elite athletes and the well documented importance of a balanced diet for overall health and athletic performance, research suggests that professional rugby players consume diets that are less than optimal [2-4]. Furthermore, nutritional knowledge of elite athletes and their coaches was shown to be inadequate [5-7]. It is argued that nutritional knowledge is strongly associated with healthy eating and healthy food choices irrespective of demographic variables [8]. In addition to this, Rugby League players generally tend to focus much less on

* Correspondence: alaunyi@hope.ac.uk
[1]Leeds Trinity University, Department of Sport, Health and Nutrition, Brownberrie Lane, Horsforth LS18 5HD, UK
[2]Liverpool Hope University, School of Health Sciences, Hope Park, Liverpool L16 9JD, UK

their diet compared to endurance athletes [9], which coupled with inadequate nutritional knowledge may result in poorer dietary choices.

The basis of adequate nutrient intake is a healthy and balanced diet, therefore, recommendations for athletes is to consume a diet, which follows current dietary guidelines for general population. The eatwell plate is used by health professionals as the national recommendation for healthy diets in the UK [10]. The main nutritional aim of the eatwell plate is to help individuals to understand the relative proportions of different food groups in a healthy and well balanced diet. Healthy adults are encouraged to consume at least five portion of fruit and vegetables a day, plenty of bread, rice, potatoes, pasta and other starchy foods (choosing wholegrain varieties where possible), some milk and dairy foods, some meat, fish (two portions a week, one of which should be oily), eggs, beans and other non-dairy sources of protein and just a small amount of foods and drinks high in fat and/or sugar [10]. The eatwell plate does not provide guidance to frequency of serving and portion sizes (with the exception of fruit, vegetables and fish) because it was developed as a tool suitable for most adults, hence, it would be misleading to include specific portion advice. Nevertheless, the eatwell plate provides food group daily proportions (starchy foods- 33%, fruit and vegetables- 33%, milk and dairy foods- 15%, meat, fish, eggs, beans and other non-dairy sources of protein- 12%, foods and drinks high in fat and/or sugar- 8%) and can be used by registered dietitians and nutritionists in giving individually tailored advice.

A number of previous studies evaluated the adequacy of the diets of elite rugby league players by comparing individual nutrients to current recommendations [3,4]. However, there is a lack of literature evaluating eating habits and diets of elite athletes using a food group analysis approach.

The aim of this study was to determine general nutritional knowledge and eating habits based on the eatwell plate food groups' categories of elite rugby league players, and to explore any associations between good or poor nutritional knowledge and eating habits in this population.

Methods

Participants

Thirty professional male Rugby League players were recruited from one team competing in English Super League. All athletes were part of the first team squad. The data was collected during the 2012–13 competition season.

The study was approved by the Ethics Committee of a UK Higher Education institution. Written consent was collected from all participants.

Table 1 summarises study subject characteristics. The age of participants ranged from 18 to 34 years with an average age of 25. All participants had educational qualifications with the majority holding GSCEs (38%), followed by A-levels (19%) and diplomas (19%). None of the participants had any special dietary needs or were on any special diet at the time of the investigation.

Table 1 Characteristics of participants

Characteristics	Participants
n	21
Age (y)	25 (*SD* = 5)
Height (m)	1.8 (*SD* = 0.1)
Weight (kg)	93 (*SD* = 12)
Game experience (years in Super League)	6 (*SD* = 4)
Position played (n):	
Back	9
Forward	12
Level of education (n):	
Secondary	3
GCSE	8
A- levels	4
Diploma	4
Degree	2
Health and/or nutrition related qualifications (n)	1
Special dietary needs/conditions (n)	0

Measures and procedure

Subject characteristics including age, position played, game experience, level of education, health or nutrition related qualifications and any current special dietary regimes were collected using a short questionnaire.

Nutritional knowledge questionnaire (NKQ) [11] consisted of 28 questions categorised into three sections:

- section A – advice - current national recommendations and heath experts' advice on nutrition;
- section B – food groups - classification of food items into the food groups, including foods low and high in sugar, fat, salt, protein, fibre;
- section C – food choice - choosing healthier food options

Food frequency questionnaire (FFQ) [12] was chosen due to the availability of local food items to account for region-specific dietary habits and consisted of 78 food and beverage items (including examples of standard portion sizes for each item), categorised into seven sections: starchy foods (breads and crackers, breakfast cereals, potatoes, rice and pasta), protein-rich foods (meat, poultry, fish, eggs and beans), dairy products (milk, yoghurt, cheese), vegetables (fresh, frozen, canned), fruits (fresh, frozen, canned, dried), foods high in sugar or/and fat, and fluids (water, tea, coffee, fresh fruit juice, juice drinks, quash, low calorie drinks and fizzy drinks).

The questionnaires were distributed to participants prior a training session and collected straight after completion.

Data analysis

Preliminary analysis screened the data for missing values, outliers, and univariate normality. Data was screened for missing values, of which there were less than 0.1% and examined for outliers using Q-Q plots. No problematic outliers were found. Most food categories demonstrated no issue with skewness (<2), though a slight negative skew was evident for starchy foods (−2.80), fluids (−2.20), and sugary foods (−2.04). All kurtosis statistics were acceptable (<7).

Nutritional knowledge was calculated as the summed total of correct answers from the NKQ, including subdimensions of expert advice, food groups, and food choice. Relationships between the subsections of the NKQ and food frequency were examined by Spearman's rank order. High and low nutritional knowledge groups were identified by a median split and a chi-square difference test was conducted to examine group differences. Similarly, we then examined the relationship between nutritional knowledge and the eatwell plate groups of starchy foods, protein, fruit and vegetables, milk and dairy, fats, and fluids.

Results

Nutritional knowledge

A response rate of 70% ($n = 21$) was achieved due to exclusion of partially completed NKQ and FFQ. The study sample comprised of male rugby league athletes (nine backs and 12 forwards) with an average professional competition experience of six years.

The average number of nutritional knowledge questions answered correctly was 52.43 ($SD = 4.40$), representing a mean nutritional knowledge score of 72.82% ($SD = 6.11$). The minimum score was 62.50% and the maximum score was 83.33%. Questions related to *advice* were answered most accurately ($M = 85.71\%$, $SD = 13.04$). Questions pertaining to food groups ($M = 71.24\%$, $SD = 7.21$) and food choice ($M = 69.52\%$, $SD = 13.96$) were answered less accurately. To further investigate nutritional knowledge, the sample was split into two groups relative to the median NFQ score. This equated to a sample of 10 players in the *poor nutritional knowledge (NK)* group and 11 players in the *good nutritional knowledge (NK)* group. These results are presented in Table 2. Overall, the good nutritional knowledge group scored significantly higher in *food groups* (76.29%) than the poor nutritional knowledge group (65.69%; $t(19) = 4.98$, $p < .01$). They also scored significantly higher in *advice* (92.56% to 78.18%; $t(19) = 2.98$, $p < .01$), and overall (77.78% to 67.36%; $t(19) = 7.78$, $p < .01$). No significant difference was observed for *choice* (73.64% to 64.00%; $t(19) = 1.46$, $p = .16$).

Table 3 shows comparisons of the frequency of consumption of food items of different food groups between good and poor nutritional knowledge groups. Starchy foods, fruit & vegetables, oily fish and milk were consumed more frequently by good nutritional knowledge group when compared to poor nutritional knowledge group. Furthermore, the latter reported more frequent consumption of fizzy drinks and squash compared to the good nutritional knowledge group. There was less variation in consumption of meat and poultry products, eggs, foods that are high in sugar and/or fat and other beverages.

Nutritional knowledge and food frequency

Spearman's rank order correlations were calculated to first examine the relationship between nutritional knowledge and food consumption. Relationships among variables were generally weak, with the exception of *advice* score, which correlated significantly with vegetable consumption ($r_s = .49$, $p < .001$).

Cross-tabulated chi-square difference tests found that the good nutritional knowledge group consumed significantly more vegetables ($p < .05$). Specifically, the good nutritional knowledge group consumed significantly ($p < .05$) more breakfast cereal, boiled/baked potatoes, meat casseroles/stews, peas/green beans, broccoli, cabbage and spring greens, cauliflower, peaches, nectarines and melons, strawberries, raspberries, mango and kiwi. In no food types did the poor nutritional knowledge group consume significantly more than the good nutritional knowledge group.

Table 2 Nutritional knowledge scores

Nutrition knowledge categories:	ALL (n = 21)		Good NK group (n = 11)		Poor NK group (n = 10)		*p* value (between groups)
	Mean (SD)	%	Mean (SD)	%	Mean (SD)	%	
A: Dietary advice (11 points)	9.43 (1.43)	85.71	10.18 (.26)	92.56	8.60 (.48)	78.18	0.01
B: Food groups (51 points)	36.33 (3.68)	71.24	38.91 (.55)	76.29	33.50 (.97)	65.69	0.01
C: Food choice (10 points)	6.95 (1.40)	69.52	7.36 (.39)	73.64	6.50 (.45)	64.00	0.16
Overall score (72 points)	52.43 (4.4)	72.82	56.00 (.69)	77.78	48.50 (.67)	67.36	0.01

Table 3 Descriptive statistics and between group comparisons for food frequency

Food group	Good Nutritional Knowledge			Poor Nutritional Knowledge		
	Never/Rarely	Occasionally	Often	Never/Rarely	Occasionally	Often
Starchy foods:						
White bread	72.7%	18.2%	9.1%	60%	30%	10%
Brown bread	18.2%	36.4%	45.5%	20%	40%	40%
Breakfast Cereals	0%	18.2%	81.8%	10%	30%	60%
Boiled and baked potatoes	18.2%	81.8%	0%	60%	40%	0%
Chips	90.9%	9.1%	0%	60%	40%	0%
Rice	72.7%	27.3%	0%	60%	40%	0%
Pasta	9.1%	36.4%	54.5%	10%	70%	20%
Protein-rich foods:						
Grilled/ baked meat or poultry	36.4%	63.6%	0%	50%	40%	10%
Meat casseroles or stews	27.3%	72.7%	0%	70%	30%	0%
White fish	90.9%	9.1%	0%	80%	20%	0%
Oily fish	0%	81.8%	18.2%	30%	60%	10%
Beans and pulses	36.4%	36.4%	27.3%	60%	30%	10%
Eggs	0%	81.8%	18.2%	20%	60%	20%
Fruits	18.2%	81.8%	0.0%	40.0%	60.0%	0.0%
Vegetables	9.1%	90.9%	0.0%	50.0%	50.0%	0.0%
Milk and dairy products:						
Milk	72.7%	0%	27.3%	100%	0%	0%
Yoghurt	18.2%	54.5%	27.3%	40%	20%	40%
Cheese	18.2%	81.8%	0%	10%	60%	30%
Foods high in fats and/or sugar:						
Chocolate	81.8%	18.2%	0%	70%	30%	0%
Crisps	90.9%	0%	9.1%	60%	40%	0%
Jam	63.6%	27.3%	9.1%	80%	10%	10%
Margarine	9.1%	18.2%	72.7%	40%	20%	40%
Fluids:						
Water	0%	9.1%	90.9%	0%	0%	100%
Fresh fruit juice	9.1%	36.4%	54.5%	20%	50%	30%
Juice drinks	45.5%	36.4%	18.2%	50%	20%	30%
Fizzy drinks	90.9%	9.1%	0%	40%	20%	40%
Squash	81.8%	18.2%	0%	70%	20%	10%
Low calorie drink	81.8%	9.1%	9.1%	80%	10%	10%
Tea	36.4%	36.4%	27.3%	40%	20%	40%

The eatwell plate analysis

Spearman's rank correlations demonstrated weak relationship between nutritional knowledge and food consumption in relation to the *eatwell* plate (Table 4). The only statistically significant relationship was the positive correlation between fruit and vegetable consumption and overall nutritional knowledge ($r_s = .52,\ p < .05$). Differences between nutritional knowledge groups were assessed through an independent samples t test, which supported the effect for fruit and vegetables ($t(19) = 3.31,\ p < .01$), which was significantly higher in the good nutritional knowledge group ($M = 30.91,\ SD = 3.08$) than the poor nutritional knowledge group ($M = 24.60,\ SD = 5.44$). Inferential statistical analysis could not detect any significant differences among other *eatwell* plate categories.

Discussion

The present study aimed to determine nutritional knowledge and eating habits based on the national healthy

Table 4 Descriptive statistics and correlations of food consumption with nutritional knowledge

Food Group	Mean frequency score	SD	Skew	Kurt	Advice	Food groups	Choice	Overall
Starchy	28.00	5.21	−2.30	5.31	.15	-.02	.11	.13
Protein-rich	14.81	1.40	.86	3.51	-.01	-.10	.01	-.03
Fruit and Vegetables	27.90	5.34	-.62	-.49	.38	.36	.33	.52*
Milk and Dairy	7.43	1.47	.10	-.71	.06	.18	.12	.18
Fats/Sugars	16.86	1.62	.80	1.40	.22	.02	-.12	.11
Fluids	11.52	1.57	1.67	2.96	-.16	-.28	-.34	-.29

*Statistically significant at p <.05.

eating recommendations tool (the eatwell plate) categories, and to evaluate the relationship between nutritional knowledge and dietary practices in elite rugby league athletes.

The mean nutritional knowledge score was 73% for elite athletes in the present study. This is higher compared to the findings observed in the population of elite Australian rugby league athletes [7]. The authors reported the mean score of 61.3% using an adapted 90-point nutritional knowledge questionnaire whilst the present study used 72-points of the same questionnaire; therefore, caution should be taken when making direct comparisons. Nevertheless, differences in nutritional knowledge scores between the studies could be explained by several factors. Firstly, athletes in the present study were notably older (25 compared to 19 years of age) and obtained higher level of education (100% of athletes had secondary and above education in the present study compared to 66% in the Australian athletes). Both variables, age and the level of education, have been previously shown to be factors in influencing nutritional knowledge [8].

Knowledge of dietary recommendations section was the most accurately completed (86% accurate answers) compared to other sections (food groups – 71%, food choice – 70%). When sample was split into good and poor nutritional knowledge groups, the trend remained the same. Consistent with the findings of another study [7], this suggests that the national health promotion campaigns, such as 5-a-day fruit and vegetables, salt reduction, and increased wholegrain intake, are successful educational public health nutrition programmes, in terms of raising public awareness and increasing nutritional knowledge. In fact, all of the participants completed the question on recommended servings of daily fruit and vegetables intake correctly.

Despite the international sports nutrition recommendations [13] and the national healthy eating guidelines [10] being based on moderate consumption of starchy staple foods, the athletes in the present study were unaware of these recommendations. All participants in the poor NK group and nearly half in the good NK group answered the questions on starchy foods consumption incorrectly ('Do you think health experts recommended that people should be eating more, the same amount, or less of starchy foods', 'Do you think experts put these in the starchy foods group?'). One plausible explanation would be the current public perception of carbohydrate-rich foods being unhealthy and in fact the majority of dietary advice provided by popular media incorporates this carbohydrate recommendation poorly [14]. This trend also translated into the eating habits of the elite athletes observed in the present study. The majority of rugby players consumed starchy carbohydrate-rich foods 'occasionally', with the exception of breakfast cereals which were reported to be consumed 'often'. Further to this, the poor NK group reported to consume significantly less starchy foods, including boiled and baked potatoes and shredded wheat breakfast cereals, compared to good NK group. It is well acknowledged that in the athlete's diet the majority of energy should come from carbohydrates as they are used as a predominant source of fuel during an intense and prolonged exercise [13]. In addition to this, a recent study highlighted inadequate carbohydrate intake in collegiate rugby players [2]. Therefore, there is a need for public health initiatives outlining the important of adequate consumption of carbohydrate-rich foods in physically active populations.

The good NK group had significantly better knowledge of high fibre foods in relation to the amount they should be consuming compared to the poor NK group. This was also reflected in their dietary practices. The good NK group included significantly more high fibre foods, such as breakfast cereals, potatoes, peas, green beans, broccoli and cauliflower, cabbage and spring greens, peaches and nectarines, melons, strawberries, raspberries, mango and kiwi, in their diets. In addition to this, the eatwell plate analysis showed the positive association between overall nutritional knowledge and consumption of fruit and vegetables ($rs = .52$, $p < .05$). Similar observations were reported in the general UK population study comprising 455 men and 584 women aged 18 to 65 years and over [8]. The highest quintile for nutritional knowledge was 25 time more likely to meet fruit and vegetables recommended daily intake than those individuals in the lowest quintile. In addition, the association between nutritional knowledge and fruit and vegetables intake was independent to gender, education and occupational class. This suggests that associations observed in the present study of elite male rugby league players follow similar patterns to the findings of general population.

Overall, there was a lack of relationship between the eatwell plate food categories and nutritional knowledge. Although a relative small sample size may explain the lack of significant associations, it may be suggested that the adequate nutritional knowledge observed may not have translated into the appropriate dietary practice in present study's cohort. Only a weak (rs <.44) positive correlation between nutritional knowledge of athletes and dietary intake was reported in five out of nine studies included in a recent systematic review [15]. In addition to this, the concept of nutritional knowledge encompasses two elements: knowledge of nutrition facts and procedural knowledge, such as planning, purchasing and preparation of foods [16]. Therefore, if declarative knowledge is adequate but procedural knowledge is poor, it is unlikely that nutritional knowledge would play a big role in the adoption of healthier food habits. Literature also indicates that female participants and athletes involved in sports with a strong emphasis on physique and those participating in endurance sports have better knowledge compared to male athletes and inactive controls [17-19]. If this is the reason for the lack of association between good knowledge and dietary practices in the cohort of male rugby league players of the present study, the future nutrition education programmes for athletes should target to improve general nutritional knowledge through incorporating procedural approaches in this population.

Conclusions

The present study assessed the level of general nutritional knowledge and eating habits of elite rugby league players.

Nutritional knowledge was adequate for dietary advice section but poorer for food groups classification and food choice sections. Further analysis of the present study suggests that the knowledge could be improved in relation to the current recommendations of increasing the consumption of carbohydrate-rich foods.

There was a lack of association observed in terms of other eatwell plate food groups and nutritional knowledge, which is most likely to be influenced by a relatively small sample size. Nevertheless, a link between knowledge and fruit and vegetables consumption was identified, which suggests that improving other domains of nutritional knowledge may be beneficial in improving the overall diet in this population.

The present study highlights the importance of qualified nutritional support at the elite level of rugby. It is recommended to appraise at the barriers of nutritional knowledge in both elite athletes and their coaches to understand why adequate nutritional knowledge may not always result in better nutrition practices.

Availability of supporting data

All the data from this research are available on your request.

Competing interests

The authors declare that they have no competing interests.

Authors' contributions

IA supervised the whole project. IA and TA formulated the research questions and designed the study. TA recruited participants and conducted data collection. JLP analyzed data and performed statistical analysis. IA wrote the manuscript. All authors amended and approved the final manuscript.

Acknowledgment

Authors wish to acknowledge the Department of Sport, Health and Nutrition (Leeds Trinity University) and the School of Health Sciences (Liverpool Hope University) for the funding support of this research project, and the help of coaches and athletes who participated in this study.

References

1. Gabbett TJ, Jenkins DG, Abernethy B. Physical demands of professional rugby league training and competition using microtechnology. J Sci Med Sport. 2012;15:80–6.
2. Imamura H, Iide K, Yoshimura Y, Kumagai K, Oshikata R, Miyahara K, et al. Nutrient intake, serum lipids and iron status of colligiate rugby players. J Int Soc Sports Nutr. 2013;10:1–9.
3. Lundy B, O'Connor H, Pelly F, Caterson I. Anthropometric characteristics and competition dietary intakes of professional rugby league players. Int J Sport Nutr Exerc Metab. 2006;16:199–213.
4. Lako JV, Sotheeswaran S, Christi KS. Food habits and nutritional status of Fiji rugby players. World Acad Sci Eng Tech. 2010;68:742–7.
5. Murphy S, Jeanes Y. Nutritional knowledge and dietary intakes of young professional football players. Nutr Food Sci. 2006;3:343–8.
6. Zinn C, Schofield G, Well C. Evaluation of sports nutrition knowledge of New Zealand premier club rugby coaches. Int J Sport Nutr Exerc Metab. 2006;16:214–25.
7. Spendlove JK, Heaney SE, Gifford JA, Prvan T, Denyer GS, O'Connor HT. Evaluation of general nutrition knowledge in elite Australian athletes. Br J Nutr. 2012;107:1871–80.
8. Wardle J, Parmenter L, Waller J. Nutrition knowledge and food intake. Appetite. 2000;34:269–75.
9. Burke LM. Dietary studies of athletes: an interview with sports dietitian bronwen lundy. Int J Sport Nutr Exerc Metab. 2006;16:226–8.
10. Public Health England: your guide to eatwell plate. 2014 available at: https://www.gov.uk/government/uploads/system/uploads/attachment_data/file/340869/2014-250_-_eatwell_plate_Final_version_2014.pdf (accessed 17 April 2015).
11. Parmenter K, Wardle J. Development of a general nutrition knowledge questionnaire for adults. Eur J Clin Nutr. 1999;53:298–308.
12. Bradford Teaching Hospitals Foundation Trust. 12-month Food Frequency Questionnaire. 2010.
13. American College of Sports Medicine, American Dietetic Association, Dietitians of Canada, Rodriguez NR, Di Marco NM, Langley S. American College of Sports Medicine position stand. Nutrition and athletic performance. Med Sci Sports Exerc. 2009;41:709–31.
14. Ellison C, White H, McElhone S. A content analysis of magazine diets in relation to the eatwell plate. J Hum Nutr Diet. 2011;24:277–310.
15. Heaney S, O'Connor H, Michael S, Gifford J, Naughton G. Nutrition knowledge in athletes: a systematic review. Int J Sport Nutr Exerc Metab. 2011;21:248–61.
16. Worsley A. Nutrition knowledge and food consumption: can nutrition knowledge change food behaviour. Asia Pac J Clin Nutr. 2002;11:S579–85.

17. Dunn D, Turner LW, Denny G. Nutrition knowledge and attitudes of college athletes. Sport J. 2007;10:1–5.
18. Raymond-Barker P, Petroczi A, Quested E. Assessment of nutritional knowledge in female athletes susceptible to the female athlete triad syndrome. J Occup Med Toxicol. 2007;2:10.
19. Douglas PD, Douglas JG. Nutrition knowledge and food practices of high school athletes. J Am Diet Assoc. 1984;84:1198–202.

29

Three and six grams supplementation of d-aspartic acid in resistance trained men

Geoffrey W Melville*, Jason C Siegler and Paul WM Marshall

Abstract

Background: Although abundant research has investigated the hormonal effects of d-aspartic acid in rat models, to date there is limited research on humans. Previous research has demonstrated increased total testosterone levels in sedentary men and no significant changes in hormonal levels in resistance trained men. It was hypothesised that a higher dosage may be required for experienced lifters, thus this study investigated the effects of two different dosages of d-aspartic acid on basal hormonal levels in resistance trained men and explored responsiveness to d-aspartic acid based on initial testosterone levels.

Methods: Twenty-four males, with a minimum of two years' experience in resistance training, (age, 24.5 ± 3.2 y; training experience, 3.4 ± 1.4 y; height, 178.5 ± 6.5 cm; weight, 84.7 ± 7.2 kg; bench press 1-RM, 105.3 ± 15.2 kg) were randomised into one of three groups: 6 $g.d^{-1}$ plain flour (D0); 3 $g.d^{-1}$ of d-aspartic acid (D3); and 6 $g.d^{-1}$ of d-aspartic acid (D6). Participants performed a two-week washout period, training four days per week. This continued through the experimental period (14 days), with participants consuming the supplement in the morning. Serum was analysed for levels of testosterone, estradiol, sex hormone binding globulin, albumin and free testosterone was determined by calculation.

Results: D-aspartic acid supplementation revealed no main effect for group in: estradiol; sex-hormone-binding-globulin; and albumin. Total testosterone was significantly reduced in D6 ($P = 0.03$). Analysis of free testosterone showed that D6 was significantly reduced as compared to D0 ($P = 0.005$), but not significantly different to D3. Analysis did not reveal any significant differences between D3 and D0. No significant correlation between initial total testosterone levels and responsiveness to d-aspartic acid was observed ($r = 0.10$, $P = 0.70$).

Conclusions: The present study demonstrated that a daily dose of six grams of d-aspartic acid decreased levels of total testosterone and free testosterone (D6), without any concurrent change in other hormones measured. Three grams of d-aspartic acid had no significant effect on either testosterone markers. It is currently unknown what effect this reduction in testosterone will have on strength and hypertrophy gains.

Keywords: D-aspartic acid, Resistance training, Testosterone, Estradiol, SHBG

Background

The anabolic hormone testosterone is considered to be a key determinant of training induced improvements in hypertrophy and strength. Circulating testosterone increases other anabolic hormones and directly interacts with androgen receptors and satellite cells, causing a cascade of events leading to protein synthesis and muscle growth [1,2]. Research has previously demonstrated correlations between testosterone levels and training related strength gains [3,4]. Furthermore exogenous elevation of testosterone to supraphysiological levels, via administration of anabolic steroids has been shown to drastically improve strength and hypertrophy [5]. Currently it is unknown whether boosting testosterone levels within normal physiological levels (mid-range to upper-range) will have a significant effect on strength and hypertrophy. Nonetheless, the supplement industry is endorsing testosterone boosters to improve training related gains. D-aspartic acid is currently recommended as a viable product to significantly raise testosterone, however research in humans only supports this recommendation

* Correspondence: g.melville@uws.edu.au
School of Science & Health, University of Western Sydney, Campbelltown Campus, Locked Bag 1797, Penrith, NSW 2751, Australia

in untrained men with below average testosterone levels. Moreover there is no information about the effect of different doses of d-aspartic acid on testosterone levels in humans.

Aspartic acid ($C_4H_7NO_4$) is an α-amino acid which is known to exist in two isoforms, l-aspartic acid and d-aspartic acid. (2R)-2-aminobutanedioic acid or d-aspartic acid (DAA), previously believed to be exclusive to brain tissue in octopus, squid and cuttlefish, has more recently been shown to exist in mammals [6]. Free DAA is found in tissues and cells related to the central nervous and endocrine systems [7,8]. DAA is believed to stimulate the production and release of testosterone through multiple pathways of the hypothalamic-pituitary-gonadal (HPG) axis. It has been shown to increase steroidogenic acute regulatory protein (StAR) gene expression in rat Leydig cells [9]. StAR is a key regulator for the transport of cholesterol from outside the mitochondrial membrane to the inner membrane [7]. By increasing levels of StAR DAA may indirectly increase testosterone, as the transportation of cholesterol is believed to be the rate limiting step in the production of testosterone [7]. *In vitro* rats studies demonstrated that DAA increased levels of testosterone, luteinizing hormone, progesterone [6] and growth hormone [10]. This is believed to occur due to the accumulation of DAA in the anterior pituitary and testes [10]. Additional *in vitro* studies on isolated rat testes [6] and Leydig cells [11] indicate that DAA increased the rate of testosterone synthesis in a dose dependent manner. In these animals the maximal effective dose of DAA, which elicited the greatest hormonal response (LH, testosterone and progesterone), was 1 $\mu mol.g^{-1}$ [6]. In humans the effects of different dosages of DAA on basal testosterone is unclear.

To date only two studies on DAA supplementation have been conducted on humans. Topo et al. [12] demonstrated that after 12 days of supplementation (3.12 $g.d^{-1}$), levels of testosterone were significantly increased by 42% (4.5–6.4 $ng.ml^{-1}$). They recruited a cohort of healthy sedentary male IVF patients (27–37 years), with low initial testosterone levels (~4.55 $ng.ml^{-1}$). Contrastingly Willoughby and Leutholtz, reported that after 29 days of supplementation (3 $g.d^{-1}$) and resistance training, levels of total testosterone and free testosterone were not significantly altered. In this study resistance trained men (age: 22.8 ± 4.67 years old; training age: > 1 year) were recruited and this cohort exhibited higher initial testosterone levels (~7.96 $ng.ml^{-1}$) [13]. The difference in outcome between these two studies may in part be explained by training status and accompanying basal testosterone levels. Basal testosterone levels of RT men range from approximately 5.8–8.6 $ng.ml^{-1}$ (20–30 $nmol.l^{-1}$), [4,14] and untrained men range from about 4.9–6.6 $ng.ml^{-1}$ (17–23 $nmol.l^{-1}$) [15-17]. Furthermore current research has only explored one dose response of DAA, 3 $g.d^{-1}$ [12,13], hence the maximum effective dose for humans is yet to be determined.

Supplement companies are currently recommending three grams of DAA once to twice a day, and these recommendations have been drawn from the only dosage studied in humans (3 $g.d^{-1}$). It is reasonable to believe that in RT males, a higher dose may be required to further increase testosterone levels. As such the primary aim of this study was to evaluate the effects of two doses of d-aspartic acid (3 g and 6 g) on basal testosterone levels in resistance trained men. A secondary aim was to establish if a relationship exists between initial testosterone levels and responsiveness to DAA. It was hypothesised that; (a) testosterone levels would be unchanged in the 3 g group; (b) testosterone levels would be increased in the 6 g group; and (c) lower initial testosterone levels would correspond with an increased responsiveness to DAA.

Methods

Subjects

The institutional review board approved the study and participants provided written informed consent prior to testing and participation. A total of twenty-four participants from the local area completed this study (Table 1). To be eligible participants had to be: male; aged 18–36; have no acute or chronic medical conditions; have the ability to bench press 100% bodyweight; and had been performing regular resistance training exercise for at least three days per week for the previous two years. None of the participants were supplementing their diet with any ergogenic or testosterone booting supplements prior to testing. All participants provided written consent and completed a medical history check. The study was approved by the University of Western Sydney human research ethics committee, and carried out in accordance with the declaration of Helsinki.

Experimental approach to the problem

This was a randomised, double-blinded, and placebo-controlled design to examine the effects of d-aspartic acid supplementation on basal testosterone levels following a two week supplementation protocol. Participants were assigned to one of three experimental groups: placebo

Table 1 Participant demographics

	Placebo ($n = 8$)	3 $g.d^{-1}$ ($n = 8$)	6 $g.d^{-1}$ ($n = 8$)
Age (years)	24.24 ± 2.26	23.16 ± 2.16	26.06 ± 4.26
Training age, (years)	2.94 ± 0.78	3.25 ± 1.04	4.00 ± 1.91
Height (m)	1.84 ± 0.03	1.74 ± 0.07	1.78 ± 0.06
Body Mass (kg)	89.41 ± 3.59	79.50 ± 6.07	85.12 ± 7.95
1 RM Bench (kg)	111.56 ± 15.17	97.50 ± 12.82	106.86 ± 15.74

Data are mean ± SD.

(D0), three grams of DAA (D3) and six grams of DAA (D6). All participants consumed 10 opaque capsules each morning with breakfast for two weeks. They contained either: six grams of flour (D0, n = 8); a mixture of three grams each of flour and DAA (D3, n = 8); or six grams of DAA (D6, n = 8). Participants were randomly allocated to treatment groups following a block randomisation procedure based on a computer-generated list of random numbers. Placebo, mixed and supplement were provided in identical opaque capsules to improve blinding. Group allocation was managed by a technical officer, whilst investigators were kept blind to group assignment throughout the intervention. All participants followed an upper/lower body split resistance training program for a full month, with the initial two weeks of training (washout period) performed without supplementation (Figure 1). Three timepoints were used to obtain testing data: T1, T2 and T3 (Figure 1).

Experimental procedures

Testing sessions consisted of a fasted blood draw, then 1-RM bench press evaluation. Initial baseline blood measures were taken at two timepoints (T1 & T2) and averaged to ensure accuracy in baseline assessment of these markers (Figure 1). After T1 prescribed training commenced for four weeks. After testing session T2 daily supplementation begun with training continuing as before. Post-measures were taken after these last two weeks of training and supplementation, at the end of week 4 (Figure 1). The supplemental period of two weeks was chosen as this has been previously shown to be a sufficient time period to see a change in total testosterone levels [12].

1-RM testing

Bench press dynamic strength one repetition max (1-RM) was measured before the standardisation period (T1), beginning of experimental period (T2) and post experiment period (T3) (Figure 1), as part of eligibility testing. Correct form included depth to the level of the chest, with feet not leaving the floor, and the backside not leaving the bench at any point during the repetition. The protocol for 1-RM testing involved one warm up set of 10 reps at approximately 50% of their estimated 1-RM, followed by two more warm ups at approximately 70% and 80% with only 1–2 reps. After the warm ups participants attempted 1-RMs with incrementally increasing weight. The weight achieved prior to the failed attempt was recorded as the 1-RM. A participant's 1-RM was achieved within five attempts and adequate rest between attempts was adhered to (3–5 mins) [18].

Fasted blood draws

All blood draws were obtained via venepuncture of the antecubital vein after a 12 hour fast. Participants were also instructed to avoid strenuous exercise and alcohol consumption the day before the draw. Blood draws were conducted by a trained phlebotomist and subsequent draws were planned for the same time of morning (7:00–10:00 am) for each particular participant, to prevent any effect of diurnal variation. Whole blood was collected using serum separator tubes (SST™ II Advance, BD Vacutainer®). They were then allowed to clot for 45 minutes and centrifuged using a fixed angle rotor centrifuge: ADAMS® Compact II Centrifuge, V:227 (Becton Dickinson & Co) (828 × g, at 2700 rpm) for 15 minutes in an air conditioned room (19°C). Serum was aliquoted and stored at −80°C until analysis (Douglas Hanly Moir Pathology, Macquarie Park, NSW, Australia). Single analysis of serum was conducted for total testosterone, estradiol, sex-hormone-binding-globulin (SHBG) and albumin. Testosterone and SHBG was measured via electrochemiluminescent (ECL) immunoassay, on a Roche E170 system (Roche Diagnostics). Albumin was measured via bromocresol green (BCG) succinate buffer method, on an Abbott 16000. Estradiol was measured via chemiluminescent microparticle immunoassay on an Abbott i2000. Free testosterone was calculated from total testosterone, SHBG and albumin.

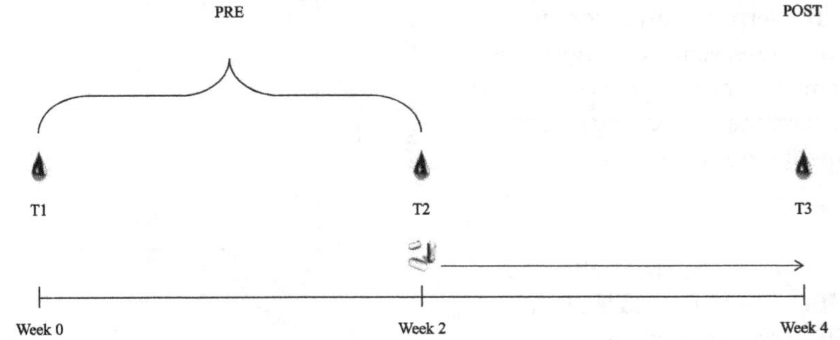

Figure 1 Timeline of the study. After completion of T1, subjects began training four days per week. Daily supplementation commenced after T2 (💊). T1-3 included fasted blood draws (💧).

Training standardisation

Participants trained for four days per week over a one month period. The prescribed training for each exercise consisted of four sets of a repetition maximum range of 8–10. If the repetition range wasn't met, participants were asked to lower or raise the weight in the next session. Exercises during the upper body session were: barbell bench press; overhand pulldown; barbell overhead press and underhand pulldown. The lower body session consisted of: back squat; good morning; leg extensions; and straight leg calf raises. Adherence was monitored via training diaries and supervised sessions (minimum 1 × per week).

Dietary intake

Participants were asked to control their diet, by avoiding any major changes throughout the study duration. To monitor their diet they were asked to weigh and recorded their food intake for three days each of the first and last week; two training days and one non-training day. These three days were averaged to get a daily mean for week one and four. The food diaries were entered into CalorieKing (Australian Edition 4.0), then analysed for caloric and macronutrient daily intakes (protein, carbohydrates and fats) and normalised to bodyweight.

Statistical analysis

Analyses were conducted using IBM SPSS Statistics for Windows version 21.0 (Armonk, NY: IBM Corp), and the level of significance was set at $P < 0.05$. Data are shown as mean ± S.D. The distribution was tested for normality using the Kolmogorov-Smirnov test. Paired sample statistics were run on total testosterone (TT), free testosterone (FT), estradiol (E_2), sex-hormone-binding-globulin (SHBG), and albumin (ALB) to determine the stability of these blood measures over the standardisation period. As these measures were found to be unchanged they were each computed (averaged) into one baseline measure. Univariate analysis of the absolute change scores: $\Delta = \left(T3 - \frac{T1+T2}{2}\right)$ was conducted, with the baseline scores: $\mathrm{PRE} = \left(\frac{T1+T2}{2}\right)$ as covariates (Figure 1). Pairwise comparisons with Bonferroni correction were performed if a group effect was observed. To explore the responsiveness of the supplement, linear regression analysis was conducted on the baseline and change scores of TT and FT, of the experimental groups ($n = 16$).

Results

Analysis of the POST values revealed no main effect for group with E_2 ($P = 0.47$), SHBG ($P = 0.07$) and ALB ($P = 0.32$). Post values of D6 TT were significantly reduced (~12.5%) as compared to the pre values ($P = 0.03$; 5.9 to 5.1 ng.ml^{-1}). FT in group D6 was significantly decreased (429.1 to 363.4 pmol.l^{-1}) as compared to D0 (439.6 to 480.9 pmol.l^{-1}) ($P = 0.005$) but not D3 (534.9 to 524.3 pmol.l^{-1}) ($P = 0.06$) (Figure 2). Diet analysis revealed no significant changes in macronutrient (CHO: $P = 0.74$; PRO: $P = 0.99$; FAT: $P = 0.54$) and caloric intakes ($P = 0.64$) during the study. Regression analysis revealed no significant correlation between baseline total testosterone levels and total testosterone change ($r = 0.10$, $P = 0.70$), and no significant correlation between baseline free testosterone and free testosterone change ($r = 0.32$, $P = 0.23$).

Discussion

The primary findings of the current study were, 1) resistance trained men consuming six grams of d-aspartic acid daily demonstrated significant reductions in total and free testosterone after 14 days of d-aspartic acid supplementation, and 2) the responsiveness to d-aspartic acid supplementation was unaffected by initial testosterone levels (total or free) in resistance trained men.

Our results demonstrate that in resistance trained men three grams daily of d-aspartic acid had no significant effect on total testosterone, estradiol, sex-hormone-binding-globulin, and albumin. This is contrary to the evidence provided by Topo et al. [12], where the cohort consumed the same dose over 12 days and reported elevated total testosterone levels (~42%). Baseline testosterone levels of the current study were higher than values found in Topo et al. [12] (6.3 and 4.5 ng.ml^{-1} respectively), presumably because the cohort in the Topo et al. study were sedentary [12]. In resistance training literature, total testosterone levels range from 5.8–8.6 ng.ml^{-1} [4,14] for trained individuals and 4.9–6.6 ng.ml^{-1} for untrained [15-17]. The increase in testosterone observed in Topo et al. [12] was likely due to the fact that testosterone levels were low enough for d-aspartic acid to have an effect. In comparison our results in the D3 group mirror the results seen in the study by Willoughby & Leutholtz [13], where

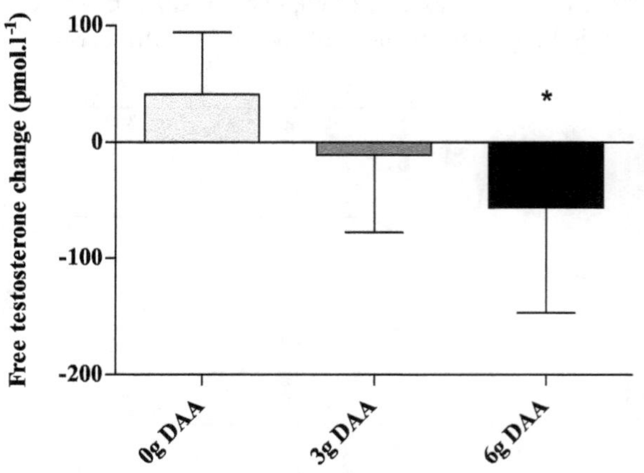

Figure 2 The absolute change of free testosterone. *statistically significant ($P < 0.05$).

the total testosterone levels fall within levels observed in resistance trained males [4,14].

It was observed in the six gram group that total testosterone was significantly reduced from baseline by ~12.5%, with a parallel decrease in free testosterone ~15.3% (see Table 2). Previous research has demonstrated that in resistance trained men, free testosterone can increase due to training [19]. A reduction in calculated free testosterone in this study is due to a reduction in total testosterone, an increase in the binding proteins or a combination of the two occurring. Within the context of increasing total testosterone a maximum effective dosage (MED) is observed in rat studies [6]. At the higher dosages there were significantly increased accumulation of d-aspartic acid observed in the pituitary and testes [6]. A dose response increase in total testosterone was observed until 1 $\mu mol.g^{-1}$. Each increase in dose past 1 $\mu mol.g^{-1}$ the rise in testosterone was reduced [6]. It could be theorised that 6 $g.d^{-1}$ may be affecting negative feedback mechanisms of the HPG axis, thus reducing pituitary initiated production of luteinizing hormone and in turn testosterone levels. Furthermore d-aspartic acid could also be over-accumulating within the testes. This may be creating a disruptive effect on the mobilisation of cholesterol from the outer membrane to the inner [7], which would attenuate testosterone production. As this was the first study to administer a six gram dosage of d-aspartic acid, these mechanisms can only be speculated due to the lack of data available on the utilisation of d-aspartic acid in humans.

Table 2 PRE (Baseline), POST (T3), and Change Scores (Δ) of hormonal markers

	Total Testosterone ($ng.ml^{-1}$)		
Time	Placebo	3 $g.d^{-1}$	6 g $g.d^{-1}$
PRE	6.03 ± 1.48	6.95 ± 1.44	5.85 ± 1.10
POST	6.07 ± 1.35	6.91 ± 1.71	5.12 ± 1.16
Δ	0.05 ± 0.80	−0.03 ± 0.68	−0.74 ± 0.95*
	Free Testosterone ($pmol.l^{-1}$)		
	Placebo	3 $g.d^{-1}$	6 g $g.d^{-1}$
PRE	439.62 ± 132.64	534.88 ± 127.65	429.13 ± 93.98
POST	480.87 ± 133.48	524.25 ± 101.67	363.38 ± 78.09
Δ	41.25 ± 52.48	−10.63 ± 66.31	−65.75 ± 79.25*
	Estradiol ($pmol.l^{-1}$)		
	Placebo	3 $g.d^{-1}$	6 g $g.d^{-1}$
PRE	118.50 ± 20.91	117.56 ± 30.58	107.50 ± 24.22
POST	125.12 ± 23.88	112.5 ± 34.51	104.75 ± 34.03
Δ	6.63 ± 14.94	−5.06 ± 19.52	−2.75 ± 23.46
	SHBG Pre ($nmol.l^{-1}$)		
	Placebo	3 $g.d^{-1}$	6 g $g.d^{-1}$
PRE	34.56 ± 16.55	32.56 ± 10.72	33.56 ± 11.82
POST	30.38 ± 12.39	32.88 ± 12.53	33.75 ± 10.98
Δ	−4.19 ± 5.90	0.31 ± 4.29	0.19 ± 1.46
	Albumin ($g.l^{-1}$)		
	Placebo	3 $g.d^{-1}$	6 g $g.d^{-1}$
PRE	46.38 ± 2.08	45.06 ± 2.60	45.50 ± 1.49
POST	44.75 ± 1.67	45.00 ± 2.33	45.50 ± 2.56
Δ	−1.63 ± 1.33	−0.06 ± 1.82	0.00 ± 2.35

Data is presented as: mean ± standard deviation.
*statistically significant ($P < 0.05$).
PRE values are an average of T1 and T2.

The reductions in testosterone observed in this study are important to consider, owing to the negative impact it could have on training gains within this population. Resistance trained men have higher levels of strength and hypertrophy compared to novice trainers and also exhibit higher basal testosterone levels [4,13-17], which suggest a link between basal total testosterone levels and training related gains. A decrease in total testosterone with a concurrent decrease in free testosterone could reduce the likelihood of interaction with androgen receptors in muscles and nerves, which would reduce the speed of testosterone initiated muscle protein synthesis [1]. Over time this could translate into reduced training gains. Conversely, alterations of testosterone within normal physiological ranges may not be clinically significant. Research indicates that when total testosterone levels are observed outside of normal healthy ranges (4.9-8.6 $ng.ml^{-1}$) it affects strength and hypertrophy. In the case of hypogonadism where testosterone levels are low this negatively affects strength and hypertrophy, and with the use of steroids a positive affect is seen [5,20]. The changes observed in the current study reflect minor alterations with respect to normal physiological ranges. It is currently unknown if these fluctuations are detrimental to training gains.

A potential limitation of this research may be the study length. The short term nature of a two week supplementation period will answer only acute hypotheses. The observed reduction in testosterone may rebound, or even decrease further and a longer term training study would be able to better explain the effects of this supplement. Moreover it would be able to delineate changes in strength and or hypertrophy, and observe whether d-aspartic acid affects training related gains positively or negatively.

Conclusion

Many testosterone boosting supplements are commercially available without sufficient research to support their efficacy. The present study has demonstrated that 3 $g.d^{-1}$ of d-aspartic acid was inadequate to affect any hormonal markers and that 6 $g.d^{-1}$ significantly reduced total testosterone and free testosterone levels, with no concurrent change in other hormones tested. It is currently unknown if any negative consequences of this reduction, with respect to strength and hypertrophy will occur over time. The need for longer-duration research utilising six grams of d-aspartic acid is clear. Future research should explore supplementation of 6 $g.d^{-1}$ over a longer period and observe any correlations between basal testosterone levels and changes in hypertrophy and strength.

Competing interests
The d-aspartic acid supplement used in this study was commercially sourced. The authors have no undisclosed professional relationships with companies or manufacturers that would benefit from the results of the present study. The authors declare that they have no competing interests.

Authors' contributions
GM, PM and JS contributed to the study conception and design, GM acquired the data, performed data analysis and interpreted the data; all authors were involved in drafting the manuscript and have given final approval of the published version.

Acknowledgments
The author's thank the volunteers who participated in the study.

References
1. Spiering BA, Kraemer WJ, Anderson JM, Armstrong LE, Nindl BC, Volek JS, et al. Resistance exercise biology: Manipulation of resistance exercise programme variables determines the responses of cellular and molecular signalling pathways. Sports Med. 2008;38(7):527–40.
2. Vingren JL, Kraemer WJ, Ratamess NA, Anderson JM, Volek JS, Maresh CM. Testosterone physiology in resistance exercise and training: The up-stream regulatory elements. Sports Med. 2010;40(12):1037–53.
3. Hakkinen K, Pakarinen A, Alen M, Kauhanen H, Komi PV. Neuromuscular and hormonal adaptations in athletes to strength training in two years. J App Physiol. 1988;65(6):2406–12.
4. Hakkinen K, Pakarinen A, Alen M, Komi PV. Serum hormones during prolonged training of neuromuscular performance. Eur J Appl Physiol Occup Physiol. 1985;53(4):287–93.
5. Bhasin S, Storer TW, Berman N, Callegari C, Clevenger B, Phillips J, et al. The effects of supraphysiologic doses of testosterone on muscle size and strength in normal men. New Eng J Med. 1996;335(1):1–7.
6. D'Aniello A, Di Cosmo A, Di Cristo C, Annunziato L, Petrucelli L, Fisher G. Involvement of D-aspartic acid in the synthesis of testosterone in rat testes. Life Sci. 1996;59(2):97–104.
7. Furuchi T, Homma H. Free D-aspartate in mammals. Biol and Pharm Bull. 2005;28(9):1566–70.
8. D'Aniello A. d-Aspartic acid: An endogenous amino acid with an important neuroendocrine role. Brain Res Rev. 2007;53(2):215–34.
9. Nagata Y, Homma H, Matsumoto M, Imai K. Stimulation of steroidogenic acute regulatory protein (StAR) gene expression by D-aspartate in rat Leydig cells. FEBS Lett. 1999;454(3):317–20.
10. D'Aniello A, Di Fiore MM, Fisher GH, Milone A, Seleni A, D'Aniello S, et al. Occurrence of D-aspartic acid and N-methyl-D-aspartic acid in rat neuroendocrine tissues and their role in the modulation of luteinizing hormone and growth hormone release. FASEB J. 2000;14(5):699–714.
11. Nagata Y, Homma H, Lee JA, Imai K. D-Aspartate stimulation of testosterone synthesis in rat Leydig cells. FEBS Lett. 1999;444(2–3):160–4.
12. Topo E, Soricelli A, D'Aniello A, Ronsini S, D'Aniello G: The role and molecular mechanism of D-aspartic acid in the release and synthesis of LH and testosterone in humans and rats. Reprod Biol Endocrinol 2009, 7.
13. Willoughby DS, Leutholtz B. D-Aspartic acid supplementation combined with 28 days of heavy resistance training has no effect on body composition, muscle strength, and serum hormones associated with the hypothalamo-pituitary-gonadal axis in resistance-trained men. Nutr Res. 2013;33(10):803–10.
14. Hakkinen K, Pakarinen A, Alen M, Kauhanen H, Komi PV. Daily hormonal and neuromuscular responses to intensive strength training in 1 week. Int J Sports Med. 1988;9(6):422–8.
15. McCall GE, Byrnes WC, Fleck SJ, Dickinson A, Kraemer WJ. Acute and chronic hormonal responses to resistance training designed to promote muscle hypertrophy. Can J App Physiol. 1999;24(1):96–107.
16. Reaburn P, Logan P, Mackinnon L. Serum testosterone response to high-intensity resistance training in male veteran sprint runners. J Strength Cond Res. 1997;11(4):256–60.
17. Staron RS, Karapondo DL, Kraemer WJ, Fry AC, Gordon SE, Falkel JE, et al. Skeletal muscle adaptations during early phase of heavy-resistance training in men and women. J App Physiol. 1994;76(3):1247–55.
18. Marshall PWM, McEwen M, Robbins DW. Strength and neuromuscular adaptation following one, four, and eight sets of high intensity resistance exercise in trained males. Eur J App Physiol. 2011;111(12):3007–16.
19. Ahtiainen JP, Pakarinen A, Alen M, Kraemer WJ, Häkkinen K. Muscle hypertrophy, hormonal adaptations and strength development during strength training in strength-trained and untrained men. Eur J App Physiol. 2003;89(6):555–63.
20. Lunenfeld B, Arver S, Moncada I, Rees DA, Schulte HM. How to help the aging male? Current approaches to hypogonadism in primary care. Aging Male. 2012;15(4):187–97.

Permissions

All chapters in this book were first published in JISSN, by BioMed Central; hereby published with permission under the Creative Commons Attribution License or equivalent. Every chapter published in this book has been scrutinized by our experts. Their significance has been extensively debated. The topics covered herein carry significant findings which will fuel the growth of the discipline. They may even be implemented as practical applications or may be referred to as a beginning point for another development.

The contributors of this book come from diverse backgrounds, making this book a truly international effort. This book will bring forth new frontiers with its revolutionizing research information and detailed analysis of the nascent developments around the world.

We would like to thank all the contributing authors for lending their expertise to make the book truly unique. They have played a crucial role in the development of this book. Without their invaluable contributions this book wouldn't have been possible. They have made vital efforts to compile up to date information on the varied aspects of this subject to make this book a valuable addition to the collection of many professionals and students.

This book was conceptualized with the vision of imparting up-to-date information and advanced data in this field. To ensure the same, a matchless editorial board was set up. Every individual on the board went through rigorous rounds of assessment to prove their worth. After which they invested a large part of their time researching and compiling the most relevant data for our readers.

The editorial board has been involved in producing this book since its inception. They have spent rigorous hours researching and exploring the diverse topics which have resulted in the successful publishing of this book. They have passed on their knowledge of decades through this book. To expedite this challenging task, the publisher supported the team at every step. A small team of assistant editors was also appointed to further simplify the editing procedure and attain best results for the readers.

Apart from the editorial board, the designing team has also invested a significant amount of their time in understanding the subject and creating the most relevant covers. They scrutinized every image to scout for the most suitable representation of the subject and create an appropriate cover for the book.

The publishing team has been an ardent support to the editorial, designing and production team. Their endless efforts to recruit the best for this project, has resulted in the accomplishment of this book. They are a veteran in the field of academics and their pool of knowledge is as vast as their experience in printing. Their expertise and guidance has proved useful at every step. Their uncompromising quality standards have made this book an exceptional effort. Their encouragement from time to time has been an inspiration for everyone.

The publisher and the editorial board hope that this book will prove to be a valuable piece of knowledge for researchers, students, practitioners and scholars across the globe.

List of Contributors

Charles L Dumke
Department of Health and Human Performance, Montana Center for Work Physiology and Exercise Metabolism, University of Montana, 32 Campus Drive, Missoula, MT 59812, USA

Dustin R Slivka
School of Health, Physical Education and Recreation, University of Nebraska at Omaha, 6001 Dodge Street, Omaha, NE 68182, USA

John S Cuddy
Department of Health and Human Performance, Montana Center for Work Physiology and Exercise Metabolism, University of Montana, 32 Campus Drive, Missoula, MT 59812, USA

Walter S Hailes
Department of Health and Human Performance, Montana Center for Work Physiology and Exercise Metabolism, University of Montana, 32 Campus Drive, Missoula, MT 59812, USA

Brent C Ruby
Department of Health and Human Performance, Montana Center for Work Physiology and Exercise Metabolism, University of Montana, 32 Campus Drive, Missoula, MT 59812, USA

Louise Deldicque
Exercise Physiology Research Group, Department of Kinesiology, KU Leuven, Leuven, Belgium

Karen Van Proeyen
Exercise Physiology Research Group, Department of Kinesiology, KU Leuven, Leuven, Belgium

Monique Ramaekers
Exercise Physiology Research Group, Department of Kinesiology, KU Leuven, Leuven, Belgium

Ivo Pischel
PhytoLab GmbH & Co. KG, Vestenbergsgreuth, Germany

Hartwig Sievers
PhytoLab GmbH & Co. KG, Vestenbergsgreuth, Germany

Peter Hespel
Exercise Physiology Research Group, Department of Kinesiology, KU Leuven, Leuven, Belgium

Surabhi Bhutani
Department of Kinesiology and Nutrition, University of Illinois at Chicago, 1919 West Taylor Street, Room 103, Chicago, IL 60612, USA

Monica C Klempel
Department of Kinesiology and Nutrition, University of Illinois at Chicago, 1919 West Taylor Street, Room 103, Chicago, IL 60612, USA

Cynthia M Kroeger
Department of Kinesiology and Nutrition, University of Illinois at Chicago, 1919 West Taylor Street, Room 103, Chicago, IL 60612, USA

Eleanor Aggour
Department of Kinesiology and Nutrition, University of Illinois at Chicago, 1919 West Taylor Street, Room 103, Chicago, IL 60612, USA

Yolian Calvo
Department of Kinesiology and Nutrition, University of Illinois at Chicago, 1919 West Taylor Street, Room 103, Chicago, IL 60612, USA

John F Trepanowski
Department of Kinesiology and Nutrition, University of Illinois at Chicago, 1919 West Taylor Street, Room 103, Chicago, IL 60612, USA

Kristin K Hoddy
Department of Kinesiology and Nutrition, University of Illinois at Chicago, 1919 West Taylor Street, Room 103, Chicago, IL 60612, USA

Krista A Varady
Department of Kinesiology and Nutrition, University of Illinois at Chicago, 1919 West Taylor Street, Room 103, Chicago, IL 60612, USA

Vandré Casagrande Figueiredo
The Liggins Institute, Faculty of Medical and Science Health, University of Auckland, 85 Park Road, Grafton, Private Bag 92019, Auckland 1023, New Zealand

David Cameron-Smith
The Liggins Institute, Faculty of Medical and Science Health, University of Auckland, 85 Park Road, Grafton, Private Bag 92019, Auckland 1023, New Zealand

Justin D Roberts
School of Life & Medical Sciences, University of Hertfordshire, College Lane, Hatfield, Hertfordshire, UK

Michael D Tarpey
School of Life & Medical Sciences, University of Hertfordshire, College Lane, Hatfield, Hertfordshire, UK

Lindsy S Kass
School of Life & Medical Sciences, University of Hertfordshire, College Lane, Hatfield, Hertfordshire, UK

Richard J Tarpey
School of Life & Medical Sciences, University of Hertfordshire, College Lane, Hatfield, Hertfordshire, UK

Michael G Roberts
School of Life & Medical Sciences, University of Hertfordshire, College Lane, Hatfield, Hertfordshire, UK

Xinying Wang
Research Institute of General Surgery, Jinling Hospital, Medical School, Nanjing University, 305 East Zhongshan Road, Nanjing 210002, Jiangsu Province, People's Republic of China

Chenglin Niu
Department of ICU, Brain Hospital, Nanjing Medical University, 264 Guangzhou Road, Nanjing 210029, Jiangsu Province, China

Jun Lu
Department of Orthopedics, Zhongda Hospital, Southeast University, 87 Dingjiaqiao, Nanjing 210009, Jiangsu Province, China

Ning Li
Research Institute of General Surgery, Jinling Hospital, Medical School, Nanjing University, 305 East Zhongshan Road, Nanjing 210002, Jiangsu Province, People's Republic of China

Jieshou Li
Research Institute of General Surgery, Jinling Hospital, Medical School, Nanjing University, 305 East Zhongshan Road, Nanjing 210002, Jiangsu Province, People's Republic of China

Daniela Chlíbková
Centre of Sports Activities, Brno University of Technology, Brno, Czech Republic

Beat Knechtle
Institute of General Practise and for Health Services Research,University of Zurich, Zurich, Switzerland
Facharzt FMH für Allgemeinmedizin, Gesundheitszentrum St. Gallen, Vadianstrasse 26, 9001 St. Gallen, Switzerland

Thomas Rosemann
Institute of General Practise and for Health Services Research,University of Zurich, Zurich, Switzerland

Alena Žákovská
Institute of Experimental Biology, Faculty of Science, Masaryk University, Brno, Czech Republic

Ivana Tomášková
Faculty of Forestry and Wood Sciences, Czech University of Life Sciences, Prague, Czech Republic

Michael T Nelson
School of Kinesiology, University of Minnesota, Minneapolis, MN, USA
Department of Pediatrics, University of Minnesota Medical School, Minneapolis, MN, USA

George R Biltz
School of Kinesiology, University of Minnesota, Minneapolis, MN, USA

Donald R Dengel
School of Kinesiology, University of Minnesota, Minneapolis, MN, USA
Department of Pediatrics, University of Minnesota Medical School, Minneapolis, MN, USA

Marc Sim
School of Sport Science, Exercise and Health, The University of Western Australia, Crawley, Western Australia, Australia

Brian Dawson
School of Sport Science, Exercise and Health, The University of Western Australia, Crawley, Western Australia, Australia

Grant J Landers
School of Sport Science, Exercise and Health, The University of Western Australia, Crawley, Western Australia, Australia

Dorine W Swinkels
Department of Laboratory Medicine, Laboratory of Genetic, Endocrine and Metabolic Disease, Radboud University Medical Centre, Nijmegen, The Netherlands

Harold Tjalsma
Department of Laboratory Medicine, Laboratory of Genetic, Endocrine and Metabolic Disease, Radboud University Medical Centre, Nijmegen, The Netherlands

Erwin T Wiegerinck
Department of Laboratory Medicine, Laboratory of Genetic, Endocrine and Metabolic Disease, Radboud University Medical Centre, Nijmegen, The Netherlands

Debbie Trinder
School of Medicine and Pharmacology, The University of Western Australia, Fremantle Hospital, Fremantle, Western Australia, Australia
Harry Perkins Institute for Medical Research, Nedlands, Western Australia, Australia

Peter Peeling
School of Sport Science, Exercise and Health, The University of Western Australia, Crawley, Western Australia, Australia

Jonathan M Oliver
Kinesiology Department, Texas Christian University, Fort Worth, TX 76129, USA

Andrew R Jagim
Sport & Exercise Science Department, Gannon University, Erie, PA 16541, USA

Ivo Pischel
Phytolab GmbH & Co. KG, Vestenbergsgreuth, Germany

Ralf Jäger
Increnovo LLC, 2138 E Lafayette Pl, Milwaukee, WI 53202, USA

Martin Purpura
Increnovo LLC, 2138 E Lafayette Pl, Milwaukee, WI 53202, USA

Adam Sanchez
Department of Health and Kinesiology, Exercise and Sport Nutrition Lab, Texas A&M University, College Station, TX 77843-4243, USA

James Fluckey
Department of Health and Kinesiology, Muscle Biology Laboratory, Texas A&M University, College Station, TX 77843-4243, USA

Steven Riechman
Department of Health and Kinesiology, Human Countermeasures Laboratory, Texas A&M University, College Station, TX 77843-4243, USA

Michael Greenwood
Department of Health and Kinesiology, Exercise and Sport Nutrition Lab, Texas A&M University, College Station, TX 77843-4243, USA

Katherine Kelly
Department of Health and Kinesiology, Exercise and Sport Nutrition Lab, Texas A&M University, College Station, TX 77843-4243, USA

Cynthia Meininger
Department of Systems Biology and Translational Medicine, Texas A&M Health Science Center, College Station, TX 77843-1114, USA

Christopher Rasmussen
Department of Systems Biology and Translational Medicine, Texas A&M Health Science Center, College Station, TX 77843-1114, USA

Richard B Kreider
Department of Health and Kinesiology, Exercise and Sport Nutrition Lab, Texas A&M University, College Station, TX 77843-4243, USA

Mai Tanabe
Department of Sports Medicine/Dentistry, Graduate School of Medical and Dental Sciences, Tokyo Medical and Dental University, Bunkyo-ku, Japan

Toshiyuki Takahashi
Department of Sports Medicine/Dentistry, Graduate School of Medical and Dental Sciences, Tokyo Medical and Dental University, Bunkyo-ku, Japan

Kazuhiro Shimoyama
Oral health care science, Tokyo Medical and Dental University, Bunkyo-ku, Japan

Yukako Toyoshima
Japanese Institute of Sports Science, Kita-ku, Japan

Toshiaki Ueno
Department of Sports Medicine/Dentistry, Graduate School of Medical and Dental Sciences, Tokyo Medical and Dental University, Bunkyo-ku, Japan

Wilson Rinaldi
Department of Physical Education, State University of Maringá, Maringá, PR, Brazil

Rodrigo Mello Gomes
Department of Physiological Sciences, State University of Maringá, Maringá, PR, Brazil

Dionízia Xavier Scomparin
Department of General Biology, State University of Ponta Grossa, Ponta Grossa, PR, Brazil

Sabrina Grassiolli
Department of General Biology, State University of Ponta Grossa, Ponta Grossa, PR, Brazil

Tatiane Aparecida Ribeiro
Department of Biotechnology, Genetics and Cell Biology, State University of Maringá, Maringá, PR, Brazil

Gabriel Sergio Fabricio
Department of Physical Education, State University of Maringá, Maringá, PR, Brazil

Luiz Felipe Barella
Department of Biotechnology, Genetics and Cell Biology, State University of Maringá, Maringá, PR, Brazil

Audrei Pavanello
Department of Biotechnology, Genetics and Cell Biology, State University of Maringá, Maringá, PR, Brazil

Amanda Bianchi Trombini
Department of Biotechnology, Genetics and Cell Biology, State University of Maringá, Maringá, PR, Brazil

Paulo Cezar de Freitas Mathias
Department of Biotechnology, Genetics and Cell Biology, State University of Maringá, Maringá, PR, Brazil

Júlio Cezar de Oliveira
Department of Biotechnology, Genetics and Cell Biology, State University of Maringá, Maringá, PR, Brazil

Mahdi Garelnabi
Department of Clinical Laboratory and Nutritional Sciences, University of Massachusetts, 3 Solomont Way, Suite 4 01854, Lowell, MA, USA

Halleh Mahini
Department of Clinical Laboratory and Nutritional Sciences, University of Massachusetts, 3 Solomont Way, Suite 4 01854, Lowell, MA, USA

Thomas Wilson
Department of Clinical Laboratory and Nutritional Sciences, University of Massachusetts, 3 Solomont Way, Suite 4 01854, Lowell, MA, USA

Edward H Robinson IV
Institute of Exercise Physiology & Wellness, University of Central Florida, 4000, Orlando, FL 32816, USA
College of Education & Human Performance, 12494 University Boulevard, Orlando, FL 32816, USA

Jeffrey R Stout
Institute of Exercise Physiology & Wellness, University of Central Florida, 4000, Orlando, FL 32816, USA
College of Education & Human Performance, 12494 University Boulevard, Orlando, FL 32816, USA

Amelia A Miramonti
Institute of Exercise Physiology & Wellness, University of Central Florida, 4000, Orlando, FL 32816, USA
College of Education & Human Performance, 12494 University Boulevard, Orlando, FL 32816, USA

David H Fukuda
Institute of Exercise Physiology & Wellness, University of Central Florida, 4000, Orlando, FL 32816, USA
College of Education & Human Performance, 12494 University Boulevard, Orlando, FL 32816, USA

Ran Wang
Institute of Exercise Physiology & Wellness, University of Central Florida, 4000, Orlando, FL 32816, USA
College of Education & Human Performance, 12494 University Boulevard, Orlando, FL 32816, USA

Jeremy R Townsend
Institute of Exercise Physiology & Wellness, University of Central Florida, 4000, Orlando, FL 32816, USA
College of Education & Human Performance, 12494 University Boulevard, Orlando, FL 32816, USA

Gerald T Mangine
Institute of Exercise Physiology & Wellness, University of Central Florida, 4000, Orlando, FL 32816, USA
College of Education & Human Performance, 12494 University Boulevard, Orlando, FL 32816, USA

Maren S Fragala
Institute of Exercise Physiology & Wellness, University of Central Florida, 4000, Orlando, FL 32816, USA
College of Education & Human Performance, 12494 University Boulevard, Orlando, FL 32816, USA

Jay R Hoffman
Institute of Exercise Physiology & Wellness, University of Central Florida, 4000, Orlando, FL 32816, USA
College of Education & Human Performance, 12494 University Boulevard, Orlando, FL 32816, USA

Yongsuk Seo
Exercise and Environmental Physiology Laboratory, Kent State University, Kent, OH, USA

Corey A Peacock
Nova Southeastern University, Fort Lauderdale, FL, USA

John Gunstad
Departments of Psychology, Kent State University, Kent, OH, USA

Keith J Burns
Exercise and Environmental Physiology Laboratory, Kent State University, Kent, OH, USA

Brandon S Pollock
Exercise and Environmental Physiology Laboratory, Kent State University, Kent, OH, USA

Ellen L Glickman
Exercise and Environmental Physiology Laboratory, Kent State University, Kent, OH, USA

James L Dorling
Department for Health, Sport, Health and Exercise Science, University of Bath, Eastwood 22-23 3.4, Bath BA2 7AY, UK

Conrad P Earnest
Department for Health, Sport, Health and Exercise Science, University of Bath, Eastwood 22-23 3.4, Bath BA2 7AY, UK

Colin Russell
Department of Kinesiology, Faculty of Applied Health Sciences, Brock University, 500 Glenridge Av., St. Catharines, Ontario L2S 3A1, Canada

Efthymios Papadopoulos
Department of Kinesiology, Faculty of Applied Health Sciences, Brock University, 500 Glenridge Av., St. Catharines, Ontario L2S 3A1, Canada

Yasmeen Mezil
Department of Kinesiology, Faculty of Applied Health Sciences, Brock University, 500 Glenridge Av., St. Catharines, Ontario L2S 3A1, Canada

Greg D Wells
Faculty of Kinesiology and Physical Education, University of Toronto, 55 Harbord St., Toronto, Ontario M5S 2W6, Canada

Michael J Plyley
Department of Kinesiology, Faculty of Applied Health Sciences, Brock University, 500 Glenridge Av., St. Catharines, Ontario L2S 3A1, Canada

Mathew Greenway
Michael G. DeGroote School of Medicine, McMaster University, 500 Glenridge Av., St. Catharines, Ontario L2S 3A1, Canada

Panagiota Klentrou
Department of Kinesiology, Faculty of Applied Health Sciences, Brock University, 500 Glenridge Av., St. Catharines, Ontario L2S 3A1, Canada

Hideki Hashimoto
Faculty of Sport Sciences, Waseda University, Saitama, Japan
Products Research & Development Laboratory, Asashi Soft Drinks Co., Ltd, Ibaraki, Japan

Toshimichi Ishijima
Faculty of Sport Sciences, Waseda University, Saitama, Japan
School of Human Culture, The University of Shiga Prefecture, Shiga, Japan

Harumi Hayashida
Faculty of Sport Sciences, Waseda University, Saitama, Japan
Faculty of Health Promotional Sciences, Tokoha University, Shizuoka, Japan

Katsuhiko Suzuki
Faculty of Sport Sciences, Waseda University, Saitama, Japan

Mitsuru Higuchi
Faculty of Sport Sciences, Waseda University, Saitama, Japan

Anna Skarpańska-Stejnborn
Department of Morphological and Health Sciences; Faculty of Physical Culture in Gorzów Wlkp, University School of Physical Education in Poznań, 13 Estkowskiego Str., 66 - 400 Gorzów Wlkp, Poland

Piotr Basta
Department of Water Sports; Branch in Gorzów Wlkp, Faculty of Physical Culture, Gorzów, Poland

Justyna Sadowska
School of Humanities, King Stanislaw Leszczynski in Leszno, Leszno, Poland

Łucja Pilaczyńska-Szcześniak
Department of Hygiene, University School of Physical Education in Poznañ, Poznañ, Poland

Corey A Rynders
Department of Human Movement Sciences, Human Performance Laboratory, Old Dominion University, Norfolk, VA, USA

Judy Y Weltman
Department of Kinesiology Exercise Physiology Core Laboratory, University of Virginia, Charlottesville, Virginia, USA

Sara D Rynders
Jordan Young Institute, Virginia Beach, VA, USA

James Patrie
Department of Kinesiology Exercise Physiology Core Laboratory, University of Virginia, Charlottesville, Virginia, USA

John McKnight
Department of Kinesiology Exercise Physiology Core Laboratory, University of Virginia, Charlottesville, Virginia, USA

Frank I Katch
Department of Kinesiology Exercise Physiology Core Laboratory, University of Virginia, Charlottesville, Virginia, USA

Jay Hertel
Department of Kinesiology Exercise Physiology Core Laboratory, University of Virginia, Charlottesville, Virginia, USA

Arthur Weltman
Department of Kinesiology Exercise Physiology Core Laboratory, University of Virginia, Charlottesville, Virginia, USA

John G Seifert
Movement Science Laboratory, Montana State University, Bozeman, MT 59717, USA

David A Connor
Movement Science Laboratory, Montana State University, Bozeman, MT 59717, USA

Karolina Łagowska
Department of Human Nutrition and Hygiene, Poznan University of Life Sciences, Poznan, Poland

Karina Kapczuk
Department of Perinatology and Gynecology, Poznan University of Medical Sciences, Poznan, Poland

Jan Jeszka
Department of Human Nutrition and Hygiene, Poznan University of Life Sciences, Poznan, Poland

Jason KW Lee
Combat Protection and Performance Programme, Defence Medical and Environmental Research Institute, DSO National Laboratories, Singapore, Republic of Singapore
Department of Physiology, National University of Singapore, Singapore, Republic of Singapore
Lee Kong Chian School of Medicine, Nanyang Technological University, Singapore, Republic of Singapore

Wee Hon Ang
Combat Protection and Performance Programme, Defence Medical and Environmental Research Institute, DSO National Laboratories, Singapore, Republic of Singapore

Jonathan WX Ng
Department of Physiology, National University of Singapore, Singapore, Republic of Singapore

Priscilla WP Fan
Combat Protection and Performance Programme, Defence Medical and Environmental Research Institute, DSO National Laboratories, Singapore, Republic of Singapore

Ya Shi Teo
Combat Protection and Performance Programme, Defence Medical and Environmental Research Institute, DSO National Laboratories, Singapore, Republic of Singapore

Heinrich W Nolte
ERGOnomics TECHnologies, Research and Development, Armscor, Pretoria, South Africa

Yvonne YW Yeo
Department of Physiology, National University of Singapore, Singapore, Republic of Singapore

Kriyot Sudsa-ard
Institute of Nutrition, Mahidol University, Salaya, Phutthamonthon, Nakhon Pathom 73170, Thailand

Kallaya Kijboonchoo
Institute of Nutrition, Mahidol University, Salaya, Phutthamonthon, Nakhon Pathom 73170, Thailand

Visith Chavasit
Institute of Nutrition, Mahidol University, Salaya, Phutthamonthon, Nakhon Pathom 73170, Thailand

Rungchai Chaunchaiyakul
College of Sports Science and Technology, Mahidol University, Salaya, Phutthamonthon, Nakhon Pathom 73170, Thailand

Amanda Qing Xia Nio
School of Sport, Cardiff Metropolitan University, Cardiff, UK

Jason Kai Wei Lee
Defence Medical and Environmental Research Institute, DSO National Laboratories, Singapore, Singapore

Matthaus Marriott
Sport and Health Sciences, College of Life and Environmental Sciences, St. Luke's Campus, University of Exeter, Exeter, UK

Peter Krustrup
Sport and Health Sciences, College of Life and Environmental Sciences, St. Luke's Campus, University of Exeter, Exeter, UK
Department of Nutrition, Exercise and Sports, Section of Human Physiology, Copenhagen Centre for Team Sport and Health, University of Copenhagen, Copenhagen, Denmark

Magni Mohr
Yong Loo Lin School of Medicine, National University of Singapore, Singapore, Singapore
Lee Kong Chian School of Medicine, Nanyang Technological University, Singapore, Singapore

Brad Jon Schoenfeld
Department of Health Science, Lehman College, Bronx, NY, USA

Alan Albert Aragon
California State University, Northridge, CA, USA

Colin D Wilborn
Exercise and Sport Science Department, University of Mary Hardin-Baylor, Belton, TX, USA

James W Krieger
Weightology, LLC, Redmond, WA, USA

Gul T Sonmez
Department of Health Science, Lehman College, Bronx, NY, USA

Thibault Brink-Elfegoun
Division of Sport Medicine and Biology of Physical Activity, University of Athens Faculty of Physical Education and Sport Science, Antistasis 41Dafni 17237 Athens, Greece

Sébastien Ratel
Clermont Université, Université Blaise Pascal, EA 3533, Laboratoire des Adaptations Métaboliques à l'Exercice en conditions Physiologiques et Pathologiques (AME2P), Bâtiment Biologie B, 24 avenue des Landais, BP 80026F-63171 Aubière Cedex, France
CRNH-Auvergne, Clermont-Ferrand -63001, France

Pierre-Marie Leprêtre
Laboratoire de Recherche Adaptations Physiologiques à l'Exercice et Réadaptation à l'Effort, EA-3300, Faculté des Sciences du Sport, Université de Picardie Jules Verne, Amiens, France

Lore Metz
Clermont Université, Université Blaise Pascal, EA 3533, Laboratoire des Adaptations Métaboliques à l'Exercice en conditions Physiologiques et Pathologiques (AME2P), Bâtiment Biologie B, 24 avenue des Landais, BP 80026F-63171 Aubière Cedex, France
CRNH-Auvergne, Clermont-Ferrand -63001, France

Gael Ennequin
Clermont Université, Université Blaise Pascal, EA 3533, Laboratoire des Adaptations Métaboliques à l'Exercice en conditions Physiologiques et Pathologiques (AME2P), Bâtiment Biologie B, 24 avenue des Landais, BP 80026F-63171 Aubière Cedex, France
CRNH-Auvergne, Clermont-Ferrand -63001, France

Eric Doré
Clermont Université, Université Blaise Pascal, EA 3533, Laboratoire des Adaptations Métaboliques à l'Exercice en conditions Physiologiques et Pathologiques (AME2P), Bâtiment Biologie B, 24 avenue des Landais, BP 80026F-63171 Aubière Cedex, France
CRNH-Auvergne, Clermont-Ferrand -63001, France

Vincent Martin
Clermont Université, Université Blaise Pascal, EA 3533, Laboratoire des Adaptations Métaboliques à l'Exercice en conditions Physiologiques et Pathologiques (AME2P), Bâtiment Biologie B, 24 avenue des Landais, BP 80026F-63171 Aubière Cedex, France
CRNH-Auvergne, Clermont-Ferrand -63001, France

David Bishop
Institute of Sport, Exercise and Active Living (ISEAL), Victoria University, Melbourne, Australia
College of Sport and Exercise Science, Victoria University, Melbourne, Australia

Nicolas Aubineau
Department of Research, Laboratoire Lescuyer, Nutratletic, Aytré, France

Jean-François Lescuyer
Department of Research, Laboratoire Lescuyer, Nutratletic, Aytré, France

Martine Duclos
Department of Sport Medicine and Functional Explorations, University-Hospital (CHU), G. Montpied Hospital, Clermont-Ferrand F-63003, France
INRA, UMR 1019, Clermont-Ferrand F-63001, France
University Clermont 1, UFR Médecine, Clermont-Ferrand F-63001, France
CRNH-Auvergne, Clermont-Ferrand -63001, France

Pascal Sirvent
Clermont Université, Université Blaise Pascal, EA 3533, Laboratoire des Adaptations Métaboliques à l'Exercice en conditions Physiologiques et Pathologiques (AME2P), Bâtiment Biologie B, 24 avenue des Landais, BP 80026F-63171 Aubière Cedex, France
CRNH-Auvergne, Clermont-Ferrand -63001, France

Sébastien L Peltier
Department of Research, Laboratoire Lescuyer, Nutratletic, Aytré, France

Ieva Alaunyte
Leeds Trinity University, Department of Sport, Health and Nutrition, Brownberrie Lane, Horsforth LS18 5HD, UK
Liverpool Hope University, School of Health Sciences, Hope Park, Liverpool L16 9JD, UK

John L Perry
Leeds Trinity University, Department of Sport, Health and Nutrition, Brownberrie Lane, Horsforth LS18 5HD, UK

Tony Aubrey
Leeds Trinity University, Department of Sport, Health and Nutrition, Brownberrie Lane, Horsforth LS18 5HD, UK

Geoffrey W Melville
School of Science & Health, University of Western Sydney, Campbelltown Campus, Locked Bag 1797, Penrith, NSW 2751, Australia

Jason C Siegler
School of Science & Health, University of Western Sydney, Campbelltown Campus, Locked Bag 1797, Penrith, NSW 2751, Australia

Paul WM Marshall
School of Science & Health, University of Western Sydney, Campbelltown Campus, Locked Bag 1797, Penrith, NSW 2751, Australia

www.ingramcontent.com/pod-product-compliance
Lightning Source LLC
LaVergne TN
LVHW080536300926
849162LV00007B/1626